GrantFinder

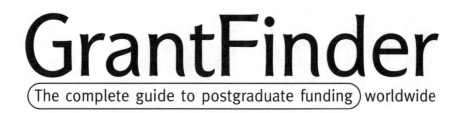

The complete guide to postgraduate funding worldwide

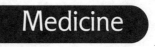

Medicine

GrantFinder

The complete guide to postgraduate funding worldwide

Medicine

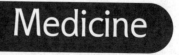

Published in the United States and Canada by

ST. MARTIN'S PRESS, INC.

175 Fifth Avenue, New York

NY 10010

ISBN 0-312-22896-1
ISSN 1526-0925

Published in Great Britain by

MACMILLAN REFERENCE LTD

25 Eccleston Place, London, SW1W 9NF

Basingstoke and Oxford

Companies and representatives throughout the world.

British Library Cataloguing in Publication Data
GrantFinder
Medicine
  1. Student aid   2. Graduate students - Scholarships, fellowships, etc.
  3. Medicine - Research grants
I. Waterlows Specialist Information Publishing
610.7'9
ISBN 0-333-777298

Typeset by Macmillan Reference Ltd

Printed and bound in Great Britain by Antony Rowe Ltd, Chippenham, Wiltshire

Visit our website: http://www.macmillan-reference.co.uk

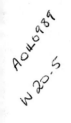

CONTENTS

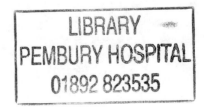

HOW TO USE GRANTFINDER

For ease of use, GrantFinder is divided into four sections:

• The Grants
• Subject and Eligibility Guide to Awards
• Index of Awards
• Index of Awarding Organisations

The Grants

Information in this section is supplied directly by the awarding organisations. Entries are arranged alphabetically by name of organisation, and awards are listed alphabetically within the awarding organisation. This section includes details on subject area, eligibility, purpose, type, numbers offered, frequency, value, length of study, study establishment, country of study, and application procedure. Full contact details appear with each awarding organisation and also appended to individual awards where additional addresses are given.

Subject and Eligibility Guide to Awards

Awards can be located through the Subject and Eligibility Guide to Awards. This section allows the user to find an award within a specific subject area. GrantFinder uses a list of subjects endorsed by the International Association of Universities (IAU), the information centre on higher education, located at UNESCO, Paris (please see pp. 332 for the complete subject list). It is further subdivided into eligibility by nationality. Thereafter, awards are listed alphabetically within their designated category, along with a page reference where full details of the award can be found.

Index of Awards

All awards are indexed alphabetically with a page reference.

Index of Awarding Organisations

A complete list of all awarding organisations, with country name and page reference.

AFRICA EDUCATIONAL TRUST

Small Grants Project
38 King Street, London, WC2E 8JS, England
Tel: (44) 171 836 5075
Fax: (44) 171 379 0090
Email: mbrophy@aet.win-uk.net
www: http://www.africaeducationaltrust.mcmail.com
Contact: Director

Africa Educational Trust Emergency Grants

Subjects: All subjects.
Eligibility: Open to students from Africa studying in the UK. The applicant must have run into unexpected difficulties at the end of his or her course for which the small level of grant will, by itself or in conjunction with other grants, solve the problem. Most awards are made on a humanitarian basis. Academic considerations are more important at the postgraduate and research levels.
Level of Study: Unrestricted.

GENERAL

Any Country

AACR Gerald B Grindley Memorial Young Investigator Award, 20
AACR Peczoller International Award for Cancer Research, 20
AACR Susan G Komen Breast Cancer Foundation Career Development Award, 21
Action Research Programme Grants, 4
Action Research Project Grants, 4

THE GRANTS

AAUW EDUCATIONAL FOUNDATION

Department 60
2201 North Dodge Street, Iowa City, IA, 52243-4030, United
States of America
Tel: (1) 319 337 1716 ext 60
www: http://www.aauw.org
Contact: Grants Management Officer

AAUW is composed of three corporations: the Association, a 150,000-member organisation with more than 1,500 branches nationwide that lobbies and advocates for education and equity; the AAUW Educational Foundation, which funds pioneering research on girls and education, community action projects, and fellowships and grants for outstanding women around the globe; and the AAUW Legal Advocacy Fund, which provides funds and a support system for women seeking judicial redress for sex discrimination in higher education.

AAUW Educational Foundation American Fellowships

Subjects: All subjects.
Eligibility: Applicants must be US citizens.
Level of Study: Doctorate, Postdoctorate.
Purpose: To offset a scholar's living expenses while she completes her final year of dissertation writing; or, to increase the number of women in tenure-track faculty positions and promote equality for women in higher education.
Type: Fellowship.
Frequency: Annual.
Value: US$15,000 for the Dissertation Award; US$27,000 for Postdoctoral Research Leave Award; and US$5,250 for the Research Publication Grant.
Length of Study: 1 year.
Country of Study: USA.
Application Procedure: Application package includes an application form, narrative autobiography, CV, statement of project, transcripts, three letters of recommendation and a filing fee.
Closing Date: November 15th.

AAUW International Fellowships Program

Subjects: All subjects.
Eligibility: Open to women who are not US citizens or permanent residents. Must hold a US bachelor's degree or equivalent. Must be planning to return to their home country upon completion of degree/research. English proficiency required.
Level of Study: Doctorate, Postdoctorate, Postgraduate, Professional development.
Purpose: To award women who are not US citizens or permanent residents studying at the graduate or postgraduate level or for research beyond the Bachelor's level.
Type: Fellowship.
No. of awards offered: 45.

Frequency: Annual.
Value: US$16,000 for the Fellowship Award; US$5,000-7,000 (limited number available) for the Community Action Grants.
Length of Study: 1 year.
Study Establishment: Any accredited institution.
Country of Study: USA.
Application Procedure: Application must be filled out for each year applying. Applications must be obtained through our customer service centre between August 1st and November 15th. Three letters of recommendation, transcripts, TOEFL scores (min 550) are also required.
Closing Date: January 15th.
Additional Information: These awards are non-renewable.

Career Development Grants

Subjects: All subjects.
Eligibility: Open to all, yet special consideration is given to AAUW members, women of colour, women pursuing their advanced degree or credentials in non-traditional fields. Applicants must be US citizens or permanent residents whose last degree was received before June 30th 1994. Candidates eligible for another AAUW Educational Foundation fellowship or grant programme are not eligible for Career Development Grants.
Purpose: To support women who currently hold a Bachelor's degree and who are preparing for a career in advancement, career change, or to re-enter the work force.
Type: Grant.
No. of awards offered: Approx. 75 in two categories: Academic Grants and Professional Development Institute Grants.
Value: US$2,000-8,000.
Closing Date: Postmark deadline January 2nd.
Additional Information: The two categories are as follows: Academic Grants - provide support for course work towards a Master's degree or specialised training in technical or professional fields. Course work must be undertaken at a fully accreditied two or four year college, university or technical school licensed, accredited, or approved by the US Department of Veterans Affairs; and Professional Development Institute Grants - support women's participation in professional institutes.

Community Action Grants

Subjects: All subjects.
Eligibility: Applicants must be women who are US citizens or permanent residents. Special consideration will be given to AAUW branch and state applicants who seek partners for collaborative projects. Collaborators can include local schools or school districts, businesses and other community based organisations.
Purpose: To provide seed money to individual women and AAUW branches and states for innovative programmes or non-degree research projects that promote education and equity for women and girls.
Type: Grant.
No. of awards offered: Approx. 40.
Value: US$2,000-$7,000 for one-year projects; US$5,000-$10,000 for two-year projects.

Length of Study: 1 or 2 years.
Application Procedure: Please write for details.
Closing Date: February 1st.
Additional Information: Two types of grants are available: one year grants for short term projects; topic areas are unrestricted but should have a clearly defined educational activity; two year grants are for longer term programmes and are restricted to projects focused on K-12 girls achievement in maths, science, and technology. Funds support planning activities and coalition building during the first year and implementation and evaluation the following year.

Selected Professions Fellowships

Subjects: Medicine, law, engineering, business administration, computer science.
Eligibility: All women are eligible to apply for fellowships in the following degree programmes, architecture (MArch); computer/information sciences (MS); engineering (ME, MS, PhD); mathematics/statistics (MS). Fellowships for the following degree programmes are restricted to women of colour to increase their participation and access in these historically under-represented fields: business administration (MBA, EMBA); law (JD); and medicine (MD,DO).
Purpose: To support women in the final year of graduate study in designated fields where women's participation has been low, and also to support engineering doctoral candidates who are in the final stages of writing their dissertations.
Type: Fellowship.
Value: Fellowship Award, $5,000-$12,000; Engineering Dissertation Award $15,000.
Application Procedure: Please write for details.
Closing Date: Application postmark deadline, January 2nd; Engineering Dissertation (only) November 15th.

ACTION RESEARCH

Vincent House, Horsham, West Sussex, RH12 2DP, England
Tel: (44) 1403 210406
Fax: (44) 1403 210541
Contact: Dr Tracy Swinfield

Action Research is a national research charity dedicated to preventing and treating disabling diseases. The charity supports a broad spectrum of research with the objective of preventing disease and disability - regardless of age group - and alleviating physical handicap, with an emphasis on clinical research, or research at the clinical and basic interface.

Action Research Programme Grants

Subjects: With the exception of cancer, cardiovascular and HIV and AIDS research, the programme supports a broad spectrum of research with the objective of preventing disease and disability, regardless of cause or age group, and alleviating physical handicap. Please note that research is on clinical research or research at the clinical or basic interface.

Eligibility: Open only to researchers in the UK.
Level of Study: Unrestricted.
Purpose: To support coherent proposals based on an established line of enquiry.
Type: Grant.
No. of awards offered: Varies.
Frequency: Every three years.
Value: Varies.
Length of Study: Normally for up to 5 years, possibly renewable.
Study Establishment: Applicants should not be based in an MRC.
Country of Study: United Kingdom.
Closing Date: March 15th, July 15th, November 15th.
Additional Information: Assessment usually takes one year. Programme Grants are only rarely awarded.

Action Research Project Grants

Subjects: With the exception of cancer, cardiovascular and HIV and AIDS research, the programme supports a broad spectrum of research with the objective of preventing disease and disability (regardless of cause or age group), and alleviating physical handicap. Please note that emphasis is on clinical research or research at the clinical or basic interface.
Eligibility: Open to researchers in the UK only. No grants are made purely for higher education.
Level of Study: Unrestricted.
Purpose: To support one precisely formulated line of research.
Type: Grant.
No. of awards offered: Varies.
Frequency: Three times each year.
Value: Varies.
Length of Study: Up to 3 years; assessed annually.
Country of Study: United Kingdom.
Application Procedure: A one page outline of the project needs to be submitted before an application form can be issued. Completed application forms must be submitted by the closing date.
Closing Date: March 15th, July 15th, November 15th.
Additional Information: Grants are not awarded to MRC units or to other charities.

Action Research Training Fellowship

Subjects: With the exception of cancer, cardiovascular and HIV/AIDS research, we support a broad spectrum of research with the objective of preventing disease and disability (regardless of cause or age group), and alleviating physical handicap. Please note that our emphasis is on clinical research or research at the clinical/basic interface.
Eligibility: Open to medical and non-medical graduates, preferably between ages of 23 and 32, as this is a training position. Although not limited to UK citizens, those who do not hold UK citizenship must be able to show that they have all the required statutory documentation (work permits etc) to cover the period of the research training fellowship.
Level of Study: Doctorate, Postgraduate, Professional development.

Purpose: To enable the training of young medical and non-medical graduates in research techniques and methodology in areas of interest to the charity.
Type: Training Fellowship.
No. of awards offered: Varies.
Frequency: Annual.
Value: Varies.
Length of Study: Up to 3 years.
Study Establishment: Arranged by the applicant.
Country of Study: United Kingdom.
Application Procedure: The appropriate application should be submitted.
Closing Date: Last Friday in January.
Additional Information: Fellowships are advertised separately each year in November.

THE ADA ENDOWMENT AND ASSISTANCE FUND, INC.

211 East Chicago Avenue, Chicago, IL, 60611-2678, United States of America
Tel: (1) 312 440 2567
Fax: (1) 312 440 2822
www: http://www.ada.org
Contact: Ms Marsha L Mountz, Manager

The purpose of the American Dental Association Endowment and Assistance Fund, Inc. is to provide a measure of financial assistance to certain groups of individuals who have a financial hardship, whether due to educational needs, chemical dependency, disability or disaster.

Allied Dental Health Scholarship (Dental Hygiene, Dental Assisting, Dental Laboratory Technology)

Subjects: Scholarships in the Allied Dental Health fields of dental hygiene, dental assisting and dental laboratory technology.
Eligibility: Open to US citizens only. Applicants must be entering first-year (Dental Assisting/Dental Laboratory Technology) or entering second year (Dental Hygiene/Dental Laboratory Technology). Students enrolled in an Allied Dental Health Programme accredited by the Commission on Dental Accreditation of the American Dental Health Association. Applicants must have a minimum GPA of 2.8 (Dental Assisting/Dental Laboroatory Technology) or 3.0 (Dental Hygiene) based on a 4.0 scale and show financial need of at least US$1,000.
Level of Study: Professional development.
Purpose: To defray study expenses which include tuition, fees, books, supplies and living expenses.
Type: Scholarship.
No. of awards offered: 20 dental hygiene, 10 dental assisting, 5 dental laboratory technology.
Frequency: Annual.
Value: US$1,000.
Country of Study: USA.

Application Procedure: Application forms are available at Allied Health Programs and are distributed by school officials. Applications must be submitted on original forms. They must be typed and completed and signed with the assistance of school officials. Applications must be embossed with the school's official seal on the academic achievement record form. Applicants must submit the completed application form, two typed letters of reference and a one page typed geographical sketch.
Closing Date: August 15th (Dental Hygiene, Dental Laboratory Technology) or September 15th (Dental Assisting).
Additional Information: Dental Laboratory student scholarships are renewable. Dental Hygiene and Dental Assisting student scholarships are not renewable.

Dental Student Scholarship

Subjects: Dentistry.
Eligibility: Open to US citizens only Applicants must be full-time entering second year students enrolled in a dental school accredited by the Commision on Dental Accreditation of the American Dental Association. Applicants must have a minimum GPA of 3.0 based on a 4.0 scale and show financial need of at least US$2,500.
Level of Study: Postgraduate.
Purpose: To defray school expenses which include tuition, fees, books, supplies and living expenses.
Type: Scholarship.
No. of awards offered: Between 15-25.
Frequency: Annual.
Value: US$2,500.
Country of Study: USA.
Application Procedure: Application forms are available at dental schools and are distributed by school officials. Applications must be submitted on original forms. They msut be typed and they must be completed and signed with the assistance of school officials. Applications must be embossed with the school's official seal on the academic achievement record form. Applicants must submit the completed application form, two typed letter of reference and a one page typed geographical sketch.
Closing Date: July 31st.
Additional Information: This scholarship is not renewable.

Minority Dental Student Scholarship

Subjects: Dentistry.
Eligibility: Open to US citizens only. Applicants must be a member of one of the following groups: Black African American, Native American or Hispanic. Open to US citizens only. Applicants must be full-time entering second year students enrolled in a dental school accredited by the Commision on Dental Accreditation of the American Dental Association. Applicants must have a minimum GPA of 3.0 based on a 4.0 scale and show financial need of at least US$2,000.
Level of Study: Postgraduate.
Purpose: To defray school expenses which include tuition, fees, books, supplies and living expenses.
Type: Scholarship.
No. of awards offered: Between 15-20.

Frequency: Annual.
Value: US$2,000.
Country of Study: USA.
Application Procedure: Application forms are available at dental schools and are distributed by school officials. Applications must be submitted on original forms. They must be typed and completed and signed with the assistance of school officials. Applications must be embossed with the school's official seal on the academic achievement record form. Applicants must submit the completed application form, two typed letters of reference and a one page typed geographical sketch.
Closing Date: July 31st.
Additional Information: This scholarship is not renewable.

ADHA INSTITUTE FOR ORAL HEALTH

Suite 3400
444 North Michigan Avenue, Chicago, IL, 60611, United States of America
Tel: (1) 312 440 8900
www: http://www.hsf.ca/research
Contact: Ms Linda Caradine, Associate Administrator

The ADHA Institute for Oral Health administers scholarship programs for full-time dental hygiene students at the certificate-associate, baccalaureate, and graduate levels. ADHA Institute Scholarship awards invest in future careers of dental hygiene students.

ADHA Institute Minority Scholarship

Subjects: Dental hygiene.
Eligibility: Eligible applicants include African Americans, Hispanics, Asians, Native Americans and males. Open to full-time students at the certificate/associate, baccalaureate graduate and doctoral levels. Scholars must currently be enrolled as full-time students in a dental hygiene programme in the USA, have completed a minimum of one year with a grade point average of at least 3.0, and be able to demonstrate financial need.
Level of Study: Postgraduate.
Purpose: Awarded to members of a minority group(s) currently under represented in dental hygiene programmes.
Type: Scholarship.
No. of awards offered: 2.
Frequency: Dependent on funds available.
Value: Up to US$2,000.
Country of Study: United Kingdom.
Application Procedure: Please write for details or visit our website.
Closing Date: June 1st.
Additional Information: This is a designated scholarship and is awarded based on how well the applicant demonstrates the goal achievement described.

ADHA Institute Scholarship Program

Subjects: Dental hygiene.
Eligibility: Open to full-time students at the certificate or associate, baccalaureate graduate and doctoral levels. Scholars must currently be enrolled as full-time students in a dental hygiene programme in the USA, have completed a minimum of one year with a grade point average of at least 3.0, and be able to demonstrate financial need. Additional requirements vary depending upon degree level.
Level of Study: Doctorate, Postgraduate.
Purpose: To invest in the future careers of dental hygiene students.
Type: Scholarship.
No. of awards offered: Approx. 20.
Frequency: Annual.
Value: Up to US$2,000.
Length of Study: 1 year; not renewable.
Country of Study: USA.
Application Procedure: Please write for details or visit our website.
Closing Date: June 1st.
Additional Information: Specific areas of this scholarship programme include Certificate/ Associate Scholarship Program, Baccalaureate Scholarship Program, and Graduate Scholarship Program.

Colgate 'Bright Smiles, Bright Futures' Minority Scholarships

Subjects: Dental Hygiene.
Eligibility: Open to male African Americans, Hispanics, Asians, and Native Americans. Open to full-time students at the certificate/associate, baccalaureate graduate and doctoral levels. Scholars must currently be enrolled as full-time students in a dental hygiene programme in the USA, have completed a minimum of one year with a grade point average of at least 3.0, and be able to demonstrate financial need.
Level of Study: Postgraduate.
Purpose: Awarded to members of minority groups currently under represented in dental hygiene programmes.
Type: Scholarship.
No. of awards offered: 2.
Frequency: Dependent on funds available.
Value: Up to US$2,000.
Country of Study: USA.
Application Procedure: Please write for details or visit our website.
Closing Date: June 1st.
Additional Information: This is a designated scholarship and is awarded based on how well the applicant demonstrates the goal achievement described.

Dr Alfred C Fones Scholarship

Subjects: Dental Hygiene.
Eligibility: Open to full-time students at the certificate/associate, baccalaureate graduate and doctoral levels. Scholars must currently be enrolled as full-time students in a dental hygiene programme in the USA, have

completed a minimum of one year with a grade point average of at least 3.0, and be able to demonstrate financial need. Additional requirements vary depending upon degree level.
Level of Study: Graduate.
Purpose: Awarded to an applicant in the baccalaureate or graduate degree categories who intends to become a dental hygiene teacher/educator.
Type: Scholarship.
No. of awards offered: 1.
Frequency: Dependent on funds available.
Value: Up to $2,000.
Country of Study: United Kingdom.
Application Procedure: Please write for details or visit our website.
Closing Date: June 1st.
Additional Information: This is a designated scholarship and is awarded based on how well the applicant demonstrates the goal achievement described.

Dr Harold Hillenbrand Scholarship

Subjects: Dental hygiene.
Eligibility: Open to full-time students at the certificate/associate, baccalaureate graduate and doctoral levels. Scholars must currently be enrolled as full-time students in a dental hygiene programme in the USA, have completed a minimum of one year with a grade point average of at least 3.0, and be able to demonstrate financial need.
Level of Study: Postgraduate.
Purpose: Awarded to an applicant who demonstrate specific academic excellence and outstanding clinical performance, in addition to having a minimum dental hygiene cumulative grade point average of 3.5.
Type: Scholarship.
No. of awards offered: 1.
Frequency: Dependent on funds available.
Value: Up to US$2,000.
Country of Study: United Kingdom.
Application Procedure: Please write for details or visit our website.
Closing Date: June 1st.
Additional Information: This is a designated scholarship and is awarded based on how well the applicant demonstrates the goal achievement described.

Irene E Newman Scholarship

Subjects: Dental hygiene.
Eligibility: Open to full-time students at the certificate/associate, baccalaureate graduate and doctoral levels. Scholars must currently be enrolled as full-time students in a dental hygiene programme in the USA, have completed a minimum of one year with a grade point average of at least 3.0, and be able to demonstrate financial need.
Level of Study: Postgraduate.
Purpose: Awarded to an applicant who demonstrates strong potential in public health or community dental health.
Type: Scholarship.
No. of awards offered: 1.
Frequency: Dependent on funds available.
Value: Up to US$2,000.

Country of Study: United Kingdom.
Application Procedure: Please write for details or visit our website.
Closing Date: June 1st.

John O Butler Graduate Scholarships

Subjects: Dental hygiene.
Eligibility: Open to full-time students at the certificate/associate, baccalaureate graduate and doctoral levels. Scholars must currently be enrolled as full-time students in a dental hygiene programme in the USA, have completed a minimum of one year with a grade point average of at least 3.0, and be able to demonstrate financial need.
Level of Study: Graduate.
Purpose: Awarded to an applicants enrolled in a Master's degree programme in dental hygiene or dental hygiene education.
Type: Scholarship.
No. of awards offered: 7.
Frequency: Dependent on funds available.
Value: Up to US$2,000.
Country of Study: USA.
Application Procedure: Please write for details or visit our website.
Closing Date: June 1st.
Additional Information: This is a designated scholarship and is awarded based on how well the applicant demonstrates the goal achievement described.

Margaret E Swanson Scholarship

Subjects: Dental hygiene.
Eligibility: Open to full-time students at the certificate/associate, baccalaureate graduate and doctoral levels. Scholars must currently be enrolled as full-time students in a dental hygiene programme in the USA, have completed a minimum of one year with a grade point average of at least 3.0, and be able to demonstrate financial need.
Level of Study: Postgraduate.
Purpose: Awarded to an applicant who demonstrates exceptional organisational leadership potential.
Type: Scholarship.
No. of awards offered: 1.
Frequency: Dependent on funds available.
Value: Up to US$2,000.
Country of Study: USA.
Application Procedure: Please write for details or visit our website.
Closing Date: June 1st.
Additional Information: This is a designated scholarship and is awarded based on how well the applicant demonstrates the goal achievement described.

Sigma Phi Alpha Graduate Scholarship

Subjects: Dental hygiene.
Eligibility: Open to full-time students at the certificate/associate, baccalaureate graduate and doctoral levels. Scholars must currently be enrolled as full-time

students in a dental hygiene programme in the USA, have completed a minimum of one year with a grade point average of at least 3.0, and be able to demonstrate financial need.
Level of Study: Graduate.
Purpose: Awarded to an outstanding applicant pursuing a degree in dental hygiene or a related field.
Type: Scholarship.
No. of awards offered: 1.
Frequency: Dependent on funds available.
Value: Up to US$2,000.
Country of Study: USA.
Application Procedure: Please write for details or visit our website.
Closing Date: June 1st.
Additional Information: This is a designated scholarship and is awarded based on how well the applicant demonstrates the goal achievement described.

AFRICA EDUCATIONAL TRUST

Small Grants Project
38 King Street, London, WC2E 8JS, England
Tel: (44) 171 836 5075
Fax: (44) 171 379 0090
Email: mbrophy@aet.win-uk.net
www: http://www.africaeducationaltrust.mcmail.com
Contact: Director

Africa Educational Trust Emergency Grants

Subjects: All subjects.
Eligibility: Open to students from Africa studying in the UK. The applicant must have run into unexpected difficulties at the end of his or her course for which the small level of grant will, by itself or in conjunction with other grants, solve the problem. Most awards are made on a humanitarian basis. Academic considerations are more important at the postgraduate and research levels.
Level of Study: Unrestricted.
Purpose: To provide one-off grants on an emergency basis to students from Africa studying in the UK.
Type: Emergency Grant.
No. of awards offered: 30.
Frequency: Monthly.
Value: £100-£600.
Length of Study: Final year.
Country of Study: United Kingdom.
Additional Information: Applications should be made by post or via a third party (such as a student welfare officer). Emergency Grants are provided at any time of year. The Trust will also consider contributions towards conference fees.

Africa Educational Trust Scholarships

Subjects: All subjects, but emphasis on those linked or relevant to development.
Eligibility: Open to people of African descent. The scholarships are aimed mainly at refugees from Africa.
Level of Study: Postgraduate, Undergraduate.

Purpose: To fund general education, mainly to refugees from Africa.
Type: Scholarship.
No. of awards offered: Varies, depending on funds available.
Frequency: Annual, if funds are available.
Value: Full and partial scholarships are awarded: full may cover fees, maintenance, transport, and fieldwork costs.
Country of Study: EC countries but mainly UK.

Emergency and Small Grants for Students from Africa

Subjects: All subjects.
Eligibility: Applicants should be studying in the UK and hold a student's visa.
Purpose: To support students in the final four months of their course who need a small amount of money to help them complete their studies.
Type: Grant.
No. of awards offered: Varies.
Value: Maximum £800.
Length of Study: Final 4 months of their course.
Application Procedure: Please write for details.

Full and Part Time Scholarships

Subjects: All subjects.
Eligibility: Criteria varies for year to year, please write for details.
Type: Scholarship.
No. of awards offered: Varies.
Frequency: As available.
Value: Covers transport costs, fees and books.
Country of Study: Europe and Africa.
Application Procedure: Criteria varies from year to year, please write for details.
Closing Date: Criteria varies from year to year, please write for details.

AFRO-ASIAN INSTITUTE IN VIENNA AND CATHOLIC WOMEN'S LEAGUE OF AUSTRIA

Student Division
Türkenstrasse 3, Vienna, A-1090, Austria
Tel: (43) 1 222 31 05 145 213
Fax: (43) 1 222 31 05 145 312
Email: aai.wien@magnet.at
Contact: Mr Markus Pleschko, Study Advisor

The AAI's major function is to aid students from third world countries. Presently the AAI provide services for more than 5,000 students from developing countries, and count as an acknowledged contribution to Austrian development aid.

One World Scholarship Program

Subjects: All subjects.
Eligibility: Open to nationals of developing countries in Africa, Asia and Latin America who are between the ages of 18 and 35, and who have had adequate previous study or vocational practice in the specific field for which the scholarship is applied.
Level of Study: Unrestricted.
Purpose: To promote cultural exchange, international development and international co-operation aid.
Type: Scholarship.
No. of awards offered: Varies.
Frequency: Annual.
Value: 2,500-7,000 Austrian Schillings each month.
Study Establishment: Universities (Vienna, Linz, Innsbruck).
Country of Study: Austria.
Application Procedure: Please contact the Institute personally, for an application form.
Closing Date: April 1st to 30th, for the following academic year.
Additional Information: It is preferred that candidates are able to speak German. Only those in financial need will be considered, and applicability of the special branch of study or training in the applicant's home country is essential. It is expected that scholars will return to their home country after studying. Good, and sometimes excellent, study results are also required. Preference is given to applicants from the least developed countries. It is one of AAI's essential aims to establish a 'partnership' contact between assisted students and the Scholarship donor which continues beyond the termination of studies. Only personal applications will be considered. Only about 10% of the applicants can be accepted. Only written applications are accepted.

AIREY NEAVE TRUST

40 Charles Street, London, W1X 7PB, England
Tel: (44) 171 495 0554
Fax: (44) 171 491 1118
Contact: Mrs Hannah Scott, Administrator

Airey Neave Trust Award

Subjects: Postgraduate education.
Eligibility: Open to refugees and those given exceptional leave to remain, recognised as such by the Home Office, and resident in Britain.
Level of Study: Doctorate, Postdoctorate, Postgraduate, Professional development.
Purpose: To help bona fide refugees in the United Kingdom, recognised by the Home Office, to re-qualify or retrain in their professions or trades.
No. of awards offered: 15-20.
Frequency: Annual.
Value: £1,000-£2,000.
Length of Study: 1 year, initially.
Study Establishment: College or university.
Country of Study: United Kingdom.

Application Procedure: Application form must be completed and submitted with a letter from the Home Office confirming status.
Closing Date: May 1st.
Additional Information: Applications should be addressed to Miss Jeanne Townsend.

For further information contact:

Calshott Cottage
Church Street
Sturminster, Newton, Dorset, DT10 1DB, England
Contact: Miss J Townsend

ALBERTA HERITAGE FOUNDATION FOR MEDICAL RESEARCH (AHFMR)

3125 Manulife Place
10180-101 Street, Edmonton, Alberta, T5J 3S4, Canada
Tel: (1) 403 423 5727
Fax: (1) 403 429 3509
Email: postmaster@ahfmr.ab.ca
www: http://www.ahfmr.ab.ca
Contact: Ms Maureen E Hagan, Grants and Awards Co-ordinator

The Alberta Heritage Foundation for Medical Research support a community of researchers who generate knowledge that improves the health and quality of life of Albertans and people throughout the world. The Foundation's long-term commitment is to fund basic patient and health research based on international standards of excellence and carried out by new and established investigators and researchers in training.

Alberta Heritage Clinical Fellowships

Subjects: Medical research.
Eligibility: Open to candidates who hold an MD or DDS and have received a significant portion of postgraduate training in Alberta.
Level of Study: Postgraduate.
Purpose: To provide an opportunity for research training to candidates who have completed clinical sub-specialty training requirements.
Type: Fellowship.
No. of awards offered: Approx. 10.
Frequency: Twice a year.
Value: C$3,000 research allowance, plus stipend.
Length of Study: 2 years; renewable for 1 additional year.
Study Establishment: An appropriate institution, normally in Alberta.
Country of Study: Canada.
Application Procedure: Application form must be completed.
Closing Date: March 1st, October 1st.

Alberta Heritage Clinical Investigatorships

Subjects: Medical research.
Eligibility: Open to candidates who hold an MD or DDS, have completed all requirements for clinical speciality recognition, and who are eligible to hold a full-time position in a clinical department of the sponsoring institution.
Level of Study: Professional development.
Purpose: To provide funding for highly qualified clinicians to further their research experience beyond the fellowship level in a setting providing guidance and supervision by an established scientist.
Type: Investigatorship.
No. of awards offered: Varies.
Frequency: Annual.
Value: A stipend plus an establishment grant; values are negotiated individually.
Length of Study: 3 years, may be extended for a further 3 years.
Study Establishment: An Alberta university or an affiliated hospital/institution.
Country of Study: Canada.
Application Procedure: Application form must be completed.
Closing Date: September 15th.
Additional Information: Candidates must be prepared to commit up to 75% of their time to medical research.

Alberta Heritage Full-Time Fellowships

Subjects: Medical research.
Eligibility: Open to graduates of science programmes relevant to AHFMR objectives or to health professional programmes, who have received a PhD not more than five years prior to application. Professional health degrees should not have been received more than ten years prior to application.
Level of Study: Postdoctorate.
Purpose: To enable doctoral graduates to prepare for careers as independent investigators.
Type: Fellowship.
No. of awards offered: Varies, approx. 30.
Frequency: Twice a year.
Value: C$2,000 research allowance, plus stipend.
Study Establishment: Normally at an Alberta university.
Country of Study: Canada.
Application Procedure: Application forms must be submitted by the deadline.
Closing Date: March 1st, October 1st.

Alberta Heritage Full-Time Studentships

Subjects: Medical research.
Eligibility: Open to academically superior students who wish to undertake full-time graduate studies in a discipline relevant to AHFMR objectives.
Level of Study: Undergraduate.
Purpose: To enable academically superior students to undertake full-time research training in a discipline relevant to the objectives of the Foundation.
Type: Studentship.

No. of awards offered: 50-70.
Frequency: Twice a year.
Value: C$16,500 stipend plus C$1,000 research allowance.
Length of Study: 1 year; renewable four times.
Study Establishment: An Alberta university.
Country of Study: Canada.
Application Procedure: Application form must be completed.
Closing Date: March 1st, October 1st.
Additional Information: Only full-time courses are health and biomedical and mental health.

Alberta Heritage Medical Scholarships

Subjects: Medical research.
Eligibility: Heritage Medical Scholars are investigators who have recently completed their postdoctoral research training and demonstrate the ability to initiate and conduct independent as well as collaborative research. They exhibit a desire and ability in training future research scientists. Heritage Senior Medical Scholarship candidates must hold a MD, DDS, DVM, PhD or the equivalent, and must have established a record of excellence in independent research over several years as a faculty member. The candidate must also show an interest in training Alberta's future research scientists.
Level of Study: Professional development.
Purpose: To assist in the recruitment and establishment of scientists in Alberta.
Type: Scholarship.
No. of awards offered: Varies.
Frequency: Annual.
Value: Stipend plus establishment grant; negotiated individually.
Length of Study: 5 years.
Study Establishment: An Alberta university or affiliate.
Country of Study: Canada.
Application Procedure: Application form must be completed.
Closing Date: September 15th.
Additional Information: Up to 75% of the candidate's time may be devoted to medical research.

Alberta Heritage Medical Scientist Awards

Subjects: Medical research.
Eligibility: Open to candidates who hold an MD, DDS, DVM or PhD (or equivalent) in a discipline important to AHFMR objectives and are eligible for a full-time appointment at the sponsoring institution.
Level of Study: Professional development.
Purpose: To assist in the recruitment and establishment of nationally or internationally recognised medical scientists in Alberta.
Type: Award.
No. of awards offered: Varies.
Frequency: Annual.
Value: Stipend plus establishment grant; negotiated individually.
Length of Study: 5 years; renewable.
Study Establishment: An Alberta university or affiliate.

Country of Study: Canada.
Application Procedure: Application form must be completed.
Closing Date: October 1st.
Additional Information: Up to 75% of the candidate's time may be devoted to medical research.

Alberta Heritage Part-Time Fellowships

Subjects: Medical research.
Eligibility: Open to graduates holding a PhD in a science relevant to AHFMR objectives or who are registered in a health professional programme in Alberta.
Level of Study: Postdoctorate.
Purpose: To enable continuing active participation in research during professional education.
Type: Fellowship.
No. of awards offered: Approx. 5.
Frequency: Twice a year.
Value: Pro-rated on full-time fellowship stipend. Dependent on the amount of time spent in research.
Length of Study: 1 year; renewable.
Study Establishment: An Alberta university.
Country of Study: Canada.
Application Procedure: Application form must be completed.
Closing Date: March 1st, October 1st.

Alberta Heritage Part-Time Studentship

Subjects: Medical research.
Eligibility: Open to students enrolled in a full-time professional degree programme who wish to continue research training on a part-time basis during the regular academic year.
Level of Study: Undergraduate.
Purpose: To enable full-time degree students to continue research training on a part-time basis.
Type: Studentship.
No. of awards offered: Approx. 5.
Frequency: Twice a year.
Value: Pro-rated on full-time stipend rate of C$16,500. Dependent on percentage of time spent in research.
Length of Study: 2 years to a maximum of 5 years support.
Study Establishment: An Alberta university.
Country of Study: Canada.
Application Procedure: Application form must be completed.
Closing Date: March 1st, October 1st.

Dr Lionel E Mcleod Health Research Scholarship

Subjects: Health.
Eligibility: Must be Canadian citizens or permanent residents at the Universities of Alberta, Calgary or British Columbia for full-time research that is relevant to human health.
Level of Study: Postgraduate.
Purpose: To enable academically superior students either engaged in, or accepted into, a full-time university program, to undertake full-time research training.

Type: Scholarship.
No. of awards offered: 1.
Frequency: Annual.
Value: Please write for details.
Country of Study: Canada.
Application Procedure: Please write for details.

Heritage Dental Fellowships

Subjects: Dentistry.
Eligibility: Candidates who possess a dental degree and who wish to pursue speciality clinical training or formal training in dental research followed by postgraduate speciality clinical training. Candidates should have obtained the degree within 5 years of application for a dental fellowship and must be licensable by the Alberta Dental Association. Candidates must be sponsored by a faculty supervisor with a record of productive health oriented research and sufficient research funding to ensure the satisfactory conduct of the research during the term of the award.
Level of Study: Postgraduate.
Purpose: To assist academically promising individuals who possess a dental degree and who wish to pursue specialist dental training.
No. of awards offered: 2.
Frequency: Twice a year.
Value: Please write for details.
Length of Study: 2 years; may be renewable.
Country of Study: Canada.
Application Procedure: The original and 10 complete copies of the application should reach the offices of the Foundation by either of the deadlines. They must be completed in full to be entered into the competition.
Closing Date: March 1st, October 1st.

Heritage Health Research Career Renewal Awards

Subjects: Epidemiology, biostatistics, psychosocial sciences, or clinical experimental method and design.
Eligibility: Must be a Canadian citizen or permanent resident.
Level of Study: Postdoctorate.
Purpose: To enable carefully selected Alberta Faculty members with demonstrated interest in clinical or health research, to obtain training.
No. of awards offered: 1.
Frequency: Twice a year.
Value: Please write for details.
Country of Study: Canada.
Application Procedure: Please write for details.
Closing Date: March 1st, October 1st.

Heritage Population Health Investigators

Subjects: Population health.
Eligibility: Applicants who have recently completed post MD or PhD research training, but who have not yet established an independent research record.
Level of Study: Postdoctorate.

Purpose: To assist in the recruitment and establishment in Alberta of well trained investigators in population health research.
No. of awards offered: 1.
Frequency: Annual.
Value: Please write for details.
Length of Study: 3 years (renewable).
Country of Study: Canada.
Application Procedure: Please write for details.
Closing Date: September 15th.

ALCOHOL BEVERAGE MEDICAL RESEARCH FOUNDATION

1122 Kenilworth Drive
Suite 407, Baltimore, MD, 21204, United States of America
Tel: (1) 410 821 7066
Fax: (1) 410 821 7065
Email: info@abmrf.org
www: http://www.abmrf.org
Contact: Dr Albert A Pawlowski, Vice President

The Foundation is a non-profit independent research organisation that provides support for scientific studies on the use of alcoholic beverages. It awards grants to study changes in drinking patterns, effects of moderate use of alcohol on health and well-being and the mechanisms underlying the behavioral and biomedical effects of alcohol.

Alcohol Beverage Medical Research Foundation Research Project Grant

Subjects: Medical and behavioral sciences.
Eligibility: Open to US and Canadian citizens.
Level of Study: Doctorate.
Purpose: To support new knowledge in order to prevent alcohol-related problems.
Type: Research Project Grant.
No. of awards offered: 30-40.
Frequency: Twice a year.
Value: Up to US$40,000.
Length of Study: Up to 2 years.
Study Establishment: Non-profit university, research institutions.
Country of Study: USA or Canada.
Application Procedure: Application form must be completed - these are available upon request.
Closing Date: February 1st and September 15th.

ALEXANDER GRAHAM BELL ASSOCIATION FOR THE DEAF

3417 Volta Place NW, Washington, DC, 20007, United States of America
Tel: (1) 202 337 5220
www: http://www.agbell.org/
Contact: Ms Elissa M Brooks, Public Relations

The Alexander Graham Bell Association for the Deaf is a nonprofit membership organisation that was established in 1890 to empower persons who are hearing impaired to function independently by promoting universal rights and optimal opportunities to learn to use, maintain, and improve all aspects of their verbal communications, including their abilities to speak, speechread, use residual hearing, and process both spoken and written language.

Alexander Graham Bell Scholarship Awards

Subjects: All subjects.
Eligibility: Open to auditory-oral students born with profound hearing loss (80 dB loss in the better ear, average), or a severe hearing loss (60 to 80 dB loss), who experienced such a loss before acquiring language. Candidates must use speech and residual hearing and/or speech-reading as their preferred customary form of communication and demonstrate a potential for leadership. In addition, applicants must have applied to, or already be enrolled full time in, a regular college or university programme for hearing students.
Level of Study: Unrestricted.
Purpose: To encourage severely or profoundly hearing-impaired students to attend regular hearing colleges.
Type: Scholarship.
No. of awards offered: Varies.
Frequency: Annual.
Value: US$250-US$1,000.
Country of Study: USA.
Application Procedure: Requests for application must be received, in writing, by December 1st. Photocopies of applications are not accepted.
Closing Date: March 15th.

ALEXANDER VON HUMBOLDT FOUNDATION

Jean-Paul Strasse 12, Bonn, Bad Godesberg, D-53173, Germany
Tel: (49) 228 833 0126
Fax: (49) 228 833 212
Email: post@avh.de
www: http://www.avh.de
Telex: 885 627
Contact: Dr Heide Radlanski

The Humboldt Foundation grants research fellowships to foreign scholars who hold doctorates and have not yet reached the age of 40, and research awards to internationally recognised foreign scholars of any age, enabling them to spend a lengthy period of research in the Federal Republic of Germany.

Federal Chancellor Scholarship

Subjects: Arts and humanities, business administration and management, fine and applied arts, mass communication and information science, medicine, recreation, welfare, protective services, religion and theology, social and behavioural sciences.
Eligibility: Open to US citizens only.
Level of Study: Postgraduate.
Purpose: To maintain and foster a close relationship between the USA and Germany by sponsoring individuals who demonstrate the potential of playing a pivotal role in the future development of this relationship.
Type: Scholarship.
No. of awards offered: 10.
Frequency: Annual.
Value: DM3,000-DM5,000 per month plus travel costs.
Length of Study: 12 months.
Study Establishment: Academic or other research institutions.
Country of Study: Germany.
Application Procedure: Application form must be completed; available from Bonn or Washington office.
Closing Date: October 31st, for next academic year.

Feodor Lynen Research Fellowships for German Scholars

Subjects: All academic fields.
Eligibility: Open to German nationals.
Level of Study: Postdoctorate.
Purpose: To enable highly-qualified German scholars (of less than 38 years of age) to conduct research of their choice at home institutions of non-German recipients of Humboldt fellowships and prizes.
Type: Fellowship.
No. of awards offered: Up to 150.
Frequency: Annual.
Value: DM4,000-DM5,000 per month (joint financing by Humboldt Foundation and host institute is required).
Length of Study: 1-4 years.
Study Establishment: Research institutions or universities.
Country of Study: Any, except Germany.
Application Procedure: Application form is required, available from Bonn and Washington addresses.
Closing Date: February 15th, June 15th, October 15th.

Humboldt Research Award for Foreign Scholars

Subjects: All subjects.
Eligibility: Open to all nationalities except Germans.
Level of Study: Postdoctorate.

Purpose: To enable internationally recognised foreign scholars to conduct research on a project of their choice in Germany.
Type: Research Prize.
No. of awards offered: Up to 200.
Frequency: Annual.
Value: Between DM20,000 and DM150,000 plus travel costs.
Length of Study: 4-12 months.
Study Establishment: Universities, research institutions.
Country of Study: Germany.
Application Procedure: Eminent German scholars propose candidates directly to the Foundation in Bonn. Direct applications are not accepted.
Closing Date: No deadline; nominations are accepted throughout the year.
Additional Information: Selection committee meetings are held twice per year, in March and October.

Japan Society for the Promotion of Science (JSPS) Research Fellowships

Subjects: All academic fields.
Eligibility: Open to German nationals only.
Level of Study: Postdoctorate.
Purpose: To enable highly-qualified German scholars (of less than 38 years of age), to carry out research projects of their own choice at universities or non-university research institutions in Japan.
Type: Fellowship.
No. of awards offered: 25.
Frequency: Annual.
Value: 270,000 Yen plus travel and housing allowance.
Length of Study: 12-24 months.
Study Establishment: University or other research institution.
Country of Study: Japan.
Application Procedure: Application form must be completed.
Closing Date: February 15th, June 15th, October 15th.

Max-Planck Award for International Co-operation

Subjects: All academic fields.
Eligibility: Open to scholars of all disciplines and nations.
Level of Study: Postdoctorate, Professional development.
Purpose: To enable internationally recognised foreign and German scholars to conduct long-term co-operative research.
Type: Research Prize.
No. of awards offered: 12.
Frequency: Annual.
Value: Up to DM250,000.
Length of Study: 3-5 years.
Country of Study: Germany.
Application Procedure: Nomination by presidents of German universities, academies of sciences, Max-Planck Society, corporations of large research establishments, Fraunhofer Society, German Research Association, former prize holders, and selection committee members.
Closing Date: April 15th.
Additional Information: Selection occurs once per year.

Postdoctoral Humboldt Research Fellowships

Subjects: Postdoctoral academic research in any subject.
Eligibility: Open to persons of any nationality other than German, up to 40 years of age, who have obtained a PhD degree or equivalent, who can furnish proof of independent research and can submit academic publications. Candidates in the arts and humanities should possess sound German language ability. Those in the natural, medical and engineering sciences should possess English language ability. (German language courses at the Goethe Institute in Germany for 2-4 months may be available prior to commencement of the Research Fellowship). Candidates should already have established relations with a German research institute where the project can be realised.
Level of Study: Postdoctorate.
Purpose: To provide opportunities for young, highly qualified scholars from abroad to carry out research projects of their own choice in Germany.
Type: Research Fellowship.
No. of awards offered: Approx. 500.
Frequency: Annual.
Value: DM3,600-DM4,400 per month, plus travel allowance for Research Fellow only, and dependant's allowance.
Length of Study: 6-12 months, with the possibility of extension for a limited number of months.
Study Establishment: Universities or research institutions in Germany.
Country of Study: Germany.
Application Procedure: Application form must be completed (available from Bonn or Washington office); submit completed forms and application documents to Bonn office at least five months before selection committee meeting, during which the decision is to be made.
Closing Date: No specified deadline, applications can be accepted at any time.
Additional Information: Applications should be forwarded directly to the Foundation or through diplomatic or consular offices of the Federal Republic of Germany in the candidates' respective countries. The Foundation also offers up to 150 Feodor Lynen Research Fellowships to German postdoctoral researchers to foster co-operation with former Humboldt Fellows and Award-holders abroad.

Science and Technology Agency (STA) Research Fellowships

Subjects: All academic fields.
Eligibility: Open to German nationals only.
Level of Study: Postdoctorate.
Purpose: To enable highly-qualified German scholars up to the age of 38 to carry out research projects of their own choice at non-university research institutions in Japan.
Type: Fellowship.
No. of awards offered: 10.
Frequency: Annual.
Value: Y270,000 plus travel and housing allowance.
Length of Study: 6-24 months.
Study Establishment: Non-university research institution.
Country of Study: Japan.

Application Procedure: Application form must be completed.
Closing Date: February 15th, June 15th, October 15th.

ALZHEIMER'S ASSOCIATION

Medical & Scientific Affairs
919 North Michigan Avenue
Suite 1000, Chicago, IL, 60611-1676, United States of America
Tel: (1) 312 335 5779
Email: grants@alz.org
www: http://www.alz.org
Contact: Grants Co-ordinator

The Alzheimer's Association aims to be a source of information, support and assistance on issues related to Alzheimer's disease. It seeks to provide leadership in attempting to eliminate Alzheimer's disease through the advancement of research, while enhancing care and support services for the individuals concerned, and their families. To this end, the Association funds select projects for biomedical, social and behavioural research, as well as promoting, developing, and disseminating educational programmes and training guidelines for health and social service professionals.

Alzheimer's Association Investigator-Initiated Research Grants

Subjects: Alzheimer's disease and related disorders.
Eligibility: Investigators from all stages of research career development are encouraged to apply.
Level of Study: Postgraduate.
Purpose: To build on the success of established investigators, by providing sustained support for independent research projects.
Type: Research Grant.
No. of awards offered: 55.
Frequency: Annual.
Value: The awards will be limited to US$60,000 per year (direct and indirect) for up to three years, for a total award of no more than US$180,000. Indirect costs are capped at 10%.
Length of Study: 2 or 3 years.
Country of Study: Any country.
Application Procedure: Please write for details.
Closing Date: October 5th.

Alzheimer's Association Pilot Research Grants

Subjects: Alzheimer's disease and related disorders.
Eligibility: Eligibility is restricted to investigators who have had less than 10 years of research experience, including postdoctoral fellowships or residencies, after receipt of the doctoral degree. The 10 year period taken from the submission date of the grant application. Applications from graduate and doctoral students for research projects, which will be used for the thesis or dissertation, will be accepted and judged by the usual scientific criteria.
Level of Study: Postgraduate.

Purpose: To stimulate interest by new investigators, to enable new and established investigators to test the feasibility of new ideas on a small scale, and to enable investigators to generate pilot data to support proposals to NIH foundations, or the Association for larger grants.

Type: Research Grant.

No. of awards offered: Varies.

Frequency: Annual.

Value: The awards will be for US$40,000 per year (direct and indirect) for up to two years, for a total award limited to US$80,000. Indirect costs are capped at 10%.

Length of Study: Up to 2 years.

Country of Study: Any country.

Application Procedure: Please write for details.

Closing Date: The letter of intent must be received by September 18th. Letters of intent will not be accepted after the receipt date. No exceptions will be made. To be considered under this research grant program, applications must be received by the close of business on October 16th.

The Alzheimer's Association Pioneer Awards for Alzheimer's Disease Research

Subjects: Alzeimer's disease.

Eligibility: Investigators who have made important, ground-breaking contributions to Alzheimer's disease are encouraged to apply. It is anticipated that the successful applicants will hold senior academic rank, have international recognition of their research contributions, have lengthy records of peer reviewed publications in major scientific journals, and have long track records of substantial funding from the National Institutes of Health or other national funding agencies. Investigators who have been Directors of Alzheimer's Disease Centers (P50 and P30), principal investigators on NIH sponsored programme projects grants (P01) or LEAD awardees are eligible. Members of the Medical and Scientific Advisory Council and of the National Board of the Alzheimer's Association are ineligible to apply to this programme.

Purpose: To offer investigators the unique opportunity of obtaining substantial research and research support funding. The goal of the award is to support a two pronged effort in the investigator's laboratory: work on a focused research project aimed at questions surrounding the interventions for Alzheimer's disease; and flexible research support which will allow rapid mid-course adjustments in the ongoing research program.

Type: Award.

No. of awards offered: 3.

Value: Each Pioneer Award is limited to a total cost of US$1,000,000, including 10% indirect cost. Requests in any year may not, exceed US$300,000 (direct and indirect).

Length of Study: Investigators may request up to 5 years of support under this program, and may allocate the funds across the 5 years as most appropriately supports their research program.

Application Procedure: Please write for details.

Closing Date: The letter of intent must be received by October 9th. Letters of intent will not be accepted after the receipt date. No exceptions will be made. To be considered under this research grant program, applications must be received by the close of business on November 20th.

The Senator Mark Hatfield Award for Clinical Research in Alzheimer's Disease

Subjects: Alzheimer's Disease and related disorders.

Eligibility: Applicants for the Hatfield Award are limited to those investigators who received their doctoral degree less than 10 years prior to submission of the application. The Hatfield Award is aimed at those investigators whose goal is to establish research careers focused on clinical issues in Alzheimer's disease.

Purpose: To honour Senator Hatfield's long commitment to Alzheimer's disease research in general, and clinical research in particular. The award is designed to focus on the Senator's interests in clinical research and support of new investigators.

Type: Award.

No. of awards offered: 1.

Value: The award will be for US$75,000 per year (direct and indirect) for up to three years, for a total award limited to US$225,000. Indirect costs are capped at 10%.

Length of Study: Up to 3 years.

Application Procedure: Please write for details.

Closing Date: The letter of intent must be received no later than October 9th. Letters of intent will not be accepted after the receipt date. No exceptions will be made. To be considered under this research grant program, applications must be received by the close of business on December 18th.

The TLL Temple Foundation Discovery Awards

Subjects: Alzheimer's disease.

Eligibility: Principal investigators must have a clear and well-demonstrated history of competitive funding. Investigators are eligible as evidenced by the following non-exclusive list (examples are for illustrative purposes only): academic appointment; peer-reviewed, external multi-year grant support on which the applicant is the principal investigator (PI); independent laboratory operation; and quality and independence of publication record. Past Temple award winners are not eligible for this competition.

Purpose: To provide support for investigators fostering new research to discover the biological basis of Alzheimer's disease and to develop effective treatments and practical methods to ease the suffering of patients and families while the search for a cure goes on.

Type: Award.

No. of awards offered: Up to 10.

Value: US$250,000 each (direct plus indirect cost) will be made under this program. Indirect costs are limited to 10%.

Application Procedure: The applications must demonstrate: a history of innovative thinking and productive research; a history of contributing significantly to Alzheimer research or related areas with the likelihood of making significant contributions to the field; and commitment and dedication to discovering the causes, effective treatments, and risk and genetic factors. Request for application material, should be sent to the attention of Nico Stanculescu via email at nico.stanculescu@alz.org or fax/mail the Association. The application kit will be sent with the instructions for completing and submitting the application.

Closing Date: To be considered under this research grant program, applications must be received by the close of business on April 2nd.

Zenith Awards

Subjects: Alzheimer's disease.
Eligibility: Open to projects that will test new and innovative ideas that are likely to lead to fundamental findings related to the biology of Alzheimer's disease.
Level of Study: Postgraduate.
Purpose: To provide major support to qualified scientists in basic biomedical research who have already made substantial contributions in the field of Alzheimer's.
Type: Award.
No. of awards offered: 5.
Frequency: Annual.
Value: The awards will be for US$100,000 per year (direct and indirect) for two years, for a total award of US$200,000. Indirect costs are capped at 10%.
Length of Study: 2 years; with possible competitive renewal upon review of research progress.
Country of Study: Any country.
Application Procedure: Please write for details.
Closing Date: The letter of intent must be received by October 23rd. Letters of intent will not be accepted after the receipt date. No exceptions will be made. To be considered under this research grant program, applications must be received by the close of business on December 4th.
Additional Information: Applications will be evaluated by an expert panel of senior scientists, already well recognised for their own accomplishments in Alzheimer's research. Detailed eligibility and application requirements are available on request.

ALZHEIMER'S DISEASE SOCIETY

Gordon House
10 Greencoat Place, London, SW1P 1PH, England
Tel: (44) 171 306 0606
Fax: (44) 171 306 0808
Email: 101762.422@compuserve.com
Contact: Mr Harry Cayton, Executive Director

The Alzheimer's Disease Society tries to relieve and treat people with Alzheimer's disease and other dementia, and to provide support for them, their families and carers.

Research Grants

Subjects: Alzheimer's research.
Eligibility: Candidates form any country are eligible to apply.
Level of Study: Postgraduate.
Purpose: Research into cause and cure of dementia.
Type: Research Grant.
No. of awards offered: Varies.
Country of Study: Any country.
Application Procedure: Please contact the Director of Research for more information.

AMERICAN ACADEMY OF CHILD AND ADOLESCENT PSYCHIATRY

3615 Wisconsin Avenue NW, Washington, DC, 20016, United States of America
Tel: (1) 202 966 7300
Fax: (1) 202 966 2891
Email: kpope@aacap.org
www: http://www.aacap.org
Contact: Ms Kayla Pope, Deputy Director of Research and Training

The American Academy of Child and Adolescent Psychiatry is a national, professional medical association established in 1953 as a non-profit corporation to support and improve the quality of life for children, adolescents and families affected by mental illnesses.

James Comer Minority Research Fellowship for Medical Students

Subjects: Psychiatry and mental health.
Eligibility: Applications are accepted from African American, Native American, Alaskan Native, Mexican American, Hispanic & Pacific Islander students in accredited US medical schools.
Level of Study: Graduate.
Purpose: To support work during the summer with a Child & Adolescent Psychiatrist-Researcher Mentor.
Type: Fellowship.
No. of awards offered: 12.
Frequency: Annual.
Value: US$2,500 plus expenses for the AACAP annual meeting.
Country of Study: USA.
Application Procedure: Applications should include: a 2-page statement from the student outlining his/her background information, career goals and specific research interests. Also require the student's résumé and a letter verifying the student's good standing in medical school.
Closing Date: April 1st.

Jeanne Spurlock Minority Medical Student Clinical Fellowship in Child and Adolescent Psychiatry

Subjects: Psychiatry and mental health.
Eligibility: Applications are accepted from African American, Asian American, Native American, Alaskan Native, Mexican American, Hispanic & Pacific Islander students in accredited US medical schools.
Level of Study: Graduate.
Purpose: To support work during the summer with a Child & Adolescent Psychiatrist Mentor.
Type: Fellowship.
No. of awards offered: 5.
Frequency: Annual.
Value: US$2,500 plus expenses for the AACAP annual meeting.
Country of Study: USA.

Application Procedure: Applications should include a 2-page statement from the student outlining his/her background information, career goals and specific research interests. Also require student's résumé and a letter verifying the student's good standing in medical school.
Closing Date: April 1st.

Jeanne Spurlock Research Fellowship in Drug Abuse and Addiction for Minority Medical Students

Subjects: Psychiatry and mental health.
Eligibility: Applications are accepted from African American, Asian American, Native American, Alaskan Native, Mexican American, Hispanic & Pacific Islander students in accredited US medical schools. All applications must relate to substance abuse research.
Level of Study: Graduate.
Purpose: To support work during the summer with a Child & Adolescent Psychiatrist Research-Mentor.
Type: Fellowship.
No. of awards offered: 5.
Frequency: Annual.
Value: US$2,500 plus expenses for the AACAP annual meeting.
Country of Study: USA.
Application Procedure: Applications should include: a 2-page statement from the student outlining his/her background information, career goals and specific research interests. Also require the student's résumé and a letter verifying the student's good standing in medical school.
Closing Date: April 1st.

THE AMERICAN ACADEMY OF FACIAL PLASTIC AND RECONSTRUCTIVE SURGERY (AAFPRS FOUNDATION)

Educational and Research Foundation for the American Academy of Facial Plastic and Reconstructive Surgery (AAFPRS Foundation)
310 Henry Street, Alexandria, VA, 22314, United States of America
Tel: (1) 703 299 9291
Fax: (1) 703 299 8898
Email: info@aadprs.org
www: http://www.aafprs.org
Contact: Ms Ann Kent Holton, Development, Research and Humanitarian Programs

The Academy represents 2,700 facial plastic and reconstructive surgeons throughout the world. Its main mission is to promote the highest quality facial plastic surgery through education, dissemination of professional information and the establishment of professional standards. The AAFPRS was created to address the medical and scientific issues confronting facial plastic surgeons.

AAFPRS Investigator Development Grant

Subjects: Facial plastic surgery, clinical or laboratory research.
Eligibility: Open to AAFPRS members.
Level of Study: Postgraduate.
Purpose: To support the work of a young faculty member conducting significant clinical or laboratory research and the training of resident surgeons in research.
Type: Research Grant.
No. of awards offered: 1.
Frequency: Annual, if funds are available.
Value: US$15,000.
Length of Study: 2 years.
Study Establishment: The recipient's institution.
Country of Study: USA.
Application Procedure: Application form and other documentation must be submitted (to include CV and research plans).
Closing Date: December 15th.
Additional Information: Application forms and guidelines are available on request.

AAFPRS Resident Research Grants

Subjects: Facial plastic surgery.
Eligibility: Open to residents who are AAFPRS members. Residents at any level may apply even if the research work will be done during their fellowship year.
Level of Study: Postgraduate.
Purpose: To stimulate resident research in projects that are well conceived and scientifically valid.
Type: Research Grant.
No. of awards offered: Up to 3.
Frequency: Annual.
Value: US$5,000 - each award.
Length of Study: 2 years.
Study Establishment: The recipient's institution.
Country of Study: USA.
Application Procedure: Application form and other documentation must be submitted (to include CV and comprehensive research proposal).
Closing Date: December 15th.
Additional Information: Residents are encouraged to enter early in their training so that their applications may be revised and resubmitted if not accepted the first time. Application forms and guidelines are available on request.

Bernstein Grant

Subjects: Original research with direct application to facial plastic and reconstructive surgery.
Eligibility: Open to AAFPRS Fellow members.
Level of Study: Professional development.
Purpose: To encourage original research projects which will advance facial plastic and reconstructive surgery.
Type: Research Grant.
No. of awards offered: 1.
Frequency: From time to time.
Value: US$25,000.
Length of Study: 3 years.

Study Establishment: The recipient's practice or institution.
Country of Study: USA.
Application Procedure: Application form and other documentation must be submitted (to include CV and research proposal).
Closing Date: December 15th.
Additional Information: Application forms and guidelines are available on request.

AMERICAN ACADEMY OF FAMILY PHYSICIANS (AAFP)

8880 Ward Parkway, Kansas City, MO, 64114-2797, United States of America
Tel: (1) 816 333 9700
www: http://www.aafp.org/
Contact: Chairman, Mead Johnson Awards Committee

The American Academy of Family Physicians (AAFP) is a national, non-profit medical association of more than 88,000 members (family physicians, family practice residents, and medical students). The AAFP was founded in 1947 to promote and maintain high quality standards for family doctors who are providing continuing comprehensive health care to the public. It has grown to become one of the largest medical organizations in the United States, with chapters in 50 states, as well as international members throughout the world.

Mead Johnson Awards for Graduate Education in Family Practice

Subjects: Residency training in family practice.
Eligibility: Open to physicians who are second year residents in an approved practice residency programme. They must express the intention to enter the Family Practice of medicine in the USA. Applicants must be resident members of the American Academy of Family Physicians.
Level of Study: Postgraduate.
Purpose: To provide financial assistance for outstanding young physicians planning careers in the family practice of medicine in the USA.
Type: Monetary.
No. of awards offered: 20.
Frequency: Annual.
Value: US$2,000 per year.
Length of Study: 12 months; not renewable.
Study Establishment: Hospital training programs accredited by the Accreditation Council for Graduate Medical Education.
Country of Study: USA.
Application Procedure: Formal application must be submitted. Application to include: CV and personal

statement, reference letter and form from residency programme director, reference letter and form from active member of AAFP.
Closing Date: March 2nd.
Additional Information: Recipients will be guest of honour at an Awards Breakfast hosted by Mead Johnson during the Annual AAFP Meeting.

THE AMERICAN ACADEMY OF FIXED PROSTHODONTICS

Department of Restorative Dentistry
The University of Illinois at Chicago, Chicago, IL, 60612-7212, United States of America
Tel: (1) 312 413 1181
Fax: (1) 312 996 3535
Email: kentk@uic.edu
www: http://www.prosthodontics.org/forum/aafp/index.html
Contact: Dr Kent Knoernschild, Chairman of the Tylman Research Programme

The Academy consists of over 500 specialists around the world, dedicated to the pursuit of knowledge, truth, and competency in research, in teaching, and in the clinical practice of crown and bridge prosthodontics.

Tylman Research Program

Subjects: Dentistry.
Eligibility: Open to full-time students enrolled in any graduate or postgraduate programme who are conducting research pertinent to fixed prosthodontics. Proposals must be endorsed by the programme director of an accredited prosthodontic programme. Priority will be given to students in prosthodontic programmes. Predoctoral dental students are not eligible.
Level of Study: Postdoctorate, Postgraduate.
Purpose: To promote and support research in the field of fixed prosthodontics by graduate students.
Type: Grant.
No. of awards offered: 6.
Frequency: Annual.
Value: US$2,000.
Country of Study: USA.
Application Procedure: Protocol of research project submitted to the Academy Research Committee. The six best protocols are funded. The student must submit progress reports and final manuscript of completed project.
Closing Date: March 1st.
Additional Information: From the finalists, three awards are given to the first three winning manuscripts. First place wins US$1,000 and trip to annual AAFP meeting to present research on programme and receive a plaque. Second place wins US$500 and third place US$300. This is a competitive process.

AMERICAN ACADEMY OF PEDIATRICS (AAP)

Department of Education
PO Box 927
141 Northwest Point Boulevard, Elk Grove Village, IL, 60009-0927, United States of America
Tel: (1) 847 981 6759
Fax: (1) 847 228 5097
www: http://www.aap.org
Contact: Ms Jackie Bucko, Sections Manager

The American Academy of Pediatrics is an organisation of 55,000 primary care paediatricians, paediatric medical subspecialists and paediatric surgical specialists dedicated to the health , safety and well-being of infants, children, adolescents and young adults. To this end the Academy publishes guidelines on issues ranging from AIDS to Welfare Reform and supports a number of research grants and scholarships.

AAP Residency Scholarships

Subjects: Pediatrics.
Eligibility: Open to legal residents of the USA, Puerto Rico or Canada who have completed, or will have completed by July 1st, a qualifying approved internship (PL-O) or have completed a PL-1 year and have a definite commitment for a first year pediatric residency (PL-1 or PL-2) accredited by the Residency Review Committee for Pediatrics, and who are pediatric residents (PL-1, PL-2, or PL-3) in a training programme and have made a definite commitment for another year of residency (not fellowship) in a programme accredited by the Residency Review Committee for Pediatrics, and who have a real need for financial assistance.
Purpose: To enable young physicians to complete their training.
Type: Scholarship.
No. of awards offered: Varies.
Frequency: Annual.
Value: Varies: US$1,000; US$3,000; US$5,000.
Country of Study: Any country.
Application Procedure: Please write for details. Applications are automatically sent to all AAP resident members.
Closing Date: February 5th.
Additional Information: Applicants must support their applications with a letter from the department head or the chief of service as well as the Residency Programme Director substantiating the requirements outlined under eligibility. The letter must address the financial need, commitment to pediatrics and performance in the programme. If a change in residency programme is contemplated (i.e. moving to another institution), a letter from the Residency Programme Director certifying acceptance into the new programme will also be necessary.

AAP Resident Research Grants

Subjects: Pediatrics.
Eligibility: Applicants must be a pediatric resident in training.

Purpose: To enhance the development of research skills among physicians in pediatric training.
Type: Research Grant.
No. of awards offered: Approx. 15.
Frequency: Annual.
Value: US$2,000-5,000 plus travel and lodging.
Length of Study: Up to 2 years.
Country of Study: Any country.
Application Procedure: Please write for details.
Closing Date: February 5th.

AMERICAN ASSOCIATION FOR CANCER RESEARCH

Public Ledger Building
Suite 816
150 South Independence Mall, Philadelphia, PA, 19106-3483, United States of America
Tel: (1) 215 440 9300
Fax: (1) 215 440 9313
Email: webmaster@aacr.org
www: http://www.aacr.org
Contact: The Research Director

The American Association for Cancer Research (AACR) a scientific society of over 13,000 laboratory and clinical cancer researchers, was founded in 1907 to facilitate communication and dissemination of knowledge among scientists and other dedicated to the cancer problem to: foster research in cancer and related biomedical sciences; encourage presentation and discussion of new and important observations in the field; foster public education, science education and training; and to advance the undertaking of cancer etiology, prevention, diagnosis, and treatment; throughout the world.

AACR Career Development Awards in Cancer Research

Subjects: Cancer research.
Eligibility: Scientists in their first or second year of a full time, tenure tracked faculty appointment, at the level of assistant professor. Candidates must have completed productive postdoctoral research and demonstrated independent, instigator initiated research. Employees of a national government and employees of private industry are not eligible.
Level of Study: Postdoctorate.
Purpose: To support research by junior tenure track scientists, at the level of assistant professor, who are engaged in meritorious cancer research at an academic institution anywhere in the world.
Type: A variable number of Grants.
No. of awards offered: Varies.
Frequency: Annual.
Value: US$50,000 per annum.
Length of Study: 2 years.
Study Establishment: Universities and research institutions worldwide.

Country of Study: Any country.
Application Procedure: Candidates must be nominated by a member of AACR and must be an AACR member or apply for membership by the time the application is submitted. AACR Associate members may not be nominators.
Closing Date: January 15th.
Additional Information: For further information, please contact: Jenny Anne Horst Martz, tel: 215 440 9300, fax: 215 440 9372, email horst@aacr.org or refer to the website.

AACR EN Young Investigator Awards for Asian Scientists

Subjects: Cancer research.
Eligibility: Full-time predoctoral students and postdoctoral fellows and physicians in training who are engaged in cancer research or have training and the potential to make contributions in this field. This award programme applies only to minority groups which have been defined by the National Cancer Institute as being traditionally under-represented in cancer and biomedical research; these groups are African Americans, Alaskan Natives, Hispanic Americans, Native Americans and Native Pacific Islanders.
Level of Study: Doctorate, Postdoctorate, Postgraduate.
Purpose: To support the attendance of medical and graduate students, physicians-in-training and postdoctoral fellows at the AACR Annual meeting.
Type: Travel Grant.
No. of awards offered: Varies.
Frequency: Annual.
Value: Varies.
Length of Study: Varies.
Study Establishment: AACR Annual Meeting.
Country of Study: USA.
Application Procedure: For details pleasse contact Ms Robin E Felder, Membership Development Co-ordinator at the AACR office.
Closing Date: December 4th.
Additional Information: Letters of reference must accompany this application. Mentors are encouraged to submit individual letters of recommendation for each candidate.

AACR Gerald B Grindley Memorial Young Investigator Award

Subjects: Cancer research.
Eligibility: Young scientists who have submitted an abstract in the field of preclinical science.
Level of Study: Doctorate, Postdoctorate, Postgraduate.
Purpose: To support the attendance of medical and graduate students, physicians-in-training and postdoctoral fellows at the AACR Annual Meeting.
Type: Travel Grant.
No. of awards offered: Varies.
Frequency: Annual.
Value: Varies.
Length of Study: AARC Annual Meeting.
Country of Study: USA.

Application Procedure: For details please contact Jenny Anne Horst-Martz, tel: 215 440 9300, fax: 215 440 9372, email: horst@aacr.org.
Closing Date: November 6th.

AACR HBCU Faculty Award in Cancer Research

Subjects: Medical sciences.
Eligibility: Scientists at the level of assistant professor or above at an HBCU who are engaged in meritorious basic, clinical or translatorial cancer research. Candidates must be citizens of the United States or Canada, or permanent residents of these countries.
Level of Study: Predoctorate.
Purpose: To increase the scientific knowledge base of faculty members at historically black colleges and universities, and to encourage them and their students to pursue careers in cancer research.
Type: Travel Grant.
No. of awards offered: Varies.
Frequency: Annual.
Value: US$1,500.
Length of Study: Varies.
Study Establishment: AACR conferences.
Country of Study: USA.
Application Procedure: Submission of an application which includes the candidate's curriculum vitae, a list of publications, a statement from the candidate describing the benefit she or he expects to derive from attending the conference and at least one letter of reference.
Closing Date: December 4th.
Additional Information: For further information about this award programme please contact Ms Robin E Felder, Membership Development Co-ordinator at the AACR office, tel: 215 440 9300, fax: 215 440 9412, email: felder@aacr.org.

AACR Peczoller International Award for Cancer Research

Subjects: Cancer research.
Eligibility: Scientists who have made a major scientific discovery in the field of cancer and whose on going work holds promise for future contributions to cancer research.
Level of Study: Postdoctorate.
Purpose: To honour a scientist who has made a major scientific discovery in the field of cancer, who continues to be active in the field and whose on going work holds promise for the future contributions to cancer research.
Type: Prize.
No. of awards offered: Varies.
Frequency: Annual.
Value: US$75,000.
Study Establishment: Universities or research institutions worldwide.
Country of Study: Any country.
Application Procedure: By nomination. Nominations can be made by any scientist who is now or has been affiliated with an institution engaged in cancer research. Nomination packages should consist of the candidates curriculum vitae and a full list of published work, an indication of the candidates most important publications, a letter of

recommendation in English explaining why the candidate is deserving of this award. This letter should summarise the candidates major scientific achievements, indicate which of the candidate's publications best describe these achievements, and explain the impact of these achievements on progress in cancer research.
Closing Date: October 1st.
Additional Information: For further information please contact: Dr Peter K Vogt, Chairperson of the Selection Committee, AACR Peczoller International Award for Cancer Research, c/o American Association for Cancer Research, Inc.

AACR Research Fellowships

Subjects: Cancer research.
Eligibility: Candidates must have completed a PhD or other doctoral degree and currently be a postdoctoral or clinical research fellow at an institution in the Americas. Preferably candidates should have been a fellow for a minimum of two years and maximum of five years prior to the award.
Level of Study: Postdoctorate.
Purpose: To foster meritorious cancer research in the Americas by young scientists currently at the postdoctoral or clinical research fellow level.
Type: A variable number of Fellowships.
No. of awards offered: Varies.
Frequency: Annual.
Value: US$30,000 per annum.
Length of Study: 1 year, with the option of renewal for a further year.
Study Establishment: Universities or research institutions in the United States or Latin America.
Country of Study: USA.
Application Procedure: Candidates must be nominated by a member of the AACR or apply for membership by the time the application is submitted.
Closing Date: January 15th.
Additional Information: Academic faculty holding the rank of assistant professor or higher, graduate and medical students, medical residents, permanent government employees and employees of private industry are not eligible. For further information please contact: Jenny Anne Horst Martz at the AACR, tel: 215 440 9300, fax: 215 440 9372, email: horst@aacr.org, or refer to the website.

AACR Susan G Komen Breast Cancer Foundation Career Development Award

Subjects: Research related to breast cancer, including epidemological and prevention studies.
Eligibility: Junior, tenure track scientist, at the level of assistant professor, who are engaged in research related to breast cancer.
Level of Study: Postdoctorate.
Purpose: To support research by junior, tenure track scientists, at the level of assistant professor, who are engaged in meritorious research related to breast cancer at an academic institution anywhere in the world.
Type: A variable number of Grants.
No. of awards offered: Varies.

Frequency: Annual.
Value: US$50,000 per annum.
Length of Study: 2 years.
Study Establishment: Universities or research institutions worldwide.
Country of Study: Any country.
Application Procedure: Candidates must be nominated by a member of AACR and must be an AACR member or apply for membership by the time the application is submitted. AACR Associate members may not not be nominators..
Closing Date: January 15th.
Additional Information: For further information, please contact: Jenny Anne Horst Martz, tel: 215 440 9300, fax: 215 440 9372, email: horst@aacr.org, or refer to the website.

American Cancer Society Award for Research Excellence in Cancer Epidemiology and Prevention

Subjects: Cancer research, epidemiology and prevention.
Eligibility: Scientists who can demonstrate outstanding acheivements in the field of epidemiology, biomarkers and prevention.
Level of Study: Postdoctorate.
Purpose: To honour outstanding acheivements in the field of epidemiology, biomarkers and prevention.
Type: Award.
No. of awards offered: 1.
Frequency: Annual.
Value: Varies.
Length of Study: Varies.
Study Establishment: Universities or research institutions worldwide.
Country of Study: Any country.
Application Procedure: By nomination.
Closing Date: September 1st.
Additional Information: For further information please contact the AACR office.

Bruce F Cain Memorial Award

Subjects: Medicinal biochemistry, biochemistry and tumour biology.
Eligibility: Outstanding scientist pursuing research in the field of design, synthesis and biological evaluation of potential anticancer drugs.
Level of Study: Postdoctorate.
Purpose: To give recognition to an individual or research team for outstanding preclinical research that has implications for the improved care of cancer patients.
Type: Award.
No. of awards offered: 1.
Frequency: Annual.
Value: Varies.
Length of Study: Varies.
Study Establishment: Universities or research institutions worldwide.
Country of Study: Any country.
Application Procedure: By nomination.
Closing Date: September 1st.

Additional Information: For further information please contact the AACR office.

G H A Clowes Memorial Award

Subjects: Cancer research including laboratory research and epidemiological investigations.
Eligibility: Scientists who can demonstrate outstanding research results.
Level of Study: Postdoctorate.
Purpose: To give recognition of outstanding research accomplishments in basic cancer research.
Type: Award.
No. of awards offered: 1.
Frequency: Annual.
Value: Varies.
Length of Study: Varies.
Study Establishment: Universities or research institutions worldwide.
Country of Study: Any country.
Application Procedure: By nomination.
Closing Date: September 1st.
Additional Information: For further information please contact the AACR office.

Gertrude B Elion Cancer Research Award

Subjects: Cancer research.
Eligibility: Tenure tracked scientist at the level of assistant professor at an institution in the United States or Canada, who have completed their postdoctoral studies or clinical research by July 1st of the award year, and ordinarily not more than five years earlier. Candidates must be members of the AACR or apply for membership by the time the applications are submitted.
Level of Study: Postdoctorate.
Purpose: To foster meritorious basic, clinical or translatorial cancer research by a non-tenured, tenure tracked scientist at the level of assistant professor.
Type: Research Grant.
No. of awards offered: Varies.
Frequency: Annual.
Value: US$30,000.
Length of Study: 1 year.
Study Establishment: Universities or research institutions in the USA or Canada.
Country of Study: USA or Canada.
Application Procedure: Nomination by a member of the AACR.
Closing Date: December 15th.
Additional Information: For further information please contact: Jenny Anne Horst Martz. AACR, tel: 215 440 9300, fax: 215 440 9372, email: horst@aacr.org, or refer to the website.

Joseph H Burchenal AACR Clinical Research Award

Subjects: Clinical cancer research.

Eligibility: Scientists who can demonstrate outstanding achievements in clinical cancer research.
Level of Study: Postdoctorate.
Purpose: To recognise outstanding acheivements in clinical cancer research.
Type: Award.
No. of awards offered: 1.
Frequency: Annual.
Value: Varies.
Length of Study: Varies.
Study Establishment: Universities or research institutions worldwide.
Country of Study: Any country.
Application Procedure: By nomination.
Closing Date: September 1st.
Additional Information: For further information please contact the AACR office.

Richard and Hinda Rosenthal Foundation Award

Subjects: Clinical cancer research.
Eligibility: Promising young investigators doing research in the field of the medical sciences. Candidates must be citizens of the United States or South America, or permanent residents of these countries.
Level of Study: Predoctorate.
Purpose: To recognise research which has made or promises to make a notable contribution to improved clinical care in the field of cancer.
Type: Award.
No. of awards offered: 1.
Frequency: Annual.
Value: Varies.
Length of Study: Varies.
Study Establishment: Universities or research institutions in The Americas.
Country of Study: USA and South America.
Application Procedure: By nomination.
Closing Date: September 1st.
Additional Information: For further information please contact the AACR office.

Women in Cancer Research Brigid G Leventhal Scholar Awards

Subjects: Cancer research.
Eligibility: Young investigators who have presented a highly rated abstract.
Level of Study: Doctorate, Postgraduate, Predoctorate.
Purpose: To support the attendance of female medical and graduate students, physicians-in-training and postdoctorate fellows at the AACR Annual Meeting.
Type: Travel Grant.
No. of awards offered: Varies.
Frequency: Annual.
Value: Travel costs and subsistence allowance.
Length of Study: Varies.
Study Establishment: AACR Annual Meeting.
Country of Study: USA.

Application Procedure: Application forms are available from Jenny Anne Horst-Martz, tel: 215 440 9300, fax: 215 440 9372, email: horst@aacr.org.
Closing Date: December 4th.

AMERICAN ASSOCIATION FOR DENTAL RESEARCH (AADR)

1619 Duke Street, Alexandria, VA, 22314-3406, United States of America
Tel: (1) 703 548 0066
Fax: (1) 703 548 1883
Email: pat@iadr.com
Contact: Ms Patricia J Reynolds, Executive Secretary

The American Association for Dental Research plan and organise research meetings where dentists and dental scientists come together to share cutting edge research. The Association also publishes research journals.

AADR Student Research Fellowships

Subjects: Basic and clinical research related to oral health.
Eligibility: Open to students enrolled in an accredited DDS/DMD or hygiene programme in a dental (health-associated) institution within the USA, who are sponsored by a faculty member at that institution. Students should not have received their degree, nor should they be due to receive their degree in the year of the award. Applicants may have an advanced degree in a basic science subject.
Level of Study: Postgraduate.
Purpose: To encourage dental students living in the United States to consider careers in oral health research.
Type: Fellowship.
No. of awards offered: Varies.
Frequency: Annual.
Value: US$2,100, plus US$300 for supplies.
Length of Study: 2 years.
Country of Study: USA.
Application Procedure: Application guidelines are available on request. Research proposals must be submitted with the application form.
Closing Date: January 15th.
Additional Information: Recipients will present their research at the AADR meeting, by submitting abstracts for poster or oral presentations.

AMERICAN ASSOCIATION OF CRITICAL-CARE NURSES (AACN)

101 Columbia, Aliso Viejo, CA, 92656-1491, United States of America
www: http://www.aacn.org
Contact: Research Department

AACN Clinical Practice Grant

Subjects: Research directly related to the AACN clinical research properties.
Eligibility: Principal investigators must be nurses holding a current AACN membership. All proposals relevant to critical care nursing practice are eligible.
Level of Study: Research.
Purpose: To support research in AACN clinical research priorities.
Type: Grant.
No. of awards offered: Varies.
Frequency: Annual.
Value: Up to US$6,000.
Application Procedure: To apply, please write for an information booklet.
Closing Date: October 1st.

AACN Critical Care Research Grant

Subjects: Critical care and nursing practice.
Eligibility: Principal investigators must be nurses holding a current AACN membership. All proposals relevant to critical care nursing practice are eligible.
Level of Study: Research.
Purpose: To fund research.
Type: Research Grant.
No. of awards offered: Varies.
Frequency: Annual.
Value: Up to US$15,000.
Application Procedure: To apply, please write for an information booklet.
Closing Date: February 1st.

AACN Sigma Theta Tau Critical Care Grant

Subjects: Critical care nursing practice.
Eligibility: Principal investigators must be nurses holding a current AACN membership. All proposals relevant to critical care nursing practice are eligible.
Level of Study: Research.
Purpose: To fund research.
Type: Grant.
No. of awards offered: Varies.

Frequency: Annual.
Value: US$10,000.
Application Procedure: To apply, please write for an information booklet.
Closing Date: October 1st.

American Nurses Foundation Research Grant

Subjects: Clinical research.
Eligibility: Principal investigators must be nurses holding a current AACN membership. All proposals relevant to critical care nursing practice are eligible.
Level of Study: Research.
Purpose: To fund research.
Type: Research Grant.
No. of awards offered: Varies.
Value: Up to US$3,500 is awarded by ANF.
Application Procedure: Information and application forms can be obtained from the American Nurses Foundation Tel: 202 651 7298.
Closing Date: May 1st.

Clinical Inquiry Fund

Subjects: Clinical research.
Eligibility: Funds will be awarded for projects that address one or more AACN research priorities and link with AACN's vision.
Level of Study: Research.
Purpose: To provide small awards to qualified individuals carrying out clinical research projects that will directly benefit patients and families.
Type: Award.
No. of awards offered: Varies.
Value: Up to US$250.
Application Procedure: To obtain an application form please call 800 899 AACN (2226).
Closing Date: January 1st, July 1st.

Data-Driven Clinical Practice Grant

Subjects: Clinical research.
Eligibility: Principal investigators must be nurses holding a current AACN membership. All proposals relevant to critical care nursing practice are eligible.
Purpose: To stimulate the use of patient focused data and/or previously generated research findings to develop, implement and evaluate changes in acute and critical care practice.
Type: Grant.
No. of awards offered: Varies.
Value: Up to US$1,000.
Application Procedure: To obtain an application form please call 800 899 AACN (2226).
Closing Date: March 1st, October 1st.

Hewlett-Packard AACN Critical Care Nursing Research Grant

Subjects: Preferred topics will address the information technology requirements of patient management in critical care.
Eligibility: Principal investigators must be nurses holding a current AACN membership. All proposals relevant to critical care nursing practice are eligible.
Level of Study: Research.
Purpose: To fund research.
Type: Grant.
No. of awards offered: Varies.
Value: US$32,000.
Application Procedure: To obtain a an application form call Hewlett-Packard at (800) 542 2351, extension AACN or visit the Hewlett-Packard website at http://www.hp.com/go/medical.
Closing Date: July 1st.

Mallincrodt, Inc. AACN Mentorship Grant

Subjects: Clinical research.
Eligibility: Principal investigators must be nurses holding a current AACN membership. All proposals relevant to critical care nursing practice are eligible.
Level of Study: Research.
Purpose: To provide research support for a novice researcher with limited or no research experience working under the direction of a mentor with expertise in the area of the proposed investigation.
Type: Grant.
No. of awards offered: Varies.
Frequency: Annual.
Value: Up to US$10,000.
Application Procedure: To apply, please write for an information booklet.
Closing Date: February 1st.
Additional Information: The mentor must show strong evidence of research in the proposed area and may not be a mentor on another AACN Mentorship Grant in two consecutive years.

Physio-Control AACN Small Projects Grants Program

Subjects: Clinical research.
Eligibility: Principal investigators must be nurses holding a current AACN membership. All proposals relevant to critical care nursing practice are eligible.
Level of Study: Research.
Purpose: To provide awards to qualified individuals carrying out projects focusing on aspects of acute myocardial infarction or resuscitation, such as the use of defibrillation, synchronised cardioversion, non-invasive pacing, or interpretive 12-lead electrocardiogram.

Type: Grant.
No. of awards offered: Varies.
Value: Up to US$500.
Application Procedure: To obtain an application form please call 800 899 AACN (2226).
Closing Date: January 15th.

For further information contact:

International Union Against Cancer
3 rue Conseil-Général, Geneva, 1205, Switzerland
Tel: (41) 22 809 1840
Fax: (41) 22 809 1081
Contact: Grants Management Officer

AMERICAN CANCER SOCIETY

1599 Clifton Road NE, Atlanta, GA, 30329-4251, United States of America
www: http://www.cancer.org/
Contact: Awards Office

The American Cancer Society is the largest non-government funder of cancer research in the United States. Since its' Research Program began in 1946, the ACS has devoted more than US$2 billion to cancer research.

American Cancer Society International Fellowships for Beginning Investigators

Subjects: Epidemiology; prevention; detection; diagnosis; treatment; psycho-oncology.
Eligibility: Eligible candidates should hold assistant professorships or similar positions at their home institutes and have a minimum of two and a maximum of seven years of postdoctoral experience after obtaining their MD or PhD degrees or equivalents. Awards are conditional on the return of the fellow to the home institute at the end of the fellowship and on the availability of appropriate facilities and resources to develop the newly acquired skills. No extensions are permitted.
Level of Study: Postdoctorate.
Purpose: To foster a bi-directional flow of knowledge, experience, expertise, and innovation to and from the USA. To enable beginning investigators and clinicians, who are in the early stages of their careers, to carry out basic or clinical research projects and to develop, acquire and apply, advanced research procedures and techniques.
Type: Fellowship.
No. of awards offered: 8-10.
Frequency: Annual.
Value: An average value of US$35,000 for travel and stipend support.
Length of Study: 12 months.
Country of Study: Any country.
Application Procedure: Application forms may be obtained from the fellowships department.
Closing Date: November 1st.
Additional Information: No allowances are made for accompanying dependants.

AMERICAN COLLEGE OF OBSTETRICIANS AND GYNECOLOGISTS (ACOG)

409 12th Street SW
PO Box 96920, Washington, DC, 20090-6920, United States of America
Tel: (1) 202 863 2577
Fax: (1) 202 554 3490
Email: lcassidy@acog.com
www: http://www.acog.org
Contact: Ms Lee Cassidy, Manager

The American College of Obstetricians and Gynecologists (ACOG) is a membership organisation of obstetrician-gynecologists dedicated to the advancement of women's health through education, advocacy, practice and research.

ACOG/3M Pharmaceuticals Research Award in Lower Genital Infections

Subjects: Gynecology and obstetrics.
Eligibility: Applicants must be ACOG Junior Fellows or Fellows who are in an approved obstetrics or gynecology residency program, or are within 3 years post-residency. Applicants must be US or Canadian citizens.
Level of Study: Postgraduate.
Purpose: To provide seed grant funds to junior investigators for clinical research in the area of lower genital infections.
Type: Research Grant.
No. of awards offered: 1.
Frequency: Annual.
Value: US$15,000 plus round-trip coach travel to the ACOG Annual Clinical Meeting.
Length of Study: 1 year.
Country of Study: USA or Canada.
Application Procedure: The proposal should address the following and not exceed six type-written pages: hypothesis; objectives; specific aims; background and significance; experimental design and methods; references. Must also include applicant's CV; letter of support from programme director, departmental chair or laboratory director; and, a one-page budget.
Closing Date: October 1st.
Additional Information: Six copies of the complete application are to be submitted.

ACOG/Cytyc Corporation Research Award for the Prevention of Cervical Cancer

Subjects: Gynecology and obstetrics.
Eligibility: Open to ACOG Junior Fellows or Fellows who are in an approved obstetrics or gynecology residency programme or within three years postresidency.
Level of Study: Postgraduate.
Purpose: To provide seed grant funds to junior investigators for clinical research in the area of cervical cancer prevention.
Type: Research Grant.
No. of awards offered: 1.
Frequency: Annual.
Value: US$15,000 plus travel expenses to attend the ACOG Annual Clinical Meeting.
Length of Study: 1 year.
Country of Study: USA or Canada.
Application Procedure: The proposal should address the following and not exceed six type-written pages: hypothesis; objectives; specific aims; background and significance; experimental design and methods; and references. Must also include applicant's CV; letter of support from programme director, departmental chair or laboratory director; and a one-page budget.
Closing Date: October 1st.
Additional Information: Six copies of the complete application should be submitted.

ACOG/Ethicon Research Award for Innovations in Gynecological Surgery

Subjects: Gynecology and obstetrics.
Eligibility: Open to ACOG Fellows or Junior Fellows who have completed at least one year of training and are considered by their residency programme director to be especially fitted for a career in academic obstetrics or gynecology.
Level of Study: Postgraduate.
Purpose: To encourage Junior Fellows or Fellows of ACOG to perform research which will advance the knowledge of gynecologic surgery.
Type: Research Grant.
No. of awards offered: 1.
Frequency: Annual.
Value: US$20,000 plus round-trip coach airfare and one night's hotel stay to attend the ACOG Annual Clinical Meeting.
Length of Study: 1 year.
Country of Study: USA or Canada.
Application Procedure: The proposal should address the following and not exceed six-type written pages: hypothesis; objectives; specific aims; background and significance; experimental design and methods; and references. Must also include applicant's CV; mentor's CV; a letter of support from the mentor agreeing to sponsor the applicant; appropriate IRB approvals; and a one-page budget.
Closing Date: October 1st.
Additional Information: Six copies of a complete application are to be submitted.

ACOG/Merck Award for Research in Migraine Management in Women's Healthcare

Subjects: Suggested areas include pathophysiology, pharmacologic and non-pharmacologic treatment and epidemiology.
Eligibility: Open to ACOG Junior Fellows or Fellows who are in an approved obstetrics or gynecology residency programme or within three years post-residency and whose project is supervised by an experienced researcher.
Level of Study: Postgraduate.
Purpose: To provide seed grant funds to support clinical research in the area of migraine management as it relates to women's healthcare.
Type: Research Grant.
No. of awards offered: 1.
Frequency: Annual.
Value: US$15,000 plus round-trip coach transportation and one night's accommodation to attend the ACOG Annual Clinical Meeting.
Length of Study: 1 year.
Country of Study: USA or Canada.
Application Procedure: The proposal should address the following and not exceed six type-written pages: hypothesis; objectives; specific aims; background and significance; experimental design and methods; and references. Must also include applicant's CV; supervisor's CV; a letter of support from the programme director, departmental chair, or laboratory director; and a one-page budget.
Closing Date: October 1st.
Additional Information: Six copies of the complete application should be submitted.

ACOG/Novartis Pharmaceuticals Fellowship for Research in Endocrinology of the Postreproductive Woman

Subjects: Gynecology and obstetrics.
Eligibility: Open to ACOG Junior Fellows or Fellows, who have completed at least one year of graduate medical education (but less than two years post-residency or fellowship), who are considered by the programme director to be especially suited to a career in obstetrics or gynecology. Applicants must be US citizens.
Level of Study: Postgraduate.
Purpose: To provide an opportunity for a Junior Fellow or Fellow of ACOG to perform research studies relating to some aspect of the endocrinology of the ageing woman.
Type: Fellowship.
No. of awards offered: 1.
Frequency: Annual.
Value: US$25,000 plus US$750 for travel to attend the ACOG Annual Clinical Meeting.
Length of Study: 1 year.
Country of Study: USA or Canada.
Application Procedure: The proposal should address the following and not exceed six typewritten pages: hypothesis; objectives; specific aims; background and significance; experimental design and methods; and references. Must also include applicant's CV; basic personal data; present position; details of institution in which Fellowship is to be held; the

name of the programme director; a description of long-range goals and how Fellowship will enhance these goals; and, letter of support from programme director, departmental chair or laboratory director.

Closing Date: October 1st.

Additional Information: Five copies of the complete application must be submitted.

ACOG/Organon, Inc. Research Award in Contraception

Subjects: Obstetrics and gynecology.

Eligibility: Applicants must be ACOG Junior Fellows or Fellows who are in an approved obstetrics or gynecology residency programme or within three years post-residency.

Level of Study: Postgraduate.

Purpose: To provide seed grant funds to junior investigators for clinical research in the area of contraception, such as oestrogen supplementation during the traditional hormone-free interval.

Type: Research Grant.

No. of awards offered: 1.

Frequency: Annual.

Value: US$25,000 plus funds for travel expenses to attend the ACOG Annual Clinical Meeting.

Length of Study: 1 year.

Country of Study: USA or Canada.

Application Procedure: The scientific research proposal should be written in eight pages or less and should include the following: hypothesis; objective; specific aims; background and significance; experimental design; and references. Application should also include a one-page budget; CV; and a letter of support from the programme director, departmental chair, or laboratory director. Six copies of the complete application are to be submitted.

Closing Date: October 1st.

ACOG/Ortho-McNeil Academic Training Fellowships in Obstetrics and Gynecology

Subjects: Gynecology and obstetrics.

Eligibility: Open to ACOG Junior Fellows or Fellows who have completed at least one year of training, and are considered by the Director of their residency programme to be especially fitted for a career in medical education or academic obstetrics and gynecology.

Level of Study: Postgraduate.

Purpose: To provide opportunities for especially-qualified obstetrics and gynecology residents or Fellows to spend an extra year involved in responsibilities which will train them for academic positions in the specialty.

Type: Research Grant.

No. of awards offered: 2.

Frequency: Annual.

Value: US$30,000 stipend plus travel expenses to attend the ACOG Annual Clinical Meeting.

Length of Study: 1 year.

Country of Study: USA or Canada.

Application Procedure: The proposal should address the following and not exceed six type-written pages: hypothesis;

objectives; specific aims; background and significance; experimental design and methods; and references. Applications should be in the form of a detailed letter including basic personal data, educational background, present position, honours, achievements and publications, name of institution in which the Fellowship will be held, the name of the programme director, a description of long range goals and how Fellowship will enhance these goals. Applications should also include a letter of support from the programme director accepting the project and a description of other duties.

Closing Date: October 1st.

Additional Information: Six copies of the complete application should be submitted.

ACOG/Parke-Davis Research Award to Advance the Management of Women's Healthcare

Subjects: One award each will be given for the following topics - impact of norethindrone acetate containing Ocs on acne in adolescent females, impact of continuous regime Ocs containing 1mg norethindrone acatate and 20ug EE on cycle control, or, impact of northindrone acetate vs. MPA on cardiovascular and metabolic parameters.

Eligibility: Applicants must be ACOG Junior Fellows or Fellows who are in an approved obstetrics or gynecology residency programme or within three years post-residency. Research project must be supervised by an experienced researcher.

Level of Study: Postgraduate.

Purpose: To provide an opportunity for junior investigators to perform research which will advance the treatment and management of women's healthcare.

Type: Research Grant.

No. of awards offered: 3.

Frequency: Annual.

Value: US$20,000 each plus travel funds to attend the ACOG Annual Clinical Meeting.

Length of Study: 1 year.

Country of Study: USA or Canada.

Application Procedure: The proposal should address the following and not exceed six typewritten pages: hypothesis; objectives; specific aims; background and significance; experimental design and methods; and references. Must also include applicant's and supervisor's CV; letter of support from the programme director, department chair or laboratory director; and a one-page budget.

Closing Date: October 1st.

Additional Information: Six copies of the application should be submitted.

ACOG/Pharmacia and Upjohn Research Award in Urogynecology of the Postreproductive Woman

Subjects: Gynecology and obstetrics.

Eligibility: Open to ACOG Junior Fellows or Fellows who are in an approved obstetrics or gynecology residency programme or within three years post-residency.

Level of Study: Postgraduate.

Purpose: To provide grant funds to junior investigators for clinical research in the area of urogynecology of the post-reproductive woman.
Type: Research Grant.
No. of awards offered: 1.
Frequency: Annual.
Value: US$15,000 plus US$1,000 travel allowance to attend the ACOG Annual Clinical Meeting.
Length of Study: 1 year.
Country of Study: USA or Canada.
Application Procedure: The proposal should address the following and not exceed six type-writeen pages: hypothesis; objectives; specific aims; background and significance; experimental design and methods; and references. Must also include applicant's CV; letter of support from programme director, departmental chair or laboratory director; and, a one-page budget.
Closing Date: October 1st.
Additional Information: Six copies of the complete application must be submitted.

ACOG/Searle Research Award in Gynecologic Infections and Their Complications

Subjects: Gynecology and obstetrics.
Eligibility: Open to ACOG Junior Fellows or Fellows who have completed an obstetrics or gynecology residency programme within the past three years.
Level of Study: Postgraduate.
Purpose: To support research in the area of gynecologic infections and their complications. These may include, but are not limited to, bacterial vaginosis, trichomoniasis, pelvic inflammatory disease, and pre-term birth.
Type: Research Grant.
No. of awards offered: 1.
Frequency: Annual.
Value: US$20,000 plus travel expenses to attend the ACOG Annual Clinical Meeting.
Length of Study: 1 year.
Country of Study: USA or Canada.
Application Procedure: The proposal should address the following and not exceed six type-writeen pages: hypothesis; objectives; specific aims; background and significance; experimental design and methods; and references. Must also include applicant's CV; letter of support from programme director, departmental chair or laboratory director; and, a one-page budget.
Closing Date: October 1st.
Additional Information: Six copies of the complete application must be submitted.

ACOG/Solvay Pharmaceuticals Research Award in Menopause

Subjects: Gynecology and obstetrics.
Eligibility: Open to ACOG Fellows or Junior Fellows who are in an approved obstetrics or gynecology residency programme or are within three years post-residency.
Level of Study: Postgraduate.

Purpose: To advance knowledge in the fields of obstetrics and gynecology through encouraging basic research on issues related to menopause. Relevant subjects include the physiological changes of the post-reproductive woman, hormonal receptor site distribution, or other investigation deemed appropriate to furthering the basic understanding of the menopause.
Type: Research Grant.
No. of awards offered: 1.
Frequency: Annual.
Value: US$20,000 plus round-trip coach transportation and one night's hotel stay to attend the ACOG Annual Clinical Meeting.
Length of Study: 1 year.
Country of Study: USA or Canada.
Application Procedure: The proposal should address the following and not exceed six typewritten pages: hypothesis; objectives; specific aims; background and significance; experimental design and methods; and references. Must also include applicant's CV; basic personal data; present position; a statement of career goals and how research will facilitate these goals; letter of support ffrom programme director, a departmental chair or laboratory director; and a one-page budget.
Closing Date: October 1st.
Additional Information: Six copies of the complete application must be submitted.

Warren H Pearse/Wyeth-Ayerst Women's Health Policy Research Award

Subjects: Gynecology and obstetrics.
Eligibility: The principal or co-principal investigator must be an ACOG Junior Fellow or Fellow. Proposals will be considered through the following: innovation, potential utility of the research, ability to generalise results, and demonstrated capability of the investigator.
Level of Study: Postgraduate.
Purpose: To provide funds to support research in health economics, health care patterns, and health care policy as it relates to the care of women.
Type: Research Grant.
No. of awards offered: 1.
Frequency: Annual.
Value: US$15,000 plus travel expenses to attend the ACOG Annual Clinical Meeting.
Length of Study: 1 year.
Country of Study: USA or Canada.
Application Procedure: The proposal should address the following and not exceed six type-written pages: hypothesis; objectives; specific aims; background and significance; experimental design and methods; and references. Must also include applicant's CV; letter of support from programme director, departmental chair or laboratory director; and, a one-page budget.
Closing Date: October 1st.
Additional Information: Six copies of the complete application must be submitted.

AMERICAN DIGESTIVE HEALTH FOUNDATION

7910 Woodmont Avenue
7th floor, Bethesda, MD, 20814 3015, United States of America
Tel: (1) 301 654 2635
Fax: (1) 301 654 1140
www: http://www.gastro.org/adhf.html
Contact: Ms Candace L Blank, Research Awards Program Co-ordinator

ADHF is the unified voice of the leading gastroenterology and hepatology societies - the American Gastroenterological Association (AGA), the American Society for Gastrointestinal Endoscopy (ASGE), and the American Association for the Study of Liver Disease (AASLD) - working together for better digestive health. ADHF's mission is to advance digestive health through financial support of research and education in the cause, prevention, diagnosis, treatment and cure of digestive and liver diseases.

Astra Merck Fellowship/Faculty Transition Awards

Subjects: Medical science, specifically gastroenterology and hepathology.
Eligibility: Applicants must be MDs currently in a gastroenterology related fellowship at an accredited North American institution, who are committed to academic careers and will have completed two years of research training at the start of this award. The additional training could be considered the equivalent of the practical training ordinarily provided in a PhD program. Therefore, individuals who hold a PhD are ineligible. Although the host institution may supplement the award, the applicant may not concurrently hold a similar training award or grant from another organisation. However, under certain circumstances, a small pool of funds may be available to support investigators as a supplement to current funding. Women and minority investigators are strongly encouraged to apply. Applicants must be a member or be sponsored by a member of any of the ADHF partner organisations.
Level of Study: Postgraduate.
Purpose: To prepare and support physicians for independent research careers in digestive diseases.
Type: Award.
No. of awards offered: 6.
Frequency: Annual.
Value: US$36,000 per year, smaller amounts may be awarded as supplement funding.
Length of Study: 2 years.
Country of Study: USA or Canada.
Application Procedure: Please write for details.
Closing Date: September 10th.

Elsevier Research Initiative Award

Subjects: Medical science, specifically gastroenterology and hepathology.

Eligibility: Investigators must possess an MD of PhD degree and must hold faculty positions at accredited North American institutions. They may not hold awards on a similar topic from other agencies. In addition, applicants must be an individual member of any of the ADHF partner organisations. Women and minority investigators are strongly encouraged to apply. Applicants for this award may not apply for the Miles & Shirley Fiterman Foundation Basic Research Award simultaneously.
Level of Study: Postgraduate.
Purpose: To provide non salary funds for new investigators to help them establish their research careers and to support pilot projects that represent new research directions for established investigators. The intent is to stimulate research in gastroenterology or hepatology related areas by permitting investigators to obtain new data that can ultimately provide the basis for subsequent grant applications of more substantial funding and duration.
Type: Award.
No. of awards offered: 1.
Frequency: Annual.
Value: US$25,000.
Length of Study: 1 year.
Country of Study: USA or Canada.
Application Procedure: Please write for details or visit the website.
Closing Date: January 8th.

Endoscopic Multicenter/Comparative Trials Award

Subjects: Medical science, specifically gastroenterology and hepathology.
Eligibility: Candidates must be MDs and established investigators currently in a gastroenterology related, endoscopic practise in an academic institution or private practice. Proposals from non MD investigators will also be considered. Applicants must be an individual member of any of the ADHF partner organisations.
Level of Study: Postgraduate.
Purpose: To provide support for established investigators performing endoscopic research.
Type: Award.
No. of awards offered: 1.
Frequency: Annual.
Value: US$50,000.
Length of Study: 1 to 2 years.
Country of Study: USA or Canada.
Application Procedure: Please write for details or visit the website.
Closing Date: September 3rd.

Endoscopic Research Awards

Subjects: Medical science, specifically gastroenterology and hepathology.
Eligibility: Candidates must be MDs currently in a gastroenterology related and endoscopic practise in academic institutions or private practise. Awards will be made

to support projects submitted by individual members or by trainees sponsored by an individual member of any of the ADHF partner organisations.
Level of Study: Postgraduate.
Purpose: To foster research in gastroenterology endoscopy both within and outside of academic centres.
Type: Award.
No. of awards offered: Varies.
Frequency: Annual.
Value: Up to US$35,000.
Length of Study: 1 year.
Application Procedure: Please write for details or visit the website.
Closing Date: September 3rd.

Industry Research Scholar Awards

Subjects: Gastroenterology and hepatology.
Eligibility: Applicants must hold full-time positions at North American Universities or professional institutes at the time of application. Applicants also must be an individual member of any of the ADHF partner organisations. The award is not intended for Fellows, but for young faculty who have demonstrated unusual promise and have some record of accomplishment in research. Candidates should be early in their careers; therefore, established investigators are not appropriate candidates. Those who have been at the assistant professor level or equivalent for more than five years are not eligible. Women and minority investigators are strongly encouraged to apply. Applicants cannot hold or have held, prior to receiving the first payment of this award, an R01, R29, K11, K08, VA Development award, or any award with similar objectives from non-federal sources. However, awards or grants obtained after receipt of an ADHF Industry Research Scholar Award need not be surrendered.
Purpose: To ensure that a major proportion of young investigators' time is protected for research. The overall objective is to enable young investigators to develop independent and productive research careers in gastroenterology and hepatology related fields.
Type: Award.
No. of awards offered: 6.
Frequency: Annual.
Value: US$50,000.
Length of Study: 3 years.
Country of Study: USA or Canada.
Application Procedure: Please write for details.
Closing Date: September 10th.

Innovative Seed Grants in Basic Research in Liver Diseases

Subjects: Liver diseases.
Eligibility: The candidate must be a faculty member at an accredited North American institution, within four years of starting his/her appointment. Applicants who hold research awards directed at salary support are also eligible. Individuals with an RO1, R2a, Merit Review or NIH First Award are ineligible. Applicants also must be an individual member of any of the ADHF partner organisations.
Level of Study: Postgraduate.

Purpose: To foster development of an original line of work by individuals who have shown commitment to excellence at an early stage of their independent research career.
Type: Grant.
No. of awards offered: 4.
Frequency: Annual.
Value: US$50,000.
Length of Study: 1 year.
Country of Study: USA or Canada.
Application Procedure: Please write for details or visit the website.
Closing Date: September 10th.

Jan Albrecht Commitment to Clonical Research Award in Liver Diseases

Subjects: Liver diseases.
Eligibility: The candidate must be a junior faculty member in an accredited North American academic institution, within four years of his/her starting appointment. At least 60 percent of effort should be devoted to research activities. Applicants who hold other research awards are not eligible. In addition, applicants must be a member or be sponsored by a member of any of the ADHF partner organisations.
Level of Study: Postgraduate.
Purpose: To foster career development for an individual performing clinical research in the liver related area who has shown commitment to excellence at an early stage of his or her research study.
Type: Award.
No. of awards offered: 1.
Frequency: Annual.
Value: US$25,000.
Length of Study: 2 years.
Country of Study: USA or Canada.
Application Procedure: Please write for details, or visit the website.
Closing Date: January 8th.

Miles and Shirley Fiterman Foundation Basic Research Awards

Subjects: Medical science, specifically gastroenterology and hepathology.
Eligibility: Applicants must hold full time faculty positions at a North American university or professional institute and may hold an MD and/or a PhD, or equivalent degree. Applicants must be an individual member of any of the ADHF partner organisations. The recipient must be at or below the level of assistant professor, and his/her initial appointment to the faculty position must have been within seven years of the time of the application. This award is not intended for fellows, but for junior faculty who have demonstrated unusual promise, have some record of accomplishment in research and have established an independent research programme at the award. Applicants may not simultaneously apply for the Industry Research Scholar Award or the Elsevier Research Initiative Award.
Level of Study: Postgraduate.

Purpose: To provide research or salary support for junior faculty members involved in basic research in any area of gastrointestinal, liver function or related diseases.
Type: Award.
No. of awards offered: 2.
Frequency: Annual.
Value: US$35,000.
Length of Study: 1 year.
Country of Study: USA or Canada.
Application Procedure: Please write for details or visit the website.
Closing Date: January 8th.

Miles and Shirley Fiterman Foundation Clinical Research in Gastroenterology or Hepatology/Nutrition Awards

Subjects: Medical science, specifically gastroenterology and hepathology.
Eligibility: The recipients of these awards should be active investigators with considerable achievements to date but whose research is ongoing. In addition, the nominee must be an individual member of any of the ADHF partner organisations.
Purpose: To recognise excellence in clinical research in hepatology or nutrition and gastroenterology and help support the clinical research of the recipients.
Type: Award.
No. of awards offered: 2.
Frequency: Annual.
Value: US$35,000.
Length of Study: N/A.
Application Procedure: Please write for details or visit the website.
Closing Date: January 8th.

Olympus Endoscopic Career Enhancement Awards

Subjects: Endoscopy.
Eligibility: Applicants must hold full time faculty positions at North American universities or profession institutions at the time of application. The award is not intended for Fellows but for faculty who have demonstrated promise and have some record of accomplishment in research. Candidates must devote at least 30 percent of their effort to research related to gastrointestinal endoscopy. In addition, the applicant must be a member of any of the ADHF partner organisations.
Level of Study: Postgraduate.
Purpose: To support investigators to acquire the skills necessary for an independent career in endoscopic research.
Type: Award.
No. of awards offered: 2.
Frequency: Annual.
Value: US$40,000.
Length of Study: 1 year.
Country of Study: USA or Canada.

Application Procedure: Please write for details or visit our website.
Closing Date: January 8th.

Outcomes Research Training Awards

Subjects: Medical science, specifically gastroenterology and hepathology.
Eligibility: Applicants must be MDs who are committed to academic careers and who, at the time of the award, have completed the clinical training necessary for board eligibility in gastroenterology at an accredited North American institution. Although the host institution may supplement the award, the applicant may not concurrently hold a similar training award or grant from another organisation. Applicants must demonstrate a coherent plan to obtain formal training in outcomes research disciplines. Women and minorities are strongly encouraged to apply. Applicants must also be a member of any ADHF partner organisations.
Level of Study: Postgraduate.
Purpose: To support physicians conducting independent research careers in digestive research careers in digestive or hepatology outcomes research.
Type: Award.
No. of awards offered: 2.
Frequency: Annual.
Value: US$50,000.
Length of Study: 2 years.
Country of Study: USA or Canada.
Application Procedure: Plaese write for details or visit our website.
Closing Date: September 10th.

R Robert and Sally D Funderburg Research Scholar Award in Gastric Biology Related to Cancer

Subjects: Gastric mucosal cell biology, regeneration and regulation of cell growth.
Eligibility: Candidates must hold faculty positions at accredited North American institutions and must have established themselves as independent investigators in the field of gastric biology. Women and minority investigators are strongly encouraged to apply. Applicants also must be individual members of any of the ADHF partner organisations.
Level of Study: Postgraduate.
Purpose: To support an active, established investigator working on novel approaches in the field of gastric biology who enhances the fundamental understanding of gastric cancer pathobiology in order to ultimately develop a cure for the disease.
Type: Award.
No. of awards offered: 1.
Frequency: Annual.
Value: US$25,000.
Length of Study: 2 years.
Country of Study: USA or Canada.
Application Procedure: Please write for details or visit the website.
Closing Date: September 10th.

Sponsored Research Symposium Awards

Subjects: Medical science, specifically gastroenterology and hepathology.

Eligibility: The symposium director must be an established investigator at a North American institution and an individual member of any of the ADHF partner organisations. Women and minority organisers are encouraged to apply. Travel support may be provided for junior investigators who are less than 40 years old and are at or below the rank of assistant professor. Up to two established investigators who are invited speakers. In the latter case, preference will be given to individuals whose expertise is outside mainstream gastroenterology-related areas, and/or investigators who have been infrequent participants at previous AGA, ASGE, or AASLD sponsored symposia. Biosketches of these individuals and a letter addressing these issues must be submitted with the application.

Level of Study: Postgraduate.

Purpose: To foster interactions and enhance the exchange of information between clinical and basic science investigators, and established and junior investigators working in gastrointestinal research.

Type: Award.

No. of awards offered: Varies.

Frequency: Three times each year.

Value: US$10,000.

Application Procedure: Please write for details.

Closing Date: September 3rd, January 8th, April 1st.

Student Research Fellowship Awards

Subjects: Medical science, specifically gastroenterology and hepathology.

Eligibility: Candidates may be medical or graduate students (not yet engaged in thesis research) at accredited North American institutions. Candidates holding advanced degrees must be enrolled as undergraduate, medical, or graduate students and they may not hold similar salary support awards from other agencies. Women and minority students are strongly encouraged to apply.

Level of Study: Postgraduate, Undergraduate.

Purpose: To stimulate interest in research careers in digestive diseases by providing salary support for research projects.

Type: Award.

No. of awards offered: 35.

Frequency: Annual.

Value: Range from US$1,500 to US$2,500.

Length of Study: Minimum of 10 weeks.

Country of Study: USA or Canada.

Application Procedure: Please write for details or see the Foundations' website.

Closing Date: March 3rd.

TAP Pharmaceuticals, Inc. Outcomes Research Awards

Subjects: Medical science, specifically gastroenterology and hepathology.

Eligibility: The applicant must be an individual member of any of the ADHF partner organisations at the time the application is submitted. There are no restrictions on faculty status or rank. Both junior and established investigators are eligible. Women and minorities are encouraged to apply.

Level of Study: Postgraduate.

Purpose: To promote digestive and liver outcomes research. Any acute or chronic condition of the digestive system or the liver is an appropriate candidate for study.

Type: Award.

No. of awards offered: 4.

Frequency: Annual.

Value: US$50,000.

Length of Study: 1 year.

Country of Study: USA or Canada.

Application Procedure: Please write for details or visit the website.

Closing Date: September 10th.

Wilson-Cook Endoscopic Research Career Development Awards

Subjects: Medical science, specifically gastroenterology and hepathology.

Eligibility: Applicants must hold full time faculty positions at North American universities or professional institutes at the time application. The award is not for Fellows but for junior faculty who have demonstrated promise and have some record of accomplishment in research. Candidates should be early in their careers and, hence, established investigators are not appropriate candidates. Those who are at or above the level of associate professor or equivalent are not eligible. The applicant must be a member of any of the ADHF partner organisations.

Level of Study: Postgraduate.

Purpose: To provide salary support for junior investigators working toward an independent research career in any area of endoscopic research.

Type: Award.

No. of awards offered: 5.

Frequency: Annual.

Value: US$36,000.

Length of Study: 1 year.

Country of Study: USA or Canada.

Application Procedure: Write for details or visit our website.

Closing Date: January 8th.

AMERICAN FOUNDATION FOR AGEING RESEARCH

North Carolina State University
Biochemistry Department
Polk Hall
Box 7622, Raleigh, NC, 27695, United States of America
Tel: (1) 919 515 5679
Fax: (1) 919 515 2047
Email: afar@bchserver.bch.ncsu.edu
www: http://www4.ncsu.edu/unity/users/a/agris/afar/afar.htm
Contact: Dr Paul F Agris, President

The American Foundation for Ageing Research aims to promote and support research that will elucidate the basic processes involved in the biology of aging and age-associated disease, by awarding scholarships and fellowships to young, motivated scientists.

Wilson-Fulton and Robertson Awards in Ageing Research, Cecille Gould Memorial Fund Award in Cancer Research, Richard Shepherd Fellowship

Subjects: Ageing and cancer research.
Eligibility: Open to students enrolled in graduate (MS, PhD, MD or DDS) degree programmes at US institutions who are working on specific projects in the fields of ageing or cancer.
Level of Study: Doctorate, Postgraduate, Undergraduate.
Purpose: To encourage young people to pursue research.
Type: Fellowship.
No. of awards offered: 5-10.
Frequency: Annual.
Value: US$500-US$1,000 per semester or summer.
Length of Study: 4 months to 1 year.
Study Establishment: Educational institutions.
Country of Study: USA.
Application Procedure: There are two levels of review: a pre-application form to determine eligibility, and a full application. Applicants should submit a request for pre-application and enclose a check or money order to AFAR for US$3.00 to cover handling and postage of both pre and full applications.
Closing Date: Please contact the Foundation for details.
Additional Information: Projects should be biological in nature. Sociological and psychological research is not accepted in this program. AFAR is a national, tax-exempt, non-profit, educational and scientific charity not associated with North Carolina State University.

AMERICAN FOUNDATION FOR VISION AWARENESS (AFVA)

243 North Lindbergh Boulevard, St Louis, MO, 63141, United States of America
Tel: (1) 800 927 2382
Fax: (1) 314 991 4101
Email: afva@aol.com
www: http://ioaweb.org/afva.html
Contact: Executive Director

The American Foundation for Vision Awareness is a national non-profit organization which provides educational programs, conducts public service projects and awards research grants and fellowship.

AFVA Research Grant

Subjects: The relationship between vision and learning.
Eligibility: Open to citizens and permanent residents of the United States.
Level of Study: Postdoctorate.
Purpose: To provide funds for projects that support the current AFVA goals and objectives with an emphasis on

projects concerning children's vision and how it relates to the learning process.
Type: Research Grant.
Frequency: Annual.
Value: Up to US$5,000.
Length of Study: 1 year.
Country of Study: Any country.
Application Procedure: Applications should include: cover sheet (Form R-1); signed agreement form (Form R-2); a statement of qualifications of the applicant and co-workers; three letters of recommendation; a brief narrative; a statement of financial needs. Five copies of the application and five copies of all attachments must be sent to: Executive Director, AFVA, 243 North Lindbergh Boulevard, St Louis, MO 63141.
Closing Date: Various cycles; apply year-round.
Additional Information: Candidates must submit research results for publication in an appropriate journal.

AMERICAN HEALTH ASSISTANCE FOUNDATION (AHAF)

15825 Shady Grove Road, Rockville, MD, 20850, United States of America
Tel: (1) 301 948 3244
Fax: (1) 301 258 9454
Email: grants@ahaf.org
www: http://www.ahaf.org
Contact: Dr John W Cross, Director of Grant Programs

The American Health Assistance Foundation is a non-profit charitable organisation that funds research and public education on age-related and degenerative diseases, and provides emergency financial assistance to Alzheimer's disease patients and their care-givers.

AHAF Macular Degeneration Research

Subjects: Opthamology, biomedicine, biochemistry, biophysics and molecular biology, pharmacology.
Eligibility: The principal investigator must hold a tenure-track or tenured position.
Purpose: To enable basic research on the causes of, or the treatment for, macular degeneration.
Type: Grant.
No. of awards offered: Varies.
Frequency: Annual.
Value: Up to US$50,000 per year for up to two years.
Length of Study: 1-2 years.
Study Establishment: At a non-profit organisation only.
Country of Study: Any country.
Application Procedure: Application form required. Current form should be requested.

AHAF National Heart Foundation

Subjects: Cardiology, biomedicine, physiology, and pharmacology.

Eligibility: Open to young investigators who are beginning independent research careers at the assistant professor level.
Level of Study: Professional development.
Purpose: To provide start-up grants for new investigators in cardiovascular disease and stroke.
Type: Grant.
No. of awards offered: Varies.
Frequency: Annual.
Value: Up to US$25,000 may be requested for one year.
Length of Study: 1 year; renewable for a further year.
Country of Study: Any country.
Application Procedure: Application form must be completed; current application form should be requested each year.

Alzheimer's Disease Research Grant

Subjects: Neurology, biomedicine, biochemistry, biophysics, molecular biology and pharmacology.
Eligibility: The principal investigator must hold the rank of assistant professor (or equivalent) or higher.
Level of Study: Biomedical research.
Purpose: To enable basic research on the causes of and treatments for Alzheimer's Disease.
Type: Grant.
No. of awards offered: Varies.
Frequency: Annual.
Value: Up to US$200,000 for the two years.
Length of Study: 1-2 years.
Country of Study: Any country.
Application Procedure: Application form required. Current application form should be requested each year.

National Glaucoma Research

Subjects: Ophthalmology, biomedicine and pharmacology.
Eligibility: The principal investigator must hold the rank of assistant professor (or equivalent) or higher.
Level of Study: Biomedical research.
Purpose: To enable basic research on the causes of, or treatments for, Glaucoma.
Type: Grant.
No. of awards offered: Varies.
Frequency: Annual.
Value: Up to US$25,000 per year for up to two years.
Length of Study: 1-2 years.
Study Establishment: At non-profit organisations only.
Country of Study: Any country.
Application Procedure: Application form required. Current application form should be requested for each year.

AMERICAN HEART ASSOCIATION, INC (AHA)

National Center
7272 Greenville Avenue, Dallas, TX, 75231-4596, United States of America
Tel: (1) 214 706 1453
Fax: (1) 214 706 1341
Email: ncrp@amhrt.org
www: http://www.americanheart.org
Contact: Ms Joanne Kauffman, Application Specialist

The American Heart Association is a non-profit, voluntary health organisation funded by private contributions. Its mission is to reduce disability and death from cardiovascular diseases and stroke. To support this goal, the Association has given almost US$1.5 billion to heart and blood vessel research since 1949.

AHA Established Investigator Grant

Subjects: Medical sciences, natural sciences, social and behavioural sciences.
Eligibility: Open to US citizens or permanent residents only.
Level of Study: Postdoctorate.
Purpose: To support the career development of highly promising clinician-scientists and PhDs who have recently acquired independent status.
Type: Salary and Project Support.
No. of awards offered: Approx. 50.
Frequency: Annual.
Value: US$75,000 each year for salary, fringe benefits, indirect costs and project costs. At least US$40,000 must be used for the project.
Length of Study: 1-4 years.
Country of Study: USA (or abroad if US citizen).
Application Procedure: Application forms may be obtained through institutions by disk after February, or they may be downloaded from the website.
Closing Date: Deadline: June 15th. Activation: January 1st.
Additional Information: Past AHA Established Investigators will not be considered. Individuals who have completed or currently hold an NIH Research Career Development Award or equivalent award from another organisation are also not eligible.

AHA Grant-in-Aid

Subjects: All basic disciplines, such as physiology, biochemistry, pathology, as well as epidemiological and clinical investigations which bear on cardiovascular problems, including stroke.
Eligibility: Open to US citizens or foreign nationals with an exchange visitor (Visa - HI, HIB, JI, TC, TN, or OI) or permanent residence visa, who hold an MD, DO, PhD, DSc, DVM or equivalent domestic or foreign degree and will be engaged in essentially full-time research.
Level of Study: Postdoctorate.

Purpose: To support research activities broadly related to cardiovascular function and disease or to related science, clinical and public health problems.
Type: Project support and salary.
No. of awards offered: Approx. 100.
Frequency: Annual.
Value: Approximately US$71,500 maximum each year; 10% indirect costs included (US$15,000 can be used for project support salary only).
Length of Study: 1-3 years.
Study Establishment: Accredited institutions.
Country of Study: USA (or abroad if US citizen).
Application Procedure: Application form must be completed; these are available on disk, or they may be downloaded from the website.
Closing Date: Deadline: June 15th. Activation: January 1st.

AHA Scientist Development Grant

Subjects: Medical sciences, natural sciences, social and behavioural sciences.
Eligibility: Open to US citizens or permanent residents only.
Level of Study: Postdoctorate.
Purpose: To support highly promising beginning scientists in their progress towards independence.
Type: Salary and Project Support.
No. of awards offered: Approx. 70.
Frequency: Annual.
Value: US$65,000 each year for salary, fringe benefits, indirect costs and project costs (at least US$35,000 must be used for the project).
Length of Study: 1-4 years.
Country of Study: USA (or abroad if US citizen).
Application Procedure: Application forms may be obtained through institutions by disk after February, or they may be downloaded from the website.
Closing Date: Deadline: June 15th. Activation: January 1st.
Additional Information: Applicants are not permitted to hold, or have held, any other national award.

AMERICAN INSTITUTE FOR CANCER RESEARCH

1759 R Street NW, Washington, DC, 20009, United States of America
Tel: (1) 202 328 7744
Fax: (1) 202 328 7226
Email: research@aicr.org
www: http://www.aicr.org
Contact: Research Department

American Institute for Cancer Research Investigator Initiator Grants

Subjects: Cancer research.
Eligibility: The principal investigator on a grant must be an assistant professor or higher position with a PhD, MD or equivalent degree.

Level of Study: Postdoctorate, Professional development.
Purpose: To support research that is on the forefront within the area of diet, nutrition and cancer.
Type: Grant.
No. of awards offered: Varies.
Frequency: Annual.
Value: Maximum of US$165,000 for two years.
Length of Study: 2 years.
Country of Study: Any country.
Application Procedure: Applications should be forwarded to the AICR.
Closing Date: July.
Additional Information: The AICR also awards Postdoctoral Award Grants and Matching Grants; interested applicants should contact the AICR for further information.

AMERICAN INSTITUTE OF NUTRITION

Suite L-4500
9650 Rockville Pike, Bethesda, MD, 20814, United States of America
Tel: (1) 301 530 7050
Fax: (1) 301 571 1892
Email: meyersa@asns.faseb.org
www: http://www.nutrition.org
Contact: Secretariat

The Bio-Serv Award in Experimental Animal Nutrition

Subjects: Nutrition research.
Eligibility: Open to investigators who have received the doctoral degree in the ten years preceding the award.
Level of Study: Postdoctorate.
Purpose: To recognise meritous research in nutrition by an investigator who has received the doctoral degree in the ten years preceding the month the award is presented.
No. of awards offered: 1.
Frequency: Annual.
Value: US$1,000 plus an engraved plaque.
Country of Study: Any country.
Application Procedure: Nominations should include: a letter stating the basis for the nomination; a selected bibliography which supports the nomination; and the reprint or series of reprints on which the nomination is based.
Closing Date: September 1st.
Additional Information: This award is made available by Bio-Serv, Inc.

The Cenrium Center for Nutritional Science Award

Subjects: Nutrition science.
Eligibility: Preference is given to scientists from the Western Hemisphere.
Level of Study: Professional development.
Purpose: To recognise investigative contributions to the understanding of human nutrition.

No. of awards offered: 1.
Frequency: Annual.
Value: US$1,500 plus an engraved plaque.
Country of Study: Any country.
Application Procedure: Nominations should include: a letter stating the significance of the work; a selected bibliography that supports the nomination; and a reprint or series of reprints reporting such research.
Closing Date: September 1st.
Additional Information: This award is made available by American Home Products Company.

The Conrad A Elvehjem Award for Public Service in Nutrition

Subjects: Nutrition science.
Eligibility: Open to qualified candidates of any nationality.
Level of Study: Unrestricted.
Purpose: To recognise distinguished service to the public through the science of nutrition.
No. of awards offered: 1.
Frequency: Annual.
Value: US$1,500 plus an engraved plaque.
Country of Study: Any country.
Application Procedure: Nominations should include: a letter stating the basis for the nomination; a selected bibliography indicating the candidate's contributions to public service; and the candidate's CV.
Closing Date: September 1st.
Additional Information: This award is made available by Nabisco, Inc.

The E L R Stokstad Award

Subjects: Nutrition science.
Eligibility: Preference is given to scientists at relatively early stages in their careers.
Level of Study: Unrestricted.
Purpose: To recognise outstanding fundamental research in nutrition.
Type: Award.
No. of awards offered: 1.
Frequency: Annual.
Value: US$2,500 plus an engraved plaque.
Country of Study: Any country.
Application Procedure: Nominations should include the following: a letter stating the basis for the nomination; a selected bibliography indicating the candidate's contributions to public service; and a reprint or series of reprints supporting the research.
Closing Date: September 1st.
Additional Information: This award is made available through an endowment from the family of E L R Stokstad.

The Mead Johnson Award

Subjects: Nutrition research.
Eligibility: Open to outstanding investigators of any nationality.
Level of Study: Postgraduate.

Purpose: To recognise a single outstanding piece of nutrition research.
No. of awards offered: 1.
Frequency: Annual.
Value: US$2,500 plus an inscribed scroll.
Country of Study: Any country.
Application Procedure: Nominations should include the following: a letter stating the significance of the work; a selected bibliography that supports the nomination; and a reprint or series of reprints reporting such research.
Closing Date: September 1st.
Additional Information: This award is made available by the Mead Johnson Nutritionals.

The Osborne and Mendel Award

Subjects: Nutrition studies.
Eligibility: Applicants need not be members of the Institute, however, the awards are usually made to professionally active nutrition scientists.
Level of Study: Unrestricted.
Purpose: To recognise outstanding basic research accomplishments in nutrition.
No. of awards offered: 1.
Frequency: Annual.
Value: US$2,500.
Country of Study: Any country.
Application Procedure: Nominations should include the following: a letter stating the significance of the work; a selected bibliography of all papers relating to the research on which the nomination is based; and a reprint or series of reprints reporting this research.
Closing Date: September 1st.
Additional Information: All material for a nomination must be submitted as an original plus five copies. This award is made available by ILSI North America.

AMERICAN LUNG ASSOCIATION

1740 Broadway, New York, NY, 10019-4374, United States of America
Tel: (1) 212 315 8793
www: http://www.lungusa.org
Contact: Ms Heather Gautney, Research Program Manager

American Lung Association Career Investigator Awards

Subjects: Research into lung disease.
Eligibility: Open to physician investigators and other scientists.
Level of Study: Postdoctorate.
Purpose: To provide support to investigators who are making the transition from junior to mid-level faculty.
No. of awards offered: 1.
Frequency: Annual.
Value: US$35,000 each year.
Length of Study: 1 year; renewable for an additional 2 years.
Country of Study: Any country.

Application Procedure: Please write for details.
Closing Date: October 1st.

American Lung Association Clinical Research Grants

Subjects: Clinical research into lung disease.
Eligibility: Open to investigators working in clinical areas relevant to lung disease. Applicants must have completed at least two years of research training and be at the instructor or assistant professor level.
Level of Study: Postdoctorate.
Type: Research Grant.
Frequency: Annual.
Value: US$25,000 each year.
Length of Study: 1 year; renewable for a second year.
Country of Study: Any country.
Application Procedure: Please write for further details.
Closing Date: November 1st.

American Lung Association Research Grants

Subjects: The area of prevention of lung disease and the promotion of lung health.
Eligibility: Awards are targeted for individuals who have completed at least two years of research training and are at the instructor or assistant professor level.
Level of Study: Postdoctorate.
Purpose: To provide starter or seed money to new investigators working in areas relevant to the prevention of lung disease and the promotion of lung health.
Type: Research Grant.
Frequency: Annual.
Value: US$25,000.
Length of Study: 1 year; renewable for an additional year.
Country of Study: Any country.
Application Procedure: Please write for further details.
Closing Date: November 1st.
Additional Information: The six individuals receiving the highest merit will be designated Edward Livingston Trudeau Scholars.

American Lung Association Research Training Fellowships

Subjects: The field of adult and pediatric pulmonary medicine and lung biology.
Eligibility: Open to individuals who have demonstrated a commitment to a career in investigative or academic medicine relevant to lung disease.
Level of Study: Postdoctorate.
Type: Fellowship.
Frequency: Annual.
Value: US$32,500 each year.
Length of Study: 1 year; renewable for a second year.
Country of Study: Any country.
Application Procedure: Please write for further details.
Closing Date: October 1st.
Additional Information: Support for applicants with a PhD will not be awarded beyond the third postdoctoral year.

Applicants must be in the 4th or 5th year of their Fellowship at the time of application.

Dalsemer Research Scholar Award

Subjects: Research into lung disease.
Eligibility: Open to physicians who have completed graduate training in pulmonary disease and are beginning a faculty track in a school of medicine.
Level of Study: Doctorate.
Purpose: To support research in interstitial lung disease.
No. of awards offered: 1.
Frequency: Annual.
Value: Up to US$25,000 each year.
Length of Study: 1 year; renewable for an additional year.
Country of Study: Any country.
Application Procedure: Please write for further details.
Closing Date: November 1st.

Lung Health Research Dissertation Grants

Subjects: Lung health research.
Eligibility: Open to doctoral students in the fields of science related to the social, behavioural, epidemiological, psychological and educational aspects of lung health as well as nurses pursuing a doctoral degree in any field.
Level of Study: Doctorate.
No. of awards offered: 1.
Frequency: Annual.
Value: Up to US$21,000 each year.
Length of Study: 1 year; renewable for 1 further year.
Country of Study: Any country.
Application Procedure: Please write for further details.
Closing Date: October 1st.
Additional Information: Individuals with an MD seeking a PhD are not eligible.

THE AMERICAN LYME DISEASE FOUNDATION, INC.

Mill Pond Offices
293 Route 100, Somers, NY, 10589, United States of America
Tel: (1) 914 277 6970
Fax: (1) 914 277 6974
Email: aldf@computer.net
www: http://www.aldf.com
Contact: Mr David L Weld, Executive Director

The American Lyme Disease Foundation is a national non-profit organisation dedicated to the diagnosis, treatment, prevention and control of Lyme Disease and other tick-borne infections. The Foundation supports research and focuses on education of the public and health care professionals.

Grants for Innovative Methods for Control of Tick-Borne Diseases

Subjects: Tick prevention and control.
Eligibility: Limited to individuals within five years of terminal degree. Studies must be undertaken in the USA.

Level of Study: Postdoctorate.
Purpose: To encourage research.
Type: Research Grant.
No. of awards offered: 3-4.
Frequency: Annual, if funds are available.
Value: US$10,000.
Length of Study: 2-3 years.
Study Establishment: Unrestricted.
Country of Study: USA.
Application Procedure: Interested parties should contact the American Lyme Disease Foundation, Inc.
Closing Date: August 1st.

AMERICAN NURSES FOUNDATION (ANF)

600 Maryland Avenue SW
Suite 100W, Washington, DC, 20024-2571, United States of America
Tel: (1) 202 651 7298
Fax: (1) 202 651 7001
Email: anf@ana.org
www: http://www.nursingworld.org/anf/
Contact: Grants Program Manager

ANF Nursing Research Grants

Subjects: Nursing.
Eligibility: Open to registered nurses of any nationality, who have obtained a Bachelor's degree or higher in Nursing.
Level of Study: Doctorate, Postdoctorate, Postgraduate.
Purpose: To support nursing research by beginning and experienced nurse researchers.
Type: Research Grant.
No. of awards offered: Approx. 30.
Frequency: Annual.
Value: US$3,500-US$10,000.
Length of Study: 1 year.
Study Establishment: Nursing Research.
Country of Study: Any country.
Application Procedure: An application form must be completed; which may be obtained by mail or via the website. A single non-refundable fee of US$50.00 must be submitted when applying for one or more award categories.
Closing Date: May 3rd.
Additional Information: Named awards included in the Grants Programme are: American Association of Critical Care Nurses; American Nurses Foundation; American Organisation of Nurse Executives; Eastern Nursing Research Society; Southern Nursing Research Society; Wyet-Ayerst Women's Health Research Institute; Germaine S Krysan, RN Scholar; Ada Sue Hinshaw; American Nurses Association Presidential Scholar; Chow-Togaski-Breitenbach Scholar; Virginia Cleland, RN Scholar; Dorothy Cornelius, RN Scholar; Julia Hardy, RN Scholar; Jean E Johnson, RN Scholar; Virginia Kelley, CRNA

Scholar; Hildegard E Peplau Scholar; Virginia Stone, RN Scholar; and Anne Zimmerman, RN Scholar. Please contact the Foundation for details.

AMERICAN OSTEOPATHIC ASSOCIATION (AOA)

142 E Ontario Street, Chicago, IL, 60611, United States of America
Tel: (1) 312 202 8109
Fax: (1) 312 202 8200
Contact: Ms Sharon L McGill, Research Services Manager

The American Osteopathic Association (AOA) is organised to advance the philosophy and practice of osteopathic medicine by promoting excellence in education, research and the delivery of quality, cost-effective healthcare in a distinct, unified profession.

AOA Research Grants

Subjects: Osteopathy.
Eligibility: Open to an osteopathic physician or biomedical researcher holding a faculty or staff appointment at an AOA accredited, affiliated, or approved osteopathic institution. Applicants must be US citizens.
Level of Study: Doctorate.
Purpose: To support clinical and basic science projects that lead to a better understanding and a more effective application of the philosophy and concepts of osteopathic medicine.
Type: Research Grant.
No. of awards offered: Dependent on funds available.
Frequency: Annual, if funds are available.
Value: Varies.
Length of Study: 1-2 years.
Study Establishment: University/hospital.
Country of Study: USA.
Application Procedure: The AOA Osteopathic Research Handbook contains grant applications and describes the programs and eligibility requirements in greater detail.
Closing Date: December 1st.

AMERICAN OSTEOPATHIC FOUNDATION (AOF)

142 E Ontario St, Chicago, IL, 60611, United States of America
Tel: (1) 312 202 8234
Fax: (1) 312 202 8216
Email: aof@aoa-net.org
www: http://www.osteopathic.org
Contact: Ms Jacqueline Weiss

Supporting education, research and the promotion of the osteopathic profession.

Zeneca Pharmaceuticals Underserved Healthcare Grant

Subjects: Osteopathy.
Eligibility: Only students in third year of study at US accredited colleges of osteopathic medicine are eligible to apply.
Level of Study: Doctorate.
Purpose: To support 4th year osteopathic medical students committed to practice in underserved or minority populations.
Type: Grant.
No. of awards offered: 2.
Frequency: Annual.
Value: Minimum of US$5,000 plus travel expenses.
Study Establishment: College of Osteopathic Medicine.
Country of Study: USA.
Application Procedure: Please submit an application form, 750 word essay, the names of three referees, and a dean's letter certifying applicant is of a good academic standard.
Closing Date: January 31st.

AMERICAN PARALYSIS ASSOCIATION

500 Morris Avenue, Springfield, NJ, 07081, United States of America
Tel: (1) 973 379 2690
Fax: (1) 973 912 9433
Email: paralysis@aol.com
www: http://www.apacure.org
Contact: Ms Aimee B McAuley, Research Assistant

The American Paralysis Association is a national non-profit organisation whose mission is to encourage and support research to find a cure for paralysis caused by a spinal cord injury.

Research Grant

Subjects: Spinal cord injury related research.
Purpose: To fund research which will lead to effective treatments, and ultimately a cure, for spinal cord injury.
Type: Research Grant.
No. of awards offered: Depends on level of science and amount of funds available. Varies from year to year.
Frequency: Twice a year.
Value: US$50,000 per year for a total maximum of US$100,000.
Length of Study: Maximum of 2 years.
Application Procedure: Application forms must be completed and 20 copies forwarded to the American Paralysis Association.
Closing Date: December 15th, June 15th.

AMERICAN PHILOSOPHICAL SOCIETY

104 S Fifth Street, Philadelphia, PA, 19106-3387, United States of America
www: http://www.amphilsoc.org
Contact: Committee on Research

Clinical Investigator Fellowships for Patient Oriented Research

Subjects: Medicine, neurology, pediatrics.
Eligibility: Candidates are expected to have held the MD, or MD/PhD degree for less than six years. The fellowship is intended to be the first post-clinical fellowship; but each case will be decided on its merits. Preference is given to candidates who have not more than two years of post-doctoral training. Applicants must expect to perform their research at an institution in the United States, under the supervision of a scientific adviser.
Purpose: To award a limited number of Clinical Investigator Fellowships for research in clinical medicine, including the fields of internal medicine, neurology, and pediatrics. For the purposes of this award, the committee emphasises patient-oriented research.
Type: Fellowship.
Value: Stipends for the fellowship are US$50,000 for the first year and US$50,000 for the second year.
Length of Study: The term of the fellowship is 1 year, with renewal for 1 year if satisfactory progress is demonstrated. Requests for renewal are due on the first Friday of January. Payments are made on July 15 and January 15..
Application Procedure: Write for forms, stating when the MD, or MD/PhD degree was awarded. Include a self-addressed mailing label. Candidates are to be nominated by their department chairman, in a letter providing assurance that the nominee will work with the guidance of a scientific adviser of established reputation who has guaranteed adequate space, supplies, etc. for the Fellow. The adviser need not be a member of the department nominating the Fellow, nor need the activities of the Fellow be limited to the nominating department. The scientific adviser need write only if the nominator cannot make the necessary guarantee. NB: As a general rule, no more than one fellowship will be awarded to a given institution in the same year of competition.
Closing Date: September 1st.
Additional Information: Foreign nationals who wish to apply may write directly to their scientific adviser, and ask the adviser to contact the Society for application forms. If they write to the Society directly for forms, their request must state when the MD, or MD/PhD degree was received, and include the name, address and telephone number of the person who will serve as the scientific adviser. Forms are available at the website.

General Research Grant Program

Subjects: Scholarly research.

Eligibility: Applicants are normally expected to have a doctorate, but applications are considered from persons whose publications display equivalent scholarly achievement. Grants are rarely made to persons who have held the doctorate less than a year, and never for predoctoral study or research. It is the Society's long-standing practice to encourage younger scholars. The Committee will seldom approve more than two grants to the same person within any five-year period. Applicants may be residents of the United States, American citizens on the staffs of foreign institutions, and foreign nationals whose research can only be carried out in the United States. Institutions are not eligible to apply. Applicants expecting to conduct interviews in a foreign language must possess sufficient competence in that language, and be able to read and translate all source materials.

Purpose: To contribute towards the cost of scholarly research in all areas of knowledge except those in which support by government or corporate enterprise is more appropriate. Scholarly research, as the term is used here, covers most kinds of scholarly inquiry by individuals leading to publication. It does not include journalistic or other writing for general readership; the preparation of textbooks, casebooks, anthologies, or other materials for use by students; or the work of creative and performing artists.

Type: Grant.

Value: The maximum grant is US$6,000. If an applicant receives an award for the same project from another granting institution, the Society will consider limiting its award to costs that are not covered by the other grant. Eligible expenses include living costs while away from home (lodging, meals and local transportation) up to a maximum of US$65 per day. Costs may exceed this amount, but the request to the Society must stay within these guidelines. Microfilms, photoreproductions which will enable the work to be done more efficiently. The Society may request that such reproductions be deposited in an appropriate institution when the research is complete. Consumable supplies, not normally available at the applicant's institution (for proposals in the natural sciences; see section E for non-eligible items). Necessary foreign and domestic travel at the lowest available rate, to a research site distant from the applicant's place of residence by more than 75 miles. US$0.25 per mile is allowed for fuel. Non-eligible expenses: the Society offers no funds for conference support, scholarships, financial aid for study, work already done, or costs of publication. The Society does not make grants to replace salary during a leave of absence, or earnings from summer teaching, pay living expenses at current place of residence, pay costs of travel to conferences, workshops or study groups, or to take up a visiting position, whether in the United States or abroad, pay consultant fees, or the cost of trips to consult with other scholars, pay for typing, secretarial services or office supplies (e.g. notebooks, computer diskettes, stationery, etc), telephone, fax charges, postage, purchase permanent equipment, such as books, cameras, laboratory apparatus, tape recorders, etc, pay research assistants, translators, or for transcription or encoding assistance, pay overhead or indirect costs to any institution.

Application Procedure: Requests for application forms must indicate eligibility of both applicant and project; state the nature of the research (e.g. laboratory, archival, fieldwork) and proposed use of the grant (e.g. travel, purchase of microfilm, etc). Foreign nationals must specify the objects of their research, only available in the United States (e.g. indigenous plants, archival materials, architectural sites, etc.). Include a self-addressed mailing label. If forms are downloaded from the website, please verify that page-format is maintained; be sure to print enough copies of the form for the letters of support.

Closing Date: October 1st for a January decision; December 1st for a March decision; October 1st for a January decision; December 1st for a March decision; March 1st for a June decision.

Additional Information: If an award is made and accepted, the recipient is required to provide the Society with a 250-word report on the research accomplished during tenure of the grant, and a one-page financial statement.

AMERICAN PHYSIOLOGICAL SOCIETY

9650 Rockville Pike, Bethesda, MD, 20814-3991, United States of America
Tel: (1) 301 530 7118
Fax: (1) 301 571 8305
Email: awards@aps.faseb.org
www: http://www.faseb.org/aps/society/html

The American Physiological Society (APS) is a non-profit scientific society devoted to fostering education, scientific research and the dissemination of information in the physiological sciences. By providing a spectrum of physiological information, the Society strives to play a role in the progress of science and the advancement of knowledge. The Society has integrated a prestigious awards programme providing funding to outstanding APS members, young investigators and scientists in need of funding to continue their research in physiology. Through its functions and activities, the society plays an important role in the progress of science and the advancement of knowledge. The Society maintains staff and offices on the campus of the Federation of American Societies for Experimental Biology (FASEB) in Bethesda, Maryland.

AAAS Travel Fellowships for Young Scientists on Problems of Environment and Health

Subjects: Epidemiologists, clinicians, health physicists and scholars who conduct research on aspects of women's health problems related to exposure to radioactivity.

Eligibility: Young scientists from Central East Europe and the former Soviet Union, who have completed their university degrees in 1998 or thereafter and who are epidemiologists, clinicians, health physicists, or conducting research on women's health problems related to exposure to radioactivity. Applicants must be able to speak English and write with a moderate degree of fluency.

Level of Study: Postgraduate, Predoctorate.
Purpose: To enable young scientists from East Central Europe and the countries of the former Soviet Union to attend the annual AAAS meeting.
Type: Travel Grant.
No. of awards offered: 5.
Frequency: Annual.
Value: Travel costs and a subsistence allowance.
Length of Study: Approx. 1 week.
Study Establishment: The AAAS Annual Meeting.
Country of Study: USA.
Application Procedure: Submission of an application which includes a letter of intent by the applicants that gives a brief summary of the applicant's research qualifications and includes the applicant's name, home university address, telephone number and email address; an abstract of the proposed paper, not to exceed 350 words; a curriculum vitae, not to exceed two pages; and two letters of support from professors or colleagues familiar with the applicant's research. Please submit applications and direct enquiries to Ms Sanoma Lee Kellogg, AAAS, 1200 New York Avenue NW, Washington, DC 20005. Tel: 1 202 326 6427.
Closing Date: October 31st.

AMERICAN PODIATRIC MEDICAL ASSOCIATION (APMA)

9312 Old Georgetown Road, Bethesda, MD, 20814, United States of America
Tel: (1) 301 571 9200
Fax: (1) 301 530 2752
www: http://www.apma.org
Contact: Research Grant Administrator

The American Podiatric Medical Association is the premier professional organisation representing the nation's podiatrists. APMA endeavours to serve both the general public and its members by gathering and presenting information valuable to people wanting to know more about afflictions and infirmities of the feet and the specialists who treat them, medically, mechanically and surgically.

APMA Research Grant Program

Subjects: Podiatric medicine - basic science and applied research. Topics change annually, please call for details.
Eligibility: Open to individual, independent investigators in predoctoral and postdoctoral podiatric medical education programmes, or in podiatric medical practice. Also open to pubic or non-profit organisations that provide podiatric medical education or services.
Level of Study: Postgraduate.
Purpose: To further develop research which contributes to the advancement of podiatric medicine.
Type: Research Grant.

No. of awards offered: Varies.
Frequency: Annual.
Value: Varies; dependent on funds available.
Length of Study: Varies.
Country of Study: Any country.
Application Procedure: Please request an application form.
Closing Date: December 1st.

AMERICAN PSYCHIATRIC ASSOCIATION

1400 K Street NW, Washington, DC, 20005, United States of America
Tel: (1) 202 682 6097
Fax: (1) 202 682 6837
Email: jtaylor@psych.org
www: http://www.psych.org
Contact: Ms Janice Taylor, Program Co-ordinator

APA/Glaxo Wellcome Fellowship

Subjects: Medical sciences, psychiatry and mental health.
Eligibility: Candidates should be in their PGY-second year of psychiatric residency training. Candidates must be either a member of the American Psychiatric Association or have applied for membership.
Level of Study: Professional development.
Purpose: To promote professional education in psychiatry. To inform psychiatric residents of the work of the association and to contribute to the professional development of the residents.
Type: Fellowship.
No. of awards offered: 10.
Frequency: Annual.
Length of Study: 2 years.
Country of Study: Any country.
Application Procedure: Application form required. Training Director's letter of recommendation must also be submitted.
Closing Date: March 31st.

AMERICAN SOCIAL HEALTH ASSOCIATION

ASHA Research Fund
PO Box 13827, Research Triangle Park, NC, 27709, United States of America
Tel: (1) 919 361 8400
Fax: (1) 919 361 8425
Email: nanher@ashastd.org
www: http://www.ashastd.org
Contact: Ms Nancy Herndon

It is the aim of the Association to stop the spread of sexually transmitted diseases and to minimise the harmful effect that they can have on individuals, families and communities.

ASHA Research Fellowship Fund

Subjects: Sexually transmitted diseases including behavioural, clinical, epidemiological and policy issues as well as basic science.
Eligibility: Open to recent recipients of a PhD, MD, or DSc degree in a relevant field, and who are resident in the USA.
Level of Study: Postdoctorate.
Purpose: To provide postdoctoral candidates with the opportunity to spend two years in a research environment under the sponsorship of an established STD researcher. The projects undertaken must make a substantive contribution to the body of medical knowledge.
No. of awards offered: Varies.
Frequency: Every two years, depending on the availability of funds.
Value: US$29,500 in the first year; US$31,000 in the second year.
Length of Study: 2 years.
Study Establishment: US research institutions.
Country of Study: USA.
Application Procedure: Application form available on request.
Closing Date: October 15th.
Additional Information: Candidates must seek the sponsorship of an established investigator at the host institution, who is willing to supervise research training during the award term.

AMERICAN SOCIETY OF HYPERTENSION

515 Madison Avenue
Ste 1212, New York, NY, 10022, United States of America
Tel: (1) 212 644 0650
Fax: (1) 212 644 0658
Email: ash@ash-us.org
www: http://www.ash-us.org
Contact: The Director

The primary goal of the American Society of Hypertension is to organise and conduct educational activities designed to promote and encourage the development, advancement, and exchange of scientific information in all aspects of research, diagnosis, and treatment of hypertension, and related cardiovascular diseases.

American Society of Hypertension/Hoechst Marion Roussel Clinical Fellowship in Hypertension

Subjects: Cardiology, endocrinology, epidemiology, nephrology.
Eligibility: Open only to physicians born in North America or those with a permanent US visa.
Level of Study: Postdoctorate.
Purpose: To support one or more years of new or ongoing research training in the field of hypertension for young clinicians planning a career in academic medicine.

Type: Fellowship.
No. of awards offered: 1.
Frequency: Annual.
Value: US$35,000.
Length of Study: 1 year.
Country of Study: USA.
Application Procedure: Application form must be submitted with project proposals.
Closing Date: December 7th.

AMERICAN SPEECH-LANGUAGE-HEARING FOUNDATION (ASLHF)

10801 Rockville Pike, Rockville, MD, 20852, United States of America
Tel: (1) 301 897 5700
Fax: (1) 301 571 0457
Email: vsmolka@asha.org
www: http://www.asha.org
Contact: Ms Gina Smolka, Executive Director

The American Speech-Language-Hearing Foundation is a private non-profit foundation, dedicated to innovation in communication sciences and disorders. It is funded, in part, by the tax-deductible contributions of individuals, corporations, and organisations. Size and quantity of funded awards are dependent on fundraising results and may vary accordingly.

ASLHF Graduate Student Scholarship

Subjects: Communication sciences.
Eligibility: Open to full-time US graduate students in communication sciences and disorders programs.
Level of Study: Postgraduate.
Purpose: To further full-time graduate students demonstrating outstanding academic achievement in communication sciences and disorders programs.
Type: Scholarship.
No. of awards offered: 7.
Frequency: Annual.
Value: US$4,000.
Length of Study: 1 year.
Country of Study: USA.
Application Procedure: Please write for application form.
Closing Date: June 5th.

ASLHF New Investigator Research Grant

Subjects: Communication sciences.
Eligibility: Open to new scientists earning their latest degree in communication sciences within the last five years to pursue research in audiology or speech-language pathology.
Level of Study: Doctorate.
Purpose: To pursue research in audiology or speech-language pathology.
Type: Grant.

No. of awards offered: Up to 7.
Frequency: Annual.
Value: US$5,000.
Length of Study: 1 year.
Country of Study: USA.
Application Procedure: Application form, abstract, research plan, management plan and budget, human subjects, bibliography, and letter of support must all be submitted.
Closing Date: June 18th.

ASLHF Student Research in Clinical Rehabilitative Audiology

Subjects: Communication sciences.
Eligibility: Open to graduate or postgraduate students in communication sciences and disorders who wish to conduct research in audiology. Applicants must be US citizens.
Level of Study: Postgraduate.
Purpose: To support research in audiology.
Type: Research Grant.
No. of awards offered: 1.
Frequency: Annual.
Value: US$2,000.
Length of Study: 1 year.
Country of Study: USA.
Application Procedure: Application form, abstract, management plan and budget, human subjects, bibliography, and a letter of support must be submitted.
Closing Date: June 12th.

ASLHF Student Research in Early Childhood Language Development

Subjects: Communication sciences.
Eligibility: Open to graduate or postgraduate students in communication sciences and disorders who wish to conduct research in early childhood language development. Applicants must be US citizens.
Level of Study: Postgraduate.
Purpose: To conduct research in early childhood language development.
Type: Grant.
No. of awards offered: 1.
Frequency: Annual.
Value: US$2,000.
Length of Study: 1 year.
Country of Study: USA.
Application Procedure: Application form, abstract, research plan, management plan and budget, human subjects, and a letter of support, must be submitted.
Closing Date: June 11th.

ASLHF Young Scholars Award for Minority Students

Subjects: Communication sciences.
Eligibility: Open to racial and ethnic college seniors who are US citizens and who are accepted for graduate study in speech-language pathology or audiology.
Level of Study: Postgraduate.
Purpose: To support graduate study in speech-language pathology or audiology.
Type: Scholarship.
No. of awards offered: 1.
Frequency: Annual.
Value: US$2,000.
Length of Study: 1 year.
Country of Study: USA.
Application Procedure: Please write for application form.
Closing Date: June 11th.

Kala Singh Graduate Scholarship

Subjects: Communication sciences.
Eligibility: Open to US applicants only.
Level of Study: Postgraduate.
Purpose: To further full-time international and minority graduate studies in communications sciences and disorders in the United States for students demonstrating outstanding academic achievement.
Type: Scholarship.
No. of awards offered: 1.
Frequency: Annual.
Value: US$2,000.
Length of Study: 1 year.
Country of Study: USA.
Application Procedure: Please contact the Foundation for further details.
Closing Date: June 11th.

Leslie Isenberg Award

Subjects: Communication sciences.
Eligibility: Open to full-time graduate students with a disability, enrolled in communications sciences and disorders programs, and demonstrating outstanding academic achievement. Applicants must be US citizens.
Level of Study: Postgraduate.
Purpose: To further full-time graduate studies in a communications sciences and disorders programme for students with a disability demonstrating outstanding academic achievement.
Type: Scholarship.
No. of awards offered: 1.
Frequency: Annual.
Value: US$2,000.
Length of Study: 1 year.
Country of Study: USA.
Application Procedure: Please write for application form.
Closing Date: June 11th.

AMERICAN TINNITUS ASSOCIATION (ATA)

PO Box 5, Portland, OR, 97207-0005, United States of America
Tel: (1) 503 248 9985
Fax: (1) 503 248 0024
Email: gloria@ata.org
www: http://www.ata.org
Contact: Dr Gloria E Reich

The American Tinnitus Association promotes relief, prevention and the eventual cure of tinnitus for the benefit of present and future generations.

ATA Scientific and Medical Research Grants

Subjects: Tinnitus.
Eligibility: Open to US nationals only.
Level of Study: Postdoctorate.
Purpose: To identify the mechanism(s) of tinnitus or improve tinnitus treatments.
Type: Research Grant.
No. of awards offered: Varies.
Frequency: Annual.
Value: Varies.
Country of Study: Any country.
Application Procedure: Please write for grant application policies and procedures brochure.
Closing Date: Proposals may be sent at any time for deadlines of June 30th and December 31st.

THE AMERICAN-SCANDINAVIAN FOUNDATION (ASF)

15 East 65th Street, New York, NY, 10021, United States of America
Tel: (1) 212 879 9779
Fax: (1) 212 249 3444
Email: grants@amscan.org
www: http://www.amscan.org
Contact: Ms Ellen B McKey, Director of Fellowships and Grants

The American-Scandinavian Foundation is a publicly supported, non-profit organisation that promotes international understanding through educational and cultural exchange between the United States and Denmark, Finland, Iceland, Norway and Sweden.

Fellowships and Grants for Study and Research in Scandinavia

Subjects: All subjects.
Eligibility: Open to US citizens or permanent residents.
Level of Study: Doctorate, Postdoctorate, Professional development.

Purpose: To encourage advanced study and research, and increase understanding between the USA and Scandinavia.
Type: Fellowship.
No. of awards offered: 25-30.
Frequency: Annual.
Value: US$3,000-US$15,000.
Length of Study: 1 year maximum.
Country of Study: Denmark, Finland, Iceland, Norway or Sweden.
Application Procedure: Please submit application form, three references, plus US$10 application fee.
Closing Date: November 1st.
Additional Information: For further information please contact Ellen McKey (Email: grants@amscan.org).

THE ANGLO-DANISH SOCIETY

Danewood
4 Daleside, Gerrards Cross, Buckinghamshire, SL9 7JF, England
Tel: (44) 1753 884846
Contact: Mrs A M Eastwood, Secretary

The Society exists to promote closer understanding between the United Kingdom and Denmark. It provides a forum in which Britons and Danes can meet one another.

The Anglo-Danish (London) Scholarships

Subjects: Other things being equal, candidates whose study topics are of specific value to Anglo-Danish cultural/scientific interests will be preferred.
Eligibility: Open to graduates of Danish nationality.
Level of Study: Doctorate, Postdoctorate, Postgraduate, Professional development.
Purpose: To promote Anglo-Danish relations.
Type: Scholarship.
No. of awards offered: 4-6.
Frequency: Dependent on funds available.
Value: £175 per month for a maximum of six months.
Length of Study: Maximum 6 month grant.
Study Establishment: UK university for Danish graduates and Danish university for British graduates.
Country of Study: United Kingdom or Denmark.
Application Procedure: Application forms are required. These are available from the Secretary, between October 1st and December 31st. Please enclose a stamped addressed envelope or international reply coupon.
Closing Date: January 12th.

The Denmark Liberation Scholarships

Subjects: Other things being equal, candidates whose study topics are of specific value to Anglo-Danish cultural/scientific interests will be preferred.
Eligibility: Open to graduates of British nationality only.
Level of Study: Doctorate, Postdoctorate, Postgraduate, Professional development.
Purpose: To promote Anglo-Danish relations.

Type: Scholarship.
No. of awards offered: 4-6.
Frequency: Annual.
Value: One major award of £9,000, and others at £6,000 each.
Length of Study: A minimum of 6 months.
Study Establishment: A Danish University or other approved institution.
Country of Study: Denmark.
Application Procedure: Application forms are required to be completed. These are available between October 1st and December 31st from the Secretary. Please enclose a stamped addressed envelope or international reply coupon.
Closing Date: January 12th.

ANGLO-JEWISH ASSOCIATION

Commonwealth House
(5th Floor)
1-19 New Oxford Street, London, WC1A 1NF, England
Tel: (44) 171 404 2111
Fax: (44) 171 404 2611
Contact: The Secretary

Anglo-Jewish Association Bursary

Subjects: All subjects.
Eligibility: Open to Jewish students of any nationality.
Level of Study: Postgraduate, Undergraduate.
Purpose: To assist students in full-time education in financial need.
Type: Bursary.
No. of awards offered: 100-120.
Frequency: Annual.
Value: Up to £2000 per year.
Country of Study: United Kingdom.
Application Procedure: Applicant must write formal letter of application in the first instance.
Closing Date: May 31st.

THE ANTI-CANCER FOUNDATION OF SOUTH AUSTRALIA

202 Grenhill Road, Eastwood, SA, 5063, Australia
Tel: (61) 8 8291 4111
Fax: (61) 8 8291 4122
www: http://www.acf.org.au
Contact: Dr Kerry Kirke, Executive Director

The Anti-Cancer Foundation is a community based charity independent of government control that has developed since 1928 with the support of South Australians. The Foundation's mission is to pursue the eradication of cancer through research and education on prevention, early detection and enhance the quality of life for people living with cancer.

Anti-Cancer Foundation Research Grants

Subjects: Any scientific or medical field directly concerned with the cause, diagnosis, prevention or treatment of cancer.
Eligibility: Open to postgraduate research workers who have established themselves in the field of cancer research or show promise of doing so.
Level of Study: Postdoctorate.
Purpose: To assist postgraduate research workers undertaking research into cancer.
Type: Cancer Research Grant.
No. of awards offered: Approx. 20.
Frequency: Annual.
Value: Varies, according to the needs of the proposed research project and available funds.
Length of Study: 1-2 years.
Study Establishment: An appropriate research organisation in South Australia.
Country of Study: Australia.
Application Procedure: Please write for details.
Closing Date: June.

THE APEX FOUNDATION FOR RESEARCH INTO INTELLECTUAL DISABILITY LTD

PO Box 311, Mount Evelyn, VIC, 3796, Australia
Tel: (61) 3 973 61261
Email: morrish@c031.aone.net.au
Contact: Mr Kevin E Morrish, Secretary

The Association of Apex Clubs raised funds some years ago to be invested in the support of research which may assist in the prevention and treatment of intellectual disability. The Foundation manages these funds and makes annual research grants in support of selected research projects.

Apex Foundation Annual Research Grants

Subjects: Disability research.
Eligibility: Open to suitably qualified researchers of any nationality. Research must be carried out in Australia.
Level of Study: Research.
Purpose: To support research projects which are concerned with the causes, diagnosis, prevention or treatment of intellectual disability.
Type: Research Grant.
No. of awards offered: Varies.
Frequency: Annual.
Value: Varies (total annual funds of around A$60,000).
Length of Study: Varies.
Country of Study: Australia.
Application Procedure: Application form may be obtained from the Secretary of the Foundation.
Closing Date: July 31st.

THE ARC OF THE UNITED STATES

500 East Border Street
Suite 300, Arlington, TX, 76010, United States of America
Tel: (1) 817 261 6003
Fax: (1) 817 277 3491
Email: thearc@metronet.com
www: http://www.thearc.org/welcome.html
Contact: Ms Ann Balson, Administrative Secretary

The Arc, a national organisation on mental retardation, is committed to securing for all people with mental retardation, the opportunity to choose and realise their goals of where and how they learn, live, work and play.

The Arc of the United States Research Grant

Subjects: Social and preventative medicine.
Eligibility: Open to US nationals only.
Level of Study: Unrestricted.
Purpose: To support research leading towards prevention, amelioration or cure of mental retardation.
Type: Research Grant.
No. of awards offered: 1-3.
Frequency: Annual.
Value: Various amounts up to US$25,000.
Length of Study: 1 year, with the option of extension.
Country of Study: USA.
Application Procedure: Applicants should submit project authorisation form, budget form, project summary, maximum of 15 double-spaced pages for narrative, and letters of support.
Closing Date: April 1st.

For further information contact:

Department of Research and Program Services
The Arc
PO Box 1047, Arlington, Texas, 76004, United States of America
Tel: (1) 817 261 6003

Distinguished Research Award

Subjects: Prevention, amelioration or mental retardation.
Eligibility: An individual or individuals whose research has had a significant impact on the prevention or amelioration of mental retardation can be nominated.
Purpose: To reward an individual or individuals whose research has had a significant impact on the prevention or amelioration or mental retardation.
Value: The recipient of the award will receive a plaque, US$1,000 and an expense-paid trip to speak at the Research and Prevention Luncheon of the Arc's National Convention.
Application Procedure: Nomination, original and five copies, must be sent to The Arc.
Closing Date: April 15th.

ARMAUER HANSEN RESEARCH INSTITUTE (AHRI)

PO Box 1005, Addis Ababa, Ethiopia
Tel: (251) 1 710288
Fax: (251) 1 711390
Email: ahri@alinks.se
Contact: Mr Sven Britton

The Armauer Hansen Research Institute is an international biomedical research institute is mainly devoted to work on bacterial infections, notably tuberculosis and leprosy. It is supported by the Ethiopian, Norweigian and Swedish Governments.

AHRI African Fellowship

Subjects: Medical sciences, parasitology, tropical medicine.
Eligibility: Open to African researchers only. Women applicants are especially encouraged to apply.
Level of Study: Doctorate.
Purpose: To promote biomedical science in Africa.
Type: Fellowship.
No. of awards offered: 1.
Frequency: Annual.
Value: Travel, accommodation and salary costs are covered.
Length of Study: 1 year.
Study Establishment: AHRI.
Country of Study: Ethiopia.
Application Procedure: Please contact the AHRI for details.
Closing Date: Usually October 1st.

ARTHRITIS FOUNDATION

1330 West Peachtree Street, Atlanta, GA, 30309, United States of America
Tel: (1) 404 872 7100 ext 6311
Fax: (1) 404 877 3170
Email: dporter@arthritis.org
www: http://www.arthritis.org
Contact: Research Administration

The mission of the Arthritis Foundation is to support research and endeavour to find the cure for arthritis, and to improve the quality of life for those affected by it.

Arthritis Foundation Biomedical Science Grant

Subjects: Arthritis and related rheumatic diseases.
Eligibility: Open to individuals with doctoral degrees (MD, PhD, or equivalent) at the assistant professor level or higher at any US non-profit institution. Evidence of independence is required.
Level of Study: Postdoctorate.
Purpose: To encourage and support high quality, original biomedical research closely related to understanding the etiology, pathogenic mechanisms and control of arthritis and related rheumatic diseases in adults and children.
Type: Grant.

No. of awards offered: Varies, 33 in 1998.
Frequency: Annual.
Value: Up to US$90,000 per year, paid quarterly to the investigator's institution.
Length of Study: 1-3 years.
Country of Study: USA.
Application Procedure: Applicants should write for details - these are available from May 1st.
Closing Date: September 1st.
Additional Information: Applications will be rated on the basis of originality, research design and the ability of the investigator(s) to carry out the proposed project. This criterion includes the past research record of the investigator(s), the involvement of critical collaborators, etc. and significance of the proposed project to the field of arthritis and rheumatic diseases. All work involving human subjects must show documented compliance with NIH guidelines as provided by the sponsoring institution's committee for clinical investigation. All work involving animal experimentation should comply with NIH guidelines for care and use of laboratory animals.

Arthritis Foundation Clinical Science Grant

Subjects: Arthritis and related rheumatic diseases.
Eligibility: Open to physicians or non-physicians with doctoral degrees or equivalent who are associated with any US non-profit institution. Ordinarily, at least one physician with expertise in the disease area being studied should be closely associated with the project.
Level of Study: Postgraduate, Professional development.
Purpose: To encourage and support high quality, original clinical research on problems closely related to the diagnosis, prognosis, management, healthcare delivery and epidemiology of adults and children with arthritis and related rheumatic diseases.
Type: Grant.
No. of awards offered: Varies, 14 in 1997.
Frequency: Annual.
Value: Up to US$90,000 per year, paid quarterly to the investigator's institution.
Length of Study: 1-5 years.
Country of Study: Any country.
Application Procedure: Applications are available from May 1st.
Closing Date: September 1st.
Additional Information: Applications are rated on the basis of potential impact on the diagnosis and management of arthritis and rheumatic diseases, research design, originality, and the researcher's background and experience as an investigator. Funds will not be provided for those aspects of studies which pharmaceutical or other commercial companies should support. All work involving human subjects must show documented compliance with NIH guidelines as provided by the sponsoring institution's committee for clinical

investigation. All work involving animal experimentation should comply with NIH guidelines for care and use of laboratory animals.

Arthritis Foundation Doctoral Dissertation Award

Subjects: The research project must be related to arthritis management and/or comprehensive patient care in rheumatology practice, research or education. Suitable studies include, but are not limited to, functional, behavioural, nutritional, occupational, or epidemiological aspects of patient care and management. Drug studies and laboratory in vitro studies are not appropriate.
Eligibility: Open to doctoral candidates entering the research phase of their programmes. The doctoral chairman must approve the project. A dissertation project is preferred. A candidate must have membership or eligibility for membership in his/her professional organisation.
Level of Study: Doctorate, Postgraduate.
Purpose: To advance the research training of men and women of promise in investigative or clinical teaching careers as they relate to the rheumatic diseases.
No. of awards offered: Varies.
Frequency: Annual.
Value: US$10,000 per year, depending on the amount of time committed to research. Payments are made monthly.
Length of Study: 1 or 2 years.
Country of Study: USA.
Application Procedure: Application is available from May 1st.
Closing Date: September 1st.
Additional Information: Individuals must pursue their research under the direction of a supervisor who possesses recognised expertise in the candidate's specific field of study. Projects are rated on the basis of proposed research environment, background and potential of the researcher, and potential significance and relevance of the project to the rheumatic diseases. All work involving human subjects must show documented compliance with NIH guidelines as provided by the sponsoring institution's committee for clinical investigation. All work involving animal experimentation should comply with NIH guidelines for care and use of laboratory animals.

Arthritis Foundation New Investigator Grant

Subjects: The research project must be related to arthritis management and/or comprehensive patient care in rheumatology practice, research or education. Suitable studies include, but are not limited to, functional, behavioural, nutritional, occupational, or epidemiological aspects of patient care and management. Drug studies and laboratory in vitro studies are not appropriate.
Eligibility: Open to holders of a PhD or equivalent doctoral degree and demonstrated research experience. These awards are meant to encourage investigators who have received a doctoral degree within the last five years. MDs are not eligible. A candidate must have membership or eligibility for membership in his/her professional organisation.
Level of Study: Postdoctorate.

Purpose: To encourage PhD-level health professionals who have research expertise to design and carry out innovative research projects related to the rheumatic diseases. The grant is intended to provide support for the period between completion of doctorate work and establishment as an independent investigator.

Type: Grant.

No. of awards offered: Varies, 1 in 1997.

Frequency: Annual.

Value: US$35,000 per year, paid quarterly to the investigator's institution.

Length of Study: 1 or 2 years (renewable for a third).

Country of Study: USA.

Application Procedure: Application forms are available from May 1st.

Closing Date: September 1st.

Additional Information: Approval of each application and research project is required from an academic institution. Endorsement of an application by the institution constitutes agreement to allow the necessary time for completion of the project within the allotted term. Principal investigators do not have to be associated with an arthritis unit. Individuals with limited research experience must apply in conjunction with a supervisor or co-investigator with demonstrated research expertise in the applicant's area of study. Projects are rated on the basis of design, originality, potential significance and relevance to the rheumatic diseases, and the principal investigator's background and experience as an investigator. All work involving human subjects must show documented compliance with NIH guidelines as provided by the sponsoring institution's committee for clinical investigation. All work involving animal experimentation should comply with NIH guidelines for care and use of laboratory animals.

Arthritis Foundation Postdoctoral Fellowship

Subjects: Research in a field related to rheumatic diseases.

Eligibility: Open to persons with an MD, PhD or equivalent doctoral degree. MDs are not eligible after six years of laboratory training (or seven years in the case of a clinical training programme which includes one year in the laboratory). PhDs are not eligible after four years of post-degree laboratory experience. Individuals at or above the Assistant Professor level, or those who have tenured positions, are ineligible to apply for the awards. If one is promoted or establishes tenure after receiving an award, he/she may continue to receive the award for the remainder of the fellowship period under the conditions of the original award.

Level of Study: Postdoctorate.

Purpose: To encourage qualified physicians and scientists to embark on careers in research broadly related to the understanding of arthritis and the rheumatic diseases. A fellowship provides the stipend support for the early years of the necessary training period.

Type: Fellowship.

No. of awards offered: Varies, 25 in 1998.

Frequency: Annual.

Value: US$35,000 per year, plus a grant of US$500 per year to the sponsoring institution to cover health insurance, supplies, travel, publication costs, etc.

Length of Study: 2 years; renewable for a third year; renewal is competitive.

Country of Study: USA.

Application Procedure: Application package available from May 1st.

Closing Date: September 1st.

Additional Information: A candidate must plan to pursue a programme under the supervision of a qualified supervisor. The written proposal may represent the joint effort of the applicant and the supervisor. Applications are rated on the basis of the environment in which the training programme will be conducted, specifically, the qualifications of the supervisor as an investigator, the unit, the facilities available and the potential for inter and extra-departmental interactions; the applicant's background, training and potential as a biomedical investigator; and the proposed research project, its scientific merit and broad relevance to arthritis. Each Postdoctoral Fellow is expected to devote 90% of his/her professional time to activities related to the fellowship programme: laboratory research, clinical investigation, field studies, or training. The Arthritis Foundation does not award part-time fellowships. A recipient of a Postdoctoral Fellowship may receive salary supplementation from other sources to a total amount consistent with the ordinary institutional level for that individual's rank and position. The extent of this supplementation must be stated on the application, and the foundation must be notified of subsequent support. All work involving human subjects must show documented compliance with NIH guidelines for human subjects, as provided by the sponsoring institution's committee for clinical investigation. All work involving animal experimentation should comply with NIH guidelines for care and use of laboratory animals.

Arthritis Investigator Award

Subjects: Research in a field related to arthritis.

Eligibility: Open to US citizens and permanent residents. Applicants must have completed a minimum of three and maximum of seven years postdoctoral research experience as of the award date. The award is not an extended postdoctoral fellowship. Applicants must hold an MD, PhD or equivalent degree, and have demonstrated distinction and productivity in research. The applicant may not hold an NIH, RO1, NSF Grant, FIRST Award, Howard Hughes Award, Pew, Wellcome, Searle, VA Merit Award or equivalent at the time of application. If such an award is made subsequently, however, the individual may retain his/her Arthritis Foundation award. Holders of NIH Physician Scientist Awards, NIH Young Investigator Awards, VA Associate Clinical Investigatorships, and similar research training awards given by other agencies will be eligible. Individuals with tenured positions are ineligible to apply. If one establishes tenure after receiving an award, he/she may continue to receive the award for the remainder of the period under the conditions of the original award.

Level of Study: Postdoctorate.

Purpose: To provide support to physicians and scientists in research fields broadly related to arthritis for the period between completion of postdoctoral fellowship training and establishment as an independent investigator. The award may provide salary and/or research support.

Type: Investigator Award.
No. of awards offered: Varies.
Frequency: Annual.
Value: US$64,000 per year for stipend only, stipend plus research, or research expenses only, plus a grant of US$1,000 to the sponsoring institution to cover health insurance, supplies, travel, publication costs, etc.
Length of Study: 3 years; up to 5 years.
Country of Study: Any country.
Application Procedure: Application is available May 1st.
Closing Date: September 1st.
Additional Information: A senior scientist familiar with the applicant's area of research should be designated as the sponsor. The sponsor and the chairman of the relevant academic department are responsible for stating the role of the applicant within the department, promising protection of time for research activities related to the award, guaranteeing space for the investigative work, and outlining future opportunities for the applicant. Applications are rated on the basis of the applicant's background, training, evidence of productivity, and potential; the proposed research project, its scientific merit and relevance to arthritis; and the environment in which the programme will be conducted, specifically, the sponsor, the academic department, the unit, available facilities, and potential for inter and extra-departmental scientific and academic interactions. Each Arthritis Investigator is expected to devote 80% of his/her professional time to activities related to laboratory research. The Arthritis Foundation does not award part-time investigators. Supplementation from the sponsoring institution or other awards for salary and research expenses are permitted up to a level consistent with institutional policies. The extent of this supplementation must be stated on the application, and the Foundation must be notified of any subsequent support. All work involving human subjects must show documented compliance with NIH guidelines for human subjects, as provided by the sponsoring institution's committee for clinical investigation. All work involving animal experimentation should comply with NIH guidelines for care and use of laboratory animals.

Physician Scientist Development Award

Subjects: Fields related to arthritis.
Eligibility: Open to MD candidates with no research background or a limited science background.
Level of Study: Postdoctorate, Professional development.
Purpose: To encourage qualified physicians without significant prior research experience to embark on careers in biomedical or clinical research related to the understanding of arthritis and the rheumatic diseases.
Type: Development Award.
No. of awards offered: Varies, 9 in 1998.
Frequency: Annual.
Value: US$27,000-US$32,000 per year, plus a US$500 grant to the institution to cover health insurance, supplies, travel and publication costs.
Length of Study: 2 years; renewable for 2 more years.
Country of Study: USA.
Application Procedure: Application is required - forms are available from May 1st.

Closing Date: September 1st.
Additional Information: A candidate must plan to pursue a programme under the supervision of a qualified supervisor. The written proposal may represent the joint effort of the applicant and the supervisor. Applications are rated on the basis of the environment in which the training programme will be conducted, specifically, the qualifications of the supervisor as an investigator, the unit, the facilities available and the potential for inter- and extra-departmental interactions; the applicant's background, training and potential as a biomedical investigator; and the proposed research project, its scientific merit and broad relevance to arthritis. Each recipient is expected to devote 90% of his/her professional time to activities related to the fellowship programme: laboratory research, clinical investigation, field studies, or training. The Arthritis Foundation does not award part-time fellowships. A recipient may receive salary supplementation from other sources to a total amount consistent with the ordinary institutional level for that individual's rank and position. The extent of this supplementation must be stated on the application, and the foundation must be notified of subsequent support. All work involving human subjects must show documented compliance with NIH guidelines for human subjects, as provided by the sponsoring institution's committee for clinical investigation. All work involving animal experimentation should comply with NIH guidelines for care and use of laboratory animals.

ARTHRITIS FOUNDATION OF AUSTRALIA (AFA)

GPO Box 121, Sydney, NSW, 2001, Australia
Tel: (61) 2 9221 2456
Fax: (61) 2 9232 2538
www: http://www.span.com.au/span/arthritis
Contact: National Executive Director

The role of the Arthritis Foundation of Australia is to provide care, education and research for people with musculoskeletal disease.

AFA Grants-in-Aid

Subjects: Rheumatology.
Eligibility: Open to medical, scientific or allied health professionals.
Level of Study: Postdoctorate.
Purpose: To support new and continuing projects in rheumatology research.
No. of awards offered: Varies.
Frequency: Annual.
Value: A$5,000 - A$10,000.
Country of Study: Australia.
Application Procedure: Please write for details.
Closing Date: Last Friday in June.
Additional Information: Includes sponsored grants such as the Allan Stephens Memorial Grant.

AFA Special Project Grants

Subjects: Arthritis research - causes and management.
Eligibility: Open to Australian citizens and permanent residents.
Level of Study: Postgraduate.
Purpose: To help establish long-term research projects in the field of rheumatic diseases which may, if they progress well, attract other support.
No. of awards offered: 4-10.
Frequency: Annual.
Value: Up to A$10,000.
Length of Study: 1 year.
Country of Study: Australia.
Application Procedure: Please write for details.
Closing Date: Last Friday in June.

AFA/ARA Heald Fellowship

Subjects: Clinical or laboratory research into the causes and treatment of rheumatic diseases.
Eligibility: Open to Australian citizens or permanent residents, no more than 35 years old, who are either science graduates with several years postdoctoral experience or medical graduates with at least six years post-MBBS experience.
Level of Study: Postdoctorate.
Type: Fellowship.
No. of awards offered: 1.
Frequency: Annual.
Value: US$25,000 plus US$1,000 or equivalent for travel.
Length of Study: 1 year; not renewable.
Country of Study: USA or Canada.
Application Procedure: Please write for details.
Closing Date: Last Friday in June.
Additional Information: A preliminary arrangement with the proposed place of work or unit with adequate facilities must have been made. A written undertaking must be made to return to work in Australia.

Frank G Spurway Scholarship and Arthritis Foundation of NSW Branches

Subjects: Rheumatology.
Eligibility: Open to Australian medical and science graduates with developed interests in, or working in units with, developed research lines. Applicants should be enrolled in studies leading to an MD or PhD degree.
Level of Study: Doctorate, Postgraduate.
Type: Scholarship.
No. of awards offered: 1.
Frequency: Annual.
Value: A$16,000 per year.
Length of Study: 1 year; renewable for a second year upon reapplication.
Country of Study: Australia.

Application Procedure: Please write for details.
Closing Date: Last Friday in June.

Mary Paxton Gibson Scholarships

Subjects: Rheumatology.
Eligibility: Open to Australian medical and science graduates with developed interests in, or working in units with, developed research lines. Applicants should be enrolled in studies leading to an MD or PhD degree.
Level of Study: Doctorate, Postgraduate.
Type: Scholarship.
No. of awards offered: Varies.
Frequency: Annual.
Value: A$22,000 per year (medical graduates) or A$15,000 (science graduates), plus A$1,000 for consumables.
Length of Study: 1 year; renewable for a second year upon reapplication.
Country of Study: Australia.
Application Procedure: Please write for details.
Closing Date: Last Friday in June.

McGill Domestic Fellowship

Subjects: Rheumatology.
Eligibility: Open to science graduates with several years postdoctoral experience, or medical graduates with at least 6 years post MBBS experience. Applicants must be Australian citizens or permanent residents. Preference is generally given to applicants under 35 years of age.
Level of Study: Postdoctorate.
Purpose: To support clinical or scientific research in rheumatology.
Type: Fellowship.
Frequency: Annual.
Value: A$32,000 per year.
Length of Study: 1 year; renewable subject to satisfactory progress for 2 years.
Country of Study: Australia.
Application Procedure: Please write for details.
Closing Date: June 20th.

Michael Mason Fellowship

Subjects: Research or clinical studies in rheumatic diseases.
Eligibility: Open to Australian citizens or permanent residents, no more than 35 years old, who are medical graduates.
Level of Study: Postgraduate.
Type: Fellowship.
No. of awards offered: 1.
Frequency: Annual.
Value: £15,000 plus £1,000 for travel expenses.
Length of Study: 1 year; not renewable.
Country of Study: United Kingdom.
Application Procedure: Please write for details.
Closing Date: Last Friday in June.
Additional Information: A preliminary arrangement with the proposed place of work or unit with adequate facilities must have been made.

Philip Benjamin Memorial Grant

Subjects: Clinical research into osteoporosis or, if no suitable application for this is received, into rheumatoid arthritis (with particular reference to Iatrogenic disease) or into histocompatibility antigens in rheumatic disease.
Eligibility: Open to suitably qualified researchers of any nationality.
Level of Study: Postdoctorate.
Type: Grant.
No. of awards offered: 1.
Frequency: Annual.
Value: A$15,000 per year.
Length of Study: 1 year; renewable for a second and possibly a third year upon reapplication.
Country of Study: Australia.
Application Procedure: Please write for details.
Closing Date: Last Friday in June.

ARTHRITIS RESEARCH CAMPAIGN (ARC)

Copeman House
St Mary's Court
St Mary's Gate, Chesterfield, S41 7TD, England
Tel: (44) 1246 558 033
Fax: (44) 1246 558 007
Email: info@arc.org.uk
www: http://www.arc.org.uk/
Contact: Research Grant Administrator

The Arthritis Research Campaign is the fifth biggest medical research charity in the UK, and the only charity in the country dedicated to finding the cause of and cure for arthritis.

ARC Clinical Research Fellowships

Subjects: Rheumatology.
Eligibility: Open to UK medical graduates at the registrar or senior registrar level.
Level of Study: Postgraduate.
Purpose: To encourage young physicians into a career in clinical rheumatology. Candidates will be expected to register for a higher degree (MD or PhD).
Type: Fellowship.
No. of awards offered: Varies.
Frequency: Twice a year.
Value: Fellow's salary plus reasonable laboratory expenses.
Length of Study: 2-3 years.
Study Establishment: Any suitable centre.
Country of Study: United Kingdom.
Application Procedure: Application forms and information regarding annual closing dates are available on request.
Closing Date: Around March and September.

ARC Postdoctoral Research Fellowships

Subjects: Rheumatology or a related subject.
Eligibility: Open to UK and Commonwealth citizens. Candidates should normally be in their first or second postdoctoral appointment.
Level of Study: Postdoctorate.
Purpose: To attract and retain talented scientists in rheumatological research.
Type: Fellowship.
No. of awards offered: Varies.
Frequency: Twice a year.
Value: Fellow's salary (usually within 1A or II range) plus reasonable running costs.
Length of Study: Up to 5 years; renewal subject to satisfactory review.
Study Establishment: A UK university department or similar research institute (preferably within a multidisciplinary research group).
Country of Study: United Kingdom.
Closing Date: Around April and November.

ARC Project Grants

Subjects: Rheumatology.
Eligibility: Open to UK and Commonwealth citizens with previous experience of investigation and research.
Level of Study: Professional development.
Purpose: To further research into rheumatic diseases.
Type: Project Grant.
Frequency: Four times each year.
Value: Varies.
Length of Study: Up to 3 years.
Study Establishment: Any suitable centre.
Country of Study: United Kingdom.
Application Procedure: Application forms are available upon request.
Closing Date: The last Monday of March, July and November.
Additional Information: Grants are made in support of specific research projects.

ARC Travelling Fellowships

Subjects: Rheumatology.
Eligibility: Open to doctors up to and including senior registrar status.
Level of Study: Professional development.
Purpose: To provide training and experience for doctors committed to a career in clinical rheumatology.
Type: Fellowship.
No. of awards offered: 2.
Frequency: Annually or when advertised.
Value: Fellow's salary and travelling costs (APEX return).
Length of Study: 1 year.
Study Establishment: A centre of the Fellow's choice, subject to the Council's approval.
Country of Study: Any country.
Closing Date: Applications are accepted at any time.

Senior ARC Fellowships

Subjects: Rheumatology or a related subject.
Eligibility: Open to UK and Commonwealth citizens with previous experience of investigation and research. Candidates should have proven ability in establishing an independent research programme.
Level of Study: Professional development.
Purpose: To further research into rheumatic diseases and to attract high-flying medical or scientific researchers into rheumatology.
Type: Fellowship.
No. of awards offered: Varies.
Frequency: Annual.
Value: Fellow's salary with lecturer B/Senior lectureship scale, plus supporting technician, running costs and essential equipment.
Length of Study: Up to 5 years, with option to renew subject to satisfactory review.
Study Establishment: Any suitable centre.
Country of Study: United Kingdom.
Application Procedure: Application forms are available on request.
Closing Date: Around February.

THE ARTHRITIS SOCIETY

393 University Avenue
Suite 1700, Toronto, ON, M5G 1E6, Canada
Tel: (1) 416 979 7228
Fax: (1) 416 979 1149
Email: kparker@arthritis.ca
www: http://www.arthritis.ca
Contact: Ms Kim Parker, Research Associate

The Arthritis Society is Canada's only not-for-profit agency dedicated solely to funding and promoting arthritis research and care.

Arthritis Society Clinical Fellowships

Subjects: Rheumatology.
Eligibility: Open to Canadian citizens or landed immigrants who have completed three years of graduate training in internal medicine or paediatrics approved by the Royal College of Physicians and Surgeons (Canada) or the Corporation of Physicians and Surgeons (Quebec). One of these three years of training should be in rheumatology.
Level of Study: Postdoctorate.
Purpose: To augment arthritis residency training programmes and enhance research skills.
Type: Fellowship.
No. of awards offered: Varies, based on the number of ministry-funded positions available.
Frequency: Annual.
Value: Fellows training in Canadian medical schools are paid at the same rate as residents of their respective schools. Fellows training abroad are paid quarterly in advance in Canadian funds, the rates being the same as those paid by the Medical Research Council of Canada.

Length of Study: 1 year, usually commencing July 1st; renewable under exceptional circumstances.
Study Establishment: Canadian Rheumatic Disease Units.
Country of Study: Canada.
Application Procedure: Application must include: letters of recommendation from three sponsors, letter of acceptance from proposed supervisor to include outline of proposed training program, and a certified transcript of undergraduate record.
Closing Date: September 15th.
Additional Information: Clinical Fellowships are intended solely for the support of rheumatology trainees and are not awarded for the support of junior faculty. Fellowships are awarded by the Society on the advice of the Clinical Fellowship Panels. The Society reserves the right to approve or decline any application without stating its reasons. Applications must be signed by the applicant's supervisor and the Rheumatic Disease Unit/Arthritis Centre Director.

Arthritis Society Industry Program

Subjects: Research relevant to arthritis.
Eligibility: Please write for details.
Level of Study: Postdoctorate.
Purpose: To foster new collaborative efforts through shared funding between The Arthritis Society and industry.
Type: Research Grant.
No. of awards offered: Varies.
Frequency: Annual.
Country of Study: Any country.
Application Procedure: Please write for details.
Closing Date: December 15th.

Arthritis Society Research Fellowships

Subjects: Arthritis.
Eligibility: Preference is given to candidates who intend to embark on a research career in Canada. Candidates must hold a PhD, MD, DDS, DVM, PharmD (or the equivalent).
Level of Study: Postdoctorate.
Purpose: To provide support for highly qualified candidates to pursue full-time research.
Type: Fellowship.
No. of awards offered: Varies.
Frequency: Annual.
Value: Based on Medical Research Council scale.
Length of Study: 2 years, usually beginning July 1st; renewable.
Study Establishment: Ordinarily Canadian Universities. Out of country training may be arranged in order to obtain specific expertise.
Country of Study: Canada.
Application Procedure: Application form must be completed and submitted with further documentation as outlined in the regulations.
Closing Date: November 1st.
Additional Information: Fellowships are awarded by the Society on the advice of the Review Panel. The Society reserves the right to approve or decline any application without stating its reasons.

Arthritis Society Research Grants

Subjects: Arthritis.
Eligibility: Open to investigators holding staff appointments at Canadian universities or other recognised Canadian institutions where the research is deemed relevant to arthritis. Must be Canadian citizens or permanent residents.
Level of Study: Postdoctorate.
Purpose: To promote and support research operations of investigators holding staff appointments at Canadian Universities.
Type: Research Grant.
No. of awards offered: Varies.
Frequency: Annual.
Value: To cover research costs. Grant funds may not be used for the remuneration of Grantees. The average grant funded in the 1998/99 competition was C$60,000; provide the society with a realistic budget and the panels will be instructed.
Length of Study: Usually 3 years; in some cases the Panel may request a progress report after 1 year.
Study Establishment: Canadian Institutions.
Country of Study: Canada.
Application Procedure: Application form and other documentation required - information can be found in regulations.
Closing Date: December 15th.

Arthritis Society Research Scholarships

Subjects: Arthritis.
Eligibility: Open to applicants who have been guaranteed appropriate academic rank (minimum Assistant Professor) in the tenure track or equivalent career development stream by the Institute. Applicants must be Canadians or permanent residents.
Level of Study: Postdoctorate.
Purpose: To provide support to newly appointed junior faculty members who are planning to pursue a career in basic or clinical research related to arthritis.
Type: Scholarship.
No. of awards offered: Varies.
Frequency: Annual.
Value: On a national salary scale, similar to other granting agencies.
Length of Study: 3 years for junior scholarship, 4 years for senior scholarship; non-renewable.
Study Establishment: Canadian institutions.
Country of Study: Canada.
Application Procedure: Completed application and other documentation as outlined in regulations.
Closing Date: December 15th.
Additional Information: Scholarships are awarded by the Society on the advice of the Grants Review Panels and the Society reserves the right to approve or decline any application without stating reasons. Applications on behalf of candidates should be made to the Chairman of the Department and countersigned by the Dean. Scholars must report annually to the Society on their professional activities.

Arthritis Society Research Scientist Awards

Subjects: Arthritis.
Eligibility: Open to applicants who have been guaranteed appropriate academic rank (minimum associate professor) in the tenure track or equivalent career development stream by their institution. Applicants must be Canadian citizens or permanent residents.
Level of Study: Postdoctorate.
Purpose: To provide support for individuals with a major interest in arthritis research and engaging in full-time academic careers in medical science, who have demonstrated their ability as independent research scientists.
Type: Scholarship Support.
No. of awards offered: Varies.
Frequency: Annual.
Value: On a national salary scale, similar to other granting agencies.
Length of Study: 3 years, subject to annual review.
Study Establishment: A Canadian institution.
Country of Study: Canada.
Application Procedure: Completed application form plus other documentation as outlined in regulations.
Closing Date: December 15th.
Additional Information: Scientist awards are awarded by the Society on the advice of the Grant Review Panels and the Society reserves the right to approve or decline any application without stating reasons. Applications on behalf of candidates should be made by the Chairman of the Department and countersigned by the Dean. Scientists must report annually to the Society on their professional activities.

Geoff Carr Lupus Fellowship

Subjects: Lupus.
Eligibility: Open to nationals of any country.
Level of Study: Postdoctorate.
Purpose: To provide advanced training to a rheumatologist specialising in lupus at an Ontario lupus clinic.
Type: Fellowship.
No. of awards offered: 1.
Frequency: Annual.
Value: C$50,000.
Length of Study: 1 year.
Study Establishment: Approved Ontario lupus clinic.
Country of Study: Canada.
Application Procedure: Application must be submitted with three letters of recommendation, a letter of acceptance from a proposed supervisor (to include an outline of proposed training program) and certified transcripts of undergraduate record.
Closing Date: November 1st.

Metro A Ogryzlo International Fellowship

Subjects: Clinical rheumatology.
Eligibility: The successful candidate will likely have completed his or her training in general medicine, and have a substantial prospect of returning to an academic position in his or her own country. Canadian citizens or landed immigrants are not eligible.

Level of Study: Postdoctorate.
Purpose: To provide advanced training to individuals from a developing country.
Type: Fellowship.
No. of awards offered: 1.
Frequency: Annual.
Value: Up to a maximum of C$31,000 per year.
Length of Study: 12 months; not renewable.
Study Establishment: A Rheumatic Disease Unit/Arthritis Centre.
Country of Study: Canada.
Application Procedure: Application must include: letters of recommendation from three sponsors, letter of acceptance from proposed supervisor to include outline of proposed training program, and a certified transcript of undergraduate record.
Closing Date: November 1st.
Additional Information: Fellows may not receive remuneration for any other work or hold a second major scholarship, except that, with the approval of their supervisors, they may engage in and accept remuneration for such departmental activities as are conducive to their development as clinicians, teachers or investigators. Ordinarily, a Fellow who is not a graduate of a medical school in the US, the UK, Republic of Ireland, Australia, New Zealand or South Africa must take the Medical Council of Canada evaluating examination to obtain the Medical Council of Canada certificate before an education licence can be issued.

ASSOCIATION FOR SPINA BIFIDA AND HYDROCEPHALUS (ASBAH)

ASBAH House
42 Park Road, Peterborough, Cambridgeshire, PE1 2UQ, England
Tel: (44) 1733 555 988
Fax: (44) 1733 555 985
Email: lynetteh@asbah.demon.co.uk
www: http://www.asbah.demon.co.uk/
Contact: Mrs Lynette Hare, Secretary to the Executive Director

The Association for Spina Bifida and Hydrocephalus (ASBAH), is a voluntary organisation which works for people with spina bifida or hydrocephalus. The charity lobbies for improvements in legislation and provides advisory and support services to clients and their families or carers, in addition to supplying information to professionals and sponsoring medical, social and educational research.

ASBAH Research Grant

Subjects: Medical sciences, natural sciences, education and teacher training, recreation, welfare, protective services.
Eligibility: Applicants must be resident in the UK.
Level of Study: Postgraduate.

Purpose: For research in an area directly related to spina bifida and/or hydrocephalus; also ways of improving the quality of life for people with spina bifida and/or hydrocephalus, ie. medical, scientific, educational and social research.
Type: Research Grant.
No. of awards offered: Varies.
Frequency: Dependent on funds available.
Value: Varies.
Length of Study: Varies.
Study Establishment: Varies.
Country of Study: Varies, but usually United Kingdom.
Application Procedure: In the first instance by letter to the Executive Director. If proposed research is considered to be interesting, the applicant will be asked to complete an application form.
Closing Date: January 1st and August 1st.
Additional Information: Applications should be made in good time for submission to the committees which meet in February and September/October. Please note that the research funds are fully committed for the next three years.

ASSOCIATION OF AFRICAN UNIVERSITIES

PO Box 5744, Accra-North, Ghana
Tel: (233) 21 77 44 95
Fax: (233) 21 77 48 21
Email: program@aau.org
www: http:// www.aau.org
Telex: 2284Adua GH
Contact: Mr Gof Ekhajuere, Senior Program Officer

DAAD/AAU Graduate Education Scholarship

Subjects: All subjects except social sciences.
Eligibility: Applicants must be junior members of African universities, be less than 36 years old, and have a bachelor's degree or equivalent.
Level of Study: Doctorate, Postgraduate.
Purpose: To contribute to the capacity building of African universities, by enabling junior staff members to undertake graduate education in African universities.
Type: Scholarship.
No. of awards offered: 10.
Frequency: Annual.
Value: Approximately US$3,000-US$10,000 per year.
Length of Study: 2-4 years.
Study Establishment: African universities.
Country of Study: Africa.
Application Procedure: The AAU invites approximately 20 universities to apply and provides them with application forms. The universities nominate one candidate each and the AAU then selects 10. Students wishing to apply have to make enquiries in their university department to establish whether their university has been selected to take part in the scheme.
Closing Date: July 31st.

ASSOCIATION OF COMMONWEALTH UNIVERSITIES

John Foster House
36 Gordon Square, London, WC1H 0PF, England
Tel: (44) 171 387 8572
Fax: (44) 171 387 2655
www: http://www.acu.ac.uk/
Contact: Awards Division

The Association of Commonwealth Universities (ACU), founded in 1913, is the oldest international association of universities in the world. It is incorporated by royal charter and Her Majesty the Queen, Head of the Commonwealth, is its patron. The aim of the Association is to promote, in various practical ways, contact and co-operation between its member institutions: by encouraging and supporting the movement of academic and administrative staff and students from one country of the Commonwealth to another; by providing information about universities; by organising meetings; and by hosting a higher education management service.

Times Higher Education Supplement Exchange Fellowship

Subjects: All subjects.
Eligibility: Open to academic, administrative, professional or library staff of ACU member universities in developing countries.
Level of Study: Professional development.
Purpose: To enable the recipient to obtain further experience at another university in a Commonwealth developing country; undertake a short study tour of at least one Commonwealth developing country; and visit another university in a Commonwealth developing country to realise a specific developmental objective.
Type: Fellowship.
No. of awards offered: 1.
Frequency: Annual.
Value: Up to £3,000.
Length of Study: Up to 3 months.
Study Establishment: Universities in Commonwealth countries.
Country of Study: Developing countries of the Commonwealth, other than the recipient's own country.
Application Procedure: Applications should be made through the Vice Chancellor's office of the candidate's university.
Closing Date: End of May.

ASSOCIATION OF INTERNATIONAL EDUCATION, JAPAN (AIEJ)

4-5-29 Komaba
Meguro-ku, Tokyo, 153, Japan
Tel: (81) 3 5454 5213
Fax: (81) 3 5454 5233
Contact: Mr Naoko Kadowaki, Student Affairs Division

The AIEJ was founded in 1957 with the aim of advancing international exchange in education. The Association is financed mainly by government services as the central organisation in carrying out projects relating to international education under the auspices of the Japanese Ministry of Education, universities and other educational institutions.

AIEJ Honors Scholarships

Subjects: All subjects.
Eligibility: Open to self-supporting foreign students studying in a university graduate school, junior college, college of technology or special training college in Japan who display excellence in their academic work and character and who are deemed to be in need of economic assistance during their stay in Japan.
Level of Study: Postgraduate, Undergraduate.
Type: Scholarship.
No. of awards offered: Approx. 8,540.
Frequency: Annual.
Value: Y70,000 per month (for graduate students); Y49,000 per month for undergraduate students).
Length of Study: 1 year.
Study Establishment: A graduate school in Japan. University, Junior College (2 year), College of Technology, Special Training College.
Country of Study: Japan.
Application Procedure: Candidates should apply through their school in Japan.
Closing Date: Specified by each school.

ASSOCIATION OF RHODES SCHOLARS IN AUSTRALIA

University of Melbourne, Parkville, VIC, 3052, Australia
Tel: (61) 3 9344 6937
Fax: (61) 3 9347 6739
Email: g.swafford@research.unimelb.edu.au
www: http://www.unimelb.edu.au
Contact: Dr Glenn Swafford, General Manager of Research

The Association of Teachers and Lecturers is the leading professional organisation and trade union for teachers and lecturers with over 150,000 members in England, Wales and Northern Ireland. The Association is committed to protecting and promoting the interests of its members and maintaining the highest quality professional support for them.

Association of Rhodes Scholars in Australia Travel Bursary

Subjects: All subjects.
Eligibility: Open to graduates of a Commonwealth university approved by the committee administering the scholarship, who are currently enrolled as a research higher degree student at their home university. Applicants must be Commonwealth citizens and may not be graduates of an Australian or New Zealand university.
Level of Study: Postgraduate.
Purpose: To enable an overseas Commonwealth student to undertake research for six months at one or more universities in Australia.
Type: Travel Bursary.
No. of awards offered: 1.
Frequency: Dependent on funds available.
Value: Currently A$9,000 including travel expenses and monthly stipend.
Length of Study: 6 months.
Study Establishment: A university.
Country of Study: Australia.
Application Procedure: Information and application forms are available through the internet site.
Closing Date: As advertised.

ASSOCIATION OF SURGEONS OF GREAT BRITAIN AND IRELAND

c/o The Royal College of Surgeons of England
35-43 Lincoln's Inn Fields, London, WC2A 3PN, England
Tel: (44) 171 973 0300
Fax: (44) 171 430 9235
Contact: Mrs Nechema Lewis, Administrative Assistant

Moynihan Travelling Fellowship

Subjects: Surgery.
Eligibility: Open to specialist registrars or consultants in general surgery within three years of appointment after the closing date for applications. Candidates must be residents of the United Kingdom or the Republic of Ireland but need not be either Fellows or Affiliate Fellows of the Association. They may be engaged in general surgery or a sub-speciality thereof. Candidates must be from the United Kingdom or Ireland.
Level of Study: Postdoctorate.
Purpose: To enable specialist registrars and consultants within three years of appointment at the closing date for applications, to broaden their education, and to present and discuss their contribution to British or Irish surgery overseas.
Type: Fellowship.
No. of awards offered: 1.
Frequency: Annual.
Value: £4,000.
Country of Study: Any country.
Application Procedure: A full CV should be submitted giving details of past and present appointments and publications,

together with a detailed account of the proposed programme of travel and the object to be achieved. Applications (11 copies) should be submitted to the Honorary Secretary at the Royal College of Surgeons.
Closing Date: October 1st.
Additional Information: Shortlisted candidates will be interviewed by the Scientific Committee of the Association who will pay particular attention to originality, scope and feasibility of the proposed journey. The successful candidate will be expected to act as an ambassador for British and Irish surgery and should be fully acquainted with the aims and objectives of the Association of Surgeons in its role in surgery. After the visit the Fellow will be asked to address the Association at its Annual General Meeting. A critical appraisal of the Centres visited should form the basis of the report.

ASSOCIATION OF UNIVERSITIES AND COLLEGES OF CANADA

International and Canadian Programs Division
350 Albert Street
Suite 600, Ottawa, ON, K1R 1B1, Canada
Tel: (1) 613 563 1236
Fax: (1) 613 563 9745
Email: mleger@aucc.ca
www: http://www.aucc.ca
Contact: Canadian Awards Program

The Association of Universities and Colleges of Canada is a non-profit, non-governmental association that represents Canadian universities at home and abroad. The Association's mandate is to foster and promote the interests of higher education in the firm belief that strong universities are vital to the prosperity and well-being of Canada.

Frank Knox Memorial Fellowships at Harvard University

Subjects: Arts and sciences (including engineering), business administration, dental medicine, design, divinity, education, law, medicine, public administration and public health.
Eligibility: Open to Canadian citizens or permanent residents who have recently graduated or are about to graduate from a university or college in Canada which is a member, or affiliated to a member, of AUCC. No application is considered from a student already in the USA, although applications will be considered from recent graduates who are working in the United States and will be applying to the MBA programme.
Level of Study: Postgraduate.
Type: Fellowship.
No. of awards offered: Up to 2.
Frequency: Annual.
Value: US$15,500 plus tuition fees and student health insurance..
Length of Study: 1 academic year.
Study Establishment: Harvard University, Cambridge, Massachusetts.
Country of Study: USA.

Application Procedure: Each candidate must apply directly to the graduate school of his or her choice. Candidates are responsible for gaining admission to Harvard University by the deadline set by the various faculties. For more information and application forms contact Alison Craig or download information and application form from the website.
Closing Date: February 1st (postmarked).
Additional Information: Fellows may not accept any other grant for the award period unless approved by the Committee on General Scholarships and the Sheldon Fund of Harvard University. Candidates applying to the School of Business Administration are required to take the Admissions Test for Graduate Study in Business in October or January. This may be arranged by contacting the Educational Testing Service, Box 966, Princeton, NJ, 08540, USA. Normally two months' notice should be given to ETS.

THE ASTHMA FOUNDATION OF NEW SOUTH WALES

Unit 1/82
Pacific Highway, St Leonards, NSW, 2065, Australia
Contact: The Executive Director

Biomedical and Medical Postgraduate Research Scholarships

Subjects: Medical, scientific and clinical research into asthma, its causes, triggers and impact.
Level of Study: Postdoctorate, Postgraduate.
Purpose: To expand the body of knowledge towards the causes of asthma and its possible cure.
Type: Scholarship.
No. of awards offered: Varies.
Frequency: Annual.
Value: A$1,500 to A$50,000.
Length of Study: 1 year.
Country of Study: Australia.
Application Procedure: Application forms, followed by interview for short-listed applicants.
Closing Date: Mid-August.

Medical Research Project Grant

Subjects: Medical, scientific and clinical research into asthma, its causes, triggers and impact.
Level of Study: Postdoctorate, Postgraduate.
Purpose: To expand the body of knowledge towards the causes of asthma and its possible cure.
Type: Project Grant.
No. of awards offered: Varies.
Frequency: Annual.
Value: A$15,00 to A$50,000.
Length of Study: 1 year.
Country of Study: Australia.
Application Procedure: Application forms, followed by interview for short-listed applicants.
Closing Date: Mid August.

ASTHMA SOCIETY OF CANADA

130 Bridgeland Avenue
Suite 425, Toronto, ON, M6A 1Z4, Canada
Tel: (1) 416 787 4050
Fax: (1) 416 787 5807
Email: asthma@myna.com
www: http://www.asthmasociety.com
Contact: Mr Chris Haromy, Executive Director

The Asthma Society of Canada is a national charitable volunteer supported organisation devoted to enhancing the quality of life of people living with asthma. The society's mandate includes public education and research funding.

Asthma Society of Canada Research Grants

Subjects: Clinical or basic research into problems related to asthma which have direct patient application; and asthma education - development of educational programs and evaluation of the benefits of such programmes.
Eligibility: Open to all researchers in asthma or related fields.
Level of Study: Postgraduate.
Purpose: To encourage and support asthma research.
Type: Research Grant.
No. of awards offered: 4.
Frequency: Annual.
Value: Up to a maximum of C$10,000.
Study Establishment: An appropriate institution.
Country of Study: Canada.
Application Procedure: Please write for details.
Closing Date: November 1st.

ASTHMA VICTORIA

69 Flemington Road, North Melbourne, VIC, 3051, Australia
Tel: (61) 3 9326 7088
Fax: (61) 3 9326 7055
Email: afv@asthma.org.au
www: http://www.asthma.org.au
Contact: Mr Garry Irving, Manager Services

Asthma Victoria is a community based organisation committed to reducing the impact of asthma. Asthma Victoria provides education, training advice, counselling and support to people with asthma, their families and community carers and educators. Asthma Victoria funds research which will have outcomes that directly benefit people living with asthma and will reduce the impact of this chronic condition.

Asthma Victoria Research Grants

Subjects: Medical or scientific research relating to increased knowledge of and improvements in asthma management, including development and evaluation of educational programmes, ideally projects should have direct patient application.

Eligibility: Open to Australian citizens or permanent residents with appropriate qualifications and experience at various levels, from honours graduates to postdoctoral level.
Level of Study: Doctorate, Postdoctorate, Postgraduate.
Purpose: To encourage and assist asthma research in Victoria, Australia.
Type: Research Grant, Research Scholarship.
No. of awards offered: Dependent on funds available.
Frequency: Annual.
Value: Varies, according to funds available.
Study Establishment: An approved institution within Victoria, Australia.
Country of Study: Australia.
Application Procedure: Application forms are available from Asthma Victoria.
Closing Date: September 30th for grants awarded for the following calendar year.
Additional Information: Specific purpose grants include: Helen M Schlt Trust Grants for General Asthma Resrach; Convoy for Kids Grant for research into asthma in children; Anna Jane Grant for research into adolescent asthma; Parker Grant for research into complimentary therapies.

Lilian Roxon Memorial Research Trust Travel Grant

Subjects: Research into the causes, prevention and treatment of asthma.
Eligibility: Open to Australian citizens or permanent residents with appropriate qualifications, currently engaged in asthma research, at the start of their career. The travel grant may be held concurrently with other awards to cover total expenditure.
Level of Study: Doctorate, Postdoctorate, Postgraduate.
Purpose: To assist a young asthma researcher to travel overseas to either continue research, or present their work at a recognised international meeting.
Type: Travel Grant.
No. of awards offered: 1.
Frequency: Annual, if funds are available.
Value: Up to A$2,000 towards travel expenses.
Country of Study: Outside Australia.
Application Procedure: Application forms are available from Asthma Victoria.
Closing Date: September 30th for grants awarded for the following calendar year.

AUSTRALIAN EARLY CHILDHOOD ASSOCIATION, INC.

PO Box 105, Watson, ACT, 2602, Australia
Tel: (61) 2 6241 6900
Fax: (61) 2 6241 5547
Email: national@aeca.org.au
www: http://www.aeca.org.au
Contact: National Director

AECA is the national non-government organisation for the interests of children aged 0-8 years of age and for older children in care. AECA promotes the provision of high quality services for young children and their families and supports the role of parents in caring for their children.

Alice Creswick and Sheila Kimpton Foundation Scholarship

Subjects: A wide range of areas of interest concerning policy, practice and research in the early childhood field.
Eligibility: Open to Australian citizens currently employed in positions which have a direct relationship with early childhood education and/or care and who have qualifications in early childhood or a related field.
Level of Study: Unrestricted.
Purpose: To provide the opportunity for travel, observation and/or major study in the early childhood field.
Type: Scholarship.
No. of awards offered: 1.
Frequency: Dependent on funds available.
Value: On application.
Country of Study: Any country.
Application Procedure: Applications will be called at appropriate times by AECA.
Closing Date: October 19th.
Additional Information: The successful applicant will be required to undertake certain commitments including the preparation of a written report and speaking engagements as required by AECA.

AUSTRALIAN FEDERATION OF UNIVERSITY WOMEN - VICTORIA

PO Box 816, Mount Eliza, VIC, 3930, Australia
www: http://www.vicnet.net.au/afuwvic/
Contact: Honorary Scholarship Secretary

AFUW Victoria Endowment Scholarship, Lady Leitch Scholarship

Subjects: All subjects.
Eligibility: Open to women graduates who are members of the Australian Federation of University Women, or its international affiliates who are graduates of Australian Universities (Endowment Scholarship). Lady Leitch is open to AFUW/IFUW members.
Level of Study: Doctorate, Postdoctorate, Postgraduate, Professional development.
Purpose: To assist advanced study or research.
Type: Scholarship.
No. of awards offered: 2.
Frequency: Annual - AFUW Victoria, every two years - Lady Leitch.
Value: Approximately A$5,000 for each award.
Length of Study: 1 year.
Country of Study: Any country.

Application Procedure: Application form must be completed, with documentation on university qualifications, names of three referees, and membership of AFUW or affiliate.
Closing Date: March 1st.
Additional Information: Application forms are available on AFUW-Vic website.

THE AUSTRALIAN FEDERATION OF UNIVERSITY WOMEN, SOUTH AUSTRALIA, INC TRUST FUND (AFUW)

GPO Box 634, Adelaide, SA, 5001, Australia
Contact: Fellowships Trustee

The AFUW's main activity is directed at assisting women in tertiary education in Australia via bursaries. Funds for the bursaries are raised through volunteer work, academic dress hire, donations and bequests.

The AFUW-SA Inc Trust Fund Bursary

Subjects: All subjects.
Eligibility: Applications are invited from women enrolled for coursework Master's degrees at an Australian university, who have a good Honours degree or equivalent, have completed at least one year of postgraduate research (not including an Honours year), and are Australian citizens who are not in full-time paid employment or on fully-paid study leave during the tenure of the bursary.
Level of Study: Postgraduate.
Purpose: To assist women to complete Master's degrees by coursework.
Type: Bursary.
No. of awards offered: 1.
Frequency: Annual.
Value: Up to A$3,000; runners-up may receive awards of less than bursary amount.
Length of Study: Bursary must be used within 12 months of date of award.
Study Establishment: A recognised Australian tertiary institution.
Country of Study: Australia.
Application Procedure: The following must accompany the completed application form: evidence of enrolment at the institution at which the qualification is to be obtained; copies of official transcripts; CV, including employment record and list of publications.
Closing Date: March 1st.

Barbara Crase Bursary

Subjects: All subjects.
Eligibility: Open to women or men of any nationality; applicants must have completed one year of postgraduate research, excluding Honours year.

Level of Study: Doctorate, Postgraduate.
Purpose: To assist in completion of a Master's or PhD research degree.
Type: Bursary.
No. of awards offered: 1.
Frequency: Annual.
Value: A$2,500.
Length of Study: Bursary must be used within 12 months of date of award.
Study Establishment: A South Australian university.
Country of Study: Australia.
Application Procedure: Please write for details.
Closing Date: March 1st.

Cathy Candler Bursary

Subjects: All subjects.
Eligibility: Open to women or men of any nationality; applicants must have completed one year of postgraduate research, excluding Honours year.
Level of Study: Doctorate, Postgraduate.
Purpose: To assist in completion of a Master's or PhD degree by research.
Type: Bursary.
No. of awards offered: 1.
Frequency: Annual.
Value: A$2,500.
Length of Study: Bursary must be used within 12 months of date of award.
Study Establishment: A South Australian university.
Country of Study: Australia.
Application Procedure: Please write for details.
Closing Date: March 1st.

Diamond Jubilee Bursary

Subjects: All subjects.
Eligibility: Open to women or men of any nationality.
Level of Study: Postgraduate.
Purpose: To assist in completion of a Master's degree by coursework.
Type: Bursary.
No. of awards offered: 1.
Frequency: Annual.
Value: A$2,000.
Length of Study: Bursary must be used within 12 months of the date of award.
Study Establishment: A South Australian university.
Country of Study: Australia.
Application Procedure: Please write for details.

Doreen McCarthy Bursary

Subjects: All subjects.
Eligibility: Open to women or men any nationality; applicants must have completed one year of postgraduate research, excluding Honours year.
Level of Study: Doctorate, Postgraduate.
Purpose: To assist in completion of a Master's or PhD degree by research.
Type: Bursary.

No. of awards offered: 1.
Frequency: Annual.
Value: A$2,500.
Length of Study: Bursary must be used within 12 months of date of award.
Study Establishment: A South Australian university.
Country of Study: Australia.
Application Procedure: Please write for details.
Closing Date: March 1st.

Padnendadlu Bursary

Subjects: All subjects.
Eligibility: Must be an Australian indigenous woman.
Level of Study: Postgraduate.
Purpose: To assist in completion of a postgraduate degree by research.
Type: Bursary.
No. of awards offered: 1 but runners up may be awarded less than the bursary amount.
Frequency: Annual.
Value: A$2,500.
Study Establishment: A South Australian university.
Country of Study: Australia.
Application Procedure: Please write for details.
Closing Date: March 1st.

Thenie Baddams Bursary and Jean Gilmore Bursary

Subjects: All subjects.
Eligibility: Open to women graduates who are enrolled at an Australian tertiary institution and have completed at least one year of postgraduate research, excluding honours year. Applicants must hold a good Honours degree or equivalent, and not be not in full-time paid employment or study leave during tenure.
Level of Study: Postgraduate.
Purpose: To assist women to complete a Master's or PhD degree, by research.
Type: Bursary.
No. of awards offered: 2.
Frequency: Annual.
Value: Up to A$6,000 each; however runners-up can be awarded a lesser amount.
Length of Study: Bursary must be used within 12 months of date of award.
Study Establishment: A recognised Australian higher education institution.
Country of Study: Any country.
Application Procedure: Applications must include: completed application form; evidence of enrolment at the institution where the qualification is to be obtained; copies of official transcripts; curriculum vitae, including employment record and list of publications. There is a A$12.00 lodgement fee.
Closing Date: March 1st.

The Winifred E Preedy Postgraduate Bursary

Subjects: Dentistry or a related field.
Eligibility: Open to women who are past or present students of the Faculty of Dentistry at the University of Adelaide and who are enrolled as graduate students in dentistry or some allied field at the University of Adelaide or such other institution of tertiary education as the Trustees may approve. The applicant must have completed one year of her postgraduate degree.
Level of Study: Postgraduate.
Purpose: To assist women in completion of a higher degree.
Type: Bursary.
No. of awards offered: 1.
Frequency: Annual.
Value: A$5,000.
Length of Study: Bursary must be used within 12 months of date of award.
Study Establishment: Anywhere if the applicant is a past student at the University of Adelaide (Australia) Dental Faculty.
Country of Study: Any country if applicant is a past student of the Faculty of Dentistry at the University of Adelaide, South Australia, otherwise the applicant must currently be enrolled in the latter faculty.
Application Procedure: Applications must include: a completed application form; evidence of enrolment at the institution where the qualification will be obtained; copies of official transcripts; curriculum vitae and list of publications.
Closing Date: March 1st.

THE AUSTRALIAN GOVERNMENT

The University of Newcastle, Callaghan, NSW, 2308, Australia
Tel: (61) 49 21 6537
Fax: (61) 49 21 6908
Contact: P H Farley, Research Branch Director

The University of Newcastle ranks ninth out of thirty-six Australian universities, in research. There are twelve special research centres, over fifty research programmes of international standing and 900 research candidates spread over ten faculties including: Architecture Building and Design, Arts and Social Science, Economics and Commerce, Education, Engineering, Law Medicine and Health Sciences, Music, Nursing Science and Mathematics.

Australian Government Postgraduate Awards

Subjects: All academic disciplines.
Eligibility: Open to Australian citizens and permanent residents who have lived in Australia for 12 months prior to application. Applicants must have completed four years of full-time undergraduate study and gained a first class Honours, or equivalent award.
Level of Study: Doctorate, Postgraduate.
Purpose: To support students undertaking full-time higher research degree programmes at Australian universities.
Type: Research Grant, Research Scholarship.

No. of awards offered: Approx. 40.
Frequency: Annual.
Value: Living allowance of approximately A$16,000 per year tax exempt and index-linked, plus allowances for relocation and thesis production and exemption of HECS payments.
Length of Study: 2 years full-time study for research Master's candidates, or 3 years full-time for PhD candidates.
Country of Study: Australia.
Application Procedure: Application form must be completed.
Closing Date: October 31st.

AUSTRALIAN INSTITUTE OF ABORIGINAL AND TORRES STRAIT ISLANDER STUDIES

GPO Box 553, Canberra, ACT, 2601, Australia
Tel: (61) 6 246 1157
Fax: (61) 6 249 7714
Email: fbb@aiatsis.gov.au
www: http://www.aiatsis.gov.au
Contact: Director of Research

AIATSIS is a federally funded organisation central in Aboriginal and Torres Strait Islander research. Its principal function is to promote Australian Aboriginal and Torres Strait Islander studies. A staff of 60, directed by the Principal, engages in a range of services through the Reseach Program, the Research Grants Program, the archives and production team, and the library.

AIATSIS Research Grants

Subjects: Health, human biology, social anthropology, linguistics, ethnomusicology, material culture, rock art, prehistory, ethnobotany, psychology, education and Aboriginal history including oral history, native title, indigenous land use agreements.
Eligibility: Open to nationals of any country.
Level of Study: Unrestricted.
Purpose: To promote research into Aboriginal and Torres Strait Islander Studies.
Type: Research Grant.
No. of awards offered: Varies according to application and availablilty of funds.
Frequency: Annual.
Value: No predetermined value.
Length of Study: 12 months maximum.
Country of Study: Australia.
Application Procedure: Application form must be completed. Application form available from Research Administrator tel: 6 246 1145 or visit the AIATSIS website.
Closing Date: January 31st.
Additional Information: Permission to conduct research project must be obtained from the appropriate Aboriginal or Torres Strait Island community or organisation.

AUSTRALIAN INSTITUTE OF MEDICAL SCIENTISTS

PO Box 1911, Milton, QLD, 4064, Australia
Tel: (61) 7 3876 2988
Fax: (61) 7 3876 2999
Email: aimsnat@medeserv.com.au
www: http://www.aims.org.au/
Contact: Grants Management Officer

AIMS is the professional association representing medical scientists working in hospital and private medical laboratories in Australia. AIMS provides medical scientists with the opportunity to continually update their professional knowledge through scientific meetings, scientific journals and postgraduate programmes.

Postgraduate Scholarship (sponsored by BioMérieux-Vitek Australia and AIMS)

Subjects: Medical laboratory science.
Eligibility: Open to Australian citizens who are members of AIMS.
Level of Study: Postgraduate.
Purpose: To support postgraduate study.
Type: Scholarship.
No. of awards offered: 1.
Frequency: Annual, if funds are available.
Value: A$3,000.
Length of Study: 1 year.
Study Establishment: Appropriate institutions.
Country of Study: Australia.
Application Procedure: Please write for details, guidelines are available. The applications should be addressed to the Executive Officer.
Closing Date: October 31st.

AUSTRALIAN NATIONAL UNIVERSITY

Canberra, ACT, 0200, Australia
Tel: (61) 6 249 2700
Fax: (61) 6 248 0054
Email: administraton.hrc@anu.edu.au
www: http://www.anu.edu.au/hrc
Contact: Humanities Research Centre

The Australian National University was founded by the Australian Government in 1946 as Australia's only completely research-oriented university. It comprises eight research schools, six teaching faculties, a graduate school and over a dozen other academic schools or centres.

Aboriginal and Torred Strait Islander Scholarship

Subjects: All subjects.
Eligibility: Awarded to an indigenous Australian who is an Aboriginal or Torres Strait Islander.

Level of Study: Doctorate, Postgraduate.
Purpose: To assist and Aboriginal or Torres Strait Islander to undertakle a graduate diploma or master degree course, or a course leading to a PhD.
Type: Scholarship.
No. of awards offered: Varies.
Frequency: Annual.
Value: A$15,888 stipend per annum.
Length of Study: Dependent on the course to which the scholarship applies.
Country of Study: Australia.
Application Procedure: Please write for details.
Closing Date: October 31st.

ANU Alumni Association Country Specific PhD Scholarships

Subjects: All subjects.
Eligibility: Open to nationals from Malaysia, Thailand and Singapore.
Level of Study: Doctorate.
Purpose: To assist students from Malaysia, Singapore and Thailand with study in Australia.
Type: Scholarship.
No. of awards offered: 3- one to a candidate from each of the eligible countries.
Value: A$15,888 basic stipend per annum, tax free.
Length of Study: Normally tenable for 3 years renewable for 6 months.
Country of Study: Australia.
Application Procedure: Please write for details.
Closing Date: August 30th.

ANU Masters Degree Scholarships (The Faculties)

Subjects: All subjects.
Eligibility: Applicants must hold a Bachelors degree with at least upper sceond class honours, and, if wishing to undertake degree by research only, must have proven capability for research.
Level of Study: Postgraduate.
Purpose: To assist study in most Graduate School programmes for courses leading to a Masters degree by research, by coursework or by coursework and research.
Type: Scholarship.
No. of awards offered: Varies.
Frequency: Annual.
Value: Basic stipend of US$15,888 per annum tax free; an additional allowanc for dependent children of married international scholars, travel to Canberra (excluding inetrnational part of the airfare for those recruited from overseas) and a grant for the reimbursement of some removal expenses.
Length of Study: 1 year.
Study Establishment: The Faculties.
Country of Study: Australia.
Application Procedure: Please write for details.

Closing Date: October 31st for citizens/permanent residents of New Zealand and Australia; August 30th for international applicants.

ANU PhD Scholarships

Subjects: All subjects.
Eligibility: Please write for details.
Level of Study: Postgraduate.
Purpose: To assist research.
Type: Scholarship.
No. of awards offered: Varies.
Value: Stipend of $A15,888 per annum tax free, and if applicable, an additional allowance for dependent children of unmarried international scholars. Economy travel to Canberra and a grant for the reimbursement of some removal expenses.
Length of Study: 3 years, renewable for six months.
Country of Study: Australia.
Application Procedure: Please write for details.
Closing Date: October 31st for citizens/permanent residents of Australia and New Zealand; August 30th for international students.

Graduate School Scholarships

Subjects: All subjects.
Eligibility: Restricted to those who are on the Order of Merit list for Australian Postgraduate Awards.
Level of Study: Graduate, Postgraduate.
Purpose: To fund graduate study.
Type: Scholarship.
Value: Stipend of A$15,888 per annum tax free, travel to Canberra from within Australia and a grant for the reimbursement of some removal expenses.
Country of Study: Australia.
Application Procedure: Please write for details.
Closing Date: October 31st.

Re-entry Scholarships for Women

Subjects: All subjects.
Eligibility: Applicants must be Australian citizens or permanent residents. The scholarship may be awarded to undertake a Master degree course or a PhD and applicants must hold qualifications appropriate to the level of course for which they wish to apply.
Level of Study: Doctorate, Postgraduate.
Purpose: To assist women graduates who wish to resume their studies after a break of at least three years since formal enrolment in a university course, the break normally being due to fulfilment of family obligations.
Type: Scholarship.
No. of awards offered: Varies.
Frequency: Annual.
Value: A$15,888 per annum.
Length of Study: Tenure is dependent upon the course to which the scholarship applies.
Country of Study: Australia.

Application Procedure: An application must be submitted along with a letter setting out the applicants case for award of the scholarship and indicating their circumstances in terms of the eligibility criteria.
Closing Date: September 30th.

Scholarships for International Students Only

Subjects: All subjects.
Eligibility: Many students come from developing countries under the Australian Government's foreign aid programme which is administered by the Australian Agency for International Development (AusAID).
Level of Study: Doctorate, Postgraduate.
Purpose: To assist international students to study in Australia.
Type: Scholarship.
No. of awards offered: Varies.
Value: Some scholarships cover full tuition, living costs and travel, others cover tuition fees only.
Country of Study: Australia.
Application Procedure: Please write for details.
Closing Date: October 30th.

Tuition Fee Scholarships

Subjects: All subjects.
Eligibility: Awarded to those on the Overseas Postgraduate Research Scholarship (OPRS) Order of Merit list.
Level of Study: Doctorate, Postgraduate.
Purpose: Tuition waiver fee scholarships awarded to candidates on the OPRS Order of Merit list.
Type: Scholarship.
No. of awards offered: Varies.
Value: Covers course fee.
Country of Study: Australia.
Application Procedure: Please write for details.

AUSTRALIAN-AMERICAN EDUCATIONAL FOUNDATION

GPO Box 1559, Canberra, ACT, 2601, Australia
Tel: (61) 2 6247 9331
Fax: (61) 2 6247 6554
Email: lindy@aaef.anu.edu.au
www: http://www.sunsite.anu.edu.au/education/fulbright
Contact: Program and Development Officer

The Australian-American Educational Foundation is a bi-national commission. The major objective of the Foundation is to further mutual understanding between the peoples of Australia and the United States through educational exchanges. The Foundation also provides information for Australians wishing to study in the United States.

Fulbright Awards

Subjects: All subjects.
Eligibility: Open to Australian postgraduate and postdoctoral students, senior scholars and professionals.
Level of Study: Doctorate, Postdoctorate, Postgraduate, Professional development.
No. of awards offered: Up to 16.
Frequency: Annual.
Value: Postgraduate students: up to A$32,530; postdoctoral fellows: up to A$38,890; senior scholars: up to A$28,350; professionals: up to A$17,600.
Length of Study: Varies.
Country of Study: USA.
Application Procedure: Application form must be completed, three referees' reports (included in the application form), documentation of citizenship and qualifications must be submitted. Additional information and an application form are available on the website.
Closing Date: September 30th.

Fulbright Postdoctoral Fellowships

Subjects: All subjects.
Eligibility: Open to Australian citizens by birth or naturalisation; naturalised citizens must provide a certificate of Australian citizenship with their application, and native-born Australians must provide a copy of their birth certificate. Those holding dual US/Australian citizenship are not eligible for this award. Applicants should have recently completed their PhD, normally less than three years prior to application, although those who have completed their PhD four to five years prior to application will be considered.
Level of Study: Postdoctorate.
Purpose: To enable those who have recently completed their PhD to conduct postdoctoral research, further their professional training, or lecture at a university.
Type: Scholarship.
No. of awards offered: Up to 2.
Frequency: Annual.
Value: Up to A$38,890.
Length of Study: 3-12 months.
Study Establishment: A university, college, research establishment or reputable private practice.
Country of Study: USA.
Application Procedure: An application form must be completed, three referees reports (included in the application form), documentation of citizenship and qualifications must be submitted. Additional Information are available on the website.
Closing Date: September 30th.

Fulbright Postgraduate Student Award for Aboriginal and Torres Strait Islander People

Subjects: All subjects.
Eligibility: Open to people of Aboriginal and Torres Strait Islander descent.
Level of Study: Postgraduate.

Purpose: To enable candidates to undertake an approved course of study for an American higher degree, or engage in research relevant to an Australian higher degree.
Type: Scholarship.
No. of awards offered: 1.
Frequency: Annually, dependent on funds available.
Value: Up to A$32,530.
Length of Study: 8-12 months funded; up to a further 4 years unfunded.
Study Establishment: An accredited institution.
Country of Study: USA.
Application Procedure: Application form, three referees' reports (included in application form), documentation of citizenship and qualifications must be submitted. Additional information and an application form can be obtained from the website.
Closing Date: September 30th.

Fulbright Postgraduate Studentships

Subjects: All subjects.
Eligibility: Open to Australian citizens by birth or naturalisation; naturalised citizens must provide a certificate of Australian citizenship with their application, and native-born Australians must provide a copy of their birth certificate. Those holding dual US/Australian citizenship are ineligible for this award. Applicants must be graduates.
Level of Study: Doctorate, Postgraduate.
Purpose: To enable students to undertake an approved course of study for an American higher degree or its equivalent, or to engage in research relevant to an Australian higher degree.
Type: Scholarship.
No. of awards offered: Up to 8.
Frequency: Annual.
Value: Up to A$32,530.
Length of Study: 8-12 months, renewable for a maximum of 5 years, but without additional allowance.
Study Establishment: An accredited US institution.
Country of Study: USA.
Application Procedure: Application form must be completed, three referees' reports (included in the application form), and documentation of citizenship and qualifications must be submitted. Additional Information and an application form are available from the website.
Closing Date: September 30th.
Additional Information: As the Award does not include any provision for maintenance payments, applicants must be able to demonstrate that they have sufficient financial resources to support themselves and any dependants during their stay in the USA.

Fulbright Professional Award

Subjects: Open to all professional fields.
Eligibility: Open to Australian citizens, resident in Australia, with a record of achievement, and are poised for

advancement to a senior management or policy role. Those who hold dual US/Australian citizenship are ineligible for this award.
Level of Study: Professional development.
Purpose: To support applicants undertaking a programme of professional development.
Type: Fellowship.
No. of awards offered: 1.
Frequency: Annual.
Value: Up to A$17,600.
Length of Study: 3-4 months between July and June; programs of longer duration may be proposed but without additional funding.
Country of Study: USA.
Application Procedure: Application form must be completed, three referees' reports (included in the application form), and documentation of citizenship and qualifications must be submitted. Additional information and an application form are available from the website.
Closing Date: September 30th.
Additional Information: Programs should include an academic as well as a practical aspect.

Fulbright Senior Awards

Subjects: All subjects.
Eligibility: Open to Australian citizens by birth or naturalisation; naturalised citizens must provide a certificate of Australian citizenship with their application, and native-born Australians must provide a copy of their birth certificate. Those holding dual US/Australian citizenship are not eligible for this award. Applicants should be either scholars of established reputation working in an academic institution who intend to teach or research in the USA; leaders in the arts (for example music, drama, visual arts); or senior members of the academically based professions who are currently engaged in the private practice of their profession.
Level of Study: Professional development.
Purpose: To teach, undertake research, be an invited speaker, or visit institutions within their field.
No. of awards offered: 2.
Frequency: Annual.
Value: Up to A$28,350.
Length of Study: 4-6 months.
Study Establishment: A university, college, research establishment or reputable private organisation.
Country of Study: USA.
Application Procedure: Application form must be completed, three referees' reports (included in application form), and documentation of citizenship and qualifications must be submitted. Additional information and an application form are available from the website.
Closing Date: September 30th.

BEIT MEMORIAL FELLOWSHIPS

c/o Molecular Immunology Group
Institute of Molecular Medicine
John Radcliffe Hospital
Headington, Oxford, OX3 9DU, England
Contact: Mrs Melanie J Goble, Administrative Secretary

Beit Memorial Fellowships

Subjects: Medical research.
Eligibility: Open to graduates of postdoctoral level or medically qualified applicants from any faculty from an approved university in the UK or in any country which is or has been since 1910 a British Dominion, Protectorate or Mandated Territory.
Level of Study: Postdoctorate.
Purpose: To promote research into medicine and allied sciences.
Type: Fellowship.
No. of awards offered: Approx. 5.
Frequency: Every two years.
Value: £15,154-£19,848 per year plus £2,134 London allowance if applicable.
Length of Study: 3 years.
Study Establishment: An approved university, research institute or medical school.
Country of Study: United Kingdom or Ireland.
Application Procedure: Please write for details.
Closing Date: March 1st.

BEIT TRUST (ZIMBABWE, ZAMBIA & MALAWI)

Beit Trust Fellowships
PO Box 76, Chisipite, Harare, Zimbabwe
Tel: (263) 4 96132
Fax: (263) 494046
Contact: Secretary to the Advisory Board

Beit Trust Postgraduate Fellowships

Subjects: All subjects.
Eligibility: Open to persons under 30 years of age (35 in the case of medical doctors) who are university graduates domiciled in Zambia (4 fellowships), Zimbabwe (4 fellowships), or Malawi (2 fellowships).
Level of Study: Postgraduate.
Purpose: To support postgraduate study or research.
Type: Fellowship.
No. of awards offered: 10.
Frequency: Annual.
Value: Personal allowance and fees (variable); plus book, clothing, thesis and departure allowances.
Length of Study: 2 years; possibly renewable for a further year.
Study Establishment: Approved universities and other institutions.

Country of Study: United Kingdom, Ireland or South Africa.
Application Procedure: Application form must be completed.
Closing Date: September 30th.

BELGIAN-AMERICAN EDUCATIONAL FOUNDATION, INC.

195 Church Street, New Haven, CT, 06510, United States of America
Tel: (1) 203 777 5765
Email: emile.boulpaep@yale.edu
Contact: The President

Belgian-American Educational Foundation Graduate Fellowships for Study in Belgium

Subjects: Agriculture, forestry and fishery, architecture and town planning, arts and humanities, business administration and management, education and teacher training, engineering, fine and applied arts, home economics, law, mass communication and information science, mathematics and computer science, medical sciences, natural sciences recreation, welfare, protective services, religion and theology, social and behavioural sciences, transport and communications.
Eligibility: Open to US citizens, preferably under 30 years of age, with a speaking and reading knowledge of Dutch, French or German. The candidate must have a Master's or equivalent degree or be working towards a PhD or equivalent degree.
Level of Study: Doctorate, Postgraduate.
Type: Fellowship.
No. of awards offered: 10.
Frequency: Annual.
Value: US$12,000, which includes round-travel expenses, lodging and living expenses, as well as tuition and enrolment fees.
Length of Study: 1 academic year.
Study Establishment: A Belgian university or other academic institution of higher learning.
Country of Study: Belgium.
Application Procedure: Application form must be completed.
Closing Date: January 31st.

Belgian-American Educational Foundation Graduate Fellowships for Study in the USA

Subjects: All subjects.
Eligibility: Open to Belgian nationals. Applicants must have a good command of the English language.
Level of Study: Doctorate, Postgraduate.
Type: Fellowship.
Frequency: Annual.
Value: US$30,000.

Length of Study: 1 year.
Study Establishment: An American University.
Country of Study: USA.
Application Procedure: Application form must be completed, and 3-5 letters of reference must be submitted.
Closing Date: October 31st.
Additional Information: The stipend consists of a fixed sum to cover living expenses, purchase of books, and similar. In addition, the Foundation pays for tuition and health insurance at the American university. Fellows are expected to stay in the USA for a full academic year.

For further information contact:

Egmonstraat 11 rue d'Egmont, Brussels, B-1050, Belgium
Tel: (32) 2 513 59 55
Fax: (32) 2 672 53 81
Contact: The Secretary

Postgraduate Fellowships for Study in the USA

Subjects: All subjects.
Eligibility: Open to Belgian nationals. Applicants must have a good command of the English language.
Level of Study: Postgraduate.
Type: Fellowship.
Frequency: Annual.
Value: US$15,000.
Length of Study: 1 year.
Study Establishment: An American university.
Country of Study: USA.
Application Procedure: Application form must be completed, and 3-5 letters of reference must be submitted.
Closing Date: October 31st.
Additional Information: The stipend consists of a fixed sum to cover living expenses, purchase of books, and similar. In addition, the Foundation pays for health insurance at the American institution. Fellows are expected to stay in the USA for a full academic year.

For further information contact:

Egmontstraat 11 rue d'Egmont, Brussels, B-1050, Belgium
Tel: (32) 2 513 59 55
Fax: (32) 2 672 53 81
Contact: The Secretary

BFWG CHARITABLE FOUNDATION (FORMERLY CROSBY HALL)

28 Great James Street, London, WC1N 3ES, England
Tel: (44) 171 404 6447
Fax: (44) 171 404 6505
Email: bfwg.charity@btinternet.com
Contact: Ms Jean V Collett, Company Secretary

Offers grants to help woman graduates with their living expenses (not fees) while registered for study or research at an approved institution of higher education in Great Britain. The criteria for awarding grants are the proven needs of the applicants and their academic calibre.

BFWG Charitable Foundation and Emergency Grants

Subjects: All subjects.
Eligibility: Open to graduate women who have completed their first year of graduate or doctoral study or research. There is no restriction on nationality.
Level of Study: Doctorate, Postdoctorate, Postgraduate.
Purpose: Main Foundation Grants are to assist women graduates who have difficulty meeting their living expenses while studying or researching at approved institutions of higher education in Great Britain; Emergency Grants are to assist graduate women facing a financial crisis which may prevent them completing an academic year's study.
Type: Grant.
No. of awards offered: Approx. 50-60 Foundation Grants and approx. 50-60 Emergency Grants.
Frequency: Foundation Grants - annually. Emergency Grants - three times per year.
Value: Foundation Grants - will not exceed £2,500; Emergency Grants - no grant is likely to exceed £500.
Length of Study: Support for courses that exceed 12 months full-time.
Study Establishment: Approved institutions in Great Britain.
Country of Study: United Kingdom.
Application Procedure: Completed application forms, two references, copy of graduate certificate, evidence of acceptance for the year, a cheque for £12, or for £5 in the case of emergency grants; and a brief summary of thesis if applicable for foundation grants.
Closing Date: Foundation Grants - March 31st; Emergency Grants - February 17th, April 16th and June 15th.

BOARD OF TRUSTEES FOR THE AWARD OF THE HEINRICH WIELAND PRIZE

Gasstrasse 18
Haus 4, Hamburg, D-22761, Germany
Tel: (49) 40 89 40 04
Fax: (49) 40 89 40 06
Email: mergarin@mediascape.de
Contact: Dr Ingo Witte

Heinrich Wieland Prize

Subjects: Medical sciences.
Eligibility: Open to nationals of any country.
Level of Study: Unrestricted.
Purpose: To encourage work on the chemistry, biochemistry, and physiology of fats and lipids, as well as on their clinical importance and their significance in the physiology of nutrition.

Type: Prize.
No. of awards offered: 1.
Frequency: Annual.
Value: DM50,000 and a Medal.
Country of Study: Any country.
Application Procedure: Application must include CV, reprints and copies of manuscripts.
Closing Date: February 28th.

BRITISH ASSOCIATION OF PLASTIC SURGEONS (BAPS)

The Royal College of Surgeons
35-43 Lincoln's Inn Fields, London, WC2A 3PN, England
Tel: (44) 171 831 5161
Fax: (44) 171 831 4041
Email: secretariat@babs.co.uk
www: http://www.babs.rcseng.ac.uk
Contact: Ms Angela Rausch, Course and Committee Administrator

A membership organisation for plastic surgeons working within the NHS.

BAPS European Travelling Scholarship

Subjects: Plastic surgery.
Eligibility: Open to members of the Association who are specialist registrars (years 4-6) or senior registrars enrolled in a recognised training programme. Applicants must be resident in the UK.
Level of Study: Professional development.
Purpose: To enable specialist registrars (year 4-6) from Britain to visit any plastic surgery centre in Europe for training purposes.
Type: Scholarship.
No. of awards offered: 2.
Frequency: Every two years.
Value: Up to £1,000.
Length of Study: Varies.
Study Establishment: Any plastic surgery centre.
Country of Study: Europe, excluding United Kingdom.
Application Procedure: An application form must be completed with proposed itinerary, giving details of costs and reasons for wanting to attend a particular unit. Also a CV of no more than two pages must be submitted.
Closing Date: September 1st, March 1st.

BAPS Fellowship

Subjects: Plastic surgery.
Eligibility: Open to senior trainees in plastic surgery, living and working in developing countries.
Level of Study: Professional development.
Purpose: To enable senior trainees from developing countries to obtain further training and experience in plastic surgery.
Type: Fellowship.
No. of awards offered: 2.

Frequency: Annual.
Value: £500 per month.
Length of Study: 6 months.
Study Establishment: Hospital plastic surgery units.
Country of Study: British Isles.
Application Procedure: Application details are available on request from the British Association of Plastic Surgeons.
Closing Date: October 1st.

BAPS Travelling Bursary

Subjects: Plastic surgery.
Eligibility: Open to members of the Association who are either specialist registrars (years 4-6) enrolled in a recognised training programme or consultant plastic surgeons of not more than three years' standing.
Level of Study: Professional development.
Purpose: To enable a plastic surgeon in the UK to study new techniques abroad.
Type: Bursary.
No. of awards offered: 2.
Frequency: Annual.
Value: Up to £4,000.
Length of Study: Varies.
Study Establishment: Hospital plastic surgery units.
Country of Study: Outside United Kingdom.
Application Procedure: An application form must be completed with proposed itinerary, giving details of costs and reasons for wanting to attend a particular unit. Also a CV of no more than two pages must be submitted.
Closing Date: September 1st, March 1st.

Paton/Maser Memorial Fund

Subjects: Plastic surgery.
Eligibility: Consultants and specialist registrars in plastic surgery working in the British Isles.
Level of Study: Research.
Purpose: To provide funds towards research projects in plastic surgery in the British Isles.
Type: Research Grant.
No. of awards offered: 1.
Frequency: Annual.
Value: £2,500.
Length of Study: Varies.
Study Establishment: Hospital or research laboratory.
Country of Study: British Isles.
Application Procedure: A letter of application with a copy of research protocol must be submitted.
Closing Date: November 1st.

Student Bursaries

Subjects: Plastic surgery.
Eligibility: Medical students in the UK.
Level of Study: Predoctorate.
Purpose: To help medical students to cover expenses of travel and research related to plastic surgery.
Type: Bursary.
No. of awards offered: 4.
Frequency: Annual.

Value: £350.
Length of Study: Varies.
Study Establishment: Hospital plastic surgery units or research laboratories.
Country of Study: Any country.
Application Procedure: A letter of application with a CV and brief outline of the proposed project must be submitted.
Closing Date: January 31st.

THE BRITISH COUNCIL

Science and Public Affairs
Hahnenstrasse 6, Koln, D-50667, Germany
Tel: (49) 221 20644 30
Fax: (49) 221 20644 55
Contact: Grants Management Officer

The purpose of the British Council is to promote a wider knowledge of the United Kingdom and the English language and to encourage cultural, scientific, technological and educational co-operation between the United Kingdom and other countries. The Council pursues its purpose through cultural relations and the provision of development assistance.

British-German Academic Research Collaboration (ARC) Programme

Subjects: All subjects.
Eligibility: Applications are invited from research groups in publicly-funded institutions in both the higher and non-higher education sectors. All areas of research are eligible, inlcuding the social sciences and humanities. Preference will be given to research projects which also provide research training opportunities for younger scientists.
Purpose: To increase collaboration between research groups in the United Kingdom and Germany.
Type: Travel Grant.
Frequency: Annual.
Country of Study: United Kingdom or Germany.
Application Procedure: Further information and application forms are available. British applicants should contact the British Council and German applicants should contact the German Academic Exchange Service, Section 313, Kennedyallee 50, D-53175 Bonn, Germany, tel (49) 228 882 0/236, fax (49) 228 882 551.
Closing Date: December 31st.
Additional Information: ARC can support research groups in the United Kingdom and Germany working in related fields for exploratory visits to establish the potential for research collaboration, and visits which are part of an agreed collaborative research project. For more information please contact the Science and Public Affairs Department , tel (49) 221 20644 15.

For further information contact:

The British Council
Science and Public Affairs
Hahnenstrasse 6, Koln, 50667, Germany
Tel: (49) 221 20644 15
Fax: (49) 221 20644 55

THE BRITISH COUNCIL

British Embassy
3100 Massachusetts Avenue NW, Washington, DC, 20008, United States of America
Tel: (1) 202 588 7830
Fax: (1) 202 588 7918
Email: study.uk@bc-washingtondc.bcouncil.org
www: http://www.britishcouncil-usa.org
Contact: Cultural Department

The British Council is Britain's international network for education, culture, and development services. It co-ordinates the Marshall Scholarships Programme in the USA.

British Marshall Scholarships

Subjects: All subjects.
Eligibility: Open only to United States citizens. Must be graduates of four-year accredited US college or university course with a minimum GPA of 3.7 and must have graduated within the last two years.
Level of Study: Postgraduate, Undergraduate.
Purpose: To enable United States college graduates of high ability to study for a degree - at either postgraduate or undergraduate level - at any UK university.
Type: Scholarship.
No. of awards offered: Up to 40.
Frequency: Annual.
Value: Covers all tuition fees, a living allowance and book allowance for two years.
Length of Study: 2-3 years.
Study Establishment: Any UK university.
Country of Study: United Kingdom.
Application Procedure: Application forms available from the British Council at the British Embassy in Washington DC, or British Consulates in Boston, Chicago, Atlanta, Houston, and San Francisco. For information on on-line applications please refer to the website.
Closing Date: October (in year preceding take up of award).

For further information contact:

Suite 2700
Marquis One Tower
245 Peachtree Centre Avenue, Atlanta, GA, 30303, United States of America
Tel: (1) 524 5856
Contact: British Consulate General

or
Federal Reserve Plaza
600 Atlantic Avenue, Boston, MA, 02210, United States of America
Tel: (1) 248 9555
Contact: British Consulate General
or
Suite 1600
The Wrigley Building
400 N Michigan Avenue, Chicago, IL, 60611, United States of America
Tel: (1) 346 1810
Contact: British Consulate General
or
First Interstate Bank Building
Suite 1900
1000 Louisiana, Houston, TX, 77002, United States of America
Tel: (1) 659 6270
Contact: British Consulate General
or
845 Third Avenue, New York, NY, 10022, United States of America
Tel: (1) 752 5747
Contact: British Information Services
or
1 Sansome Street
Suite 850, San Francisco, CA, 94104, United States of America
Tel: (1) 981 3030
Contact: British Consulate General

BRITISH DENTAL ASSOCIATION

64 Wimpole Street, London, W1M 8AL, England
Tel: (44) 171 935 0875
Fax: (44) 171 487 5232
Email: enquiries@bda-dentistry.org.uk
www: http://www.bda-dentistry.org.uk
Contact: Dentsply Scholarship Fund Secretary

The British Dental Association is the National Professional Association for Dentists. With over 18,000 members, the Association strives to enhance the science, arts and ethics of dentistry, improve the nations oral health, and promote the interests of its members.

Dentsply Scholarship Fund

Subjects: Dentistry.
Eligibility: Open to British citizens studying in the UK or abroad, or citizens of any country studying in the UK.
Level of Study: Postgraduate, Undergraduate.
Purpose: To give financial assistance to undergraduate or postgraduate students of dentistry to enable them to undertake or continue studies in schools in the UK.
Type: Mostly interest-free loans, some grants.
No. of awards offered: Varies.
Frequency: Annual.

Value: A few hundred pounds.
Country of Study: United Kingdom.
Application Procedure: Application forms must be completed and submitted by May 31st, along with an academic reference or supporting letter.
Closing Date: May 31st.

BRITISH DIABETIC ASSOCIATION

10 Queen Anne Street, London, W1M 0BD, England
Tel: (44) 171 462 2693
Fax: (44) 171 637 3644
Email: marir@diabetes.org.uk
www: http://www.diabetes.org.uk
Contact: Dr Jayne East, Research Administrator

The British Diabetic Association's overall aim is to help and to care for people with diabetes and those closest to them; to represent and campaign for their interests; and to fund research into diabetes. The BDA continues to encourage research into all areas of diabetes.

British Diabetic Association Equipment Grant

Subjects: Endocrinology.
Eligibility: Open to suitably qualified members of the medical or scientific professions, who are resident in the UK.
Level of Study: Postdoctorate.
Purpose: To enable the purchase of equipment which is required only for a single project or programme which is solely concerned with diabetes research.
Type: Equipment Grant.
No. of awards offered: Varies.
Frequency: Three times each year.
Value: A minimum of £5,000.
Country of Study: United Kingdom.
Application Procedure: Application form must be submitted by the closing date, for assessment by the peer review. Please write to Dr M Murphy.
Closing Date: May 1st, September 1st, December 1st.

British Diabetic Association Project Grants

Subjects: Endocrinology.
Eligibility: Open to suitably qualified members of the medical or scientific professions, who are resident in the UK.
Level of Study: Postdoctorate.
Purpose: To provide funding for a well-defined research proposal of timeliness and promise which, in terms of the application, may be expected to lead to a significant advance in our knowledge of diabetes.
Type: Project Grant.
No. of awards offered: Varies.
Frequency: Annual.
Value: Not usually more than £40,000 per year.
Length of Study: 1-3 years.
Country of Study: United Kingdom.

Application Procedure: Application form submitted by closing dates will be assessed by peer review. Please write to Dr M Murphy.
Closing Date: May 1st, September 1st, December 1st.

British Diabetic Association Research Fellowships

Subjects: Diabetes mellitus research.
Eligibility: Open to suitably qualified members of the medical or scientific professions who are resident in the UK.
Level of Study: Postdoctorate.
Type: Varies.
Frequency: As advertised.
Value: Varies.
Length of Study: 2-3 years.
Country of Study: United Kingdom.
Application Procedure: Application form must be completed. Please write to Dr M Murphy.
Closing Date: Advertised annually with a deadline in Autumn. Please write for details.
Additional Information: Availability is advertised annually in scientific/medical press.

British Diabetic Association Research Studentships

Subjects: Endocrinology.
Eligibility: Applications are invited from potential supervisors in single departments or in collaborative projects between departments, pre-clinical or clinical. Applicants must be resident in the UK.
Level of Study: Postgraduate.
Purpose: To train basic scientists in diabetes research.
Type: Studentship.
No. of awards offered: Varies.
Frequency: Annual.
Value: London: £11,500 maintenance and £5,000 expenses (lab); out of London: £10,500 maintenance and £5,000 expenses (lab).
Length of Study: 3 years.
Country of Study: United Kingdom.
Application Procedure: Application form must be submitted. Please write to Dr M Murphy.
Closing Date: Advertised in scientific/medical press in September each year. Deadline in Autumn each year. Please write for details.

British Diabetic Association Small Grant Scheme

Subjects: Endocrinology.
Eligibility: Open to suitably qualified members of the medical or scientific professions who are resident in the UK.
Level of Study: Postdoctorate.
Purpose: To enable research workers to progress new ideas in the field of diabetes research.
Type: Grant.
No. of awards offered: Varies.
Frequency: All year round.
Value: Up to £5,000.

Length of Study: Usually 1 year.
Country of Study: United Kingdom.
Application Procedure: An application form must be completed, which will be assessed by the peer review within 6-8 weeks. Please write to Dr M Murphy.
Closing Date: Applications are accepted at any time.

Diabetes Development Project

Subjects: Endocrinology.
Eligibility: Open to suitably qualified members of the medical or scientific professions, and health care professionals, who are resident in the UK.
Level of Study: Postdoctorate.
Purpose: To benefit the diabetic community by improving care and services.
Type: Development Project.
No. of awards offered: Varies.
Frequency: Twice a year.
Value: Not usually more than £30,000 per year.
Length of Study: 1-3 years.
Country of Study: United Kingdom.
Application Procedure: Application form must be submitted. Please write to Dr M Murphy.
Closing Date: Contact the BDA for dates; usually in March and October.

BRITISH FEDERATION OF WOMEN GRADUATES (BFWG)

4 Mandeville Courtyard
142 Battersea Park Road, London, SW11 4NB, England
Tel: (44) 171 498 8037
Fax: (44) 171 498 8037
www: http://homepages.wyenet.co.uk/bfwg
Contact: The Secretary

BFWG promotes women's opportunities in education and public life; works as part of an international organisation to improve the lives of women and girls; fosters local, national, and international friendship; and offers scholarships for postgraduate research.

AAUW/IFUW International Fellowships

Subjects: Research in any subject. Preference will be given to women who show prior commitment to the advancement of women and girls through civic, community, or professional work.
Eligibility: Women applicants must be a member of BFWG or another national federation or association of IFUW. It is a condition that the candidate will have started her second year of research at least (to which her application refers) at the time of the application and must be studying for three or more years. Taught Master's degrees do not count as research, though research done for a MPhil may count on the assumption that it will be upgraded to a PhD.
Level of Study: Postgraduate.

Type: Fellowship.
No. of awards offered: 6.
Frequency: Annual.
Value: Approximately US$15,000. The fellowships do not cover travel.
Length of Study: 12 months.
Country of Study: USA.
Application Procedure: Applicants studying in the UK should write for details enclosing a C5 stamped addressed envelope. Applicants must apply through their respective federation or association. A list of IFUW national federations can be sent on request.
Closing Date: December 1st in the year preceding the competition.

For further information contact:

AAUW Educational Foundation
Fellowships and Grants
PO Box 4030, Iowa City, IA, 52243-4030, United States of America

AFUW Georgina Sweet Fellowship

Subjects: Research in any subject.
Eligibility: Women applicants must be members of BFWG. It is a condition that the candidate will have started her second year of research at least (to which her application refers) at the time of application and must be studying for three years or more. Taught Master's degrees do not count as research, though research done for a MPhil may count on the assumption that it will be upgraded to a PhD.
Level of Study: Postgraduate, Research.
Type: Fellowship.
No. of awards offered: 1.
Frequency: Every two years.
Value: Approximately A$4,500. The fellowship does not cover travel.
Length of Study: 4-12 months.
Study Establishment: An Australian university.
Country of Study: Australia.
Application Procedure: Please write for details including a C5 stamped addressed envelope.
Closing Date: Early September in the year preceding the competition.
Additional Information: Recipients must submit a written report within six months of concluding the research.

For further information contact:

AFUW
PO Box 14
Bullcreek, WA, 6149, Australia

Australian Capital Territory Bursary

Subjects: All subjects.
Eligibility: Women applicants must be a member of BFWG or another national federation or association or IFUW. It is a condition that the candidate will have started her second year of research (to which her application refers) at least at the time of the application, and must be studying for three or

more years. Taught Master's degrees do not count as research, though research done for a MPhil may count on the assumption that it will be upgraded to a PhD.
Level of Study: Postgraduate, Research.
Type: Bursary.
No. of awards offered: 1.
Frequency: Annual.
Value: AUS$1,000.
Length of Study: 3 months.
Study Establishment: Canberra.
Country of Study: Australia.
Application Procedure: Applicants should write for details enclosing a C5 stamped addressed envelope. Applicants must apply through their respective Federation or Association, and members of BFWG may apply for consideration by BFWG. A list of IFUW national federations can be sent upon request.
Closing Date: July 31st.

For further information contact:

AFUW-ACT Inc
GPO Box 520, Canberra, ACT, 201, Australia
Contact: The Fellowship Convener

BFWG Scholarships

Subjects: All subjects.
Eligibility: Candidates not of UK nationality but whose studies take place in the UK are eligible. They would not be eligible however, if they lived outside the UK and planned to continue to study out of the UK. It is a condition that the candidate will have started her second year of research (to which her application refers) at least at the time of the application and must be studying for three or more years. Taught Master's degrees do not count as research, although research completed for a MPhil may count on the assumption that it will be upgraded to a PhD.
Level of Study: Postgraduate, Research.
Purpose: To assist postgraduate research.
Type: Scholarship.
No. of awards offered: 1+.
Frequency: Annual.
Value: £750-£1,000.
Country of Study: United Kingdom.
Application Procedure: Applicants studying in the UK should write for details enclosing a C5 stamped addressed envelope. Overseas applicants must include two international reply coupons.
Closing Date: Early September in the year preceding the competition.
Additional Information: Recipients must submit a written report within six months of concluding the research.

IFUW International Fellowships

Subjects: Research in any subject.
Eligibility: Woman applicants must be a member of BFWG or another national federation or Association of IFUW. It is a condition that the candidate will have started her second year of research at least (to which her application refers) at the

time of the application and must be studying for three or more years. Taught Master's degrees do not count as research, although research undertaken may count on the assumption that it will be updated to a PhD.

Level of Study: Postgraduate.

Type: Fellowship.

No. of awards offered: 7+.

Frequency: Every two years.

Value: Varies. The award does not cover travel.

Length of Study: 8 months.

Country of Study: Any country.

Application Procedure: Applicants studying in the UK should write for details enclosing a C5 stamped addressed envelope to BFWG. Applicants must apply through their respective federation or association. A list of national federations can be sent on request.

Closing Date: Early September in the year preceding the competition.

Additional Information: Recipients must submit a written report within 6 months of concluding the research.

For further information contact:

IFUW Headquarters
8 rue de l'Ancien-Port, Geneva, CH 1201, Switzerland
Tel: (41) 22 731 23 80
Fax: (41) 22 738 04 40
Contact: Grants Management Officer

JAUW International Fellowships

Subjects: Research in any subject.

Eligibility: Women applicants must be a member of BFWG or another national federation or association or IFUW. It is a condition that the candidate will have started her second year of research at least (to which her application refers) at the time of the application and must be studying for three or more years. Taught Master's degrees do not count as research, though research done for a MPhil may count on the assumption that it will be upgraded to a PhD.

Level of Study: Postgraduate, Research.

Type: Fellowship.

No. of awards offered: 1+.

Frequency: Annual.

Value: Y600,000. The fellowships do not cover travel.

Length of Study: 3 months.

Study Establishment: A Japanese institution.

Country of Study: Japan.

Application Procedure: Applicants should write for details enclosing a C5 stamped addressed envelope. Applicants must apply through their respective Federation or Association, and members of BFWG may apply for consideration by BFWG. A list of IFUW national federations can be sent upon request.

Closing Date: Early September in the year preceding the competition.

Additional Information: Recipients must submit a written report within six months of concluding their research.

For further information contact:

8 rue de l'Ancien Port, Geneva, CH 1201, Switzerland
Contact: International Federation of University Women

Kathleen Hall Memorial Fellowships

Subjects: Research in any subject.

Eligibility: People from countries with a low per capita income are eligible. They should be candidates not of UK nationality but whose studies take place in the UK. It is a condition that the candidate will have started her second year of research (to which her application refers) at least at the time of application and must be studying for three or more years. Taught Master's degrees do not count as research, although research undertaken for a MPhil may count on the assumption that it will be upgraded to a PhD.

Level of Study: Postgraduate, Research.

Type: Fellowship.

No. of awards offered: 1+.

Frequency: Annual.

Value: Approx. £1,000.

Country of Study: United Kingdom.

Application Procedure: Applicants studying in the UK should write for details enclosing a C5 stamped addressed envelope, while overseas applicants must include two international reply coupons.

Closing Date: Early September in the year including the competition.

Additional Information: The recipient must submit a written report within six months of concluding the research.

Margaret K B Day Memorial Scholarships

Subjects: Research in any subject.

Eligibility: Candidates not of UK nationality but whose studies take place in the UK are eligible. (They would not be eligible however, if they lived out of the UK and planned to continue to study out of the UK). It is a condition that the candidate will have started her second year of research at least (to which her application refers) at the time of application and must be studying for at least three or more years. Taught Master's degrees do not count as research, though research undertaken for a MPhil may count on the assumption that it will be upgraded to a PhD.

Level of Study: Postgraduate, Research.

Purpose: To assist postgraduate research.

Type: Scholarship.

No. of awards offered: 1+.

Frequency: Annual.

Value: £1,000.

Country of Study: United Kingdom.

Application Procedure: Applicants studying in the UK should write for details enclosing a C5 stamped addressed envelope. Overseas applicants must include two international reply coupons.

Closing Date: Early September in the year preceding the competition.

Rose Sidgwick Memorial Fellowship

Subjects: Preference will be given to women who show prior committment to the advancement of women and girls through civic, community, or professional work.

Eligibility: Open to British candidates below 35 years of age who are members of BFWG. It is a condition that the candidate will have started her second year of research (to which her application refers) at least at the time of application and must be studying for three or more years. Taught Master's degrees do not count as research, although research undertaken for a MPhil may count on the assumption that it will be upgraded to a PhD.

Level of Study: Postgraduate, Research.

Type: Fellowship.

No. of awards offered: 1.

Frequency: Annual.

Value: Approximately US$15,000. The fellowship does not cover travel.

Length of Study: 12 months.

Country of Study: USA.

Application Procedure: Applicants studying in the UK should write for details enclosing a C5 stamped addressed envelope. Overseas applicants must include two international reply coupons.

Closing Date: Early September in the year preceding the competition.

Additional Information: Recipients must submit a written report within six months of concluding the research.

Victorian Beatrice Fincher Scholarship

Subjects: Research in any subject that will benefit mankind.

Eligibility: Women applicants must be members of BFWG or another national federation or association of IFUW. A list of IFUW national federations can be sent upon request. It is a condition that the candidate will have started her second year of research at least (to which her application refers) at the time of application and must be studying for three or more years. Taught Master's degrees do not count as research, although research done for a MPhil may count on the assumption that it will be upgraded to a PhD.

Level of Study: Postgraduate, Research.

Type: Scholarship.

No. of awards offered: 1.

Frequency: Annual.

Value: Approximately A$5,000. The scholarship does not cover travel.

Country of Study: Any country.

Application Procedure: Applicants should write for details enclosing two international reply coupons.

Closing Date: March 1st in the year preceding the competition.

Additional Information: Recipients must submit a written report within six months of concluding the research.

For further information contact:

AFUW (Vic) Inc
PO Box 816, Mount Eliza, VIC, 3930, Australia
Contact: The Scholarship Secretary

Western Australian Bursaries

Subjects: Research in any subject.

Eligibility: Woman applicants must be members of BFWG or another national federation or association of IFUW. A list of IFUW national federations is available upon request. It is a condition that the candidate will have started her second year of research at least (to which her application refers) at the time of application and must be studying for three or more years. Taught Master's degrees do not count as research, though research done for a MPhil may count on the assumption that it will be upgraded to a PhD.

Level of Study: Postgraduate, Research.

Type: Bursary.

No. of awards offered: 1+.

Frequency: Annual.

Value: Approximately A$1,500-A$2,750. The bursaries do not cover travel.

Length of Study: 12 months.

Country of Study: Australia.

Application Procedure: Applicants should write for details enclosing two international reply coupons.

Closing Date: July 31st in the year preceding the competition.

Additional Information: Recipients must submit a written report within six months of concluding the research.

For further information contact:

AFUW (WA) Inc
PO Box 48, Nedlands, WA, 6909, Australia
Contact: The Bursary Liason Officer

BRITISH HEART FOUNDATION (BHF)

14 Fitzharding Street, London, W1H 4DH, England
Tel: (44) 171 935 0185
Contact: Ms Valerie Mason, Research Funds Manager

The British Heart Foundation exists to encourage research into the causes, diagnosis, prevention and advances of cardiovascular disease; to inform doctors throughout the country of advances in the diagnosis, cure and treatment of heart diseases; and to improve facilities for treatment of heart patients where the National Health Service is unable to help.

BHF Clinical Science Fellowships

Subjects: Research relevant to the cardiovascular system.

Eligibility: Open to British citizens and persons who have been resident in the UK for a minimum of three years at the time of application. Candidates should be clinicians (aged approximately 25-30 years).

Level of Study: Professional development.
Purpose: To enable clinicians who have demonstrated an interest in and potential for research to be trained.
Type: Fellowship.
No. of awards offered: Varies.
Frequency: Three times each year.
Value: The award reimburses for salary (commensurate with seniority within the health service) and carries a consumables allowance of up to £5,000 per year.
Length of Study: Up to 7 years.
Study Establishment: The first 3 years are spent in a basic science department, preferably, but not necessarily, away from the sponsoring department.
Country of Study: Based in United Kingdom, but research training period can be spent overseas.
Application Procedure: Application should be made by the proposed Fellow on the appropriate form and with the approval of the head of department. The application must include a full research protocol and/or training programme together with the curriculum vitae of the proposed Fellow. Shortlisted applicants will normally be required to attend for interview. Application forms and further information are available on request.
Closing Date: Available on request.

BHF Intermediate Research Fellowships

Subjects: Research projects in the field of basic or applied clinical cardiology.
Eligibility: Open to British citizens or those who have been resident in the UK for a minimum of three years at the time of application.
Level of Study: Professional development.
Purpose: To enable highly qualified independent researchers to pursue their research objectives.
Type: Fellowship.
No. of awards offered: Varies.
Frequency: Three times each year.
Value: A salary commensurate with seniority within the university and health service at registrar/first-year senior registrar level (or academic equivalent), and up to £7,000 per year may be applied for to cover running expenses which must be fully justified.
Length of Study: A maximum of 3 years.
Country of Study: United Kingdom.
Application Procedure: Application may be made on the appropriate form by the proposed Fellows or the supervisor, with the approval of the head of department. The application must include a full research protocol, together with the curriculum vitae of the proposed Fellow.
Closing Date: Available on request.
Additional Information: These Fellowships are unlikely to be awarded to those who are unable to obtain advancement within the health services.

BHF Junior Research Fellowships

Subjects: Research projects in the field of basic or applied clinical cardiology.
Eligibility: Open to postgraduates who wish to be trained in academic research under the direct supervision of senior and experienced research workers. Candidates must be British citizens or have been resident in the UK for a minimum of three years at the time of application.
Level of Study: Postgraduate.
Purpose: To enable postgraduates to be trained in academic research.
Type: Fellowship.
No. of awards offered: Varies.
Frequency: Three times each year.
Value: A salary, not to be higher than the top of the registrar scale or equivalent, and up to £5,000 per year to cover running expenses.
Length of Study: A total of 2 years, but Junior Research Fellows may proceed to the second year only after the head of department has submitted, and the Foundation has approved, a progress report on the first year's work.
Country of Study: United Kingdom.
Application Procedure: Applications should be made on the approved form by the planned supervisor and with the approval of the head of department. The application must include a full research protocol together with the curriculum vitae of the proposed Fellow. The head of department must confirm that no additional financial support is necessary in order to carry out the project.
Closing Date: Available on request.

BHF Overseas Visiting Fellowships

Subjects: Basic or applied clinical cardiology.
Eligibility: Open to established research workers of proven outstanding talent able to contribute to the work of the host department.
Level of Study: Professional development.
Purpose: To enable senior overseas research workers to undertake research in the UK.
Type: Fellowship.
No. of awards offered: Varies.
Frequency: Three times each year.
Value: Funds to cover the Fellow's salary and up to £5,000 per year as a contribution towards research expenses. The applicant must confirm that no additional financial support is necessary in order to carry out the project. Application may be made for funds to cover economy travel fares for the Fellow and one dependant (the latter only being eligible for travel funds if the Fellow is to be resident in the UK for one year or more).
Length of Study: Up to 2 years.
Study Establishment: A recognised research centre in the UK.
Country of Study: United Kingdom.
Application Procedure: Application must be made by the head of department in the UK institution on behalf of the Fellow and should include a full research protocol. The role of the Visiting Fellow in the research should be clearly stated. A curriculum vitae of the proposed Fellow and two letters of recommendation from the Fellow's country of origin should be included.
Closing Date: Available on request.
Additional Information: These Fellowships are not given for training.

BHF PhD Studentships

Subjects: Basic or applied clinical cardiology.
Eligibility: Open to candidates who have obtained a minimum of an upper second class honours degree.
Level of Study: Doctorate.
Purpose: To enable graduates to proceed to a PhD degree.
Type: Studentship.
No. of awards offered: Varies.
Frequency: Three times each year.
Value: The level of stipend is set by the British Heart Foundation. Applicants may apply for funds to cover university fees. Up to £5,000 per year may also be applied for to cover research consumables.
Length of Study: 3 years.
Study Establishment: An appropriate university.
Country of Study: United Kingdom.
Application Procedure: Applications are actually made by heads of department and may be made for named or unnamed candidates, although priority will be given to named candidates. Application should be made on the appropriate form and should include a full research protocol and curriculum vitae of the candidate (if known).
Closing Date: Available on request.

BHF Research Awards

Subjects: Cardiovascular research.
Level of Study: Postdoctorate.
Purpose: Research into cardiovascular disease (basic or clinical).
Type: Research Grant.
No. of awards offered: Limited by funding.
Frequency: Varies, according to committee.
Value: Varies.
Length of Study: Varies.
Study Establishment: Universities, medical schools.
Country of Study: United Kingdom.
Application Procedure: Please contact BHF for details.
Closing Date: Varies, according to committee.
Additional Information: Annual report available upon request.

BHF Senior Research Fellowships

Subjects: Research projects in the field of basic or applied clinical cardiology.
Eligibility: Open to British citizens or persons who have been resident in the UK for a minimum of three years at the time of application. The applicant should have been engaged in original research for at least two years and have published results, and should show outstanding ability both in original thought and practical application. This ability should already have been recognised outside the applicant's institution by invitations to talk to societies both at home and abroad. The applicant's career plans should be academic medicine and research. Senior Research Fellowships are awarded to those thought likely to gain high office in teaching and research institutions.
Level of Study: Professional development.

Purpose: To enable researchers with an international reputation of outstanding ability to pursue their research interests.
Type: Fellowship.
No. of awards offered: Varies.
Frequency: Annual.
Value: Salary commensurate with seniority within the university and health service up to consultant level. Up to £10,000 per year may be applied for to cover running expenses which should be fully justified.
Length of Study: 3 years initially; may be extended to 5 years after submission of a progress report which has been judged to be satisfactory by the Foundation.
Country of Study: United Kingdom.
Application Procedure: Applications should be made by the proposed Fellow on the appropriate form and with the approval of the head of department. The application must include a full research protocol together with the curriculum vitae of the proposed Fellow. Shortlisted applicants will be required to attend for interview.
Closing Date: Available on request.
Additional Information: A Senior Research Fellow may apply to the Committee for a second 5-year period by the end of which it would be expected that the Fellow would have secured a permanent and more senior position. In this case an interview will be required.

BHF Travelling Fellowships

Subjects: Basic or applied clinical cardiology.
Eligibility: Open to established research workers who are UK citizens and who are of proven outstanding talent. At the time of application the proposed Fellow should hold a post in a research institution of university with tenure of not less than five years.
Level of Study: Professional development.
Purpose: To enable established research workers to undertake research abroad, or acquire special knowledge which would assist them in their research in the UK after their return.
Type: Fellowship.
No. of awards offered: Varies.
Frequency: Three times each year.
Value: The proposed Fellow may apply for funds to cover the cost of economy travel and a reasonable subsistence allowance at the place of work. It is expected that the Fellow's salary would continue to be paid by the university or institution in the UK during his or her absence abroad.
Length of Study: Up to 6 months.
Country of Study: Outside United Kingdom.
Application Procedure: Application must be made on the appropriate form together with details of the purpose of the visit and what the Fellow expects to gain as a result of the visit. The applicant's curriculum vitae and a letter of acceptance by the host institution must be included in the application.
Closing Date: Available on request.

John Fyffe Memorial Fellowship

Subjects: Research in the field of collagen disease and, in particular, the causes, diagnosis, treatment including surgical techniques, and the eventual elimination of the disease known as Marfan's Syndrome.
Eligibility: Open to British citizens and persons who have been resident in the UK for a minimum of three years at the time of application.
Level of Study: Professional development.
Purpose: To enable researchers to visit other centres working in the field in order to acquire first-hand knowledge and techniques so that they may be applied to research being undertaken in the UK.
Type: Fellowship.
No. of awards offered: Varies.
Frequency: Three times each year.
Value: Up to £3,000 per year.
Country of Study: Any country.
Application Procedure: Application forms and further information are available on request.
Closing Date: Available on request.

BRITISH INSTITUTE OF RADIOLOGY

36 Portland Place, London, W1N 4AT, England
Tel: (44) 171 580 4085
Fax: (44) 171 255 3209
Contact: Chief Executive

The British Institute of Radiology being an independent forum has as its aim to bring together all the professions in radiology, medical and scientific disciplines, to share knowledge, and educate the public, thereby improving the prevention and detection of disease and the management and treatment of patients.

British Institute of Radiology Travel Bursary

Subjects: Radiology.
Eligibility: Open to members of the BIR who are under 35 years of age.
Level of Study: Postgraduate.
Purpose: To present a paper at a national or international forum.
No. of awards offered: 1.
Frequency: Annual.
Value: Up to £1,000.
Country of Study: Any country.
Application Procedure: Application form and supporting documentation must be submitted.
Closing Date: August 1st.

Flude Memorial Prize

Subjects: Radiology.
Eligibility: Open to members of the Institute.
Level of Study: Postgraduate.

No. of awards offered: 1.
Frequency: Annual.
Value: £250.
Country of Study: Any country.
Application Procedure: Application form and supporting documentation must be submitted.
Closing Date: August 1st.

Nic McNally Memorial Prize

Subjects: Radiology.
Eligibility: Open to young scientists under 35 years of age at the time of application and employed in a scientific post. Applicants need not be members of the Institute.
Level of Study: Unrestricted.
Type: Travel Grant.
No. of awards offered: 1.
Frequency: Annual.
Value: £250.
Study Establishment: Travel to either a scientific meeting or a laboratory.
Country of Study: Any country.
Application Procedure: Application form and supporting documents must be submitted.
Closing Date: February 1st.

Nycomed Amersham Fellowship

Subjects: Radiology - Pharmaceuticals in diagnostic imaging.
Eligibility: Open to diagnostic radiologists of senior registrar or junior consultant status. Preference is given to members of the Institute.
Level of Study: Postgraduate.
Purpose: To enable a diagnostic radiologist to gain in-depth experience abroad.
Type: Fellowship.
No. of awards offered: 1.
Frequency: Annual.
Value: Up to £5,000.
Length of Study: Up to 2 months.
Study Establishment: One or more academic departments of radiology.
Country of Study: Anywhere outside the UK.
Application Procedure: Application form and supporting documentation must be submitted.
Closing Date: End of February.
Additional Information: The successful scholar will be required to produce a report of up to 1000 words for publication in the British Journal of Radiology bulletin.

Stanley Melville Memorial Award

Subjects: Radiology.
Eligibility: Open to members of the Institute who are under 35 years of age.
Level of Study: Unrestricted.
Purpose: To enable a member of the Institute to visit clinics and institutions abroad.
No. of awards offered: 1.
Frequency: Triennially (next 2002).
Value: Approximately £250.

Country of Study: Any country.
Application Procedure: Application form and supporting documentation must be submitted.
Closing Date: December 31st of the year preceding the year of the award.
Additional Information: While the successful applicant will not be obliged to write a formal report on his or her visit, it is hoped that he or she will submit a description of the work seen during the visit in a form suitable for publication in the Journal.

BRITISH LUNG FOUNDATION

78 Hatton Garden, London, EC1N 8JR, England
Tel: (44) 171 831 5831
Fax: (44) 171 831 5832
Contact: Mr Alex Mazzetta, Research Grants Manager

The British Lung Foundation exists to fund medical research into all lung diseases in the UK. To help achieve this the Foundation provides information on lung diseases and lung health and supports people with a lung condition through the Breathe Easy Club.

British Lung Foundation Project Grants

Subjects: Respiratory diseases.
Eligibility: Open to graduates working within the UK who have some experience of research. The principal applicant must be based in a research centre in the United Kingdom.
Level of Study: Postdoctorate, Postgraduate, Predoctorate, Professional development, Research.
Purpose: To promote medical research into the prevention, diagnosis and treatment of all lung diseases.
Type: Project Grant.
No. of awards offered: Approx. 3.
Frequency: Annual.
Value: Up to £95,000.
Study Establishment: UK research centre.
Country of Study: United Kingdom.
Application Procedure: Application forms are available from the British Lung Foundation.
Closing Date: Last week in February.

BRITISH MEDICAL AND DENTAL STUDENTS' TRUST

Mackintosh House
120 Blythswood Street, Glasgow, G2 4EH, Scotland
Tel: (44) 141 221 5858
Fax: (44) 141 228 1208
Contact: Secretary

British Medical and Dental Students' Trust provides awards to help medical and dental students studying at UK medical and dental schools, and also finances elective periods spent overseas during the clinical years of study.

British Medical and Dental Students' Trust Scholarships and Travel Grants

Subjects: Medicine and dental medicine.
Eligibility: Open to clinical students of any nationality, from British medical and dental schools and hospitals.
Level of Study: Undergraduate.
Purpose: To enable medical and dental students to study and travel outside the UK.
Type: Scholarship.
No. of awards offered: Approx. 160 scholarships and travel grants per year.
Frequency: Twice a year.
Value: £100-£500.
Length of Study: From 2 weeks to 3 months.
Country of Study: Any country.
Application Procedure: Application form, protocol for elective, and confirmation of elective from hospital to be visited, must be submitted.
Closing Date: January 31st and July 31st.

BRITISH MEDICAL ASSOCIATION (BMA)

Board of Science and Education
Tavistock Square, London, WC1H 9JP, England
Tel: (44) 171 383 6351
Fax: (44) 171 383 6399
Email: hglanville@bma.org.uk
www: http://www.bma.org.uk
Contact: Ms H J Glanville, Principal Executive Officer

The British Medical Association is a professional association of doctors, representing their interests and providing services for its 111,000 plus members. It is an independent trade union, a scientific and educational body, and a publishing house.

Albert McMaster and Helen Tomkinson Research Awards

Subjects: Cancer research, including health education.
Eligibility: Open to members of the BMA.
Level of Study: Postdoctorate.
Purpose: To assist research.
Type: Research Grant.
No. of awards offered: 2.
Frequency: Annual.
Value: Approximately £4,250 (McMaster Award); approximately £6,250 (Tomkinson Award).
Length of Study: 1 year.
Country of Study: Any country.
Application Procedure: Application forms are available in January.
Closing Date: End of March.
Additional Information: Advertised in January.

Brackenbury Research Award

Subjects: Research of immediate practical importance to public health, to a medico-political or medico-sociological problem, or to an educational question, whether general, medical or postgraduate.
Eligibility: Open to members of the BMA.
Level of Study: Postdoctorate.
Purpose: To assist research.
Type: Research Grant.
No. of awards offered: 1.
Frequency: Every three years (1999).
Value: Approximately £1,000.
Length of Study: 1 year.
Country of Study: Any country.
Application Procedure: Application form must be completed; these are available in January of the award year.
Closing Date: End of March.

C H Milburn Research Award

Subjects: Medical jurisprudence and/or forensic medicine.
Eligibility: Open to registered medical practitioners.
Level of Study: Postdoctorate.
Purpose: To assist research.
Type: Research Grant.
No. of awards offered: 1.
Frequency: Every two years.
Value: Approximately £600.
Length of Study: 1 year.
Country of Study: Any country.
Application Procedure: Application forms are available in January.
Closing Date: End of March.

Doris Hillier Research Award

Subjects: Rheumatism, arthritis and/or Parkinson's disease.
Eligibility: Open to registered medical practitioners.
Level of Study: Postdoctorate.
Purpose: To assist research.
Type: Research Grant.
No. of awards offered: 1.
Frequency: Annual.
Value: Approximately £16,000.
Length of Study: 3 years.
Country of Study: Any country.
Application Procedure: Application forms are available in January.
Closing Date: End of March.
Additional Information: Advertised in January.

Doris Odlum Research Award

Subjects: Mental health.
Eligibility: Open to medical practitioners registered in the British Commonwealth or the Republic of Ireland.
Level of Study: Postdoctorate.
Purpose: To assist research.
Type: Research Grant.
No. of awards offered: 1.

Frequency: Every two years.
Value: Approximately £500.
Length of Study: 1 year.
Country of Study: Any country.
Application Procedure: Application forms are available in January.
Closing Date: End of March.

Elizabeth Wherry Research Award

Subjects: Kidney treatment.
Eligibility: Open to registered medical practitioners.
Level of Study: Postdoctorate.
Purpose: To assist research.
Type: Research Grant.
No. of awards offered: 1.
Frequency: Annual.
Value: Approximately £450.
Length of Study: 1 year.
Country of Study: Any country.
Application Procedure: Application forms are available in January.
Closing Date: End of March.
Additional Information: Advertised in January.

Geoffrey Holt, Ivy Powell and Edith Walsh Research Awards

Subjects: Cardiovascular disease.
Eligibility: Open to members of the BMA.
Level of Study: Postdoctorate.
Purpose: To assist research.
Type: Research Grant.
No. of awards offered: 3.
Frequency: Annual.
Value: Approx. £1,500 (Holt and Walsh Awards); approx. £200 (Powell Award).
Length of Study: 1 year.
Country of Study: Any country.
Application Procedure: Application forms are available in January.
Closing Date: End of March.
Additional Information: Advertised in January.

H C Roscoe Fellowship

Subjects: Elimination of the common cold and/or other viral diseases of the human respiratory system.
Eligibility: Open to members of the BMA and non-medical scientists working in association with a BMA member.
Level of Study: Postdoctorate.
Purpose: To assist research.
Type: Fellowship.
No. of awards offered: 1.
Frequency: Annual.
Value: Approx. £80,000.
Length of Study: 3 years.
Country of Study: Any country.
Application Procedure: Application forms are available in January.

Closing Date: End of March.
Additional Information: Advertised in January.

Insole Research Award

Subjects: The causation, prevention or treatment of disease.
Eligibility: Open to members of the BMA.
Level of Study: Postdoctorate.
Purpose: To assist research.
Type: Research Grant.
No. of awards offered: 1.
Frequency: Every two years (1999).
Value: Approx. £600.
Length of Study: 1 year.
Country of Study: Any country.
Application Procedure: Application forms are available in January.
Closing Date: End of March.

Joan Dawkins Fellowship

Subjects: Biomedicine - preference is given to particular areas which are defined on an annual basis.
Eligibility: Projects must relate to the UK only.
Level of Study: To be defined.
Purpose: To encourage, foster and maintain the highest possible standards in medical practice, medical learning and research.
Type: Fellowship.
No. of awards offered: To be defined.
Frequency: Annual.
Value: Approx. £50,000.
Length of Study: 3 years.
Country of Study: United Kingdom.
Application Procedure: Application forms are available in January.
Closing Date: End of March.

John William Clark Research Award

Subjects: The causes of blindness.
Eligibility: Open to members of the BMA.
Level of Study: Postdoctorate.
Purpose: To assist research.
Type: Research Grant.
No. of awards offered: 1.
Frequency: Annual.
Value: Approx. £6,000.
Length of Study: 1 year.
Country of Study: Any country.
Application Procedure: Application forms are available for completion.
Closing Date: End of March.
Additional Information: Advertised in January.

Katherine Bishop Harman Research Award

Subjects: Research into the diminution and avoidance of risks to health and life in pregnancy and childbearing.

Eligibility: Open to medical practitioners registered in the UK or any country at any time forming part of the British Empire.
Level of Study: Postdoctorate.
Purpose: To assist research.
Type: Research Grant.
No. of awards offered: 1.
Frequency: Every two years.
Value: Approx. £600.
Length of Study: 1 year.
Country of Study: Any country.
Application Procedure: Application forms are available in January.
Closing Date: End of March.

Margaret Temple Fellowship

Subjects: Psychiatry and mental health.
Eligibility: Projects must relate to the UK.
Level of Study: Unrestricted.
Purpose: For research into schizophrenia.
Type: Fellowship.
No. of awards offered: 1.
Frequency: Annual.
Value: Approx. £40,000.
Length of Study: 3 years.
Country of Study: United Kingdom.
Application Procedure: Application forms are available in January.
Closing Date: End of March.

Middlemore Research Award

Subjects: Any branch of ophthalmic medicine or surgery.
Eligibility: Open to registered medical practitioners.
Level of Study: Postdoctorate.
Purpose: To assist research.
Type: Research Grant.
No. of awards offered: 1.
Frequency: Every three years (1999).
Value: Approx. £1,000.
Length of Study: 1 year.
Country of Study: Any country.
Application Procedure: Application forms are available in January.
Closing Date: End of March.

Nathaniel Bishop Harman Research Award

Subjects: Hospital practice.
Eligibility: Open to registered medical practitioners on the staff of a hospital in Great Britain or Northern Ireland who are not members of the staff of a recognised undergraduate or postgraduate medical school.
Level of Study: Postdoctorate.
Purpose: To assist research.
Type: Research Grant.
No. of awards offered: 1.
Frequency: Every two years.
Value: Approx. £675.
Length of Study: 1 year.
Country of Study: Any country.

Application Procedure: Application forms are available in January.
Closing Date: End of March.

Sir Charles Hastings and Charles Oliver Hawthorne Research Awards

Subjects: General practice, observation, research and record-keeping.
Eligibility: Open to members of the BMA engaged in general practice.
Level of Study: Postdoctorate.
Purpose: To assist research.
Type: Research Grant.
No. of awards offered: 2.
Frequency: Every two years.
Value: Approx. £1,600 (Hastings Award); approx. £500 (Hawthorne Award).
Length of Study: 1 year.
Country of Study: Any country.
Application Procedure: Application forms are available in January.
Closing Date: End of March.

T P Gunton Research Award

Subjects: Health education with special regard to the earlier diagnosis and treatment of cancer.
Eligibility: Open to both medical and non-medical scientists.
Level of Study: Unrestricted.
Purpose: To assist research.
Type: Research Grant.
No. of awards offered: 1.
Frequency: Annual.
Value: Approx. £12,100.
Length of Study: 3 years.
Country of Study: Any country.
Application Procedure: Application forms are available in January.
Closing Date: End of March.
Additional Information: Advertised in January.

T V James Research Fellowship

Subjects: The nature, causation, prevention or treatment of bronchial asthma.
Eligibility: Open to members of the BMA.
Level of Study: Postdoctorate.
Purpose: To assist research.
Type: Fellowship.
No. of awards offered: 1.
Frequency: Annual.
Value: Approx. £20,000.
Length of Study: 3 years.
Country of Study: Any country.
Application Procedure: Application forms are available in January.
Closing Date: End of March.
Additional Information: Advertised in January.

Vera Down Research Award

Subjects: Neurological disorders.
Eligibility: Open to registered medical practitioners.
Level of Study: Postdoctorate.
Purpose: To assist research.
Type: Research Grant.
No. of awards offered: 1.
Frequency: Annual.
Value: Approx. £10,000.
Length of Study: 3 years.
Country of Study: Any country.
Application Procedure: Application forms are available in January.
Closing Date: End of March.
Additional Information: Advertised in January.

THE BRITISH NUTRITION FOUNDATION (BNF)

High Holborn House, London, WC1V 6RQ, England
Tel: (44) 171 404 6504
Fax: (44) 171 404 6747
Email: 100634.445@compuserve.com
www: http://british_nutrition.org.uk
Contact: Ms Caroline Lee

The Foundation promotes the nutritional well being of society through the impartial interpretation and effective dissemination of scientifically based nutritional knowledge and advice. It works in partnership with academic and research institutes, the food industry, educators and government. The Foundation influences all in the food chain, government, the professions and the media. The Foundation is a charitable organisation which receives funds from the food industry, government and other sources.

The BNF/Nestlé Bursary Scheme

Subjects: Nutritional problems associated with adults in apparent health and disease states, including special areas of maternal health and infant nutrition.
Eligibility: Open to medical students at UK medical schools.
Level of Study: Undergraduate.
Purpose: To help selected medical students to undertake an elective concerned with nutritional problems encountered in developing countries.
Type: Bursary.
No. of awards offered: Up to 12.
Frequency: Annual.
Value: Up to £500 to reimburse travel and accommodation.
Country of Study: Developing countries.
Application Procedure: Application form needs to be completed, with an outline of the proposed study and a reference from the medical school.
Closing Date: Normally January 31st.
Additional Information: Two copies of a detailed report of the study are required within five months of returning to the UK.

The Denis Burkitt Study Awards

Subjects: Public health and hygiene, social/preventive medicine, dietetics.
Eligibility: Open to candidates from any country but they must be studying in the UK.
Level of Study: Postgraduate, Undergraduate.
Purpose: To help medical and nutrition science students, who wish to undertake elective or other studies in developing nations on food and nutrition, and their relationship to health and disease within any age group.
Type: Bursary.
No. of awards offered: Up to 10.
Frequency: Annual.
Value: £750.
Country of Study: Developing countries.
Application Procedure: Application form must be completed - details are sent to medical schools in the autumn. They can also be obtained from the British Nutrition Foundation at that time.
Closing Date: About January 20th - although it varies from year to year.

BRITISH ORTHODONTIC SOCIETY

BOS Office
Eastman Dental Hospital
256 Gray's Inn Road, London, WC1X 8LD, England
Tel: (44) 171 837 2193
Fax: (44) 171 837 2193
Contact: Honorary Secretary

The aim of the British Orthodontic Society is to promote the science of orthodontics and its good practice in the UK. The Society holds regular meetings and courses and actively encourages research and audit in the field. It also publishes The British Journal of Orthodontics four times per year.

BOS Research and Audit Fund

Subjects: Orthodontics.
Eligibility: Only open to full members of the British Orthodontic Society.
Level of Study: Postgraduate.
Purpose: To provide sponsorship for a BOS member to carry out a clinically related orthodontic project of value to the orthodontic speciality.
Type: Research Grant.
Frequency: Annual.
Value: Up to £3,000.
Country of Study: Any country.
Application Procedure: Application to be made on the standard form.
Closing Date: April 1st.

Chapman Prize

Subjects: An essay on orthodontics or an allied subject which must contain original material not previously published.
Eligibility: Open to members of BOS holding a recognised dental degree and within fifteen years of initial qualification.
Level of Study: Postgraduate.
Purpose: To promote research in orthodontics.
No. of awards offered: 1.
Frequency: Annual.
Value: £1,200.
Country of Study: Any country.
Closing Date: April 30th.
Additional Information: The essay shoud be no more than 8,000 words.

Houston Research Scholarship

Subjects: Orthodontics.
Eligibility: Open to members of BOS within fifteen years of initial dental qualification.
Level of Study: Postgraduate.
Purpose: To allow the scholar to pursue an academic or clinically based research project which will promote the specialty of orthodontics.
Type: Scholarship.
No. of awards offered: 1.
Frequency: Annual.
Value: Up to £5,000.
Country of Study: United Kingdom or abroad as approved.
Application Procedure: Application must be made on the standard form, with a 200 word abstract of the proposed research.
Closing Date: June 1st.
Additional Information: There may be a significant travel component to enable the scholar to study in another centre in the UK or overseas but the most significant factor will be the quality of the research proposed.

THE BRITISH SCHOOLS AND UNIVERSITIES FOUNDATION, INC. (BSUF)

6 Windmill Hill
Hampstead, London, NW3 6RU, England
Tel: (44) 171 435 4648
Contact: Mrs S Wiltshire, UK Representative BSUF

The British Schools and Universities Foundation makes grants to educational, scientific or literary institutes in the UK and in member nations of the British Commonwealth. The Foundation also fosters the education and academic work of American scholars and students at British institutions and vice versa. It also provides a way for the US tax payer to make tax deductable gifts to the UK for colleges and schools.

British Schools and Universities Foundation, Inc. Scholarships

Subjects: All subjects.
Eligibility: Open to scholars from US, UK, Australia, Canada, and New Zealand.
Level of Study: Doctorate, Postgraduate, Professional development.
Purpose: To promote, foster and assist the education and academic work of British scholars and students at American educational institutions, and of American scholars and students at British educational institutions.
Type: Scholarship.
No. of awards offered: 4-6.
Frequency: Annual.
Value: US$12,500 maximum.
Length of Study: 2 years maximum.
Study Establishment: US educational institutions (UK candidates) or UK educational institutions (US candidates).
Country of Study: USA or United Kingdom.
Application Procedure: Application form can be obtained from representative. Please enclose SAE with request.
Closing Date: March 1st, for an award to commence the following September.

May and Ward

Subjects: All subjects.
Eligibility: Applicants must provide a strong rationale for attending an institution abroad and give evidence if possible. They must be attending or be graduates (usually) of an accredited institute of learning.
Level of Study: Doctorate, Graduate, Postgraduate, Predoctorate, Professional development, Research.
Purpose: To support US scholars at UK educational, literary and scientific institutions and vice versa.
Type: Scholarship.
No. of awards offered: 4-6.
Frequency: Annual.
Value: $12,500 annually.
Length of Study: 1-2 years.
Study Establishment: College, University or Research establishment.
Country of Study: USA or UK.
Application Procedure: For application form and guidelines apply to BSVF representative if in the UK at the London address and if in the USA at the New York address.
Closing Date: March 1st.

For further information contact:

BSVF
Suite 1006
575 Madison Ave, New York, NY, 10022-2511, United States of America

BUNAC

16 Bowling Green Lane, London, EC1R 0BD, England
Tel: (44) 171 251 3472
Fax: (44) 171 251 0215
Email: bunac@easynet.co.uk
www: http://www.bunac.org.uk/
Contact: Ms Jenna Peters

BUNAC Educational Scholarship Trust (BEST)

Subjects: Any subject. Some awards are specifically for sports and geography-related courses.
Eligibility: Open to British citizens who have recently (within the last five years) graduated from a British university. Candidates must have a first degree.
Level of Study: Postgraduate.
Purpose: To help further Anglo-American understanding.
Type: Scholarship.
No. of awards offered: 10.
Frequency: Annual.
Value: From a total of US$25,000. Usually approx. US$2,000.
Length of Study: From 3 months to 3 years.
Study Establishment: A North American university or college.
Country of Study: USA or Canada.
Application Procedure: Application forms are available on request (from January each year).
Closing Date: March 25th.

THE BUNTING INSTITUTE OF RADCLIFFE COLLEGE

34 Concord Avenue, Cambridge, MA, 02138, United States of America
Tel: (1) 617 495 8212
Fax: (1) 617 495 8136
Email: bunting_fellowships@radcliffe.harvard.edu
www: http://www.radcliffe.edu
Contact: Fellowships Co-ordinator

The Mary Ingraham Bunting Institute was founded in 1960 as the Radcliffe Institute for Independent Study. The Institute is a multidisciplinary research centre for women scholars, scientists, artists, and writers and is one of the major centres for advanced study in the United States.

Bunting Fellowship

Subjects: Any discipline, including creative writing, visual and performing arts.
Eligibility: Open to women scholars in any field, with receipt of a doctorate or appropriate terminal degree at least two years prior to appointment, women creative writers, and visual or performing artists with a record of significant accomplishment and equivalent professional experience (special eligibility requirements apply to creative artists).
Level of Study: Postdoctorate.

Purpose: The programme seeks to support women of exceptional promise and demonstrated accomplishment who wish to pursue independent work in professional and academic fields and in the creative arts.
Type: Fellowship.
No. of awards offered: 8-10.
Frequency: Annual.
Value: US$36,500 for a year appointment starting September 15th. Bunting Fellows may not simultaneously hold another major fellowship which provides more than US$20,000.
Length of Study: 1 year.
Country of Study: USA.
Closing Date: October 1st.
Additional Information: Applications are judged on the quality and significance of the proposed project, the applicant's record of accomplishment, and the difference the fellowship might make in advancing the applicant's career. The Bunting Institute is a multidisciplinary programme for women scholars, scientists, artists, and writers. Office or studio space, auditing privileges, and access to libraries and most other resources of Radcliffe and Harvard are provided. Residence in the Boston area is required during the fellowship appointment. Fellows are expected to present their work in progress at public colloquia or in exhibitions.

Bunting Institute Affiliation

Subjects: All subjects.
Eligibility: Open to women scholars in any field, with receipt of a doctorate or appropriate terminal degree at least two years prior to appointment, and with a record of significant accomplishment. Women holding or seeking grants or fellowships from other sources are invited to apply. Radcliffe College and the Bunting Institute are unable to serve as the fiscal agent of, or assist in the development and management of, other awards. We issue a special invitation for proposals with public policy implications.
Level of Study: Postdoctorate.
Purpose: The programme seeks to support women of exceptional promise and demonstrated accomplishment.
Type: Affiliations.
No. of awards offered: 10-20.
Frequency: Annual.
Value: This appointment is without stipend, includes office space and other resources available to all Fellows.
Length of Study: 1 semester, or 1 academic year.
Country of Study: USA.
Closing Date: October 1st.
Additional Information: Applications are judged on the quality and significance of the proposed project, the applicant's record of accomplishment, and the difference the fellowship might make in advancing the applicant's career. The Bunting Institute is a multidisciplinary programme for women scholars, scientists, artists, and writers. Office or studio space, auditing privileges, and access to libraries and most other resources of Radcliffe and Harvard are provided. Residence in the Boston area is required during the fellowship appointment. Fellows are expected to present their work in progress.

BUSINESS AND PROFESSIONAL WOMEN'S FOUNDATION

Scholarships and Loans Office
2012 Massachusetts Avenue NW, Washington, DC, 20036, United States of America
Tel: (1) 202 293 1200 ext 169
Fax: (1) 202 861 0298
www: http://www.bpwusa.org
Contact: Grants Management Officer

The Buiness and Professional Women's Foundation was established in 1956 by the members of BPW/USA to promote equity for women through education, research and training. This non-profit, non partisan public foundation is headquartered in Washington DC.

New York Life Foundation Scholarship for Women in the Health Professions Program

Subjects: Healthcare, including nursing in particular.
Eligibility: Open to women who are US citizens, 25 years of age or older, who can demonstrate critical financial need, are officially accepted into a programme of study at an accredited US institution, and are graduating within 24 months of the time of application for a scholarship. Candidates must be receiving a degree or certificate at the conclusion of their studies, acquiring marketable skills that will increase their economic security, and be entering the workforce after they receive their degree or certificate. Applicants should be women seeking the education necessary for a career in a healthcare field.
Level of Study: Postgraduate.
Purpose: To assist women seeking the education necessary for entry or re-entry into the workforce, or career advancement in a business-related field.
Type: Scholarship.
No. of awards offered: Varies, approx. 50.
Frequency: Annual.
Value: US$750-US$1,000.
Length of Study: 1 year.
Study Establishment: An accredited institution.
Country of Study: USA.
Application Procedure: Application forms are available from January 1st to April 1st. Please submit a business-size, self-addressed, double-stamped envelope.
Closing Date: Postmark on or before April 15th.

Wyeth Ayerst Scholarship for Women in Graduate Medical and Health Business Programs

Subjects: Emerging health fields such as biomedical engineering, biomedical research, medical technology, pharmaceutical marketing, public health and public health policy.
Eligibility: Open to women who are US citizens, 25 years of age or older, who can demonstrate critical financial need, are officially accepted into a programme of study at an accredited US institution, and are graduating within 24 months of the time of application for a scholarship. Candidates must be

receiving a degree or certificate at the conclusion of their studies, be acquiring marketable skills that will increase their economic security, and be entering the workforce after they receive their degree or certificate. Applicants should be women seeking the education necessary for a career in a healthcare field.

Level of Study: Postgraduate.

Purpose: To assist women in gaining entry into under-represented and under-utilised health related occupations, especially in the medical and health business professions.

Type: Scholarship.

No. of awards offered: Varies.

Frequency: Annual.

Value: US$2,000.

Study Establishment: An accredited institution.

Country of Study: USA.

Application Procedure: Application forms are available from January 1st to April 1st. Please submit a business-size, self-addressed, double-stamped envelope.

Closing Date: Postmark on or before April 15th.

THE CALEDONIAN RESEARCH FOUNDATION

The Carnegie Trust for the Universities of Scotland
Cameron House
Abbey Park Place, Dunfermline, Fife, KY12 7PZ, Scotland
Tel: (44) 1383 622148
Fax: (44) 1383 622149
Email: carnegie.trust@ed.ac.uk
www: http://www.geo.ed.ac.uk/carnegie/carnegies.html
Contact: The Secretary and Treasurer

Caledonian Scholarship

Subjects: All subjects in the university curriculum. At least one scholarship each year is made in a non-scientific discipline.

Eligibility: Open to persons possessing a first class honours degree from a Scottish University.

Level of Study: Postgraduate.

Purpose: To support postgraduate research in any subject.

Type: Scholarship.

No. of awards offered: 2-3.

Frequency: Annual.

Value: £6,877 (in 1998/99) plus tuition fees and allowances.

Length of Study: A maximum of 3 years, subject to annual review.

Study Establishment: Any university in Scotland.

Country of Study: United Kingdom.

Application Procedure: Please write for details.

Closing Date: March 15th.

Additional Information: Considered along with Carnegie Scholarships.

CAMBRIDGE COMMONWEALTH TRUST, CAMBRIDGE OVERSEAS TRUST AND ASSOCIATED TRUSTS

PO Box 252, Cambridge, CB2 1TZ, England
Tel: (44) 1223 323322
Fax: (44) 1223 351449
Email: egs10@cam.ac.uk

Arab-British Chamber Charitable Foundation Scholarships

Subjects: All subjects.

Eligibility: The Trusts cannot admit students to the University or any of its Colleges. Applicants for awards from the Trusts must therefore also apply to the University of Cambridge and be offered a place at Cambridge in the normal way. All applicants must have a first class or high second class honours degree, or equivalent and normally be under 26. For citizens of Algeria, Comoro Islands, Djibouti, Egypt, Jordan, Mauritania, Morocco, Palestine, Somalia, Sudan, Syria, Tunisia and the Yemen.

Type: Scholarship.

No. of awards offered: 5.

Frequency: Annual.

Value: The scholarships will cover the University Composition Fee at the overseas rate, approved College fees, a maintenance allowance sufficient for a single student, a contribution top a return economy airfare.

Length of Study: 1 year.

Study Establishment: Cambridge University.

Country of Study: United Kingdom.

Application Procedure: Candidates must complete a Preliminary Application Form, which can be obtained from local universities, offices of the British Council or, the main address. Completed application forms must be returned to the main address. Candidates short-listed will be sent forms for admission to the University of Cambridge and a scholarship application form. These forms must be returned to The Board of Graduate Studies.

Closing Date: September 21st, a full year in advance of the proposed entry date to Cambridge for preliminary application, January 31st for actual application.

For further information contact:

The Board of Graduate Studies
4 Mill Lane, Cambridge, CB2 1TZ, England
Contact: The Secretary

Blue Circle Cambridge Scholarship

Subjects: All subjects.

Eligibility: The Trusts cannot admit students to the University or any of its Colleges. Applicants for awards from the Trusts must therefore also apply to the University of Cambridge and be offered a place at Cambridge in the normal way. All applicants must have a first class or high second class

honours degree, or equivalent and normally be under 26. This scholarship is for students from Nigeria.
Level of Study: Doctorate.
Type: Scholarship.
No. of awards offered: 1.
Frequency: Annual.
Length of Study: Tenable for up to 3 years.
Study Establishment: Cambridge University.
Country of Study: United Kingdom.
Application Procedure: Preliminary application forms for these scholarships can be obtained from Blue Circle Industries PLC, PO Box 1001, Lagos and should be returned to this address by September 1st.

Britain-Australia Bicentennial Scholarships

Subjects: All subjects.
Eligibility: The Trusts cannot admit students to the University or any of its Colleges. Applicants for awards from the Trusts must therefore also apply to the University of Cambridge and be offered a place at Cambridge in the normal way. All applicants must have a first class or high second class honours degree, or equivalent and normally be under 26. Open to students from Australia.
Level of Study: Postgraduate.
Purpose: To assist one year taught postgraduate courses.
Type: Scholarship.
No. of awards offered: 2.
Frequency: Annual.
Study Establishment: Jesus College, Cambridge.
Country of Study: United Kingdom.
Application Procedure: Application form for the scholarship will be sent out to eligible candidates once the completed form for admission to the University of Cambridge has reached the Board of Graduate Studies.
Closing Date: Scholarship forms must be returned by April 30th.

For further information contact:

The Board for Graduate Studies
4 Mill Lane, Cambridge, CB2 1TZ, England
Contact: The Secretary

British Chevening Cambridge Scholarship - Namibia

Subjects: All subjects.
Eligibility: The Trusts cannot admit students to the University or any of its Colleges. Applicants for awards from the Trusts must therefore also apply to the University of Cambridge and be offered a place at Cambridge in the normal way. All applicants must have a first class or high second class honours degree, or equivalent and normally be under 26. For students from Namibia.
Level of Study: Postgraduate.
Type: Scholarship.
No. of awards offered: 1.
Frequency: Annual.
Value: Scholarships will cover the University Composition Fee at the overseas rate; approved College fees; a maintenance

allowance sufficient for a single student.
Length of Study: 1 year.
Study Establishment: Cambridge University.
Country of Study: United Kingdom.
Application Procedure: Candidates must complete a Preliminary Application Form, which can be obtained from local universities, offices of the British Council or, the main address. Completed application forms must be returned to the main address. Candidates short-listed will be sent forms for admission to the University of Cambridge and a scholarship application form. These forms must be returned to The Board of Graduate Studies.
Closing Date: September 21st, a full year in advance of the proposed entry date to Cambridge for preliminary application, January 31st for actual application.

For further information contact:

The Board of Graduate Studies
4 Mill Lane, Cambridge, CB2 1TZ, England
Contact: The Secretary

British Chevening Cambridge Scholarship for PhD Study - Mexico

Subjects: All subjects.
Eligibility: The Trusts cannot admit students to the University or any of its Colleges. Applicants for awards from the Trusts must therefore also apply to the University of Cambridge and be offered a place at Cambridge in the normal way. All applicants must have a first class or high second class honours degree, or equivalent and normally be under 26. Successfully nominated for an ORS award which pays the difference between the home and overseas rate of the University Composition Fee.
Level of Study: Doctorate.
Purpose: To assist study towards a PhD.
Type: Scholarship.
No. of awards offered: 1.
Frequency: Annual.
Value: Scholarships will cover the University Composition Fee at the overseas rate; approved College fees; a maintenance allowance sufficient for a single student.
Length of Study: Tenable for up to 3 years.
Study Establishment: Cambridge University.
Country of Study: United Kingdom.
Application Procedure: All candidates for this scholarship must complete a Preliminary Application Form which can only be obtained from the British Council, Mexico City.

For further information contact:

British Council
Maestro Antonio Caso 127
Col San Rafael
Delegacion Cuauhtemoc
Apartado postal 30-588, Mexico City, 06470 DF, Mexico

British Chevening Cambridge Scholarship for Postgraduate Study - Australia

Subjects: All subjects.
Eligibility: The Trusts cannot admit students to the University or any of its Colleges. Applicants for awards from the Trusts must therefore also apply to the University of Cambridge and be offered a place at Cambridge in the normal way. All applicants must have a first class or high second class honours degree, or equivalent and normally be under 26. For students from Australia.
Level of Study: Postgraduate.
Purpose: To assist with one year taught postgraduate courses.
Type: Scholarship.
No. of awards offered: 4.
Frequency: Annual.
Study Establishment: Cambridge University.
Country of Study: United Kingdom.
Closing Date: Scholarship forms must be returned by April 30th.

For further information contact:

The Board for Graduate Studies
4 Mill Lane, Cambridge, CN2 1TZ, England
Contact: The Secretary

British Chevening Cambridge Scholarship for Postgraduate Study - Cyprus

Subjects: All subjects.
Eligibility: The Trusts cannot admit students to the University or any of its Colleges. Applicants for awards from the Trusts must therefore also apply to the University of Cambridge and be offered a place at Cambridge in the normal way. All applicants must have a first class or high second class honours degree, or equivalent and normally be under 26. Applicants must pass a medical examination, and sign an undertaking with the Cyprus Scholarship Board to return to work in Cyprus for a minimum of three years which may be deferred if, for example, the scholar obtains a subsequent award for further studies. Candidates who are currently receiving, or who have received a British Award within the past three years, are not normally eligible for this scholarship.
Level of Study: Postgraduate.
Purpose: To assist study towards one year taught postgraduate courses of study.
Type: Scholarship.
No. of awards offered: 3.
Frequency: Annual.
Value: Scholarships will cover the University Composition Fee at the overseas rate; approved College fees; a maintenance allowance sufficient for a single student; a contribution to a return economy airfare.
Length of Study: 1 year.
Study Establishment: Cambridge University.
Country of Study: United Kingdom.
Application Procedure: Candidates must complete a Preliminary Application Form, which can be obtained from local universities, offices of the British Council or the main address. Completed application forms must be returned to the main address. Candidates short-listed will be sent forms for admission to the University of Cambridge and a scholarship application form. These forms must be returned to The Board of Graduate Studies.
Closing Date: September 21st, a full year in advance of the proposed entry date to Cambridge for preliminary application, January 31st for actual application.

For further information contact:

The Board of Graduate Studies
4 Mill Lane, Cambridge, CB2 1TZ, England
Contact: The Secretary

British Chevening Cambridge Scholarship for Postgraduate Study - East and West Africa

Subjects: All subjects.
Eligibility: The Trusts cannot admit students to the University or any of its Colleges. Applicants for awards from the Trusts must therefore also apply to the University of Cambridge and be offered a place at Cambridge in the normal way. All applicants must have a first class or high second class honours degree, or equivalent and normally be under 26. For students from Ghana, Sierra Leone, Tanzania and Uganda.
Level of Study: Postgraduate.
Type: Scholarship.
No. of awards offered: Up to 7: 3 to Ghana, 1 to Sierra Leone, 1 to Tanzania, 1 to Uganda.
Frequency: Annual.
Study Establishment: Cambridge University.
Country of Study: United Kingdom.
Application Procedure: Candidates must complete a Preliminary Application Form, which can be obtained from local universities, offices of the British Council or the main address. Completed application forms must be returned to the main address. Candidates short-listed will be sent forms for admission to the University of Cambridge and a scholarship application form. These forms must be returned to The Board of Graduate Studies.
Closing Date: September 21st, a full year in advance of the proposed entry date to Cambridge for preliminary application, January 31st for actual application.

For further information contact:

The Board of Graduate Studies
4 Mill Lane, Cambridge, CB2 1TZ, England
Contact: The Secretary

British Chevening Cambridge Scholarship for Study Towards a PhD - Uganda

Subjects: All subjects.
Eligibility: The Trusts cannot admit students to the University or any of its Colleges. Applicants for awards from the Trusts must therefore also apply to the University of Cambridge and be offered a place at Cambridge in the normal way. All applicants must have a first class or high second class honours degree, or equivalent and normally be under 26. This scholarship is for students from Uganda.
Level of Study: Doctorate.

Purpose: To assist students for study towards a PhD.
Type: Scholarship.
No. of awards offered: 1.
Frequency: Annual.
Study Establishment: Cambridge University.
Country of Study: United Kingdom.
Application Procedure: Candidates must complete a Preliminary Application Form, which can be obtained from local universities, offices of the British Council or, the main address. Completed application forms must be returned to the main address. Candidates short-listed will be sent forms for admission to the University of Cambridge and a Scholarship application form. These forms must be returned to The Board of Graduate Studies.
Closing Date: September 21st, a full year in advance of the proposed entry date to Cambridge for preliminary application, January 31st for actual application.

For further information contact:

The Board of Graduate Studies
4 Mill Lane, Cambridge, CB2 1RZ, England
Contact: The Secretary

British Chevening Cambridge Scholarships - Chile

Subjects: All subjects.
Eligibility: The Trusts cannot admit students to the University or any of its Colleges. Applicants for awards from the Trusts must therefore also apply to the University of Cambridge and be offered a place at Cambridge in the normal way. All applicants must have a first class or high second class honours degree, or equivalent and normally be under 26. For a student from Chile.
Level of Study: Postgraduate.
Type: Scholarship.
No. of awards offered: 1.
Frequency: Annual.
Value: Scholarships will cover the University Composition Fee at the overseas rate; approved College fees; a maintenance allowance sufficient for a single student.
Length of Study: 1 year.
Study Establishment: Cambridge University.
Country of Study: United Kingdom.
Application Procedure: Candidates for this scholarship must apply directly to the British Council, Chile.
Closing Date: July 15th of the year before the year of entry.

For further information contact:

British Council
Eliodoro Yanez 832, Santiago de Chile, Chile

British Chevening Cambridge Scholarships - Eastern Europe

Subjects: All subjects.
Eligibility: The Trusts cannot admit students to the University or any of its Colleges. Applicants for awards from the Trusts must therefore also apply to the University of Cambridge and be offered a place at Cambridge in the normal way. All

applicants must have a first class or high second class honours degree, or equivalent and normally be under 26. For students from Poland, Romania and Yugoslavia.
Level of Study: Postgraduate.
Purpose: To assist students studying for one year taught postgraduate courses.
Type: Scholarship.
No. of awards offered: Up to 6.
Frequency: Annual.
Value: Scholarships will cover the University Composition Fee at the overseas rate; approved College fees; a maintenance allowance sufficient for a single student.
Length of Study: 1 year.
Study Establishment: Cambridge University.
Country of Study: United Kingdom.
Application Procedure: Candidates must complete a Preliminary Application Form, which can be obtained from local universities, offices of the British Council or the main address. Completed application forms must be returned to the main address. Candidates short-listed will be sent forms for admission to the University of Cambridge and a scholarship application form. These forms must be returned to The Board of Graduate Studies.
Closing Date: September 21st, a full year in advance of the proposed entry date to Cambridge for preliminary application, January 31st for actual application.

For further information contact:

The Board of Graduate Studies
4 Mill Lane, Cambridge, CB2 1TZ, England
Contact: The Secretary

British Chevening Cambridge Scholarships - Hong Kong

Subjects: All subjects.
Eligibility: The Trusts cannot admit students to the University or any of its Colleges. Applicants for awards from the Trusts must therefore also apply to the University of Cambridge and be offered a place at Cambridge in the normal way. All applicants must have a first class or high second class honours degree, or equivalent and normally be under 26. For students from Hong Kong.
Level of Study: Postgraduate.
Purpose: To assist one year taught postgraduate study.
Type: Scholarship.
No. of awards offered: Up to 8.
Frequency: Annual.
Value: Scholarships will cover the University Composition Fee at the overseas rate; approved College fees; a maintenance allowance sufficient for a single student.
Length of Study: 1 year.
Study Establishment: Cambridge University.
Country of Study: United Kingdom.
Application Procedure: Candidates must complete a Preliminary Application Form, which can be obtained from local universities, offices of the British Council or the main address. Completed application forms must be returned to the main address. Candidates short-listed will be sent forms for admission to the University of Cambridge and a

scholarship application form. These forms must be returned to The Board of Graduate Studies.
Closing Date: September 21st, a full year in advance of the proposed entry date to Cambridge for preliminary application, January 31st for actual application.

For further information contact:

The Board of Graduate Studies
4 Mill Lane, Cambridge, CB2 1TZ, England
Contact: The Secretary

British Chevening Cambridge Scholarships - Indonesia

Subjects: All subjects.
Eligibility: The Trusts cannot admit students to the University or any of its Colleges. Applicants for awards from the Trusts must therefore also apply to the University of Cambridge and be offered a place at Cambridge in the normal way. All applicants must have a first class or high second class honours degree or equivalent and normally be under 26. For students from Indonesia.
Level of Study: Postgraduate.
Purpose: To assist students with one year taught postgraduate courses of study.
Type: Scholarship.
No. of awards offered: 3.
Frequency: Annual.
Value: Scholarships will cover the University Composition Fee at the overseas rate; approved College fees; a maintenance allowance sufficient for a single student.
Length of Study: 1 year.
Study Establishment: Cambridge University.
Country of Study: United Kingdom.
Application Procedure: Candidates for these scholarships must apply directly to the British Embassy in Indonesia.
Closing Date: September 21st, a full year in advance of the proposed entry date to Cambridge for preliminary application, January 31st for actual application.

For further information contact:

British Embassy
Jalan M H Thamrin 75, Jakarta, 10310, Indonesia

British Chevening Cambridge Scholarships - Malta

Subjects: All subjects.
Eligibility: The Trusts cannot admit students to the University or any of its Colleges. Applicants for awards from the Trusts must therefore also apply to the University of Cambridge and be offered a place at Cambridge in the normal way. All applicants must have a first class or high second class honours degree or equivalent and normally be under 26. For students from Malta.
Level of Study: Postgraduate.
Purpose: To assist study for one year taught postgraduate courses.
Type: Scholarship.
No. of awards offered: 2.

Frequency: Annual.
Value: The scholarships will cover the University Composition Fee at the overseas rate and approved College fees.
Length of Study: 1 year.
Study Establishment: Cambridge University.
Country of Study: United Kingdom.
Application Procedure: Candidates must complete a Preliminary Application Form, which can be obtained from local universities, offices of the British Council or the main address. Completed application forms must be returned to the main address. Candidates short-listed will be sent forms for admission to the University of Cambridge and a scholarship application form. These forms must be returned to The Board of Graduate Studies.
Closing Date: September 21st, a full year in advance of the proposed entry date to Cambridge for preliminary application, January 31st for actual application.

For further information contact:

The Board of Graduate Studies
4 Mill Lane, Cambridge, CB2 1TZ, England
Contact: The Secretary

British Chevening Cambridge Scholarships - Mozambique

Subjects: All subjects.
Eligibility: The Trusts cannot admit students to the University or any of its Colleges. Applicants for awards from the Trusts must therefore also apply to the University of Cambridge and be offered a place at Cambridge in the normal way. All applicants must have a first class or high second class honours degree, or equivalent and normally be under 26. For students from Mozambique.
Level of Study: Postgraduate.
Type: Scholarship.
No. of awards offered: Up to 4.
Frequency: Annual.
Value: Scholarships will cover the University Composition Fee at the overseas rate; approved College fees; a maintenance allowance sufficient for a single student.
Length of Study: 1 year.
Study Establishment: Cambridge University.
Country of Study: United Kingdom.
Application Procedure: Candidates must complete a Preliminary Application Form, which can be obtained from local universities, offices of the British Council or the main address. Completed application forms must be returned to the main address. Candidates short-listed will be sent forms for admission to the University of Cambridge and a scholarship application form. These forms must be returned to The Board of Graduate Studies.
Closing Date: September 21st, a full year in advance of the proposed entry date to Cambridge for preliminary application, January 31st for actual application.

For further information contact:

The Board of Graduate Studies
4 Mill Lane, Cambridge, CB2 1TZ, England
Contact: The Secretary

British Chevening Cambridge Scholarships - Thailand

Subjects: All subjects.
Eligibility: The Trusts cannot admit students to the University or any of its Colleges. Applicants for awards from the Trusts must therefore also apply to the University of Cambridge and be offered a place at Cambridge in the normal way. All applicants must have a first class or high second class honours degree, or equivalent and normally be under 26. For students from Thailand.
Level of Study: Postgraduate.
Type: Scholarship.
No. of awards offered: 2.
Frequency: Annual.
Value: Scholarships will cover the University Composition Fee at the overseas rate; approved College fees; a maintenance allowance suffcient for a single student.
Length of Study: 1 year.
Study Establishment: Cambridge University.
Country of Study: United Kingdom.
Application Procedure: Candidates must complete a Preliminary Application Form, which can be obtained from local universities, offices of the British Council or the main address. Completed application forms must be returned to the main address. Candidates short-listed will be sent forms for admission to the University of Cambridge and a scholarship application form. These forms must be returned to The Board of Graduate Studies.
Closing Date: September 21st, a full year in advance of the proposed entry date to Cambridge for preliminary application, January 31st for actual application.

For further information contact:

The Board of Graduate Studies
4 Mill Lane, Cambridge, CB2 1TZ, England
Contact: The Secretary

British Chevening Cambridge Scholarships - The Philippines

Subjects: All subjects.
Eligibility: The Trusts cannot admit students to the University or any of its Colleges. Applicants for awards from the Trusts must therefore also apply to the University of Cambridge and be offered a place at Cambridge in the normal way. All applicants must have a first class or high second class honours degree or equivalent and normally be under 26. For students from the Philippines.
Level of Study: Postgraduate.
Type: Scholarship.
No. of awards offered: 3.
Frequency: Annual.
Length of Study: 1 year.
Study Establishment: Cambridge University.

Country of Study: United Kingdom.
Application Procedure: Candidates must complete a Preliminary Application Form, which can be obtained from local universities, offices of the British Council or the main address. Completed application forms must be returned to the main address. Candidates short-listed will be sent forms for admission to the University of Cambridge and a scholarship application form. These forms must be returned to The Board of Graduate Studies.
Closing Date: September 21st, a full year in advance of the proposed entry date to Cambridge for preliminary application, January 31st for actual application.

For further information contact:

The Board of Graduate Studies
4 Mill Lane, Cambridge, CB2 1TZ, England
Contact: The Secretary

British Chevening Cambridge Scholarships - Vietnam

Subjects: All subjects.
Eligibility: The Trusts cannot admit students to the University or any of its Colleges. Applicants for awards from the Trusts must therefore also apply to the University of Cambridge and be offered a place at Cambridge in the normal way. All applicants must have a first class or high second class honours degree, or equivalent and normally be under 26. For students from Vietnam.
Level of Study: Postgraduate.
Purpose: To assist towards one year taught postgraduate courses of study.
Type: Scholarship.
No. of awards offered: 2.
Frequency: Annual.
Length of Study: 1 year.
Study Establishment: Cambridge University.
Country of Study: United Kingdom.
Application Procedure: Candidates for these scholarships should apply directly to the British Embassy, Vietnam.
Closing Date: October 1st.

For further information contact:

British Embassy
16 Ly Thuong Kiet, Hanoi, Vietnam

British Chevening Cambridge Scholarships for Postgraduate Study - Cuba

Subjects: All subjects.
Eligibility: The Trusts cannot admit students to the University or any of its Colleges. Applicants for awards from the Trusts must therefore also apply to the University of Cambridge and be offered a place at Cambridge in the normal way. All applicants must have a first class or high second class honours degree, or equivalent and normally be under 26. Applicants must be from Cuba.
Level of Study: Postgraduate.
Purpose: To assist one year taught postgraduate courses.
Type: Scholarship.

No. of awards offered: 2.
Frequency: Annual.
Study Establishment: Cambridge University.
Country of Study: United Kingdom.
Application Procedure: Candidates must complete a Preliminary Application Form, which can be obtained from local universities, offices of the British Council or the main address. Completed application forms must be returned to the main address. Candidates short-listed will be sent forms for admission to the University of Cambridge and a scholarship application form. These forms must be returned to The Board of Graduate Studies.
Closing Date: September 21st, a full year in advance of the proposed entry date to Cambridge for preliminary application, January 31st for actual application.

For further information contact:

The Board of Graduate Studies
4 Mill Lane, Cambridge, CB2 1TZ, England
Contact: The Secretary

British Chevening Cambridge Scholarships for Postgraduate Study - Mexico

Subjects: All subjects.
Eligibility: The Trusts cannot admit students to the University or any of its Colleges. Applicants for awards from the Trusts must therefore also apply to the University of Cambridge and be offered a place at Cambridge in the normal way. All applicants must have a first class or high second class honours degree, or equivalent and normally be under 26. For students from Mexico.
Level of Study: Postgraduate.
Type: Scholarship.
No. of awards offered: 1.
Frequency: Annual.
Value: Scholarships will cover the University Composition Fee at the overseas rate; approved College fees; a maintenance allowance suffcient for a single student.
Length of Study: 1 year.
Study Establishment: Cambridge University.
Country of Study: United Kingdom.
Application Procedure: All candidates for this scholarship must complete a Preliminary Application Form which can only be obtained from the British Council, Mexico City.

For further information contact:

British Council
Maestro Antonio Caso 127
Col San Rafael
Delegacion Cuauhtemoc
Apartado postal 30-588, Mexico City, 06470 DF, Mexico

British Chevening Scholarships for Postgraduate Study - Pakistan

Subjects: All subjects.
Eligibility: The Trusts cannot admit students to the University or any of its Colleges. Applicants for awards from the Trusts must therefore also apply to the University of Cambridge and

be offered a place at Cambridge in the normal way. All applicants must have a first class or high second class honours degree, or equivalent and normally be under 26. For students of outstanding academic merit from Pakistan.
Level of Study: Postgraduate.
Type: Scholarship.
No. of awards offered: 5.
Frequency: Annual.
Study Establishment: Cambridge University.
Country of Study: United Kingdom.
Application Procedure: Candidates must complete a Preliminary Application Form, which can be obtained from local universities, offices of the British Council or the main address. Completed application forms must be returned to the main address. Candidates short-listed will be sent forms for admission to the University of Cambridge and a scholarship application form. These forms must be returned to The Board fof Graduate Studies.
Closing Date: September 21st, a full year in advance of the proposed entry date to Cambridge for preliminary application, January 31st for actual application.

For further information contact:

The Board of Graduate studies
4 Mill Lane, Cambridge, CB2 1TZ, England
Contact: The Secretary

British Prize Scholarships

Subjects: All subjects.
Eligibility: The Trusts cannot admit students to the University or any of its Colleges. Applicants for awards from the Trusts must therefore also apply to the University of Cambridge and be offered a place at Cambridge in the normal way. All applicants must have a first class or high second class honours degree, or equivalent and normally be under 26.
Level of Study: Postgraduate.
Purpose: To assist study for one year taught postgraduate courses.
Type: Scholarship.
No. of awards offered: 2.
Frequency: Annual.
Study Establishment: Cambridge University.
Country of Study: United Kingdom.
Application Procedure: Candidates must complete a Preliminary Application Form, which can be obtained from local universities, offices of the British Council or the main address. Completed application forms must be returned to the main address. Candidates short-listed will be sent forms for admission to the University of Cambridge and a scholarship application form. These forms must be returned to The Board of Graduate Studies.
Closing Date: September 21st, a full year in advance of the proposed entry date to Cambridge for preliminary application, January 31st for actual application.
Additional Information: One scholarship annually to a student from Barbados and one from the Eastern Caribbean (Antigua and Barbuda, Dominica, Grenada, St Kitts-Nevis, St Lucia, St Vincent and the Grenadines).

For further information contact:

The Board of Graduate Studies
4 Mill Lane, Cambridge, CB2 1TZ, England
Contact: The Secretary

Cambridge Livingstone Trust Scholarships for Postgraduate Study

Subjects: All subjects.
Eligibility: The Trusts cannot admit students to the University or any of its Colleges. Applicants for awards from the Trusts must therefore also apply to the University of Cambridge and be offered a place at Cambridge in the normal way. All applicants must have a first class or high second class honours degree, or equivalent and normally be under 26. For students from Botswana, Lesptho, Malawi, Namibia, Swaziland, Zambia and Zimbabwe.
Level of Study: Doctorate.
Purpose: To assist students with study for a one year taught postgraduate course.
Type: Scholarship.
No. of awards offered: Varies.
Frequency: Annual.
Length of Study: 1 year.
Study Establishment: Cambridge University.
Country of Study: United Kingdom.
Application Procedure: Candidates must complete a Preliminary Application Form, which can be obtained from local universities, offices of the British Council or the main address. Completed application forms must be returned to the main address. Candidates short-listed will be sent forms for admission to the University of Cambridge and a scholarship application form. These forms must be returned to The Board of Graduate Studies.
Closing Date: September 21st, a full year in advance of the proposed entry date to Cambridge for preliminary application, January 31st for actual application.

For further information contact:

The Board of Graduate Studies
4 Mill Lane, Cambridge, CB2 1TZ, England
Contact: The Secretary

Cambridge Livingstone Trust Scholarships for Study Towards a PhD

Subjects: All subjects.
Eligibility: The Trusts cannot admit students to the University or any of its Colleges. Applicants for awards from the Trusts must therefore also apply to the University of Cambridge and be offered a place at Cambridge in the normal way. All applicants must have a first class or high second class honours degree, or equivalent and normally be under 26. For students from Botswana, Lesotho, Malawi, Namibia, Swaziland, Zambia and Zimbabwe.
Level of Study: Doctorate.
Type: Scholarship.
No. of awards offered: Varies.
Frequency: Annual.

Value: The scholarships will cover the University Composition Fee at the home rate; approved college fees; a maintenance allowance sufficient for a single student; a contribution to a return economy airfare.
Length of Study: Tenable for up to 3 years.
Study Establishment: Cambridge University.
Country of Study: United Kingdom.
Application Procedure: Candidates must complete a Preliminary Application Form, which can be obtained from local universities, offices of the British Council or the main address. Completed application forms must be returned to the main address. Candidates short-listed will be sent forms for admission to the University of Cambridge and a scholarship application form. These forms must be returned to The Board of Graduate Studies.
Closing Date: September 21st, a full year in advance of the proposed entry date to Cambridge for preliminary application, January 31st for actual application.

For further information contact:

The Board of Graduate Studies
4 Mill Lane, Cambridge, CB2 1TZ, England
Contact: The Secretary

Cambridge Nehru Scholarships

Subjects: All subjects.
Eligibility: The Trusts cannot admit students to the University or any of its Colleges. Applicants for awards from the Trusts must therefore also apply to the University of Cambridge and be offered a place at Cambridge in the normal way. All applicants must have a first class or high second class honours degree, or equivalent and normally be under 26. For students from India.
Level of Study: Doctorate.
Purpose: To assist study towards a PhD.
Type: Scholarship.
No. of awards offered: 8.
Frequency: Annual.
Value: The scholarships will cover the University Composition Fee at the home rate; approved college fees; a maintenance allowance sufficient for a single student; a contribution to a return economy airfare.
Length of Study: Tenable for up to 3 years.
Study Establishment: Cambridge University.
Country of Study: United Kingdom.
Application Procedure: Candidates from India may obtain further details and a Preliminary Application Forms by writing before August 17th of the year before entry to The Joint Secretary, Nehru Trust for Cambridge University, Teen Murti House, Teen Murti Marg, New Delhi, 110011, giving details of academic qualifications. Completed forms must be returned to the same address no later than September 9th. Those candidates who are successfully short-listed will be sent forms for admission to the University of Cambridge as a graduate student which should be completed and returned to The Secretary, Board of Graduate Studies, 4 Mill Lane, Cambridge, CB2 1TZ no later than January 31st.
Closing Date: September 9th for preliminary application; January 31st for actual application.

Cambridge Raffles Scholarships

Subjects: All subjects.
Eligibility: The Trusts cannot admit students to the University or any of its Colleges. Applicants for awards from the Trusts must therefore also apply to the University of Cambridge and be offered a place at Cambridge in the normal way. All applicants must have a first class or high second class honours degree, or equivalent and normally be under 26. For students from Singapore.
Level of Study: Postgraduate.
Type: Scholarship.
No. of awards offered: 2.
Frequency: Annual.
Length of Study: 1 year.
Study Establishment: Cambridge University.
Country of Study: United Kingdom.
Application Procedure: Candidates must complete a Preliminary Application Form, which can be obtained from local universities, offices of the British Council or the main address. Completed application forms must be returned to the main address. Candidates short-listed will be sent forms for admission to the University of Cambridge and a scholarship application form. These forms must be returned to The Board of Graduate Studies.
Closing Date: September 21st, a full year in advance of the proposed entry date to Cambridge for preliminary application, January 31st for actual application.

For further information contact:

The Board of Graduate Studies
4 Mill Lane, Cambridge, CB2 1TZ, England
Contact: The Secretary

Cambridge Shared Scholarships

Subjects: All subjects.
Eligibility: The Trusts cannot admit students to the University or any of its Colleges. Applicants for awards from the Trusts must therefore also apply to the University of Cambridge and be offered a place at Cambridge in the normal way. All applicants must have a first class or high second class honours degree or equivalent (if applying for a postgraduate course), be under the age of 35 on October 1st of the year they are applying for, return to their own country to work or study after completing the course, not be employed by a government department or by a parastatal organisation, not at present be living in a developed country, and not have taken studies lasting a year or more in a developed country. Candidates wishing to pursue a course of study related to the economic and social development of their country will be given priority. Citizens from developing countries of the Commonwealth are eligible - The Falkland Islands, St Helena, Tristan de Cunha, Bangladesh, Pakistan, Sri Lanka, The Maldives, Brunei, Cameroon, Gambia, Ghana, Kenya, Sierra Leone, Tanzania, Uganda, India, Malta, Mauritius, Seychelles, Kiribati, Pitcairn, Tuvalu, Nauru, Solomon Islands, Vanuatu, Papua New Guinea, Tonga, Western Samoa, South Africa, Botswana, Namibia, Lesotho, Malawi, Swaziland and commonwealth countries of the Caribbean, Zambia, Mozambique, Zimbabwe.

Level of Study: Postgraduate, Undergraduate.
Type: Scholarship.
No. of awards offered: 50.
Frequency: Annual.
Value: Scholarships will cover up to the University Composition Fee at the overseas rate; approved College fees; a maintenance allowance sufficient for a single student; a contribution to a return economy airfare.
Length of Study: 1 year.
Study Establishment: Cambridge University.
Country of Study: United Kingdom.
Application Procedure: Please apply to the address relevant to your country. If there is no specfic address for your country then apply to the main address.
Closing Date: September 1st for preliminary form, January 31st for actual form for India; September 21st for the preliminary form, January 31st for the actual form for rest of world.
Additional Information: The shared scholarships for undergraduate study are only available when the course is not available at the student's local or regional university. Preliminary application forms should be sent to the address applicable to that particular country. The final application forms should be sent to The Secretary, Board of Graduate Studies.

For further information contact:

Board of Graduate Studies
4 Mill Lane, Cambridge, CB2 1TZ, England
Contact: The Secretary
or
Cambridge Commonwealth Trust (TPG)
c/o Nehru Trust for Cambridge University
Teen Murti House
Teen Murti Marg, New Delhi, 110011, India

Cambridge Thai Foundation Scholarships

Subjects: All subjects.
Eligibility: The Trusts cannot admit students to the University or any of its Colleges. Applicants for awards from the Trusts must therefore also apply to the University of Cambridge and be offered a place at Cambridge in the normal way. All applicants must have a first class or high second class honours degree, or equivalent and normally be under 26. For PhD study applicants must be successfully nominated for an ORS award which pays the difference between the home and overseas rate of the University Composition Fee. For students from Thailand.
Level of Study: Doctorate, Postgraduate.
Type: Scholarship.
No. of awards offered: 1 PhD, 2 postgraduate study.
Frequency: Annual.
Value: Scholarships will cover the university Composition Fee at the home rate, approved College fees, a maintenance allowance sufficient for a single student, a contribution to a return economy airfare.
Length of Study: Tenable for up to 3 years-PhD; 1 year Postgraduate study.
Study Establishment: Cambridge University.
Country of Study: United Kingdom.

Application Procedure: Candidates must complete a Preliminary Application Form, which can be obtained from local universities, offices of the British Council or the main address. Completed application forms must be returned to the main address. Candidates short-listed will be sent forms for admission to the University of Cambridge and a scholarship application form. These forms must be returned to The Board of Graduate Studies.

Closing Date: September 21st, a full year in advance of the proposed entry date to Cambridge for preliminary application, January 31st for actual application.

For further information contact:

The Board of Graduate Studies
4 Mill Lane, Cambridge, CB2 1TZ, England
Contact: The Secretary

Cambridge-Malaysia Scholarship for Study Towards the Degree Of PhD

Subjects: All subjects.
Eligibility: The Trusts cannot admit students to the University or any of its Colleges. Applicants for awards from the Trusts must therefore also apply to the University of Cambridge and be offered a place at Cambridge in the normal way. All applicants must have a first class or high second class honours degree, or equivalent and normally be under 26. For students from Malaysia.
Level of Study: Doctorate.
Purpose: To assist study towards a PhD.
Type: Scholarship.
No. of awards offered: 1.
Frequency: Annual.
Value: The scholarships will cover the university Composition Fee at the home rate, approved College fees, a maintenance allowance sufficient for a single student, a contribution to a return economy airfare.
Length of Study: Up to 3 years.
Study Establishment: Cambridge University.
Country of Study: United Kingdom.
Application Procedure: Candidates must complete a Preliminary Application Form, which can be obtained from local universities, offices of the British Council or the main address. Completed application forms must be returned to the main address. Candidates short-listed will be sent forms for admission to the University of Cambridge and a scholarship application form. These forms must be returned to The Board of Graduate Studies.
Closing Date: September 21st, a full year in advance of the proposed entry date to Cambridge for preliminary application, January 31st for actual application.

For further information contact:

The Board of Grdauate Studies
4 Mill Lane, Cambridge, CB2 1TZ, England
Contact: The Secretary

Cambridge-Malaysia Scholarships for One Year Taught Postgraduate Courses of Study

Subjects: All subjects.
Eligibility: The Trusts cannot admit students to the University or any of its Colleges. Applicants for awards from the Trusts must therefore also apply to the University of Cambridge and be offered a place at Cambridge in the normal way. All applicants must have a first class or high second class honours degree, or equivalent and normally be under 26. For students from Malaysia.
Level of Study: Postgraduate.
Type: Scholarship.
No. of awards offered: 4.
Frequency: Annual.
Value: Scholarships will cover up to the University Composition Fee at the overseas rate; approved College fees; a maintenance allowance sufficient for a single student; a contribution to a return economy airfare.
Length of Study: 1 year.
Study Establishment: Cambridge University.
Country of Study: United Kingdom.
Application Procedure: Candidates must complete a Preliminary Application Form, which can be obtained from local universities, offices of the British Council or, the main address. Completed application forms must be returned to the main address. Candidates short-listed will be sent forms for admission to the University of Cambridge and a Scholarship application form. These forms must be returned to The Board of Graduate Studies.
Closing Date: September 21st, a full year in advance of the proposed entry date to Cambridge for preliminary application, January 31st for actual application.

For further information contact:

The Board of Graduate Studies
4 Mill Lane, Cambridge, CB2 1TZ, England
Contact: The Secretary

Canada Cambridge Scholarships

Subjects: All subjects.
Eligibility: The Trusts cannot admit students to the University or any of its Colleges. Applicants for awards from the Trusts must therefore also apply to the University of Cambridge and be offered a place at Cambridge in the normal way. All applicants must have a first class or high second class honours degree, or equivalent and normally be under 26. For students from Canada.
Level of Study: Doctorate.
Type: Scholarship.
No. of awards offered: 5.
Frequency: Annual.
Value: The scholarships will pay the University Composition Fee at the home rate and approved College fees.
Study Establishment: Cambridge University.
Country of Study: United Kingdom.
Application Procedure: Application form for the scholarship will be sent out to eligible candidates once the completed form for admission to the University of Cambridge has reached the Board of Graduate Studies.

Closing Date: Scholarship forms must be returned by April 30th.

For further information contact:

The Board of Graduate Studies
4 Mill Lane, Cambridge, CB2 1TZ, England
Contact: The Secretary

CEU Soros Cambridge Scholarships

Subjects: For study in the subjects relevant to the needs of Central and Eastern Europe, the former Soviet Union and Mongolia.
Eligibility: For graduates from the Central European University. Applicants must be successfully nominated for an ORS award, which covers the difference between the home and overseas rate of the University Composition Fee, pursue research in the same subject area they followed at the CEU, and pursue a course of research which requires one academic year of fieldwork away from Cambridge in Central and Eastern Europe and the former Soviet Union or at the CEU.
Level of Study: Doctorate.
Purpose: To assist study towards a PhD.
Type: Scholarship.
No. of awards offered: 3.
Frequency: Annual.
Value: Scholarships will cover the University Composition Fee at the home rate; approved College fees; a maintenance allowance sufficient for a single student; a return economy airfare; fieldwork costs in the region.
Length of Study: Tenable for up to 3 years.
Study Establishment: Cambridge University.
Country of Study: United Kingdom.
Application Procedure: Applicants for the CEU Soros Cambridge Scholarship must complete a application form for admission to the University of Cambridge as a graduate student which can be obtained from, and must be returned to, the Scholarships Office at the Central European University, no later than December 16th.
Additional Information: There are also five awards available to enable candidates pursuing a course of research leading to the degree of PhD at the Central European University to undertake short periods of study at Cambridge as part of their PhD at the CEU. Potential candidates should make application through the Scholarships Office at the CEU, in consultation with their academic advisors.

Coles Myer Cambridge Scholarship

Subjects: All subjects.
Eligibility: The Trusts cannot admit students to the University or any of its Colleges. Applicants for awards from the Trusts must therefore also apply to the University of Cambridge and be offered a place at Cambridge in the normal way. All applicants must have a first class or high second class honours degree, or equivalent and normally be under 26. For students from Australia.
Level of Study: Doctorate.
Type: Scholarship.

No. of awards offered: 1.
Frequency: As available.
Study Establishment: Cambridge University.
Country of Study: United Kingdom.
Application Procedure: Application forms for the scholarship will be sent out to eligible candidates once the completed form for admission to the University of Cambridge has reached the Board of Graduate Studies.
Closing Date: Scholarship forms must be returned by April 30th.

For further information contact:

The Board of Graduate Studies
4 Mill Lane, Cambridge, CB2 1TZ, England
Contact: The Secretary

Corpus Christi ACE Scholarship

Subjects: All subjects (with preference given to candidates wishing to pursue a MPhil in Environment and Development).
Eligibility: The Trusts cannot admit students to the University or any of its Colleges. Applicants for awards from the Trusts must therefore also apply to the University of Cambridge and be offered a place at Cambridge in the normal way. All applicants must have a first class or high second class honours degree, or equivalent and normally be under 26. For students from the Developing World with preference for applicants wishing to pursue the MPhil in environment and development.
Level of Study: Postgraduate.
Type: Scholarship.
No. of awards offered: 1.
Frequency: Annual.
Length of Study: 1 year.
Study Establishment: Corpus Christi College, Cambridge.
Country of Study: United Kingdom.
Application Procedure: Candidates must complete a Preliminary Application Form, which can be obtained from local universities, offices of the British Council or the main address. Completed application forms must be returned to the main address. Candidates short-listed will be sent forms for admission to the University of Cambridge and a scholarship application form. These forms must be returned to The Board of Graduate Studies.
Closing Date: September 21st, a full year in advance of the proposed entry date to Cambridge for preliminary application, January 31st for actual application.

For further information contact:

The Board of Graduate Studies
4 Mill Lane, Cambridge, CB2 1TZ, England
Contact: The Secretary

Cyprus Cambridge Scholarships

Subjects: All subjects.
Eligibility: The Trusts cannot admit students to the University or any of its Colleges. Applicants for awards from the Trusts must therefore also apply to the University of Cambridge and be offered a place at Cambridge in the normal way. All

applicants must have a first class or high second class honours degree, or equivalent and normally be under 26. For students from Cyprus. Candidates must be successfully nominated for an ORS award, which covers the difference between the home and overseas rate of the University Composition Fee.

Level of Study: Doctorate.
Purpose: To assist study towards a PhD.
Type: Scholarship.
No. of awards offered: 1.
Frequency: As available.
Value: The scholarships will take into account the financial resources of the applicant and will cover up to the University Composition Fee at the overseas rate; approved College fees; a maintenance allowance sufficient for a single student; a contribution to a return economy airfare.
Length of Study: Tenable for up to 3 years.
Study Establishment: Cambridge University.
Country of Study: United Kingdom.
Application Procedure: Candidates must complete a Preliminary Application Form, which can be obtained from local universities, offices of the British Council or the main address. Completed application forms must be returned to the main address. Candidates short-listed will be sent forms for admission to the University of Cambridge and a scholarship application form. These forms must be returned to The Board of Graduate Studies.
Closing Date: September 21st, a full year in advance of the proposed entry date to Cambridge for preliminary application, January 31st for actual application.

For further information contact:

The Board of Graduate Studies
4 Mill Lane, Cambridge, CB 2 1TZ, England
Contact: The Secretary

Developing World Education Fund Cambridge Scholarships for One Year Taught Postgraduate Courses of Study

Subjects: All subjects.
Eligibility: The Trusts cannot admit students to the University or any of its Colleges. Applicants for awards from the Trusts must therefore also apply to the University of Cambridge and be offered a place at Cambridge in the normal way. All applicants must have a first class or high second class honours degree, or equivalent and normally be under 26. For students from China.
Level of Study: Postgraduate.
Type: Scholarship.
No. of awards offered: 2.
Frequency: Annual.
Study Establishment: Cambridge University.
Country of Study: United Kingdom.
Application Procedure: Candidates must complete a Preliminary Application Form, which can be obtained from local universities, offices of the British Council or the main address. Completed application forms must be returned to the main address. Candidates short-listed will be sent forms for admission to the University of Cambridge and a

scholarship application form. These forms must be returned to The Board of Graduate Studies.
Closing Date: September 21st, a full year in advance of the proposed entry date to Cambridge for preliminary application, January 31st for actual application.

For further information contact:

The Board of Graduate Studies
4 Mill Lane, Cambridge, CB2 1TZ, England
Contact: The Secretary

Developing World Education Fund Cambridge Scholarships for Study Towards the Degree of PhD

Subjects: All subjects.
Eligibility: The Trusts cannot admit students to the University or any of its Colleges. Applicants for awards from the Trusts must therefore also apply to the University of Cambridge and be offered a place at Cambridge in the normal way. All applicants must have a first class or high second class honours degree, or equivalent and normally be under 26. For students from Bangladesh, Pakistan, Sri Lanka and China. Applicants must be successfully nominated for and ORS award, which covers the difference between the home and overseas rate of the University Composition Fee.
Level of Study: Doctorate.
Purpose: To support study towards a PhD.
Type: Scholarship.
No. of awards offered: Varies.
Frequency: Annual.
Value: Scholarships will cover up to the University Composition Fee at the overseas rate; approved College fees; a maintenance allowance sufficient for a single student; a contribution to a return economy airfare.
Length of Study: Tenable for up to 3 years.
Study Establishment: Cambridge University.
Country of Study: United Kingdom.
Application Procedure: Candidates must complete a Preliminary Application Form, which can be obtained from local universities, offices of the British Council or the main address. Completed application forms must be returned to the main address. Candidates short-listed will be sent forms for admission to the University of Cambridge and a scholarship application form. These forms must be returned to The Board of Graduate Studies.
Closing Date: September 21st, a full year in advance of the proposed entry date to Cambridge for preliminary application, January 31st for actual application.

For further information contact:

The Board of Graduate Studies
4 Mill Lane, Cambridge, CB2 1TZ, England
Contact: The Secretary

Dharam Hinduja Cambridge Scholarships

Subjects: All subjects.
Eligibility: The Trusts cannot admit students to the University or any of its Colleges. Applicants for awards from the Trusts

must therefore also apply to the University of Cambridge and be offered a place at Cambridge in the normal way. All applicants must have a first class or high second class honours degree, or equivalent and normally be under 26. For students from India.

Level of Study: Doctorate.
Purpose: To assist with study towards a PhD.
Type: Scholarship.
No. of awards offered: 2.
Frequency: Annual.
Value: The scholarships will cover the University Composition Fee at the home rate; approved college fees; a maintenance allowance sufficient for a single student; a contribution to a return economy airfare.
Length of Study: Tenable for up to 3 years.
Study Establishment: Cambridge University.
Country of Study: United Kingdom.
Application Procedure: Candidates from India may obtain further details and a Preliminary Application Forms by writing before August 17th of the year before entry to The Joint Secretary, Nehru Trust for Cambridge University, Teen Murti House, Teen Murti Marg, New Delhi, 110011, giving details of academic qualifications. Completed forms must be returned to the same address no later than September 9th. Those candidates who are successfully short-listed will be sent forms for admission to the University of Cambridge as a graduate student which should be completed and returned to The Secretary, Board of Graduate Studies, 4 Mill Lane, Cambridge, CB2 1TZ no later than January 31st.
Closing Date: September 9th, preliminary application; January 31st actual application.

Dharam Hinduja Cambridge Shared Scholarships

Subjects: All subjects.
Eligibility: The Trusts cannot admit students to the University or any of its Colleges. Applicants for awards from the Trusts must therefore also apply to the University of Cambridge and be offered a place at Cambridge in the normal way. All applicants must have a first class or high second class honours degree, or equivalent and normally be under 26. For students from India.
Level of Study: Postgraduate.
Type: Scholarship.
No. of awards offered: 4.
Frequency: Annual.
Study Establishment: Cambridge University.
Country of Study: United Kingdom.
Application Procedure: Candidates from India may obtain further details and a Preliminary Application Forms by writing before August 17th of the year before entry to The Joint Secretary, Nehru Trust for Cambridge University, Teen Murti House, Teen Murti Marg, New Delhi, 110011, giving details of academic qualifications. Completed forms must be returned to the same address no later than September 9th. Those candidates who are successfully short-listed will be sent forms for admission to the University of Cambridge as a graduate student which should be completed and returned to The Secretary, Board of Graduate Studies, 4 Mill Lane, Cambridge, CB2 1TZ no later than January 31st.

Closing Date: September 9th, preliminary application; January 31st actual application.

Downing Müller Cambridge Scholarships

Subjects: All subjects.
Eligibility: The Trusts cannot admit students to the University or any of its Colleges. Applicants for awards from the Trusts must therefore also apply to the University of Cambridge and be offered a place at Cambridge in the normal way. All applicants must have a first class or high second class honours degree, or equivalent and normally be under 26. For students from a Third World country, Eastern Europe or from a German speaking country liable to pay fees at the overseas rate.
Level of Study: Doctorate.
Purpose: To assist study towards a PhD.
Type: Scholarship.
No. of awards offered: 2.
Frequency: Annual.
Value: The scholarships will cover the University Composition Fee at the home rate; approved college fees; a maintenance allowance suffiecient for a single student; a contribution to a return economy airfare.
Length of Study: Tenable for up to 3 years.
Study Establishment: Downing College, Cambridge.
Country of Study: United Kingdom.
Application Procedure: Candidates must complete a Preliminary Application Form, which can be obtained from local universities, offices of the British Council or the main address. Completed application forms must be returned to the main address. Candidates short-listed will be sent forms for admission to the University of Cambridge and a scholarship application form. These forms must be returned to The Board of Graduate Studies.
Closing Date: September 21st, a full year in advance of the proposed entry date to Cambridge for preliminary application, January 31st for actual application.

For further information contact:

The Board of Graduate Studies
4 Mill Lane, Cambridge, CB2 1TZ, England
Contact: The Secretary

Downing Müller Cambridge Shared Scholarships

Subjects: All subjects.
Eligibility: For students from a developing country of the Commonwealth. Applicants must be under the age of 35 on October 1st of the year of entry, undertake to return to their own country to work or study after completing the course at Cambridge, not be employed by a government department or be a parastatal organisation, not be at present living or studying in a developed country, and not have undertaken studies lasting a year or more in a developed country. Priority will be given to candidates wishing to pursue a course of study related to the economic and social development of their country.
Level of Study: Postgraduate.
Type: Scholarship.

No. of awards offered: 2.
Frequency: Annual.
Value: The scholarships will cover the University Composition Fee at the home rate; approved college fees; a maintenance allowance sufficient for a single student; a contribution to a return economy airfare.
Length of Study: 1 year.
Study Establishment: Dowing College.
Country of Study: United Kingdom.
Application Procedure: Candidates must complete a Preliminary Application Form, which can be obtained from local universities, offices of the British Council or the main address. Completed application forms must be returned to the main address. Candidates short-listed will be sent forms for admission to the University of Cambridge and a scholarship application form. These forms must be returned to The Board of Graduate Studies.
Closing Date: September 21st, a full year in advance of the proposed entry date to Cambridge for preliminary application, January 31st for actual application.
Additional Information: From time to time, a Downing Müller Cambridge Scholarship will be offered to a candidate from Eastern Europe.

For further information contact:

The Board of Graduate Studies
4 Mill Lane, Cambridge, CB2 1TZ, England
Contact: The Secretary

FCO-China Chevening Fellowships

Subjects: All subjects.
Eligibility: The Trusts cannot admit students to the University or any of its Colleges. Applicants for awards from the Trusts must therefore also apply to the University of Cambridge and be offered a place at Cambridge in the normal way. All applicants must have a first class or high second class honours degree, or equivalent and normally be under 26.
Level of Study: Postgraduate.
Type: Fellowship.
No. of awards offered: 3.
Frequency: Annual.
Study Establishment: Cambridge University.
Country of Study: United Kingdom.
Application Procedure: Candidates must complete a Preliminary Application Form, which can be obtained from local universities, offices of the British Council or the main address. Completed application forms must be returned to the main address. Candidates short-listed will be sent forms for admission to the University of Cambridge and a scholarship application form. These forms must be returned to The Board of Graduate Studies.
Closing Date: September 21st, a full year in advance of the proposed entry date to Cambridge for preliminary application, January 31st for actual application.

For further information contact:

The Board of Graduate Studies
4 Mill Lane, Cambridge, CB2 1TZ, England
Contact: The Secretary

Guy Clutton-Brock Scholarship

Subjects: All subjects.
Eligibility: The Trusts cannot admit students to the University or any of its Colleges. Applicants for awards from the Trusts must therefore also apply to the University of Cambridge and be offered a place at Cambridge in the normal way. All applicants must have a first class or high second class honours degree, or equivalent and normally be under 26. For a student from Zimbabwe who has been offered a place at Magdelene College, Cambridge.
Level of Study: Doctorate, Postgraduate.
Type: Scholarship.
No. of awards offered: 1 PhD, 1 postgraduate study.
Frequency: As available.
Value: Scholarships will cover the University Composition Fee at the overseas rate; approved College fees; a maintenance allowance sufficient for a single student; a contribution to a return economy airfare.
Length of Study: Up to 3 years PhD; 1year postgraduate study.
Study Establishment: Magdelene College, Cambridge.
Country of Study: United Kingdom.
Application Procedure: Candidates must complete a Preliminary Application Form, which can be obtained from local universities, offices of the British Council or the main address. Completed application forms must be returned to the main address. Candidates short-listed will be sent forms for admission to the University of Cambridge and a scholarship application form. These forms must be returned to The Board of Graduate Studies.
Closing Date: September 21st, a full year in advance of the proposed entry date to Cambridge for preliminary application, January 31st for actual application.

For further information contact:

The Board of Graduate Studies
4 Mill Lane, Cambridge, CB2 1TZ, England
Contact: The Secretary

Hamilton Cambridge Scholarship

Subjects: All subjects.
Eligibility: The Trusts cannot admit students to the University or any of its Colleges. Applicants for awards from the Trusts must therefore also apply to the University of Cambridge and be offered a place at Cambridge in the normal way. All applicants must have a first class or high second class honours degree, or equivalent and normally be under 26.
Level of Study: Doctorate.
Type: Scholarship.
No. of awards offered: 1.
Frequency: As available.

Value: Scholarships will cover the University Composition Fee at the overseas rate; approved College fees; a maintenance allowance sufficient for a single student; a contribution to a return economy airfare.
Length of Study: Tenable for up to 3 years.
Study Establishment: Selwyn College.
Country of Study: United Kingdom.
Application Procedure: Candidates must complete a Preliminary Application Form, which can be obtained from local universities, offices of the British Council or the main address. Completed application forms must be returned to the main address. Candidates short-listed will be sent forms for admission to the University of Cambridge and a scholarship application form. These forms must be returned to The Board of Graduate Studies.
Closing Date: September 21st, a full year in advance of the proposed entry date to Cambridge for preliminary application, January 31st for actual application.

For further information contact:

The Board of Graduate Studies
4 Mill Lane, Cambridge, CB2 1TZ, England
Contact: The Secretary

Hong Kong Cambridge Scholarships

Subjects: All subjects.
Eligibility: The Trusts cannot admit students to the University or any of its Colleges. Applicants for awards from the Trusts must therefore also apply to the University of Cambridge and be offered a place at Cambridge in the normal way. All applicants must have a first class or high second class honours degree, or equivalent and normally be under 26. With preference for graduates of the Chinese University of Hong Kong and the University of Hong Kong.
Level of Study: Doctorate.
Type: Scholarship.
No. of awards offered: Up to 5.
Frequency: Annual.
Length of Study: Up to 3 years.
Study Establishment: Cambridge University.
Country of Study: United Kingdom.
Application Procedure: Candidates must complete a Preliminary Application Form, which can be obtained from local universities, offices of the British Council or the main address. Completed application forms must be returned to the main address. Candidates short-listed will be sent forms for admission to the University of Cambridge and a scholarship application form. These forms must be returned to The Board of Graduate Studies.
Closing Date: September 21st, a full year in advance of the proposed entry date to Cambridge for preliminary application, January 31st for actual application.

For further information contact:

The Board of Graduate Studies
4 Mill Lane, Cambridge, CB2 1TZ, England
Contact: The Secretary

International Renaissance Foundation/FCO Scholarships

Subjects: All subjects.
Eligibility: The Trusts cannot admit students to the University or any of its Colleges. Applicants for awards from the Trusts must therefore also apply to the University of Cambridge and be offered a place at Cambridge in the normal way. All applicants must have a first class or high second class honours degree, or equivalent and normally be under 26. For students from the Ukraine.
Level of Study: Postgraduate.
Type: Scholarship.
No. of awards offered: 3.
Frequency: Annual.
Study Establishment: Cambridge University.
Country of Study: United Kingdom.
Application Procedure: Candidates must complete a Preliminary Application Form, which can be obtained from local universities, offices of the British Council or the main address. Completed application forms must be returned to the main address. Candidates short-listed will be sent forms for admission to the University of Cambridge and a scholarship application form. These forms must be returned to The Board of Graduate Studies.
Closing Date: September 21st, a full year in advance of the proposed entry date to Cambridge for preliminary application, January 31st for actual application.

For further information contact:

The Board for Graduate Studies
4 Mill Lane, Cambridge, CB2 1TZ, England
Contact: The Secretary

Jawaharlal Nehru Memorial Trust Cambridge Scholarships

Subjects: All subjects.
Eligibility: The Trusts cannot admit students to the University or any of its Colleges. Applicants for awards from the Trusts must therefore also apply to the University of Cambridge and be offered a place at Cambridge in the normal way. All applicants must have a first class or high second class honours degree, or equivalent and normally be under 26. Applicants for all scholarships for study towards the degree of PhD must be successful in winning an ORS award, which pays the difference between the home and overseas rate of the University Composition Fee. Those who have, in addition to a first class honours degree, a first class Master's degree, or its equivalent, may be given preference. For students from India.
Level of Study: Doctorate.
Purpose: To assist study towards a PhD.
Type: Scholarship.
No. of awards offered: 1.
Frequency: Annual.
Value: The scholarships will cover the University Composition Fee at the home rate; approved college fees; a maintenance allowance sufficient for a single student; a contribution to a return economy airfare.
Length of Study: Tenable for up to 3 years.

Study Establishment: Trinity College, Cambridge.
Country of Study: United Kingdom.
Application Procedure: Candidates from India may obtain further details and a Preliminary Application Forms by writing before August 17th of the year before entry to The Joint Secretary, Nehru Trust for Cambridge University, Teen Murti House, Teen Murti Marg, New Delhi, 110011, giving details of academic qualifications. Completed forms must be returned to the same address no later than September 9th. Those candidates who are successfully short-listed will be sent forms for admission to the University of Cambridge as a graduate student which should be completed and returned to The Secretary, Board of Graduate Studies, 4 Mill Lane, Cambridge, CB2 1TZ no later than January 31st.
Closing Date: September 9th, preliminary application; January 31st actual application.

Jawaharlal Nehru Memorial Trust Cambridge Shared Scholarships

Subjects: All subjects.
Eligibility: The Trusts cannot admit students to the University or any of its Colleges. Applicants for awards from the Trusts must therefore also apply to the University of Cambridge and be offered a place at Cambridge in the normal way. All applicants must have a first class or high second class honours degree, or equivalent and normally be under 26. For students from India.
Level of Study: Postgraduate.
Type: Scholarship.
No. of awards offered: 2.
Frequency: Annual.
Study Establishment: Cambridge University.
Country of Study: United Kingdom.
Application Procedure: Candidates from India may obtain further details and a Preliminary Application Forms by writing before August 17th of the year before entry to The Joint Secretary, Nehru Trust for Cambridge University, Teen Murti House, Teen Murti Marg, New Delhi, 110011, giving details of academic qualifications. Completed forms must be returned to the same address no later than September 9th. Those candidates who are successfully short-listed will be sent forms for admission to the University of Cambridge as a graduate student which should be completed and returned to The Secretary, Board of Graduate Studies, 4 Mill Lane, Cambridge, CB2 1TZ no later than January 31st.
Closing Date: September 9th, preliminary application; January 31st actual application.

Kalimuzo Cambridge Scholarship

Subjects: All subjects.
Eligibility: The Trusts cannot admit students to the University or any of its Colleges. Applicants for awards from the Trusts must therefore also apply to the University of Cambridge and be offered a place at Cambridge in the normal way. All applicants must have a first class or high second class honours degree, or equivalent and normally be under 26. For a student from Uganda.
Level of Study: Doctorate.
Purpose: To support study towards a PhD.

Type: Scholarship.
No. of awards offered: 1.
Frequency: Annual.
Study Establishment: Cambridge University.
Country of Study: United Kingdom.
Application Procedure: Candidates must complete a Preliminary Application Form, which can be obtained from local universities, offices of the British Council or the main address. Completed application forms must be returned to the main address. Candidates short-listed will be sent forms for admission to the University of Cambridge and a scholarship application form. These forms must be returned to The Board of Graduate Studies.
Closing Date: September 21st, a full year in advance of the proposed entry date to Cambridge for preliminary application, January 31st for actual application.
Additional Information: The scholarship is awarded in the memory of Professor Frank Kalimuzo former Vice-Chancellor of Makerere University.

For further information contact:

The Board of Graduate Studies
4 Mill Lane, Cambridge, CB2 1TZ, England
Contact: The Secretary

Kalimuzo Cambridge Shared Scholarships

Subjects: All subjects.
Eligibility: The Trusts cannot admit students to the University or any of its Colleges. Applicants for awards from the Trusts must therefore also apply to the University of Cambridge and be offered a place at Cambridge in the normal way. All applicants must have a first class or high second class honours degree, or equivalent and normally be under 26. For students from Uganda.
Type: Scholarship.
No. of awards offered: 3.
Frequency: Annual.
Study Establishment: Cambridge University.
Country of Study: United Kingdom.
Application Procedure: Candidates must complete a Preliminary Application Form, which can be obtained from local universities, offices of the British Council or the main address. Completed application forms must be returned to the main address. Candidates short-listed will be sent forms for admission to the University of Cambridge and a scholarship application form. These forms must be returned to The Board of Graduate Studies.
Closing Date: September 21st, a full year in advance of the proposed entry date to Cambridge for preliminary application, January 31st for actual application.
Additional Information: Scholarships offered in the memory of Professor Frank Kalimuzo former Vice-Chancellor of Makerere University.

For further information contact:

The Board of Graduate Studies
4 Mill Lane, Cambridge, CB2 1TZ, England
Contact: The Secretary

Karim Rida Said Cambridge Scholarships

Subjects: All subjects.
Eligibility: The Trusts cannot admit students to the University or any of its Colleges. Applicants for awards from the Trusts must therefore also apply to the University of Cambridge and be offered a place at Cambridge in the normal way. All applicants must have a first class or high second class honours degree, or equivalent and normally be under 26. Applicants must be successfully nominated for an ORS award which pays the difference between the home and overseas rate of the University Composition Fee. For students from Egypt, Jordan, Lebanon, Palestine and Syria.
Level of Study: Doctorate, Postgraduate.
Type: Scholarship.
No. of awards offered: 2 PhD, 4 postgraduate study.
Frequency: Annual.
Value: Scholarships will cover the University Composition Fee at the overseas rate; approved College fees; a maintenance allowance sufficient for a single student; a contribution to a return economy airfare.
Length of Study: Tenable for up to 3 years-PhD; 1 year Postgraduate study.
Study Establishment: Cambridge University.
Country of Study: United Kingdom.
Application Procedure: Candidates must complete a Preliminary Application Form, which can be obtained from local universities, offices of the British Council or the main address. Completed application forms must be returned to the main address. Candidates short-listed will be sent forms for admission to the University of Cambridge and a scholarship application form. These forms must be returned to The Board of Graduate Studies.
Closing Date: September 21st, a full year in advance of the proposed entry date to Cambridge for preliminary application, January 31st for actual application.
Additional Information: Scholars must undertake to return to their home country, or to another member state of the Arab League, on completion of studies at Cambridge.

For further information contact:

The Board of Graduate Studies
4 Mill Lane, Cambridge, CB2 1TZ, England
Contact: The Secretary

Kater Cambridge Scholarship

Subjects: All subjects.
Eligibility: The Trusts cannot admit students to the University or any of its Colleges. Applicants for awards from the Trusts must therefore also apply to the University of Cambridge and be offered a place at Cambridge in the normal way. All applicants must have a first class or high second class honours degree, or equivalent and normally be under 26. Open to students from Australia.
Level of Study: Doctorate.
Purpose: For study towards a PhD.
Type: Scholarship.
No. of awards offered: 1.
Frequency: As available.

Value: Scholarships will cover up to the University Composition Fee at the overseas rate; approved College fees; a maintenance allowance sufficient for a single student; a contribution to a return economy airfare.
Length of Study: Tenable for up to 3 years.
Study Establishment: Cambridge University.
Country of Study: United Kingdom.
Application Procedure: Application form for the scholarship will be sent out to eligible candidates once the completed form for admission to the University of Cambridge has reached the Board of Graduate Studies.
Closing Date: Studentship forms must be returned by April 30th.

For further information contact:

The Board of Graduate Studies
4 Mill Lane, Cambridge, CB2 1TZ, England
Contact: The Secretary

Kenya Cambridge Scholarship

Subjects: All subjects.
Eligibility: The Trusts cannot admit students to the University or any of its Colleges. Applicants for awards from the Trusts must therefore also apply to the University of Cambridge and be offered a place at Cambridge in the normal way. All applicants must have a first class or high second class honours degree, or equivalent and normally be under 26. For a student from Kenya.
Level of Study: Doctorate.
Type: Scholarship.
No. of awards offered: 1.
Frequency: Annual.
Length of Study: Tenable for up to 3 years.
Study Establishment: Cambridge University.
Country of Study: United Kingdom.
Application Procedure: Candidates must complete a Preliminary Application Form, which can be obtained from local universities, offices of the British Council or the main address. Completed application forms must be returned to the main address. Candidates short-listed will be sent forms for admission to the University of Cambridge and a scholarship application form. These forms must be returned to The Board of Graduate Studies.
Closing Date: September 21st, a full year in advance of the proposed entry date to Cambridge for preliminary application, January 31st for actual application.

For further information contact:

The Board of Graduate Studies
4 Mill Lane, Cambridge, CB2 1TZ, England
Contact: The Secretary

Kenya Cambridge Shared Scholarship

Subjects: All subjects.
Eligibility: The Trusts cannot admit students to the University or any of its Colleges. Applicants for awards from the Trusts must therefore also apply to the University of Cambridge and be offered a place at Cambridge in the normal way. All

applicants must have a first class or high second class honours degree, or equivalent and normally be under 26. For a student from Kenya.
Level of Study: Postgraduate.
Type: Scholarship.
No. of awards offered: 1.
Frequency: Annual.
Study Establishment: Cambridge University.
Country of Study: United Kingdom.
Application Procedure: Candidates must complete a Preliminary Application Form, which can be obtained from local universities, offices of the British Council or the main address. Completed application forms must be returned to the main address. Candidates short-listed will be sent forms for admission to the University of Cambridge and a scholarship application form. These forms must be returned to The Board of Graduate Studies.
Closing Date: September 21st, a full year in advance of the proposed entry date to Cambridge for preliminary application, January 31st for actual application.

For further information contact:

The Board of Graduate Studies
4 Mill Lane, Cambridge, CB2 1TZ, England
Contact: The Secretary

Kopke Cambridge Scholarship

Subjects: All subjects.
Eligibility: The Trusts cannot admit students to the University or any of its Colleges. Applicants for awards from the Trusts must therefore also apply to the University of Cambridge and be offered a place at Cambridge in the normal way. All applicants must have a first class or high second class honours degree, or equivalent and normally be under 26. Open to candidates from Australia.
Level of Study: Doctorate.
Purpose: To assist towards the study for a PhD.
Type: Scholarship.
No. of awards offered: 1.
Frequency: As available.
Value: Scholarships will cover up to the University Composition Fee at the overseas rate; approved College fees; a maintenance allowance sufficient for a single student; a contribution to a return economy airfare.
Length of Study: Tenable for up to 3 years.
Study Establishment: Cambridge University.
Country of Study: United Kingdom.
Application Procedure: Application form for the scholarship will be sent out to eligible candidates once the completed form for admission to the University of Cambridge has reached the Board of Graduate Studies.
Closing Date: Scholarship forms must be returned by April 30th.

For further information contact:

The Board of Graduate Studies
4 Mill Lane, Cambridge, CB2 1TZ, England
Contact: The Secretary

Lady Noon Cambridge Shared Scholarships

Subjects: All subjects.
Eligibility: The Trusts cannot admit students to the University or any of its Colleges. Applicants for awards from the Trusts must therefore also apply to the University of Cambridge and be offered a place at Cambridge in the normal way. All applicants must have a first class or high second class honours degree, or equivalent and normally be under 26. For students from Pakistan.
Level of Study: Postgraduate.
Type: Scholarship.
No. of awards offered: 1.
Frequency: Annual.
Length of Study: 1 year.
Study Establishment: Cambridge Unibersity.
Country of Study: United Kingdom.
Application Procedure: Candidates must complete a Preliminary Application Form, which can be obtained from local universities, offices of the British Council or the main address. Completed application forms must be returned to the main address. Candidates short-listed will be sent forms for admission to the University of Cambridge and a scholarship application form. These forms must be returned to The Board fof Graduate Studies.
Closing Date: September 21st, a full year in advance of the proposed entry date to Cambridge for preliminary application, January 31st for actual application.

For further information contact:

The Board of Graduate Studies
4 Mill Lane, Cambridge, CB2 1TZ, England
Contact: The Secretary

Link Foundation/FCO Chevening Cambridge Scholarships

Subjects: All subjects.
Eligibility: The Trusts cannot admit students to the University or any of its Colleges. Applicants for awards from the Trusts must therefore also apply to the University of Cambridge and be offered a place at Cambridge in the normal way. All applicants must have a first class or high second class honours degree, or equivalent and normally be under 26. For students from New Zealand.
Level of Study: Postgraduate.
Purpose: The fund taught postgraduate courses.
Type: Scholarship.
No. of awards offered: 3.
Frequency: Annual.
Value: The scholarships will make a substantial contribution of up to £10,000 towards the costs of study and a contribution of £1,000 towards the return airfare to the UK.
Length of Study: 1 year.
Study Establishment: Cambridge University.
Country of Study: United Kingdom.
Application Procedure: Application form for the scholarship will be sent out to eligible candidates once the completed form for admission to the University of Cambridge has reached The Board of Graduate Studies.

Closing Date: Scholarship forms must be returned by April 30th.

For further information contact:

The Board of Graduate Studies
4 Mill Lane, Cambridge, CB2 1TZ, England
Contact: The Secretary

Malaysian Commonwealth Scholarships

Subjects: All subjects.
Eligibility: The Trusts cannot admit students to the University or any of its Colleges. Applicants for awards from the Trusts must therefore also apply to the University of Cambridge and be offered a place at Cambridge in the normal way. All applicants must have a first class or high second class honours degree, or equivalent and normally be under 26. For students from Commonwealth countries.
Level of Study: Doctorate, Postgraduate.
Type: Scholarship.
No. of awards offered: A number of full-cost scholarships for PhD students, a number of scholarships for postgraduate study students.
Frequency: Annual.
Value: Full-cost, PhD; postgraduate scholarships will cover the University Composition Fee at the overseas rate; approved College fees; a maintenance allowance sufficient for a single student; a contribution to a return economy airfare.
Length of Study: 3 years PhD; 1 year postgraduate study.
Study Establishment: Cambridge University.
Country of Study: United Kingdom.
Application Procedure: Candidates must complete a Preliminary Application Form, which can be obtained from local universities, offices of the British Council or the main address. Completed application forms must be returned to the main address. Candidates short-listed will be sent forms for admission to the University of Cambridge and a scholarship application form. These forms must be returned to The Board of Graduate Studies.
Closing Date: September 21st, a full year in advance of the proposed entry date to Cambridge for preliminary application, January 31st for actual application.

For further information contact:

The Board of Graduate Studies
4 Mill Lane, Cambridge, CB2 1TZ, England
Contact: The Secretary

Mandela Cambridge Scholarships

Subjects: All subjects.
Eligibility: The Trusts cannot admit students to the University or any of its Colleges. Applicants for awards from the Trusts must therefore also apply to the University of Cambridge and be offered a place at Cambridge in the normal way. All applicants must have a first class or high second class honours degree, or equivalent and normally be under 26. Applicants for study towards a PhD must be successfully nominated for an ORS award which pays the difference

between the home and overseas rate of the University Composition Fee. For students from South Africa.
Level of Study: Doctorate, Postgraduate.
Purpose: To assist study towards a PhD and one year taught postgraduate courses.
Type: Scholarship.
No. of awards offered: 10 PhD, 20 Postgraduate study.
Frequency: Annual.
Value: Scholarships will cover up to the University Composition Fee at the overseas rate; approved College fees; a maintenance allowance sufficient for a single student; a contribution to a return economy airfare.
Length of Study: Up to 3 years PhD, 1year taught postgraduate courses.
Study Establishment: Cambridge University.
Country of Study: United Kingdom.
Application Procedure: Candidates must complete a Preliminary Application Form, which can be obtained from local universities, offices of the British Council or the main address. Completed application forms must be returned to the main address. Candidates short-listed will be sent forms for admission to the University of Cambridge and a scholarship application form. These forms must be returned to The Board of Graduate Studies.
Closing Date: September 21st, a full year in advance of the proposed entry date to Cambridge for preliminary application, January 31st for actual application.
Additional Information: Offered by the Malaysian Commonwealth Studies Centre, the Cambridge Local Examinations Syndicate, Trinity College, Cambridge and the Cambridge University Press in honour of President Mandela.

For further information contact:

The Board of Graduate Studies
4 Mill Lane, Cambridge, CB2 1TZ, England
Contact: The Secretary

Mandela Magdalene College Scholarships

Subjects: All subjects.
Eligibility: The Trusts cannot admit students to the University or any of its Colleges. Applicants for awards from the Trusts must therefore also apply to the University of Cambridge and be offered a place at Cambridge in the normal way. All applicants must have a first class or high second class honours degree, or equivalent and normally be under 26. For students who have been offered a place at Magdalene College, Cambridge.
Level of Study: Postgraduate.
Type: Scholarship.
No. of awards offered: Up to 3.
Frequency: Annual.
Value: Scholarships will cover the University Composition Fee at the overseas rate; approved College fees; a maintenance allowance sufficient for a single student; a contribution to a return economy airfare.
Length of Study: 1 year.
Study Establishment: Magdalene College, Cambridge.
Country of Study: United Kingdom.

Application Procedure: Candidates must complete a Preliminary Application Form, which can be obtained from local universities, offices of the British Council or the main address. Completed application forms must be returned to the main address. Candidates short-listed will be sent forms for admission to the University of Cambridge and a scholarship application form. These forms must be returned to The Board of Graduate Studies.

Closing Date: September 21st, a full year in advance of the proposed entry date to Cambridge for preliminary application, January 31st for actual application.

For further information contact:

The Board Of Graduate Studies
4 Mill Lane, Cambridge, CB2 1TZ, England
Contact: The Secretary

Ministry of Education, Malaysia, Scholarships

Subjects: All subjects.
Eligibility: The Trusts cannot admit students to the University or any of its Colleges. Applicants for awards from the Trusts must therefore also apply to the University of Cambridge and be offered a place at Cambridge in the normal way. All applicants must have a first class or high second class honours degree, or equivalent and normally be under 26. Candidates must be nominated by the Ministry of Education.
Level of Study: Postgraduate.
Type: Scholarship.
No. of awards offered: 4.
Frequency: Annual.
Value: Scholarships will cover up to the University Composition Fee at the overseas rate; approved College fees; a maintenance allowance sufficient for a single student; a contribution to a return economy airfare.
Length of Study: 1 year.
Study Establishment: Cambridge University.
Country of Study: United Kingdom.
Application Procedure: Candidates must complete a Preliminary Application Form, which can be obtained from local universities, offices of the British Council or the main address. Completed application forms must be returned to the main address. Candidates short-listed will be sent forms for admission to the University of Cambridge and a scholarship application form. These forms must be returned to The Board of Graduate Studies.
Closing Date: September 21st, a full year in advance of the proposed entry date to Cambridge for preliminary application, January 31st for actual application.

For further information contact:

The Board of Graduate Studies
4 Mill Lane, Cambridge, CB2 1TZ, England
Contact: The Secretary

Ministry of Science, Technology and the Environment Cambridge Scholarships

Subjects: All subjects.

Eligibility: The Trusts cannot admit students to the University or any of its Colleges. Applicants for awards from the Trusts must therefore also apply to the University of Cambridge and be offered a place at Cambridge in the normal way. All applicants must have a first class or high second class honours degree, or equivalent and normally be under 26. Candidates must be nominated by the Ministry of Science, Technology and the Environment. For students from Malaysia.
Level of Study: Postgraduate.
Type: Scholarship.
No. of awards offered: 10.
Frequency: Annual.
Value: Scholarships will cover up to: the University Composition Fee at the overseas rate; approved College fees a maintenance allowance sufficient for a single student; a contribution to a return economy airfare.
Length of Study: 1 year.
Study Establishment: Cambridge University.
Country of Study: United Kingdom.
Application Procedure: Candidates must complete a Preliminary Application Form, which can be obtained from local universities, offices of the British Council or the main address. Completed application forms must be returned to the main address. Candidates short-listed will be sent forms for admission to the University of Cambridge and a scholarship application form. These forms must be returned to The Board of Graduate Studies.
Closing Date: September 21st, a full year in advance of the proposed entry date to Cambridge for preliminary application, January 31st for actual application.

For further information contact:

The Board of Graduate Studies
4 Mill Lane, Cambridge, CB2 1TZ, England
Contact: The Secretary

Nepal Cambridge Scholarships

Subjects: All subjects.
Eligibility: The Trusts cannot admit students to the University or any of its Colleges. Applicants for awards from the Trusts must therefore also apply to the University of Cambridge and be offered a place at Cambridge in the normal way. All applicants must have a first class or high second class honours degree, or equivalent and normally be under 26. For students from Nepal.
Level of Study: Postgraduate.
Type: Scholarship.
No. of awards offered: 1.
Frequency: Annual.
Value: The scholarships will cover the University Composition Fee at the overseas rate, approved College fees, a maintenance allowance sufficient for a single student, a contribution to a return economy airfare.
Length of Study: 1 year.
Study Establishment: Cambridge University.
Country of Study: United Kingdom.
Application Procedure: Candidates must complete a Preliminary Application Form, which can be obtained from local universities, offices of the British Council or the main address. Completed application forms must be returned to

the main address. Candidates short-listed will be sent forms for admission to the University of Cambridge and a scholarship application form. These forms must be returned to The Board of Graduate Studies.
Closing Date: September 21st, a full year in advance of the proposed entry date to Cambridge for preliminary application, January 31st for actual application.

For further information contact:

The Board of Graduate Studies
4 Mill Lane, Cambridge, CB2 1TZ, England
Contact: The Secretary

Oxford and Cambridge Society of Bombay Cambridge Shared Scholarship

Subjects: All subjects.
Eligibility: The Trusts cannot admit students to the University or any of its Colleges. Applicants for awards from the Trusts must therefore also apply to the University of Cambridge and be offered a place at Cambridge in the normal way. All applicants must have a first class or high second class honours degree, or equivalent and normally be under 26. For a resident of Bombay City or the state of Maharashtra whose application is supported by the Oxford and Cambridge Society of Bombay.
Level of Study: Postgraduate.
Type: Scholarship.
No. of awards offered: 1.
Frequency: Annual.
Study Establishment: Cambridge University.
Country of Study: United Kingdom.
Application Procedure: Candidates from India may obtain further details and a Preliminary Application Forms by writing before August 17th of the year before entry to The Joint Secretary, Nehru Trust for Cambridge University, Teen Murti House, Teen Murti Marg, New Delhi, 110011, giving details of academic qualifications. Completed forms must be returned to the same address no later than September 9th. Those candidates who are successfully short-listed will be sent forms for admission to the University of Cambridge as a graduate student which should be completed and returned to The Secretary, Board of Graduate Studies, 4 Mill Lane, Cambridge, CB2 1TZ no later than January 31st.
Closing Date: September 9th, preliminary application; January 31st actual application.

Packer Cambridge Scholarships

Subjects: All subjects.
Eligibility: The Trusts cannot admit students to the University or any of its Colleges. Applicants for awards from the Trusts must therefore also apply to the University of Cambridge and be offered a place at Cambridge in the normal way. All applicants must have a first class or high second class honours degree, or equivalent and normally be under 26. For students from Australia.
Level of Study: Doctorate.
Purpose: To support study towards a PhD.
Type: Scholarship.

No. of awards offered: 5.
Frequency: As available.
Value: Scholarships will cover up to the University Composition Fee at the overseas rate; approved College fees; a maintenance allowance sufficient for a single student; a contribution to a return economy airfare.
Length of Study: Tenable for up to 3 years.
Study Establishment: Cambridge University.
Country of Study: United Kingdom.
Application Procedure: Application form for the scholarship will be sent out to eligible candidates once the completed form for admission to the University of Cambridge has reached The Board of Graduate Studies.
Closing Date: Scholarship forms must be returned by April 30th.

For further information contact:

The Board of Graduate Studies
4 Mill Lane, Cambridge, CB2 1TZ, England
Contact: The Secretary

Part-Cost Bursaries - India

Subjects: All subjects.
Eligibility: The Trusts cannot admit students to the University or any of its Colleges. Applicants for awards from the Trusts must therefore also apply to the University of Cambridge and be offered a place at Cambridge in the normal way. All applicants must have a first class or high second class honours degree, or equivalent and normally be under 26. For applicants who are not successful at winning a scholarship.
Level of Study: Unrestricted.
Type: Bursary.
No. of awards offered: Varies.
Value: Determined in the light of the financial circumstances of the applicant.
Study Establishment: Cambridge University.
Country of Study: United Kingdom.

Pok Rafeah Cambridge Scholarship

Subjects: All subjects.
Eligibility: The Trusts cannot admit students to the University or any of its Colleges. Applicants for awards from the Trusts must therefore also apply to the University of Cambridge and be offered a place at Cambridge in the normal way. All applicants must have a first class or high second class honours degree, or equivalent and normally be under 26. Applicants for scholarships for study towards the degree of PhD must be successfully nominated for an ORS award, which covers the difference between the home and overseas rate of the University Composition Fee. For students from Indonesia.
Level of Study: Doctorate, Postgraduate.
Type: Scholarship.
No. of awards offered: 1 for study towards a PhD, 2 for postgraduate study.
Frequency: Annual.

Value: The scholarships will cover the University Composition Fee at the home rate, approved College fees, a maintenance allowance sufficient for a single student, a contribution to a return economy airfare.
Length of Study: Up to 3 years for PhD; 1 year for taught postgraduate course.
Study Establishment: Cambridge University.
Country of Study: United Kingdom.
Application Procedure: Candidates must complete a Preliminary Application Form, which can be obtained from local universities, offices of the British Council or the main address. Completed application forms must be returned to the main address. Candidates short-listed will be sent forms for admission to the University of Cambridge and a scholarship application form. These forms must be returned to The Board of Graduate Studies.
Closing Date: September 21st, a full year in advance of the proposed entry date to Cambridge for preliminary application, January 31st for actual application.

For further information contact:

The Board of Graduate Studies
4 Mill Lane, Cambridge, CB2 1TZ, England
Contact: The Secretary

Poynton Cambridge Scholarships

Subjects: All subjects.
Eligibility: The Trusts cannot admit students to the University or any of its Colleges. Applicants for awards from the Trusts must therefore also apply to the University of Cambridge and be offered a place at Cambridge in the normal way. All applicants must have a first class or high second class honours degree, or equivalent and normally be under 26. For students from Australia.
Level of Study: Doctorate.
Purpose: To assist study towards a PhD.
Type: Scholarship.
No. of awards offered: 5.
Frequency: Annual.
Length of Study: Tenable for up to 3 years.
Study Establishment: Cambridge University.
Country of Study: United Kingdom.
Application Procedure: Application form for the scholarship will be sent out to eligible candidates once the completed form for admission to the University of Cambridge has reached The Board of Graduate Studies.
Closing Date: Scholarship forms must be returned by April 30th.

For further information contact:

The Board of Graduate Studies
4 Mill Lane, Cambridge, CB2 1TZ, England
Contact: The Secretary

President Árpád Göncz Scholarship

Subjects: All subjects.
Eligibility: The Trusts cannot admit students to the University or any of its Colleges. Applicants for awards from the Trusts

must therefore also apply to the University of Cambridge and be offered a place at Cambridge in the normal way. All applicants must have a first class or high second class honours degree, or equivalent and normally be under 26. For a student from Hungary.
Level of Study: Postgraduate.
Purpose: To assist with one year taught postgraduate courses of study. Originally set up to commemorate the visit of the President of Hungary to the University of Cambridge.
Type: Scholarship.
No. of awards offered: 1.
Frequency: Annual.
Value: Scholarships will cover the University Composition Fee at the overseas rate; approved College fees; a maintenance allowance sufficient for a single student; a contribution to a return economy airfare.
Length of Study: 1 year.
Study Establishment: Cambridge University.
Country of Study: United Kingdom.
Application Procedure: Candidates must complete a Preliminary Application Form, which can be obtained from local universities, offices of the British Council or the main address. Completed application forms must be returned to the main address. Candidates short-listed will be sent forms for admission to the University of Cambridge and a scholarship application form. These forms must be returned to The Board of Graduate Studies.
Closing Date: September 21st, a full year in advance of the proposed entry date to Cambridge for preliminary application, January 31st for actual application.

For further information contact:

The Board of Graduate Studies
4 Mill Lane, Cambridge, CB2 1TZ, England
Contact: The Secretary

President Aylwin Studentship

Subjects: All subjects.
Eligibility: The Trusts cannot admit students to the University or any of its Colleges. Applicants for awards from the Trusts must therefore also apply to the University of Cambridge and be offered a place at Cambridge in the normal way. All applicants must have a first class or high second class honours degree, or equivalent and normally be under 26. Applicants must be successfully nominated for an ORS award, which covers the difference between the home and overseas rate of the University Composition Fee. For students from Chile.
Level of Study: Doctorate.
Type: Studentship.
No. of awards offered: 1.
Frequency: Annual.
Value: These studentships will cover the University Composition Fee at the home rate, approved college fees, a maintenance allowance sufficient for a single student, a contribution to a return economy airfare.
Length of Study: Tenable for up to 3 years.
Study Establishment: Cambridge University.
Country of Study: United Kingdom.

Application Procedure: Candidates for these studentships should apply in the first instance to the Agencia de Cooperacion International (AGCI), Providencia 1017, 1er Piso, Santiago from whom Preliminary Application Forms can be obtained.

Closing Date: September 21st, a full year in advance of the proposed entry date to Cambridge for preliminary application, January 31st for actual application.

President's Cambridge Scholarships for One Year Taught Postgraduate Study

Subjects: All subjects.
Eligibility: The Trusts cannot admit students to the University or any of its Colleges. Applicants for awards from the Trusts must therefore also apply to the University of Cambridge and be offered a place at Cambridge in the normal way. All applicants must have a first class or high second class honours degree, or equivalent and normally be under 26. For students from Ghana.
Level of Study: Postgraduate.
Type: Scholarship.
No. of awards offered: Up to 5.
Frequency: Annual.
Length of Study: 1 year.
Study Establishment: Cambridge University.
Country of Study: United Kingdom.
Application Procedure: Candidates must complete a Preliminary Application Form, which can be obtained from local universities, offices of the British Council or the main address. Completed application forms must be returned to the main address. Candidates short-listed will be sent forms for admission to the University of Cambridge and a scholarship application form. These forms must be returned to The Board of Graduate Studies.
Closing Date: September 21st, a full year in advance of the proposed entry date to Cambridge for preliminary application, January 31st for actual application.

For further information contact:

The Board of Graduate Studies
4 Mill Lane, Cambridge, CB2 1TZ, England
Contact: The Secretary

President's Cambridge Scholarships for Study Towards a PhD

Subjects: All subjects.
Eligibility: The Trusts cannot admit students to the University or any of its Colleges. Applicants for awards from the Trusts must therefore also apply to the University of Cambridge and be offered a place at Cambridge in the normal way. All applicants must have a first class or high second class honours degree, or equivalent and normally be under 26. For students from Ghana.
Level of Study: Doctorate.
Type: Scholarship.
No. of awards offered: Up to 5.

Frequency: Annual.
Length of Study: Tenable for up to 3 years.
Study Establishment: Cambridge University.
Country of Study: United Kingdom.
Application Procedure: Candidates must complete a Preliminary Application Form, which can be obtained from local universities, offices of the British Council or the main address. Completed application forms must be returned to the main address. Candidates short-listed will be sent forms for admission to the University of Cambridge and a scholarship application form. These forms must be returned to The Board of Graduate Studies.
Closing Date: September 21st, a full year in advance of the proposed entry date to Cambridge for preliminary application, January 31st for actual application.

For further information contact:

The Board of Graduate Studies
4 Mill Lane, Cambridge, CB2 1TZ, England
Contact: The Secretary

Prince of Wales Scholarships

Subjects: All subjects.
Eligibility: The Trusts cannot admit students to the University or any of its Colleges. Applicants for awards from the Trusts must therefore also apply to the University of Cambridge and be offered a place at Cambridge in the normal way. All applicants must have a first class or high second class honours degree, or equivalent and normally be under 26. For students from New Zealand. All applicants must be successfully nominated for an ORS award, which covers the difference between the home and overseas rate of the University Composition Fee.
Level of Study: Doctorate.
Purpose: To support study towards a PhD.
Type: Scholarship.
No. of awards offered: 5.
Frequency: Annual.
Value: Scholarships will cover the University Composition Fee at the overseas rate; approved College fees; a maintenance allowance sufficient for a single student; a contribution to a return economy airfare.
Length of Study: Tenable for up to 3 years.
Study Establishment: Cambridge University.
Country of Study: United Kingdom.
Application Procedure: Candidates should apply directly to the Scholarships Officer at their own university. Otherwise they should apply directly to the Scholarships Officer at the New Zealand Vice Chancellor's Committee.
Closing Date: October 1st.

For further information contact:

New Zealand Vice Chancellors' Committee
PO Box 11-915
Manners Street, Wellington, New Zealand
Contact: Scholarships Officer

Prince Philip Graduate Exhibitions

Subjects: All subjects.
Eligibility: The Trusts cannot admit students to the University or any of its Colleges. Applicants for awards from the Trusts must therefore also apply to the University of Cambridge and be offered a place at Cambridge in the normal way. All applicants must have a first class or high second class honours degree, or equivalent and normally be under 26. One scholarship will go to a student who has graduated from the Chinese University of Hong Kong and one will go to a student who has graduated from the University of Hong Kong. Applicants must be successfully nominated for an ORS award.
Level of Study: Doctorate.
Type: Scholarship.
No. of awards offered: 2.
Frequency: Annual.
Value: Scholarships will cover the University Composition Fee at the overseas rate; approved College fees; a maintenance allowance sufficient for a single student; a contribution to a return economy airfare.
Length of Study: Up to 3 years.
Study Establishment: Cambridge University.
Country of Study: United Kingdom.
Application Procedure: Candidates must complete a Preliminary Application Form, which can be obtained from local universities, offices of the British Council or the main address. Completed application forms must be returned to the main address. Candidates short-listed will be sent forms for admission to the University of Cambridge and a scholarship application form. These forms must be returned to The Board of Graduate Studies.
Closing Date: September 21st, a full year in advance of the proposed entry date to Cambridge for preliminary application, January 31st for actual application.

For further information contact:

The Board of Graduate Studies
4 Mill Lane, Cambridge, CB2 1TZ, England
Contact: The Secretary

Sally Mugabe Memorial Shared Cambridge Scholarship

Subjects: Preference given to candidates studying subjects relevant to the needs of Zimbabwe, in particular the broad area of social studies relating to the welfare, education and health of women and children.
Eligibility: All applicants must be under the age of 35 on October 1st of the year they are applying for, undertake to return to their own country to work or study after completing the course, not be employed by a government department or by a parastatal organisation, not be at present living or studying in a developed country, and not have undertaken studies lasting a year or more in a developed country. Priority will be given to candidates wishing to pursue a course of study related to the economic and social development of their country. For a woman graduate from Zimbabwe.
Level of Study: Postgraduate.
Type: Scholarship.

No. of awards offered: 1.
Frequency: Annual.
Value: Scholarships will cover the University Composition Fee at the overseas rate; approved College fees; a maintenance allowance sufficient for a single student; a contribution to a return economy airfare.
Length of Study: 1 year.
Study Establishment: Cambridge University.
Country of Study: United Kingdom.
Application Procedure: Candidates must complete a Preliminary Application Form, which can be obtained from local universities, offices of the British Council or the main address. Completed application forms must be returned to the main address. Candidates short-listed will be sent forms for admission to the University of Cambridge and a scholarship application form. These forms must be returned to The Board of Graduate Studies.
Closing Date: September 21st, a full year in advance of the proposed entry date to Cambridge for preliminary application, January 31st for actual application.

For further information contact:

The Board of Graduate Studies
4 Mill Lane, Cambridge, CB2 1TZ, England
Contact: The Secretary

Schlumberger Cambridge Scholarships

Subjects: All subjects.
Eligibility: The Trusts cannot admit students to the University or any of its Colleges. Applicants for awards from the Trusts must therefore also apply to the University of Cambridge and be offered a place at Cambridge in the normal way. All applicants must have a first class or high second class honours degree or equivalent and normally be under 26. For students from a developing country.
Level of Study: Doctorate.
Type: Scholarship.
No. of awards offered: 1.
Frequency: Annual.
Value: Scholarships will cover the University Composition Fee at the overseas rate; approved College fees; a maintenance allowance sufficient for a single student; a contribution to a return economy airfare.
Length of Study: Tenable for up to 3 years.
Study Establishment: Cambridge University.
Country of Study: United Kingdom.
Application Procedure: Candidates must complete a Preliminary Application Form, which can be obtained from local universities, offices of the British Council or the main address. Completed application forms must be returned to the main address. Candidates short-listed will be sent forms for admission to the University of Cambridge and a scholarship application form. These forms must be returned to The Board of Graduate Studies.
Closing Date: September 21st, a full year in advance of the proposed entry date to Cambridge for preliminary application, January 31st for actual application.

For further information contact:

The Board of Graduate Studies
4 Mill Lane, Cambridge, CB2 1TZ, England
Contact: The Secretary

South African College Bursaries

Subjects: All subjects.
Eligibility: The Trusts cannot admit students to the University or any of its Colleges. Applicants for awards from the Trusts must therefore also apply to the University of Cambridge and be offered a place at Cambridge in the normal way. All applicants must have a first class or high second class honours degree, or equivalent and normally be under 26. For students from South Africa.
Purpose: To enable citizens of South and Southern Africa to take up college places at Cambridge.
Type: Bursary.
No. of awards offered: Varies.
Study Establishment: Cambridge University.
Country of Study: United Kingdom.
Application Procedure: Candidates must complete a Preliminary Application Form, which can be obtained from local universities, offices of the British Council or the main address. Completed application forms must be returned to the main address. Candidates short-listed will be sent forms for admission to the University of Cambridge and a scholarship application form. These forms must be returned to The Board of Graduate Studies.
Closing Date: September 21st, a full year in advance of the proposed entry date to Cambridge for preliminary application, January 31st for actual application.
Additional Information: The bursaries are normally held in conjunction with other awards from Cambridge Commonwealth Trust and other sources.

For further information contact:

The Board of Graduate Studies
4 Mill Lane, Cambridge, CB2 1TZ, England
Contact: The Secretary

Tan Sri Lim Goh Tong Cambridge Bursaries

Subjects: All subjects.
Eligibility: The Trusts cannot admit students to the University or any of its Colleges. Applicants for awards from the Trusts must therefore also apply to the University of Cambridge and be offered a place at Cambridge in the normal way. All applicants must have a first class or high second class honours degree, or equivalent and normally be under 26. For students from Malaysia.
Level of Study: Unrestricted.
Type: Bursary.
Frequency: Annual.
Value: The value will normally be at a fixed rate of up to £2,000 per annum to be held in conjunction with other awards from the Cambridge Commonwealth Trust or other sources. Candidates will be means tested.
Study Establishment: Cambridge University.
Country of Study: United Kingdom.

Application Procedure: Candidates must complete a Preliminary Application Form, which can be obtained from local universities, offices of the British Council or the main address. Completed application forms must be returned to the main address. Candidates short-listed will be sent forms for admission to the University of Cambridge and a scholarship application form. These forms must be returned to The Board of Graduate Studies.
Closing Date: September 21st, a full year in advance of the proposed entry date to Cambridge for preliminary application, January 31st for actual application.

For further information contact:

The Board of Graduate Studies
4 Mill Lane, Cambridge, CB2 1TZ, England
Contact: The Secretary

Tanzania Cambridge Scholarship

Subjects: All subjects.
Eligibility: The Trusts cannot admit students to the University or any of its Colleges. Applicants for awards from the Trusts must therefore also apply to the University of Cambridge and be offered a place at Cambridge in the normal way. All applicants must have a first class or high second class honours degree, or equivalent and normally be under 26. For a student from Tanzania. Applicants must be successfully nominated for an ORS award, which covers the difference between the home and overseas rate of the University Composition Fee.
Level of Study: Doctorate.
Type: Scholarship.
No. of awards offered: 1.
Frequency: Annual.
Value: Scholarships will cover the University Composition Fee at the overseas rate; approved College fees; a maintenance allowance sufficient for a single student; a contribution to a return economy airfare.
Length of Study: Tenable for up to 3 years.
Study Establishment: Cambridge University.
Country of Study: United Kingdom.
Application Procedure: Candidates must complete a Preliminary Application Form, which can be obtained from local universities, offices of the British Council or the main address. Completed application forms must be returned to the main address. Candidates short-listed will be sent forms for admission to the University of Cambridge and a scholarship application form. These forms must be returned to The Board of Graduate Studies.
Closing Date: September 21st, a full year in advance of the proposed entry date to Cambridge for preliminary application, January 31st for actual application.

For further information contact:

The Board of Graduate Studies
4 Mill Lane, Cambridge, CB2 1TZ, England
Contact: The Secretary

Tanzania Cambridge Shared Scholarships

Subjects: All subjects.
Eligibility: The Trusts cannot admit students to the University or any of its Colleges. Applicants for awards from the Trusts must therefore also apply to the University of Cambridge and be offered a place at Cambridge in the normal way. All applicants must have a first class or high second class honours degree, or equivalent. For students from Tanzania. Applicants must be under the age of 35 on October 1st of the year they are applying for; return to their own country to work or study after completing the course at Cambridge; not be employed by a government department or by a parastatal organisation; not at present be living or studying in a developed country; not have undertaken studies lasting a year or more in a developed country. Priority will be given to candidates wishing to pursue a course of study related to the economic and social development of their country.
Level of Study: Postgraduate.
Type: Scholarship.
No. of awards offered: Up to 4.
Frequency: Annual.
Value: Scholarships will cover the University Composition Fee at the overseas rate; approved College fees; a maintenance allowance sufficient for a single student; a contribution to a return economy airfare.
Length of Study: 1 year.
Study Establishment: Cambridge University.
Country of Study: United Kingdom.
Application Procedure: Candidates must complete a Preliminary Application Form, which can be obtained from local universities, offices of the British Council or the main address. Completed application forms must be returned to the main address. Candidates short-listed will be sent forms for admission to the University of Cambridge and a scholarship application form. These forms must be returned to The Board of Graduate Studies.
Closing Date: September 21st, a full year in advance of the proposed entry date to Cambridge for preliminary application, January 31st for actual application.

For further information contact:

The Board of Graduate Studies
4 Mill Lane, Cambridge, CB2 1TZ, England
Contact: The Secretary

Tate and Lyle/FCO Cambridge Scholarships

Subjects: All subjects.
Eligibility: The Trusts cannot admit students to the University or any of its Colleges. Applicants for awards from the Trusts must therefore also apply to the University of Cambridge and be offered a place at Cambridge in the normal way. All applicants must have a first class or high second class honours degree, or equivalent and normally be under 26. Successful applicants will be expected to return to their home country at the end of the course of study at Cambridge. Open to students from Barbados, Belize, the Eastern Caribbean States, Fiji, Guyana, Jamaica and Trinidad and Tobago, Hungary, Slovakia, Ukraine, Mauritius, Mexico, Saudi Arabia, the Philippines, Swaziland, Zambia, Zimbabwe, Vietnam.

Level of Study: Postgraduate.
Purpose: To assist one year taught postgraduate courses of study.
Type: Scholarship.
No. of awards offered: Up to 10.
Frequency: Annual.
Value: Scholarships will cover the University Composition Fee at the overseas rate; approved College fees; a maintenance allowance sufficient for a single student; a contribution to a return economy airfare.
Study Establishment: Cambridge University.
Country of Study: United Kingdom.
Application Procedure: Candidates must complete a Preliminary Application Form, which can be obtained from local universities, offices of the British Council or the main address. Completed application forms must be returned to the main address. Candidates short-listed will be sent forms for admission to the University of Cambridge and a scholarship application form. These forms must be returned to The Board of Graduate Studies.
Closing Date: September 21st, a full year in advance of the proposed entry date to Cambridge for preliminary application, January 31st for actual application.

For further information contact:

The Board of Graduate Studies
4 Mill Lane, Cambridge, CB2 1TZ, England
Contact: The Secretary

Tidmarsh Cambridge Scholarship

Subjects: All subjects.
Eligibility: The Trusts cannot admit students to the University or any of its Colleges. Applicants for awards from the Trusts must therefore also apply to the University of Cambridge and be offered a place at Cambridge in the normal way. All applicants must: have a first class or high second class honours degree or equivalent and normally be under 26. For students from Canada who have been successfully nominated for an ORS award, which covers the difference between the home and overseas rate of the University Composition Fee.
Level of Study: Doctorate.
Purpose: To assist study towards a PhD.
Type: Scholarship.
No. of awards offered: 1.
Frequency: As available.
Value: The scholarship will pay the University Composition Fee at the home rate, approved College fees and a maintenance allowance sufficient for a single student.
Study Establishment: Cambridge University.
Country of Study: United Kingdom.
Application Procedure: Application form for the scholarship will be sent out to eligible candidates once the completed form for admission to the University of Cambridge has reached the Board of Graduate Studies.
Closing Date: Scholarship forms must be returned by April 30th.

For further information contact:

The Board for Graduate Studies
4 Mill Lane, Cambridge, CB2 1TZ, England
Contact: The Secretary

Zambia Cambridge Scholarships

Subjects: All subjects.
Eligibility: The Trusts cannot admit students to the University or any of its Colleges. Applicants for awards from the Trusts must therefore also apply to the University of Cambridge and be offered a place at Cambridge in the normal way. All applicants must have a first class or high second class honours degree, or equivalent and normally be under 26. For a student from Zambia.
Level of Study: Doctorate, Postgraduate.
Type: Scholarship.
No. of awards offered: 1 PhD, 1 postgraduate study.
Frequency: As available.
Value: Scholarships will cover the University Composition Fee at the overseas rate; approved College fees; a maintenance allowance sufficient for a single student; a contribution to a return economy airfare.
Length of Study: Tenable for up to 3 years; 1 year for postgraduate study.
Study Establishment: Cambridge University.
Country of Study: United Kingdom.
Application Procedure: Candidates must complete a Preliminary Application Form, which can be obtained from local universities, offices of the British Council or the main address. Completed application forms must be returned to the main address. Candidates short-listed will be sent forms for admission to the University of Cambridge and a scholarship application form. These forms must be returned to The Board of Graduate Studies.
Closing Date: September 21st, a full year in advance of the proposed entry date to Cambridge for preliminary application, January 31st for actual application.

For further information contact:

The Board of Graduate Studies
4 Mill Lane, Cambridge, CB2 1TZ, England
Contact: The Secretary

Zimbabwe Cambridge Scholarships

Subjects: All subjects.
Eligibility: The Trusts cannot admit students to the University or any of its Colleges. Applicants for awards from the Trusts must therefore also apply to the University of Cambridge and be offered a place at Cambridge in the normal way. All applicants must have a first class or high second class honours degree, or equivalent and normally be under 26. All applicants for the PhD must be successfully nominated for an ORS award which pays the difference between home and overseas rate of the University Composition Fee. For a student from Zimbabwe.
Level of Study: Doctorate, Postgraduate.
Type: Scholarship.
No. of awards offered: 1 PhD, 1 postgraduate study.

Frequency: As available.
Value: Scholarships will cover: the University Composition Fee at the overseas rate; approved College fees; a maintenance allowance sufficient for a single student; a contribution to a return economy airfare.
Length of Study: 3 years- PhD; 1 year postgraduate study.
Study Establishment: Cambridge University.
Country of Study: United Kingdom.
Application Procedure: Candidates must complete a Preliminary Application Form, which can be obtained from local universities, offices of the British Council or the main address. Completed application forms must be returned to the main address. Candidates short-listed will be sent forms for admission to the University of Cambridge and a scholarship application form. These forms must be returned to The Board of Graduate Studies.
Closing Date: September 21st, a full year in advance of the proposed entry date to Cambridge for preliminary application, January 31st for actual application.

For further information contact:

The Board of Graduate Studies
4 Mill Lane, Cambridge, CB2 1TZ, England
Contact: The Secretary

THE CANADIAN BLOOD SERVICES

1800 Alta Vista Drive, Ottawa, ON, K1G 4J5, Canada
www: http://www.bloodservices.ca
Contact: The Research Director

Canadian Blood Services Career Development Fellowship Awards

Subjects: Blood services testing.
Eligibility: Candidates must hold a recent PhD (or equivalent research degree) or an MD/DDS/DVM, plus a recent research degree in an appropriate health field (minimum MSc) or equivalent research experience, must not be registered for a higher degree at the time of acceptance of the award, nor undertake formal studies for such a degree during the period of appointment.
Purpose: To support highly qualified candidates who have recently completed their formal research training and wish to acquire further experience in a blood services setting. It is expected that candidates will be interested in a career in research related to blood and blood products, including the impact of infectious diseases, upon completion of their award, but this is not a condition of the award.
Type: Fellowship.
No. of awards offered: 2.
Value: The value of each fellowship is related to the major degree(s) and experience the applicant holds. The Fellowship offers a stipend based on current Medical Research Council rates for each of one of three years, as well as a first year rersearch allowance of C$10,000.
Length of Study: 1-3 years.

Application Procedure: Candidates are required to complete a an application form (RD40). Applications must be made through and with the support of the Medical Officer of the Blood Centre at which the applicant intends to work. Complete details are contained in the guide and application forms which may be obtained form the Medical Office of the closest Canadian Blood Services Centre or from Manager, Research and Development at the main address.
Closing Date: January 15th.

Canadian Blood Services Research and Development Programme - Individual Grants

Subjects: Research into blood.
Eligibility: Available to Principal Investigators who are staff members at one of the CBS centres.
Purpose: To carry out research in all areas on the collection, testing, processing and therapeutic use of blood and blood products in order to maximise effectiveness, to minimise risk to the health of donor and recipient, to minimise cost of products and service and to ensure that all applicable and validated scientific advances in blood transfusion therapy and related fields are incorporated in a timely fashion for the benefit of the public.
Type: Grant.
Value: To cover materials, supplies, equipment, travel and laboratory personnel.
Length of Study: 1, 2 or 3 year period of research.
Application Procedure: Applications must be submitted on CBS Form RD10. Applications and guidelines may be obtained from any of the Canadian Blood Services Centres across the country or from the Manager, Research and Development, at the main address.
Closing Date: Deadline for letter of intent December 15th, deadline for full application February 15th.

Canadian Blood Services Research and Development Programme - Major Equipment Grants

Subjects: Research into blood.
Purpose: To carry out research in all areas on the collection, testing, processing and therapeutic use of blood and blood products in order to maximise effectiveness, to minimise risk to the health of donor and recipient, to minimise cost of products and service and to ensure that all applicable and validated scientific advances in blood transfusion therapy and related fields are incorporated in a timely fashion for the benefit of the public.
Type: Grant.
Frequency: Annual.
Value: For the purchase of specific items of permanent and otherwise unavailable equipment costing US$10,000 or more, necessary for research relevant to the CBS R&D Program. Less expensive items of equipment are provided for under the Individual and Group Grants and the Request for Proposal.
Application Procedure: Applications must be submitted on CBS Form RD30. Applications and guidelines may be obtained from any of the Canadian Blood Services Centres across the country or from the Manager, Research and Development, at the main address.
Closing Date: Deadline for letter of intent December 15th, deadline for full application February 15th.

Canadian Blood Services Transfusion Medicine Fellowship Awards

Subjects: Transfusion medicine.
Eligibility: Candidates must be in the final year of preparation for certifying examinations by the Royal College of Physicians and Surgeons, or should be newly qualified in a speciality of the Royal College. Priority will be given to those with interest and experience in areas of infectious diseases, epidemiology, public health and blood utilisation.
Purpose: Support for physicians in Canada to require training in transfusion medicine through exposure to the work carried out in the Canadian Blood Services Centres. It is intended that successful candidates will have some commitment to transfusion medicine in their future career plans.
Type: Fellowship.
No. of awards offered: 2.
Value: The fellowship offers a stipend based on the current level of house staff salaries appropriate to the level of training, provided for in the provincial scale of the province in which the Fellowship is awarded, as well as a first year research and travel allowance of C$10,000.
Length of Study: 1 or 2 years.
Application Procedure: Application form TM-95 must be completed. Applications must be made through and with the support of the Medical Officer of the Blood Centre at which the applicant intends to work. Application forms are available from the Medical Officers at one of the fifteen Canadian Blood Services Centres acroos Canada, or at the main address.
Closing Date: January 15th.

CANADIAN BUREAU FOR INTERNATIONAL EDUCATION (CBIE)

220 Laurier Avenue West
Suite 1100, Ottawa, ON, K1P 5Z9, Canada
Tel: (1) 613 237 4820
Fax: (1) 613 237 1073
Email: gbeauoloirn@cbie.ca
www: http://www.cbie.ca
Contact: Grants Management Officer

The Canadian Bureau for International Education (CBIE) is a national non-profit association comprising educational institutions, organisations and individuals dedicated to internal education and intercultural training. CBIE's mission is to promote the free movement of learners and trainees across national boarders. Activities include advocacy, research and information services, training programmes, scholarship management, professional development for international educators and a host of other services for members and learners.

Celanese Canada Internationalist Fellowships

Subjects: All subjects.
Eligibility: Applications are considered in an annual competition. Application is open to Canadians and permanent residents of Canada who hold at least one university degree, or are in the final year of a degree programme. College graduates (post-secondary level) holding a recognised bachelor's degree are also eligible. The latest degree must have been awarded no longer than five years from the date of application Applicants must have achieved a high academic standing. The fellowshgips are tenable anywhere in the world outside Canada.
Type: Fellowship.
No. of awards offered: 25.
Frequency: Annual.
Value: C$10,000 non-renewable.
Length of Study: A minimum of 8 consecutive months including at least 4 taught months of study courses.
Country of Study: Any country.
Application Procedure: Application forms are available at CBIE's website. To receive printed or electronic versions please write to the main address or email flepage@cbie.ca or gbeaudoin@cbie.ca. Applicants must submit a completed application form, a letter of intent outlining the proposed study programme abroad, curriculum vitae, academic transcripts, and two letters of reference, (one academic and one personal).
Closing Date: March 1st (date subject to change so check before applying).

CANADIAN CYSTIC FIBROSIS FOUNDATION

2221 Yonge Street 601, Toronto, ON, M4S 2B4, Canada
Tel: (1) 416 485 9149
Fax: (1) 416 485 0960
Email: kethier@ccff.ca
www: http://www.ccfa/~cfwww/index.html
Contact: Ms Karen Ethier, Research Programmes Co-ordinator

Since 1960, the Canadian Cystic Fibrosis Foundation has worked to provide a brighter future for every child born with CF. Through its research and clinical programmes, the Foundation helps to provide outstanding care for affected individuals, while pursuing the quest for a cure or control.

Canadian Cystic Fibrosis Foundation Fellowships

Subjects: Biomedical or behavioural science pertinent to cystic fibrosis.
Eligibility: Open to individuals who are graduates of a medical school or who hold a PhD degree. Medical graduates

should have already completed their basic core years of residency training. Applications for a Fellowship in a clinical area must have a strong component of research in the proposed programme. Clinical, non-research residency-type fellowships will not be awarded. Canadian Fellowship applicants of exceptional quality requesting funding to study abroad will be considered. Applications will be strengthened by an indication of intention to return to Canada.
Level of Study: Doctorate, Postdoctorate.
Purpose: To encourage research training, basic research or clinical research.
Type: Fellowship.
No. of awards offered: Varies.
Frequency: Annual.
Value: Varies.
Length of Study: 2 years; renewable for 1 further year.
Study Establishment: Any approved university, hospital or research institute.
Country of Study: Canada.
Application Procedure: Please write for details.
Closing Date: October 1st, April 1st.

Canadian Cystic Fibrosis Foundation Research Grants

Subjects: Scientific research concentrating on cystic fibrosis.
Eligibility: Please write for details.
Level of Study: Postgraduate.
Purpose: To provide research grants that are intended to facilitate the scientific investigation of all aspects of cystic fibrosis.
Type: Research Grant.
Frequency: Annual.
Value: The amount of a grant will be determined by the medical/scientific advisory committee, following a detailed review of the applicant's proposed budget.
Length of Study: Research grants are awarded for a term of 1, 2, or in a limited number of instances, 3 years.
Study Establishment: A Canadian Institution.
Country of Study: Canada.
Application Procedure: Please write for details.
Closing Date: Applications must be received by the Foundation no later than October 1st. Incomplete or late applications will be returned to the applicant.
Additional Information: Investigators are eligible to hold more than one research grant. No more than one initial application may be submitted to a single competition; and it is a requirement that the focus of a second grant be clearly delineated form the first one. The specific aims of a second grant should represent new approaches to the CF problem, and not an extension of an existing research program.

Canadian Cystic Fibrosis Foundation Research Grants Scholarships for Research in Cystic Fibrosis

Subjects: Cystic fibrosis.
Eligibility: Open to holders of an MD or PhD degree who may recently have completed training or who are established investigators wishing to devote major research effort to cystic

fibrosis. The beginning investigator should have demonstrated promise of ability to initiate and carry out independent research; the established investigator should have a published record of excellent scientific research.
Level of Study: Doctorate, Postgraduate.
Purpose: To allow investigators the opportunity to develop outstanding research programmes unhampered by heavy teaching or clinical loads.
Type: Scholarship.
No. of awards offered: Varies.
Frequency: Annual.
Value: Salary support, dependent on the qualifications and experience of the Scholar and determined according to prevailing rates.
Length of Study: 3 years; renewable for a further 2 years on receipt of a satisfactory progress report.
Study Establishment: Any approved university, hospital or research institute.
Country of Study: Canada.
Application Procedure: Please write for details.
Closing Date: October 1st.

Canadian Cystic Fibrosis Foundation Studentships

Subjects: Biomedical and behavioural sciences relevant to the study of cystic fibrosis.
Eligibility: Studentships are awarded for studies at the Master's or doctoral levels.
Level of Study: Doctorate, Postgraduate.
Purpose: To support highly qualified graduate students who are registered for a higher degree, and who are undertaking full-time research training in areas of the biomedical or behavioural sciences relevant to cystic fibrosis.
Type: Studentship.
No. of awards offered: Varies.
Frequency: Annual.
Value: The value of a CCFF Studentship is reviewed on an annual basis, and is commensurate with prevailing Canadian rates.
Length of Study: Initial studentships are awarded for a term of 2 years. Routine notification will be required from the supervisor by October 1st indicating that the student has taken up the award and that he or she plans to proceed through the second year.
Study Establishment: Awards are tenable only at Canadian universities.
Country of Study: Canada.
Application Procedure: Please write for details. Applications must be received by the Foundation no later than October 1st/April 1st. Incomplete or late applications will be returned to the applicant.
Closing Date: October 1st, April 1st.

Visiting Scientist Awards

Subjects: Biomedical and behavioural sciences relevant to the study of cystic fibrosis.
Eligibility: Please write for details.

Level of Study: Postgraduate, Professional development.
Type: Travel Grant.
No. of awards offered: A limited number.
Frequency: Dependent on funds available.
Value: Varies.
Length of Study: Varies.
Country of Study: Any country.
Application Procedure: Please write for details.
Closing Date: Applications may be submitted at any time, but the Foundation should be consulted in advance with respect to the availablilty of funds.

CANADIAN FEDERATION OF UNIVERSITY WOMEN (CFUW)

251 Bank Street
Suite 600, Ottawa, ON, K2P1X3, Canada
Tel: (1) 613 234 2732
Email: cfuw.ho@sympatico.ca
www: http://www.cfuw.ca
Contact: Ms Dorothy Howland, Chair of the Fellowships Committee

Founded in 1919, the Canadian Federation of University Women is a voluntary, non-partisan, non-profit, self-funded bilingual organisation of 10,000 women university graduates. CFUW members are active in public affairs, working to raise the social, economic, and legal status of women, as well as to improve education, the environment, peace, justice, and human rights.

Alice E Wilson Awards

Subjects: All subjects.
Eligibility: Open to women who are Canadian citizens or have held landed immigrant status for at least one year prior to submitting application. Candidates should have a Bachelor's degree or its equivalent from a recognised university, not necessarily in Canada. Special consideration is given to candidates returning to study after at least three years. Candidates must have been accepted into the proposed programme of study.
Level of Study: Postgraduate.
Purpose: To assist women's study. Special consideration is given to candidates returning to study after at least three years.
No. of awards offered: Varies.
Frequency: Annual.
Value: C$1,000.
Study Establishment: Recognised university.
Country of Study: Any country.
Application Procedure: Application forms are available from the Federation.
Closing Date: November 15th.

Beverley Jackson Fellowship

Subjects: All subjects.
Eligibility: Open to women over the age of 35 at the time of application who are enrolled in graduate work at an Ontario university. Candidates should hold at least a Bachelor's degree or equivalent from a recognised university and be Canadian citizens or have held landed immigrant status for at least one year prior to submission of application and must have been accepted into the proposed programme of study.
Level of Study: Postgraduate.
Purpose: To provide partial funding for graduate study.
Type: Fellowship.
No. of awards offered: 1.
Frequency: Annual.
Value: C$3,000.
Study Establishment: A recognised university in Ontario.
Country of Study: Canada.
Application Procedure: Please write for details.
Closing Date: November 15th.
Additional Information: The Fellowship is funded by UWC North York.

CFUW 1989 Polytechnique Commemorative Award

Subjects: Any subject, with special consideration given to study of issues related to women.
Eligibility: Open to women who hold at least a Bachelor's degree or equivalent from a recognised university, who are Canadian citizens or have held landed immigrant status for at least one year, and who are able to justify the relevance of their work to women.
Level of Study: Postgraduate.
Purpose: To provide partial funding for graduate study.
No. of awards offered: 1.
Frequency: Annual.
Value: C$2,400.
Study Establishment: Recognised University.
Country of Study: Any country.
Application Procedure: Please write for details.
Closing Date: November 15th.

CFUW Professional Fellowship

Subjects: All subjects.
Eligibility: Open to women who are Canadian citizens or who have held landed immigrant status for at least one year prior to submitting application. Candidates should hold a bachelor's degree or its equivalent from a recognised Canadian university and wish to pursue graduate work at Master's degree level.
Level of Study: Postgraduate.
Purpose: To provide partial funding for graduate study at Master's degree level.
Type: Fellowship.
No. of awards offered: 1.
Frequency: Annual.
Value: C$5,000 paid in two half-yearly instalments.
Study Establishment: A recognised university.
Country of Study: Any country.

Application Procedure: Please write for details.
Closing Date: November 15th.
Additional Information: The Fellowship is not renewable. Application forms are available from the Federation.

The Dr Marion Elder Grant Fellowship

Subjects: All subjects.
Eligibility: Open to women who have a Bachelor's degree or equivalent from a recognised university, who are Canadian citizens or have held landed immigrant status for at least one year prior to submission of application and who have been accepted into the proposed programme of study. All things being equal, preference will be given to the holder of an Acadia University degree.
Level of Study: Postgraduate.
Purpose: To provide partial funding for full-time graduate study.
Type: Fellowship.
No. of awards offered: 1.
Frequency: Annual.
Value: C$8,000.
Study Establishment: Recognised University.
Country of Study: Any country.
Application Procedure: Please write for details.
Closing Date: November 15th.

Georgette Lemoyne Award

Subjects: All subjects.
Eligibility: Open to women who have a Bachelor's degree or equivalent from a recognised university and who are Canadian citizens or have held landed immigrant status for at least one year prior to submission of application and who have been accepted into the proposed programme of study.
Level of Study: Postgraduate.
Purpose: To provide partial funding for graduate study.
No. of awards offered: 1.
Frequency: Annual.
Value: C$1,000.
Study Establishment: A Canadian university where one language of administration and instruction is French.
Country of Study: Canada.
Application Procedure: Application forms are available from the Federation.
Closing Date: November 15th.

Margaret McWilliams Predoctoral Fellowship

Subjects: All subjects.
Eligibility: Open to women who are Canadian citizens or who have held landed immigrant status for at least one year prior to submission of application. A candidate should hold a Bachelor's degree or its equivalent from a recognised university, not necessarily in Canada, and be a full-time student at an advanced stage (at least one year) in her doctoral programme.
Level of Study: Doctorate.
Purpose: To provide funding for doctoral study.
Type: Fellowship.
No. of awards offered: 1.

Frequency: Annual.
Value: C$10,000 paid in two half-yearly instalments.
Country of Study: Any country.
Application Procedure: Please write for details.
Closing Date: November 15th.
Additional Information: The Fellowship is not renewable. Application forms are available from the Federation.

CANADIAN FOUNDATION FOR THE STUDY OF INFANT DEATHS

586 Eglinton Avenue East
Suite 308, Toronto, ON, M4P 1P2, Canada
Tel: (1) 416 488 3260
Fax: (1) 416 488 3864
Email: sidscanada@inforamp.net
www: http://www.sidscanada.org/sids.html
Contact: Executive Director

The Canadian Foundation for the Study of Infant Deaths is a federally incorporated charitable organisation which was set up in 1973 to respond to the needs of families experiencing a sudden and unexpected infant death. It is the only organisation in Canada solely dedicated to finding the cause(s) of Sudden Infant Death Syndrome, its effect on families, and to the education of the public.

Dr Sydney Segal Research Grants

Subjects: Any discipline (medical, psychological, nursing, biological, sociological) which is concerned with the causes, effects and/or prevention of Sudden Infant Death Syndrome.
Eligibility: Open to suitably qualified graduate students who are undertaking full-time training in research in the health sciences leading to an MSc or PhD or the equivalent (studentship level) and to suitably qualified persons who are undertaking higher-level training in research into Sudden Infant Death Syndrome (fellowship level).
Level of Study: Doctorate, Postdoctorate, Postgraduate.
Purpose: To enable students to pursue full-time higher degree studies researching into the possible causes, effects and/or prevention of Sudden Infant Death Syndrome.
Type: Research Grant.
No. of awards offered: up to 20.
Frequency: Annual.
Value: In accordance with current MRC stipends for studentships and fellowships.
Length of Study: Normally 1 year.
Study Establishment: A Canadian university.
Country of Study: Canada.
Application Procedure: Application forms are available from the Foundation. Completed forms should be submmitted together with references from the Head of Department of the university where the applicant wishes to conduct research and other documents which are listed in more detail on the application form.
Closing Date: June 1st.

CANADIAN LIVER FOUNDATION

365 Bloor Street East
Suite 200, Toronto, ON, M4W 3L4, Canada
Tel: (1) 416 964 1953
Fax: (1) 416 964 0024
Email: clf@liver.ca
www: http://www.liver.ca
Contact: The Executive Director

The Canadian Liver Foundation provides support for research and education into the causes, diagnosis, prevention and treatment of diseases to the liver.

Canadian Liver Foundation Establishment Grants

Subjects: Hepatology.
Eligibility: Open to clinical investigators and basic scientists who hold an MD or PhD degree or equivalent and have a proven interest in the structure and function of the liver or its diseases. Applicants must have completed a minimum of two and preferably three years' formal research training (post-medical speciality training in the case of MDs) and have obtained additional research experience as a clinical investigator.
Level of Study: Doctorate, Postgraduate.
Purpose: To help young investigators to become established within three years of their first academic appointment with the clear intent for ongoing research in liver disorders.
Type: Grant.
Frequency: Annual.
Value: Up to C$60,000 per year.
Length of Study: 2 years.
Study Establishment: At the recipient's own laboratory in a Canadian university.
Country of Study: Canada.
Application Procedure: Please write for details.
Closing Date: November 1st.

Canadian Liver Foundation Fellowships

Subjects: Hepatic function or disease.
Eligibility: Open to holders of an MD or PhD who are Canadian citizens normally resident in Canada or researchers resident in Canada at the time of application. Canadian citizens and landed immigrants will receive first consideration, others will be considered if the situation permits.
Level of Study: Doctorate, Postgraduate.
Purpose: To provide support for specialised clinical or experimental training for those who have already completed the basic graduate programme.
Type: Fellowship.
Frequency: Annual.
Value: Equivalent to current scales of other national Fellowship awards.
Length of Study: 1 year; renewable once.
Country of Study: Any country.
Application Procedure: Please write for details.
Closing Date: November 1st.

Canadian Liver Foundation Graduate Studentships

Subjects: Any discipline relevant to the objectives of the Canadian Liver Foundation.
Eligibility: Candidates must be accepted into a full-time university graduate science programme in a medically related discipline related to a Master's or Doctoral degree and hold a record of superior academic performance in studies relevant to the proposed training.
Level of Study: Doctorate, Postgraduate.
Purpose: To enable academically superior students to undertake full-time studies in a Canadian university.
Type: Studentship.
No. of awards offered: Up to 4.
Frequency: Annual.
Value: A stipend equivalent to that awarded by a Medical Research Council of Canada studentship award.
Length of Study: 1 year; renewable up to 3 times.
Country of Study: Canada.
Application Procedure: Please write for details.
Closing Date: February 15th.
Additional Information: A student supported by the Foundation must not hold a current stipend award from another granting agency.

Canadian Liver Foundation Operating Grant

Subjects: Hepatology.
Eligibility: Open to hepatobiliary research investigators who hold an academic appointment in a Canadian institution.
Level of Study: Professional development.
Purpose: To support research projects directed towards a defined objective.
Type: Grant.
Frequency: Dependent on funds available.
Value: C$60,000 per year.
Country of Study: Canada.
Application Procedure: Application forms plus supporting documentation must be submitted.
Closing Date: December 15th.

THE CANADIAN NATIONAL INSTITUTE FOR THE BLIND (CNIB)

1929 Bayview Avenue, Toronto, ON, M4G 3E8, Canada
Tel: (1) 416 480 7707
Fax: (1) 416 480 7000
Email: millins@east.cnib.ca
www: http://www.cnib.ca
Contact: Ms Sandra Millington, Executive Assistant

The Canadian National Institute for the Blind is a voluntary, non-profit rehabilitation agency that provides services for people who are blind, visually impaired or deafblind. The CNIB provides consultation in safe and efficient travel training, braille, tape and electronic information, employment, environmental accessibility, government and community entitlements, technology, sight enhancement, eye banks and community integration.

E A Baker Fellowship/Grant

Subjects: Ophthalmology.
Eligibility: Open to Canadians for research or study in Canada or abroad if returning to practice in Canada, with priority given to university teaching.
Level of Study: Professional development.
Purpose: To further the prevention of blindness in Canada.
Type: Fellowship, Grant.
No. of awards offered: Varies.
Frequency: Annual.
Value: C$40,000.
Length of Study: 2 years.
Country of Study: Any country.
Application Procedure: Please visit the website for information and an application form.
Closing Date: December 1st.

CANADIAN NURSES FOUNDATION

50 Driveway, Ottawa, ON, K2P 1E2, Canada
Tel: (1) 613 237 2133
Fax: (1) 613 237 3520
Email: cnf@cnursesfdn.ca
www: http://www.can-nurses.ca/cnf
Contact: Ms Beverly Campbell

The Canadian Nurses Foundation (CNF) is a registered charity founded in 1962. It is the only national foundation committed to promoting the health of Canadians through the advancement of the nurses profession by financially supporting Canadian nurses in pursuing further education, research, or certification in their speciality. The CNF is funded through donations from corporations, nursing associations, and individuals - it does not receive support from any level of government.

CNF Scholarships and Fellowships

Subjects: All nursing specialities, several awards are identified for neuro-surgical, oncology, community health nursing, epidemiology, gerontology, child/family health care, nursing administration, occupational health, northern nursing, dialysis nursing.
Eligibility: Open to Canadian nurses who are members of the Canadian Nurses Foundation.
Level of Study: Doctorate, Postgraduate, Baccalaureate.
Purpose: To assist Canadian nurses pursuing further education and research.
Type: Scholarship, Fellowship.
No. of awards offered: Varies.
Frequency: Annual.

Value: C$3,000-C$3,500 for a Master's programme; C$4,500-C$6,000 for a doctoral programme; C$1,500-C$2,000 for a baccalaureate programme.
Length of Study: 1 year.
Country of Study: Any country.
Application Procedure: Please write for details or visit our website.
Closing Date: April 15th.
Additional Information: In accepting an award from the Foundation, a recipient agrees to serve in a nursing position in Canada for a period of one year for each year of financial assistance and to submit to CNF a copy of any thesis, study or major paper undertaken as part of the course.

CANADIAN PHARMACISTS ASSOCIATION

1785 Alta Vista Drive, Ottawa, ON, K1G 3Y6, Canada
Tel: (1) 613 523 7877
Fax: (1) 613 523 0445
Email: exec@cdnpharm.ca
www: http://www.cdnpharm.ca
Contact: Mr Leroy Fevang

The Canadian Pharmacists Association is the national voluntary organisation of pharmacists committed to providing leadership for the profession of pharmacy. CPA represents more than 9,000 pharmacists and pharmacy students.

CPhA Canada Centennial Scholars Award

Subjects: Pharmacy.
Eligibility: Open to students at Canadian university faculties of pharmacy with satisfactory standing during the first three years of their pharmacy course and who show active leadership in student activities.
Level of Study: Graduate.
Purpose: To encourage good student citizenship and student-body leadership and to provide students with the opportunity to participate in the annual Canadian Pharmacists Association conference.
No. of awards offered: 9.
Frequency: Annual.
Value: C$300, which is often matched by the provincial pharmaceutical association; travel expenses and registration to the CPhA Pharmacy Conference.
Study Establishment: Each of the nine university faculties of pharmacy.
Country of Study: Canada.
Additional Information: Awardees are selected each February by their respective faculties of pharmacy. The award is activated in May for the duration of the annual Pharmaceutical Conference.

CANADIAN SOCIETY FOR MEDICAL LABORATORY SCIENCE

PO 2830
LCD1, Hamilton, ON, L8N 3N8, Canada
Tel: (1) 905 528 8642
Fax: (1) 905 528 4968
Email: memserv@cslt.com
www: http://www.cslt.com
Contact: Ms Alicia Maurer, Administration Director

The Canadian Society for Medical Laboratory Science is the certifying body and professional association for laboratory technologists in Canada. Its purpose is to promote and maintain a nationally accepted standard of medical laboratory technology by which other health professionals and the public are assured of effective and economical laboratory services and to promote, maintain and protect the professional identity and interest of medical laboratory technologists and of the profession.

CSMLS Founders' Fund Award

Subjects: Medical laboratory technology.
Eligibility: Open to certified members in good standing at the time of application.
Level of Study: Professional development.
Purpose: To assist members with costs of professional continuing education.
Type: Study Grant.
No. of awards offered: Varies.
Frequency: Dependent on funds available.
Value: Varies, at the discretion of the Founders' Fund Committee.
Country of Study: Canada.
Additional Information: Applications may be submitted at any time during the year and will be dealt with at the next scheduled meeting of the Founders' Fund Committee. These are held in conjunction with the meetings of the Board of Directors, usually in February, June, September and November/December. The decision on whether to grant an award and the amount of the award shall be at the discretion of the Founders' Fund Committee. Applicants may only apply for one award for any activity.

Quebec CE Fund Grants

Subjects: Medical technology.
Eligibility: Open to any person or group who is able to establish or co-ordinate the establishment of continuing education programmes for Francophone members of the CSMLS. This would include individual CSMLS members, an affiliated Society or Branch, the Ordre Professionnelle des Technologistes Médicaux du Québec (OPTMQ) and institutions which teach medical technology.
Level of Study: Postgraduate.
Purpose: To promote continuing education among medical laboratory technologists who are francophones.
Type: Grant.

No. of awards offered: Varies.
Value: Varies.
Country of Study: Canada.
Application Procedure: Please write for application forms.
Additional Information: It is CSMLS policy that continuing education programmes should normally be financially self-supporting through the fees charged for the programme. However, there are some situations in which a programme is needed in a particular location, but the programme cannot be self-supporting without charging unacceptably high fees. There may also be a need to fund development costs for certain types of programmes. All requests for the use of the Quebec CE funds shall be reviewed and approved or rejected by the Quebec CE Fund Committee and then considered for ratification at the next CSMLS Board of Directors meeting. There is no standardised application form, but all applications must include the following documentation: the amount of the grant requested from the Quebec CE fund; an outline of the proposed programme; a comprehensive budget including a breakdown of expenses; a statement of other support to be received or being applied for, e.g. a subsidy from a provincial Society; expected revenues; who will hold control of the programme and the proposed method of administration; development times and the dates that progress reports will be submitted during development; evidence of the need for the programme; and a signed statement declaring that CSMLS members will be permitted to participate in the finished programme at no increased differential fee.

CANADIAN-SCANDINAVIAN FOUNDATION

c/o Office of the Director of Libraries
McGill University
3459 McTavish Street, Montreal, PQ, H3A 1Y1, Canada
Tel: (1) 514 398 4740
Fax: (1) 514 398 7356
Email: moller@libi.lan.mcgill.ca
Contact: Dr Hans Moller, Vice President

The Canadian-Scandinavian Foundation was established in 1950 and offers research and study support to qualified young, talented Canadians of university age and aspiring scholars.

CSF Special Purpose Grants

Subjects: All subjects.
Eligibility: Open to qualified Canadians and landed immigrants.
Level of Study: Postgraduate.
Purpose: To provide travel support for shorter study or research visit to a Scandinavian or Nordic country destination.
Type: Grant.
No. of awards offered: 2-3.
Frequency: Annual.

Value: Approx. C$600-C$1,000.
Length of Study: A short period of time.
Country of Study: Scandinavia and Finland.
Application Procedure: Application form must be completed.
Closing Date: January 31st.

CANCER ASSOCIATION OF SOUTH AFRICA

PO Box 2000, Johannesburg, 2000, South Africa
Tel: (27) 11 616 7662
Fax: (27) 11 622 3424
Email: rbotha@cansa.org.za
Contact: Mr Ristie Botha, Research Administrator

The Cancer Association of South Africa is dedicated to prevent and fight cancer and its consequences in partnership with all South African communities by providing direction for and supporting health promotion, patient service and research. Research is focused on problems of national importance and is conducted by consortiums of researchers.

Cancer Association of South Africa Research Grants

Subjects: All aspects of the cancer problem, particularly those aspects which have a South African significance and can be investigated locally.
Eligibility: Open to medical graduates, biochemists, graduates in social science, etc, who are in full-time employment and can show distinct evidence of a capacity for original research or, in the case of BSc graduates, have won distinctions during their undergraduate studies. Candidates should be resident in South Africa.
Level of Study: Postgraduate.
Purpose: To assist professional staff with major or specialised equipment, laboratory running expenses, skilled or unskilled laboratory or other assistants; also to assist with printing and/or publishing the results of all types of research which fall within the Association's scope.
Type: Research Grant.
No. of awards offered: Varies.
Frequency: Annual.
Value: Varies, according to merit.
Length of Study: 1-3 calendar years.
Study Establishment: University or research institution.
Country of Study: South Africa.
Application Procedure: Application form must be completed.
Closing Date: May 31st.
Additional Information: All major equipment will remain the property of the Association. Specific details of the types of research which fall within the Association's scope and additional information are available from the Association.

Cancer Association of South Africa Travel and Subsistence (Study) Grants

Subjects: Cancer projects.
Eligibility: Open to suitably qualified applicants in some aspect of the cancer field who are in full-time employment. Applicants must be South African citizens.
Level of Study: Postgraduate.
Purpose: To assist workers in the cancer field in improving their academic and/or technical qualifications and experience for the furtherance of cancer research and education, and for the improvement of diagnostic and/or treatment services to cancer patients in South Africa.
No. of awards offered: Varies.
Frequency: Twice a year, dependent on funds available.
Value: Not to exceed 50% of the minimum costs (on condition that the applicant, through his own institution or by other means, pays the balance of the minimum costs). Minimum costs are calculated on the basis of an economy class air fare to the furthest point of travel with such deviations as may be approved by the Association, plus a subsistence allowance appropriate to the geographical area concerned.
Country of Study: Any country.
Application Procedure: Travel Grant application form to be completed and forwarded to executive committee for approvals.
Closing Date: January 31st, July 31st.
Additional Information: Travel Grants are awarded to suitable applicants to enable them to attend national or international conferences in the cancer field. Study Grants are awarded to suitable applicants who, by study at specialised centres, will be able to increase their knowledge in the cancer field with a view to its subsequent application in South Africa. Grantees are required to return to South Africa within a period of six months after expiration of the period for which the Grant was awarded (an extension will be considered on application) and to continue for a period of two years in the service in which they were employed at the time of the award. Grants may not be used for the purpose of studying for or obtaining degrees or diplomas. The Association also offers support to certain foreign medical scientists in the cancer field who are invited to visit South Africa to participate in scientific meetings and congresses, or for particular purposes as the need may arise.

Lady Cade Memorial Fellowship

Subjects: Research into the causation, diagnosis and/or treatment of cancer.
Eligibility: Open to medical graduates of senior status who are resident in South Africa, or South African nationals who are domiciled in the British Commonwealth, or in some cases, elsewhere. Preference is given to those holding senior posts at approved universities or other institutions to which the Fellows will be expected to return within six months of the termination of the Fellowship and work there for a period of not less than two years.
Level of Study: Postgraduate, Professional development.
Purpose: To encourage professional development in cancer research.

Type: Fellowship.
No. of awards offered: 1.
Frequency: Occasionally, dependent on funds available.
Value: R80,000 plus return economy air fare to the United Kingdom for the Fellow and his/her family.
Length of Study: 1-3 years.
Study Establishment: University or research institution.
Country of Study: United Kingdom.
Application Procedure: Application form must be completed and submitted with curriculum vitae.
Closing Date: Approximately six months prior to commencement of the Fellowship.
Additional Information: South Africans in the United Kingdom may apply through Cancer Research Campaign, 2 Carlton House Terrace, London SW1Y 5AR.

THE CANCER RESEARCH CAMPAIGN

10 Cambridge Terrace, London, NW1 4JL, England
Tel: (44) 171 224 1333
Fax: (44) 171 487 4302
Contact: Ms Katherine Weight, Science Department

The Cancer Research Campaign was founded in 1923 and is one of the largest cancer charities in the UK. A leading European charity in anti-cancer drug development, Cancer Research aim to provide around one third of the total UK funding into all types of cancer research.

Cancer Research Campaign Research Grant

Subjects: Cancer research, the Campaign only considers research proposals which are cancer related and contain a definite research aspect. Cancer education and psychosocial research projects are also available.
Eligibility: Applications will be accepted from scientists, clinicians or healthcare workers who possess suitable academic qualifications, and have the support of the head of department in the proposed place of work. Grants are normally available to applicants who have been resident in the UK for at least three years.
Level of Study: Doctorate, Postdoctorate.
Purpose: To support cancer research.
Type: Research Grant.
No. of awards offered: Varies.
Frequency: Annual.
Value: Salaries, running expenses and equipment.
Length of Study: 3-5 years.
Study Establishment: Appropriate universities, medical schools, hospitals and some research institutions. The host institution is responsible for administering the grant.
Country of Study: United Kingdom.
Application Procedure: Applications can be obtained from the Scientific Department of The Cancer Research Campaign. Contact the Scientific Secretary, Project Grants, for an application form and deadlines.
Closing Date: Project grant applications are considered in January, April, July and October.

Additional Information: Funding is also available for cancer education and psychosocial research projects. Contact the Education Department for details. The Campaign also awards a limited number of Fellowships and PhD Studentships. These are advertised annually. Contact the Scientific Secretary (fellowships) for details.

THE CANCER RESEARCH SOCIETY, INC.

1 Place Ville Marie
Suite 2332, Montreal, PQ, H3B 5C3, Canada
Tel: (1) 514 861 9227
Fax: (1) 514 861 9220
Email: crs@cam.org
www: http://www.cancer-research-society.ca
Contact: Ms Ivy Steinberg, President

The Cancer Research Society, founded in 1945, is a national organisation which devotes its funds exclusively to research on cancer. The Society is committed to funding basic cancer research or "seed" money for original ideas. The funds are allocated in the form of grants and fellowships to universities and hospitals across Canada.

Cancer Research Society, Inc. (Can) Postdoctoral Fellowships

Subjects: Basic medical sciences.
Eligibility: Open to holders of a PhD or MD degree, of any nationality.
Level of Study: Postdoctorate.
Purpose: To provide financial support to recent PhD and MDs to acquire a more complete formation in research.
Type: Fellowship.
No. of awards offered: 7, including renewals.
Frequency: Annual.
Value: C$28,510.
Study Establishment: Canadian universities and their affiliated institutions.
Country of Study: Canada.
Application Procedure: Please write for details.
Closing Date: February 15th.

Cancer Research Society, Inc. (Can) Predoctoral Fellowships

Subjects: Biology, physiology, biochemistry, molecular biology, genetics, microbiology and immunology, medical sciences.
Eligibility: Open to persons of any nationality. The candidate must be registered in a Canadian graduate school.
Level of Study: Doctorate, Postgraduate.
Purpose: To provide financial support for candidates registered in graduate programs leading to the MSc or PhD degrees.
Type: Fellowship.
No. of awards offered: 18 including renewals.

Frequency: Annual.
Value: C$15,050.
Study Establishment: Canadian universities and their affiliated institutions, for MSc or PhD programmes in a recognised Canadian graduate school.
Country of Study: Canada.
Application Procedure: Please write for details.
Closing Date: February 15th.

Cancer Research Society, Inc. (Can) Research Grants

Subjects: Fundamental research on cancer.
Eligibility: Candidates must hold an academic position on the staff of a Canadian university.
Level of Study: Professional development.
Purpose: To provide support for new or continuing research activities by independent scientists or group of investigators in the field of cancer.
Type: Research Grant.
No. of awards offered: 98.
Frequency: Annual.
Value: C$30,000-C$60,000 to cover the cost of research. No equipment or travel permitted.
Study Establishment: Canadian universities and their affiliated institutions.
Country of Study: Canada.
Application Procedure: Please write for details.
Closing Date: February 15th.

THE CANON FOUNDATION

Rijnsburgerweg 3, Leiden, NL-2334 BA, Netherlands
Tel: (31) 71 5156555
Fax: (31) 71 5157027
Email: foundation@canon-europa.com
Contact: Executive Officer

The Canon Foundation is a non-profit, grant making philanthropic organisation founded to promote, develop and spread science, knowledge and understanding, in particular between Europe and Japan.

Canon Foundation Visiting Research Fellowships/Professorships

Subjects: All subjects.
Eligibility: Open to Japanese and European nationals only.
Level of Study: Doctorate, Postdoctorate, Postgraduate.
Purpose: To contribute to scientific knowledge and international understanding, particularly between Japan and Europe.
Type: Monetary.
No. of awards offered: 10-12.
Frequency: Annual.
Value: Maximum award of DFL60,000.
Length of Study: 1 year maximum.
Country of Study: Europeans to Japan only, and Japanese to Europe.

Application Procedure: Applications must be completed and submitted with two reference letters, CV, list of papers, two photographs, and copies of certificates of higher education.
Closing Date: October 15th.

CARNEGIE TRUST FOR THE UNIVERSITIES OF SCOTLAND

Cameron House
Abbey Park Place, Dunfermline, Fife, KY12 7PZ, Scotland
Tel: (44) 1383 622148
Fax: (44) 1383 622149
Email: carnegie.trust@ed.ac.uk
www: http://www.geo.ed.ac.uk/carnegie/carnegie.html
Contact: Secretary

The Carnegie Trust for the Universities of Scotland, founded in 1901, is one of the many philantrophic agencies established by Andrew Carnegie. The trust aims to offer assistance to students, to aid the expansion of the Scottish universities and to stimulate research.

Carnegie Grants

Subjects: Any subject in the university curriculum.
Eligibility: Open to graduates of a Scottish university, or full-time members of staff of a Scottish university.
Level of Study: Postgraduate, Professional development.
Purpose: To support personal research projects or aid in the publication of books in certain fields, where likely to benefit the universities of Scotland.
Type: Grant.
No. of awards offered: Varies.
Frequency: Throughout the year.
Value: Varies according to requests; candidates must provide a detailed estimate of anticipated costs, but the normal maximum is £2,000.
Length of Study: Up to 3 months.
Country of Study: Any country.
Application Procedure: Application form must be completed; these are available from the Trust office.
Closing Date: February 1st, June 1st, November 1st; prior to Executive Committee meetings in those months.

Carnegie Scholarships

Subjects: Most subjects in the university curriculum.
Eligibility: Open to persons possessing a first class honours degree from a Scottish university.
Level of Study: Postgraduate.
Purpose: To support postgraduate research.
Type: Scholarship.
No. of awards offered: 16.
Frequency: Annual.
Value: £6,788 (in 1998/99) per year, plus tuition fees and allowances.
Length of Study: A maximum of 3 years, subject to annual review.

Study Establishment: Any university in the UK.
Country of Study: United Kingdom.
Application Procedure: Candidates should be nominated by a senior member of staff of a Scottish university. Application forms are available from the Trust office.
Closing Date: March 15th.

THE CATHOLIC UNIVERSITY OF LOUVAIN (UCL)

Secrétariat à la Coopération Internationale
Halles Universitaires
Place de l'Université 1, Louvain-la-Neuve, B-1348, Belgium
Tel: (32) 10 47 30 93
Fax: (32) 10 47 40 75
Email: baeyens@sco.ucl.ac.be
www: http://www.ucl.ac.be
Contact: Mr Duque Christian

The French-speaking Catholic University of Louvain (UCL) organises a yearly scholarship contest for postgraduate studies, medical specialisation and PhD.

Catholic University of Louvain Cooperation Fellowships

Subjects: Any subject relevant to third world development.
Eligibility: Open to nationals of developing countries, who hold all the requirements to be admitted at postgraduate level at UCL. Applicants should have an excellent academic background and some professional experience, they should demonstrate that their study programme is able to promote the development of their home country and they should have a good command of French (DELF). Applicants must be less than 35 years for a PhD or 40 years for a specialisation.
Level of Study: Doctorate, Postgraduate.
Purpose: To promote economic, social, cultural and political progress in the developing countries by postgraduate training of graduates from these countries.
Type: Fellowship.
No. of awards offered: Up to 20.
Frequency: Annual.
Value: Tuition, living expenses, family allowance, medical insurance, transportation costs to home country at the end of studies.
Length of Study: A maximum of 4 years.
Study Establishment: The Catholic University of Louvain.
Country of Study: Belgium.
Application Procedure: Application form must be completed; additional documentation is required (motivated letter and CV).
Closing Date: December 31st.
Additional Information: Application forms available on request.

CENTER FOR INDOOR AIR RESEARCH (CIAR)

1099 Winterson Road
Suite 280, Linthicum, MD, 21090, United States of America
Tel: (1) 410 684 3777
Fax: (1) 410 684 3729
Email: ciarinc@aol.com
Contact: Grants Management Officer

The mission of the Center for Indoor Air Research is to sponsor high quality research on indoor air-related issues to facilitate communication of research findings to the broad scientific community.

CIAR Postdoctoral Fellowships

Subjects: Indoor air research and related sciences.
Eligibility: Applicants must hold a PhD degree, an MD degree, or an equivalent degree at the time of the award, and have demonstrated an ability to conduct independent research.
Level of Study: Postdoctorate.
Purpose: To develop the scientific productivity of outstanding young people pursuing careers in indoor air research, and to stimulate interest in entering the field of indoor air research among individuals with strong backgrounds in related or allied sciences.
Type: Fellowship.
Frequency: Annual.
Value: The total budget each year is limited to US$25,000 for stipend and fringe benefits and up to US$5,000 for research supplies and other approved expenses.
Length of Study: 1 year; possibility of renewal for a further year.
Country of Study: Any country.
Application Procedure: Applicants should submit a three-page research proposal, applicant's CV, sponsoring investigator's CV, three letters of recommendation, and a letter of endorsement of the applicant by the sponsor indicating sources and level of research support for this project.
Closing Date: October 31st.
Additional Information: Following completion of the fellowship, the Center will request periodic updates of the fellow's academic accomplishments.

CIAR Research Contract

Subjects: Indoor air research.
Eligibility: There are no eligibility restrictions.
Level of Study: Doctorate.
Purpose: To support scientific research according to the needs and interests of the awarding body as described in the research agenda.
No. of awards offered: Varies.
Frequency: Annual.
Value: Approx US$50,000-US$200,000 per year.
Length of Study: Up to 3 years.
Country of Study: Any country.

Application Procedure: Please write, email or call for an application. Application procedures are described in the Request for Applications booklet, and application forms are provided with this booklet.
Closing Date: June 1st.
Additional Information: Awards are made initially for one year. Continuing support is dependent on approval of continuing applications submitted by the awardee for each approved year beyond the first.

CENTER FOR MENTAL HEALTH SERVICES

American Psychiatric Association
1400 K Street N W, Washington, DC, 20005, United States of America
Tel: (1) 202 682 6096
Fax: (1) 202 682 6837
Email: mking@psych.org
Contact: Ms Marilyn King, Program Co-ordinator

APA/CMHS and Zeneca Minority Fellowship Programme in Psychiatry

Subjects: Psychiatry and mental health.
Eligibility: Open to psychiatric residents in at least their PGY-2 of training. Applicants must be US citizens.
Level of Study: Postgraduate.
Purpose: To provide enriching training experiences through participation in APA Fall Components and Annual meetings; and to stimulate interest in pursuing training in areas of psychiatry where minority groups are underrepresented, such as research, child psychiatry, and addiction psychiatry.
Type: Fellowship.
No. of awards offered: Varies.
Frequency: Dependent on funds available.
Value: Dependent on funds available; support takes the form of a partial stipend.
Length of Study: 9 months.
Country of Study: Any country.
Application Procedure: Application form must be completed.
Closing Date: January 31st.
Additional Information: Fellows are selcted on the basis of: 1) their commitment to serve minority and underserved populations, 2) their demonstrated leadership abilities, and 3) their interest in the interrelationship between mental health and transcultural factors.

APA/Zeneca Fellowship

Subjects: Psychiatry and mental health.
Eligibility: Open to psychiatric residents in at least their PGY-2 of training. Applicants must be US citizens or permanent residents.
Level of Study: Postgraduate.

Purpose: To provide recipients with enriching training experiences through participation in the APA Fall Components and Annual Meetings; to provide resources to support activities that enhance culturally relevant aspects of their training program; and to stimulate their interest in pursuing training in areas of psychiatry where minority groups are underrepresented, such as research, child psychiatry, and addiction psychiatry.
Type: Fellowship.
No. of awards offered: Up to 10.
Frequency: Annual.
Value: Travel expenses (transportation, hotel, incidentals) to the APA fall meeting in September, the annual meeting in May, and other component related meetings as appropriate.
Length of Study: 2 years.
Country of Study: Any country.
Application Procedure: An application packet can be obtained from the APA/Office of Minority and National Affairs.
Closing Date: Applications are accepted between November and January for notifcation in the spring.
Additional Information: Fellows are selected on the basis of their commitment to serve minority and underserved populations, their demonstrated leadership abilities, and their interest in the inter-relationship between mental health and transcultural factors.

CENTRE DE RECHERCHE EN SCIENCES NEUROLOGIQUES

Faculté De Médecine
Université De Montréal
CP 6128
Succ Centre-ville, Montreal, PQ, H3C 3J7, Canada
Tel: (1) 514 343 6366
Fax: (1) 514 343 6113
Email: naulc@physio.umontreal.ca
www: http://www.crsn.umontreal.ca/
Contact: Dr Serge Rossignol, Director

Founded in 1975, the Centre de Recherche en Sciences Neurologiques is a multidisciplinary unit based in the Department Of Physiology, Faculty of Medicine, University of Montreal. Educational activities at the Centre include an international symposium each spring, open to all neuroscientists; weekly research seminars in neuroanatomy, neurophysiology, and neurochemistry, and the HH Jasper and the JP Cordeau Postdoctoral Fellowships.

Herbert H Jasper Fellowship

Subjects: Neurology, neurosciences.
Eligibility: Open to Canadian citizens or permanent residents.
Level of Study: Postdoctorate.

Purpose: To provide the opportunity for the recipient to work closely with the investigator of his or her choice within a large active group of neuroscientists who are members of the Center.
Type: Fellowship.
No. of awards offered: 1.
Frequency: Annual.
Value: C$25,000 to C$30,000 per year.
Length of Study: 1 year.
Study Establishment: Centre de Recherche en Sciences Neurologiques, Université de Montréal.
Country of Study: Canada.
Application Procedure: An application form is required and can be obtained by writing to the Fellowship Committee.
Closing Date: December 31st.

JP Cordeau Fellowship

Subjects: Neurology, neurosciences.
Eligibility: Open to Canadian citizens or permanent residents.
Level of Study: Postdoctorate.
Purpose: Offers the use of the exceptional research facilities of the Center for Research in Neurological Sciences of the Université de Montréal. The fellowship also provides the opportunity for the recipient to work closely with the investigator of his or her choice within a large active group of neuroscientists who are members of the Center.
Type: Fellowship.
No. of awards offered: 1.
Frequency: Annual.
Value: C$25,000 - C$30,000.
Length of Study: 1 year.
Study Establishment: Centre de Recherche en Sciences Neurologiques, Université de Montréal.
Country of Study: Canada.
Application Procedure: A completed application form is required and can be obtained by writing to the Fellowship Committee.
Closing Date: December 31st.

CENTRE FOR ADDICTION AND MENTAL HEALTH

250 College Street, Toronto, ON, M5T 1R8, Canada
Tel: (1) 416 979 4747 ext 2432
Fax: (1) 416 979 4695
Email: broughtonj@cs.clarke-inst.on.ca
www: http://www.camh.net
Contact: Ms Janice Broughton-Cafazzo, Research Grants Officer

The Centre for Addiction and Mental Health was formed in early 1998 and involves the amalgamation of the Addiction Research Foundation, Clarke Institute, Donwood Institute and Queen Street Mental Health Centre. As a teaching hospital and research institute fully affiliated with the University of Toronoto, the Centre is in a unique position to contribute to one common goal - better understanding, prevention and care for mental health.

Postdoctoral Training Programme in Addiction and Mental Health

Subjects: Addiction and mental health.
Eligibility: Candidates must have a PhD or MD (or equivalent) at the time of taking up the appointment. Preference is given to Canadian citizens and permanent residents (other successful applicants must obtain an appropriate visa). The successful applicant is expected to be located at the CAMH during the period of appointment. Applicants must obtain sponsorship of a supervisor at the Centre who holds an appointment as associate or full professor.
Level of Study: Postdoctorate.
Purpose: To provide fellows with a comprehensive training programme in the fields of addiction and mental health with training in research techniques.
Type: Fellowship.
No. of awards offered: Varies.
Frequency: Annual, if funds are available.
Value: Postdoctoral salary varies depending on experience: C$29,155-C$32,070 (bases on MRC salary scale).
Length of Study: 1 year subject to renewal for a second year.
Study Establishment: Centre for Addiction and Mental Health.
Country of Study: Canada.
Application Procedure: Applicants hould include 10 copies of each of the following: application cover sheet, description of the propsed programme of research relevant to the mission of the centre of agreed upon by the proposed supervisor (not to exceed 2 pages, single space), a curriculum vitae and 2 letters of reference to be sent directly to Janice Broughton-Cafazzo Grants Officer, Centre for Addiction and Mental Health, Graduate School transcripts and 2 papers of sample writing, a 2 page biosketch of the proposed supervisor including current funding.
Closing Date: March 1st.

CENTRE FOR INTERNATIONAL MOBILITY (CIMO)

PO Box 343
Hakaniemenkatu 2, Helsinki, SF-00531, Finland
Tel: (358) 9 7 747 7033
Fax: (358) 9 7 747 7064
Email: cimoinfo@cimo.fi
www: http://www.cimo.fi
Contact: Grants Management Officer

The Centre for International Mobility, CIMO, is a service-sector organisation whose expertise is geared to the promotion of cross-cultural communication in education, training and international mobility with the focus on education and training, work and young people. CIMO gathers, processes and distributes information, and co-ordinates international education and training programmes.

CIMO Bilateral Scholarships

Subjects: Various subjects.
Eligibility: Open to applicants from: Australia, Austria, Belgium, Bulgaria, Canada, China, Cuba, Czech Republic, Denmark, Egypt, France, Germany, Great Britain, Greece, Hungary, Iceland, India, Republic of Ireland, Israel, Italy, Japan, Luxembourg, Mexico, Mongolia, the Netherlands, Norway, Poland, Portugal, Republic of Korea, Romania, Slovakia, Spain, Sweden, Switzerland, Turkey and the USA.
Level of Study: Postgraduate.
Type: Scholarship.
Frequency: Annual.
Value: The bilateral scholarships usually consist of a monthly allowance of FIM4,100. For short-term visitors there is a daily allowance, the amount of which is determined annually. Accommodation is provided for short-term visitors. There are no travel grants to or from Finland.
Length of Study: Postgraduate research of 3-9 months; study visits of 1-2 weeks.
Study Establishment: A Finnish university.
Country of Study: Finland.
Application Procedure: Applications should be made to the appropriate authority in the applicant's country, which selects the candidates to be proposed to CIMO.
Closing Date: Depends on the country.

CIMO Nordic Scholarship Scheme for the Baltic Countries and Northwest Russia

Subjects: Education and research in all fields. Priority is given to fields that promote further development in the region, as well as to fields where the special competence and experience of Nordic countries can be made use of.
Eligibility: Open to applicants from the five Nordic countries and the three Baltic Republics as well as areas in Northwest Russia.
Level of Study: Unrestricted.
Purpose: To promote collaboration between the five Nordic countries and the three Baltic Republics as well as areas in northwest Russia, within the fields of education and research.
Type: Scholarship.
Frequency: Twice a year.
Length of Study: 1-6 months.
Study Establishment: A Finnish university.
Country of Study: Finland.
Application Procedure: Application form must be completed and can be obtained by writing to the Nordic Information Offices and to CIMO.
Closing Date: October 1st, March 1st.
Additional Information: Priority will be given to applications where contact or co-operation has been established.

CIMO Scholarships for Young Researchers and University Teaching Staff

Subjects: Education and research in all subjects.
Eligibility: Open to nationals of any county. The applicant should not be older than 35.
Level of Study: Doctorate, Postdoctorate, Postgraduate.

Purpose: To promote international co-operation in teaching and research.
Type: Scholarship.
Frequency: Every three months.
Value: FIM4,000-6,000 per month.
Length of Study: 3-12 months.
Study Establishment: University.
Country of Study: Finland.
Application Procedure: Application form must be completed. The Finnish receiving university department must apply for the grant.
Closing Date: Applications are accepted at any time.
Additional Information: Established contact with the receiving institute prior to application is required.

THE CHARLES A AND ANNE MORROW LINDBERGH FOUNDATION

708 South 3rd Street
Suite 110, Minneapolis, MN, 55415-1141, United States of America
Tel: (1) 612 338 1703
Fax: (1) 612 338 6826
Email: lindfdtn@mtn.org
www: http://www.mtn.org/lindfdtn
Contact: Ms Marlene White, Grants Administrator

The Foundation is dedicated to furthering a balance between technological advancement and environmental preservation which was the Lindbergh's shared vision.

Lindbergh Grants

Subjects: Adaptive technology, waste minimisation and management, agriculture, aviation/aerospace, conservation of natural resources, humanities/education, arts, intercultural communication, exploration, biomedical research, health and population sciences.
Eligibility: Open to nationals of any country.
Level of Study: Unrestricted.
Purpose: To provide grants to individuals whose initiative in a wide spectrum of disciplines seeks to actively further a better balance between technology and the natural environment.
Type: Research Grant.
No. of awards offered: Approx. 10.
Frequency: Annual.
Value: Maximum of US$10,580.
Country of Study: Any country.
Application Procedure: Application form must be completed.
Closing Date: Second Tuesday in June.

CHARLES AND JULIA HENRY FUND

University Registry
The Old Schools, Cambridge, CB2 1TN, England
Tel: (44) 122 333 2317
Fax: (44) 122 333 2332
Email: mrf25@admin.cam.ac.uk
www: http://www.admin.cam.ac.uk
Contact: Ms Melanie Foster, Scholarships Clerk

Henry Fellowships (Harvard and Yale)

Subjects: Unrestricted, but subject to approval and feasibility.
Eligibility: Open to unmarried citizens, under 26 years of age, of the UK and Commonwealth. They should be undergraduates of a UK university who have completed six terms of residence by January 1st preceding the fellowship, or graduates of a UK university who are in their first year of postgraduate study at a UK university.
Level of Study: Postgraduate.
Purpose: To strengthen bonds between Britain and the USA.
Type: Fellowship.
No. of awards offered: 2.
Frequency: Annual.
Value: US$16,300 plus a travel grant of £1,250,(reviewed annually), tuition fees and health insurance.
Length of Study: 1 year.
Study Establishment: Harvard University, Cambridge, Massachusetts, or Yale University, New Haven, Connecticut.
Country of Study: USA.
Application Procedure: Application form must be completed and referee's reports submitted.
Closing Date: Early December.
Additional Information: Applicants must produce evidence of intellectual ability and must also submit a scheme of study or research not consisting of a degree course. The Fellowships are awarded in conjunction with other awards to finance a continuing course of study and are not tenable for degree courses. Fellows must undertake to return to the British Isles or some other part of the Commonwealth on the expiration of their term of tenure. The Fellowship must be vacated if the Fellow marries.

CHARLES H HOOD FOUNDATION

95 Berkeley Street
Suite 201, Boston, MA, 02116, United States of America
Tel: (1) 617 695 9439
Fax: (1) 617 423 4619
Contact: Mr Raymond Considine

Charles H Hood Foundation Child Health Research Grant

Subjects: Emphasis is on the initiation and furtherance of medical research which will help to diminish health problems affecting large numbers of children.

Eligibility: Funds may only be paid to a New England (6-states) medical or academic institution.
Level of Study: Faculty.
Purpose: Designed for junior faculty who are initiating independent research in new areas of inquiry, and have limited federal grant experience.
Type: Research Grant.
No. of awards offered: 10-12.
Frequency: Annual.
Value: US$50,000.
Length of Study: 2 year.
Country of Study: Any country.
Application Procedure: Write for application forms. These must be completed and submitted along with letters of recommendation, curriculum vitae, non-technical summary, scientific summary and itemised budget.
Closing Date: April and October. Exact dates vary each year.

CHINESE AMERICAN MEDICAL SOCIETY (CAMS)

281 Edgewood Avenue, Teaneck, NJ, 07666, United States of America
Tel: (1) 201 833 1506
Fax: (1) 201 833 8252
Email: hw5@columbia.edu
www: http://www.camsociety.org
Contact: Dr H H Wang, Executive Director

The Chinese American Medical Society is a non-profit, charitable, educational and scientific society which aims to promote the scientific association of medical professionals of Chinese descent, to advance medical knowledge and scientific research with emphasis on aspects unique to the Chinese and to promote the health status of Chinese Americans. The Society makes scholarships available to medical dental students and provides endowments to medical schools and hospitals of good standing.

CAMS Scholarship

Subjects: Medical or dental studies.
Eligibility: Open to Chinese Americans, or Chinese residing in the USA. Applicants must be full-time medical or dental students in approved schools in the USA and be able to show academic proficiency and financial hardship.
Level of Study: Doctorate.
Purpose: To help defray the cost of study.
Type: Scholarship.
No. of awards offered: 3-5.
Frequency: Annual.
Value: US$1,000-US$1,500.
Country of Study: USA.
Application Procedure: Complete application form, send it together with letter for the Dean of Students verifying good standing, 2-3 letters of recommendation, personal statement and CV, plus financial statement.
Closing Date: March 31st.

CLIVE AND VERA RAMACIOTTI FOUNDATIONS

c/o Perpetual Trustee Company Limited
39 Hunter Street, Sydney, NSW, 2000, Australia
Tel: (61) 2 9229 9000
Fax: (61) 2 9221 3286
Email: foundations@perpetual.com.au
www: http://www.perpetual.com.au
Contact: The Administrator

Perpetual is Australia's largest and oldest trustee company with over A$450 million in charitable trusts and foundations.

Ramaciotto Travel Awards

Subjects: Medical research or such related fields of experimental science as are approved by the Ramaciotti Board of Trustees.
Eligibility: Open only to workers engaged in research. Travel undertaken solely to attend meetings or congresses or purely for educational or vocational purposes does not come within the scope of this scheme. The awards are not available for predoctoral workers or medical students during their elective period. Postdoctoral candidates must be able to demonstrate independent research experience.
Level of Study: Postdoctorate, Professional development.
Purpose: To enable medical researchers from Australia to visit countries other than the UK or Ireland, in order to undertake short-term collaborative research or to learn a new technique.
Type: Travel Grant.
Frequency: Quarterly.
Value: Decided by the Board of Trustees in the light of the candidate's experience and current practice.
Length of Study: 21-91 days.
Country of Study: Any country other than the UK or Ireland.
Application Procedure: Please write for application details.
Closing Date: At least two months prior to departure date.
Additional Information: Candidates wishing to consult with colleagues, or to work at a research centre overseas, should find out in advance that their visits will be welcomed by the colleagues in question, and that appropriate facilities can be made available, and should state this in their application. A letter from the institution to be visited, supporting the proposal, must be submitted with the application. If the host institution requires the research expenses to be covered, a note outlining these should be included in this letter. It is expected that recipients of a grant will return to their country of origin on completion of the period of the grant, and should submit a brief report of their visit. Applications must be supported by the Head or a Senior Member of the applicant's Department who should be requested by the applicant to assess the value of the visit, to certify that the applicant is engaged in bona fide research and that local resources are insufficient. Applications submitted without such support will not be considered.

COLLEGE OF OCCUPATIONAL THERAPISTS

106-114 Borough High Street
Southwark, London, SE1 1LB, England
Tel: (44) 171 357 6480
Fax: (44) 171 207 9612
Contact: I Ilott, Research & Development Group Head

The College of Occupational Therapists is the professional body for occupational therapy in the United Kingdom. The college promotes the profession and standards of good practice and occupational therapy, education and research.

Agnes Storar/Constance Owens Fund

Subjects: Occupational therapy.
Eligibility: Open to occupational therapy teachers in recognised schools of occupational therapy. Applicants must be members of the British Association of Occupational Therapists.
Level of Study: Unrestricted.
Purpose: To provide travel bursaries for occupational therapy teachers in recognised schools of occupational therapy to travel abroad to observe the practice and teaching of occupational therapy or to attend relevant international conferences.
Frequency: Annual.
Value: £600.
Country of Study: Outside United Kingdom.
Application Procedure: Announced annually in OT News and BJOT.
Closing Date: Last day of November, March or July.

Farrer-Brown Professional Development Fund

Subjects: Occupational therapy, including awards for work-based projects, research or evaluation of aspects of occupational therapy, awards to enable the publication of relevant papers or for such other purposes of a similar nature.
Eligibility: Open to occupational therapists who are members of the British Association of Occupational Therapists.
Level of Study: Professional development.
Purpose: The development and improvement of professional aspects of occupational therapy.
No. of awards offered: Varies, 2-3.
Frequency: Annual.
Value: Varies.
Country of Study: Any country.
Application Procedure: Application procedure is announced annually from August in OT News and BJOT.
Closing Date: End of November.

Margaret Dawson Fund

Subjects: Occupational therapy.
Eligibility: Open to occupational therapists in clinical practice who are members of the British Association of Occupational Therapists, and final year occupational therapy students.
Level of Study: Professional development.

Purpose: To provide travel bursaries for occupational therapists or final year occupational therapy students to travel abroad to observe the practice of occupational therapy or to attend relevant international conferences.
Frequency: Annual.
Value: £400.
Country of Study: Outside United Kingdom.
Application Procedure: Announced annually in OT News.
Closing Date: Last Friday in November, March or July.

COLOMBO PLAN

The Colombo Plan Bureau
12 Melbourne Avenue
PO Box 596, Colombo, 4, Sri Lanka
Tel: (94) 1 581813
Fax: (94) 1 580754
Email: cplan@slt.lk

Colombo Plan Scholarships, Fellowships and Training Awards

Subjects: Colombo Plan awards are usually, but not necessarily, restricted to areas of study that are of significant interest to developing countries.
Eligibility: A request for an award usually originates from a recipient developing country on the basis of its priority needs, and the donor country to which the request is directed may grant it if training facilities and resources in the requested field are available. In some cases, however, offers of training originate from the donor countries themselves. Individuals wishing to apply for Colombo Plan Scholarships must be sponsored by their own governments.
Level of Study: Postgraduate.
No. of awards offered: Varies.
Frequency: Annual.
Value: Varies.
Country of Study: Colombo Plan member countries.
Application Procedure: Candidates should apply to the Ministry in their home country. The Colombo Plan office does not handle applications.
Additional Information: Please contact the Colombo Plan office for further details on the application procedure.

COMMISSION OF THE EUROPEAN COMMUNITIES - DG XXII/A/2

Rue De La Loi 200, Brussels, B-1040, Belgium
Fax: (32) 2 299 4153
www: http://europa.eu.int/en/com/dg22/socrates/erasinf.html
Telex: comeu b 21877
Contact: Mr Massimo Gaudina, Administrator

This unit deals with the ERASMUS chapter of the Socrates programme. Its objectives are the development of the European dimension of higher education and the improvement of quality.

ERASMUS Grants

Subjects: Any field of studies.
Eligibility: Condition: Agreement between home and host university.
Level of Study: Postgraduate.
Purpose: The encourage the mobility of university and postgraduate students in Europe.
Type: Partial Fellowship.
No. of awards offered: Approx. 100,000.
Frequency: Annual.
Value: Varies.
Length of Study: 3-12 months.
Country of Study: European countries.
Application Procedure: Through the home university (International Relation Office).
Closing Date: Varies.

COMMONWEALTH FUND

Harkness House
1 East 75th Street, New York, NY, 10021-2692, United States of America
Tel: (1) 212 606 3809
Fax: (1) 212 606 3875
Email: ro@cmwf,org
www: http://www.cmwf.org
Contact: The Awards Committee

The Commonwealth Fund is a philanthropic foundation established in 1918 with the broad charge to enhance the common good. The fund carries out its mandate through its efforts to help Americans live healthy and productive lives and to assist scientific groups with serious and neglected problems.

Atlantic Fellowships in Public Policy

Subjects: Education and training, welfare reform, health care, youth and families, reinventing government, workplace and employment issues, information technology, local government, criminal justice and crime prevention, environment, race relations, tax policy, science and technology, community development, public utilities, banking policy and regulations, arts policy, telecommunications, transportation, urban policy.
Eligibility: Applicants must be US citizens with at least five years experience in their professions. There are no formal age limits, but the focus of the fellowship is on mid-career development, and successful candidates are likely to be in their late twenties to early forties. Open to mid-career professionals active in any part of the public, business or philanthropic sectors.
Level of Study: Professional development.
Purpose: To reinforce Anglo-American relations by enabling highly qualified US domestic policy experts to undertake policy research in Britain and benefit from British ideas and best practice, thereby enhancing their ability to make an innovative contribution to policymaking in the US. Also to help improve the theory and practice of public policy in the UK and US by fostering the cross-fertilisation of ideas and

experience in both countries; and to help create a transatlantic network of public policy experts and practitioners concerned with society's most pressing needs and encourage ongoing collaboration and exchange.
Type: Fellowship.
Value: Where possible candidates are expected to obtain paid leave. The basic award is not intended to match fellows US salaries. Fellows on paid leave will receive an allowance of £500 per month (£600 in London) on top of their salaries and will also be entitled to family allowances. Fellows unable to obtain paid leave will receive a monthly living allowance of £1,300 (£1,700 in London), intended to cover basic expenses of residence. Further allowances are as follows: travel from home to UK base and return, for a Fellow, spouse and children under 18 years; direct payment will be made to host institutions for provision of office space use of telephone, fax, computer and office equipment; spouse's allowance of £150 per month (not payable to Fellows whose spouses are employed or receiving a grant or fellowship), and £50 per month for each of two children under 18 years. Please note: eligibility for family allowances is based on a Fellow's family status at the time of interview and will remain unchanged throughout tenure. UK travel allowances: Fellows are expected to travel extensively in the UK to further their study programmes therefore is provided with up to £250 per month for this. A setting up allowance of £600 will be provided for household goods. A baggage allowance of £300 for a single Fellow, £425 for a married Fellow, and £600 for a married Fellow with children will be available to cover the costs of shipping personal items. Fellows will not be responsible for paying UK income tax on the allowances and awards. They will however be liable for US income tax.
Study Establishment: An institution in the United Kingdom, typically a university, research institute or "think tank", but it could be a public agency or other body.
Country of Study: United Kingdom.
Application Procedure: A formal application must be completed, including a project proposal.
Closing Date: November 16th.
Additional Information: Applications are welcome equally from men and women, from members of any ethnic group, and regardless of physical disabilities.

THE COMMONWEALTH FUND OF NEW YORK

1 East 75th Street, New York, NY, 10021, United States of America
Tel: (1) 212 535 0400
Fax: (1) 212 249 1276
Email: ro@cmwf.org
Contact: Ms Robin Osborn, International Programs in Health Policy Director

Harkness Fellowships in Health Care Policy

Subjects: Health policy and health services research.
Eligibility: Open to individuals who: have completed a Master's degree or PhD in health services or health policy research and showing significant promise as a policy-oriented researcher or practitioner (for example physicians or health

administrators) with a strong interest in policy issues; are at the research fellow to senior lecturer level, if academically based; are in their late 20s to early 40s; have been nominated by their department chair or the director of their institution.

Level of Study: Professional development.

Purpose: To encourage the professional development of junior health care policy researchers whose multinational experience and outlook will contribute to innovation in health care policy and practice in America and their home countries.

Type: Fellowship.

No. of awards offered: 10.

Frequency: Annual.

Value: To cover basic expenses of travel, residence and research. Up to US$75,000.

Length of Study: 1 year (4 months minimum is spent in the USA).

Study Establishment: An academic or other institution.

Country of Study: USA.

Application Procedure: Completion of formal application is required. Please write to the correct country address.

Closing Date: October 1st.

Additional Information: Successful candidates will have a policy-oriented research project, ideally involving cross-national comparisons, on a topic relevant to the Fund's national programme areas. Projects will be supervised by senior researchers in the home country and at the US institution, and each Fellow will be expected to produce a publishable report contributing to a better understanding of health policy issues in both the home country and the USA.

For further information contact:

(Australia)
Center for Health Economics Research and Evaluation
University of Sydney
Mallett Street Campus
88 Mallett Street
Level 6
Building F, Camperdown, New South Wales, 2050, Australia
Tel: (61) 2 9351 0900
Fax: (61) 2 9351 0930
Contact: Dr Jane Hall, Associate Professor and Director
or
(New Zealand)
New Zealand-United States Educational Foundation
PO Box 3465, Wellington, New Zealand
Tel: (64) 472 2065
Fax: (64) 499 5364
Contact: Ms Jennifer M Gill, Policy Representative/Executive Director
or
(United Kingdom)
The Commonwealth Fund
One East 75th Street, New York, NY, 10021, United States of America
Tel: (1) 212 606 3809
Fax: (1) 212 606 3875
Contact: Ms Robin Osbourn, International Program in Health Policy Director

COMMONWEALTH SCHOLARSHIP COMMISSION IN THE UNITED KINGDOM

c/o Association of Commonwealth Universities
John Foster House
36 Gordon Square, London, WC1H 0PF, England
Tel: (44) 171 387 8572
Fax: (44) 171 387 2655
Contact: Ms Mary C Denyer, Awards Administrator

Commonwealth Academic Staff Scholarships

Subjects: All subjects.

Eligibility: Open to Commonwealth citizens or British protected persons permanently resident in a developing country of the Commonwealth, who should hold, or be about to obtain, a degree or an equivalent qualification, and should already hold a teaching appointment in a university or similar institution or have the assurance of such an appointment on his or her return. Candidates should be under 42 years of age at the time the award is taken up. All candidates must have sufficient competence in English to profit from the proposed study. These awards are not given to Indian nationals.

Level of Study: Postgraduate.

Purpose: To help universities in the developing countries of the Commonwealth build up the numbers and enhance the experience of their locally born staff. The scholarships are intended to enable promising staff members from universities and similar institutions in the developing Commonwealth to obtain experience in a university or other appropriate institution in the UK.

Type: Scholarship.

No. of awards offered: 45-50.

Frequency: Annual.

Value: To cover cost of return air fare to the UK, approved tuition, laboratory and examination fees, personal maintenance allowance at the rate of £493 per month or £592 a month for those studying at institutions in the London Metropolitan area, grant for books and equipment, and grant towards the expense of preparing a thesis or dissertation, where applicable, grant for approved travel within the UK, an initial clothing allowance in special cases, and in certain circumstances a marriage and child allowance. The emoluments are not subject to UK income tax.

Length of Study: 1-3 years.

Study Establishment: A university or comparable institution.

Country of Study: United Kingdom.

Application Procedure: Candidates must be nominated by one of the following: the vice-chancellor of a UK university, the vice-chancellor of the university on whose permanent staff the applicant serves or is to serve, (heads of Bangladeshi universities should send their nominations to the University Grants Commission in Dhaka); the Commonwealth Scholarship agency in the candidate's own country (for addresses, see the entry for the Commonwealth Scholarship and Fellowship Plan); in special cases, the head of an autonomous non-university institution in the Commonwealth, or the vice-chancellor of a UK university.

Closing Date: December 31st.
Additional Information: Scholars are required to sign an undertaking to return to resume their academic post in their own country on completion of the scholarships.

Commonwealth Fellowships

Subjects: All subjects.
Eligibility: Open to Commonwealth citizens and to British protected persons permanently resident in a developing Commonwealth country. Preference is given to candidates between 28 and 50 years of age. Candidates must have completed a Doctoral degree more than five but not more than ten years ago, and should have had at least two years' experience as a staff member of a university or similar institution in their own country.
Level of Study: Postdoctorate.
Purpose: To help universities in the developing countries of the Commonwealth build up the numbers and enhance the experience of their locally born staff. The fellowships are intended to enable promising staff members from universities and similar institutions in the developing Commonwealth to obtain experience in a university or other appropriate institution in the UK.
Type: Fellowship.
No. of awards offered: Approx. 50.
Frequency: Annual.
Value: £705 per month or £846 for those studying at institutions in the London Metropolitan area (reviewed annually) plus approved air fares to and from the UK and in certain circumstances a marriage and child allowance. A grant for approved travel within the UK and a book grant are also paid and, where recommended, an initial clothing allowance is offered. The emoluments are not subject to UK income tax.
Length of Study: 6 or 12 months.
Study Establishment: A university or comparable institution.
Country of Study: United Kingdom.
Closing Date: December 31st.
Additional Information: Fellows are required to sign an undertaking to return to resume their academic post in their country on completion of the Fellowships. Candidates must be nominated by one of the following: the vice-chancellor of a UK university, the vice-chancellor of the university on whose permanent staff the applicant serves or is to serve (heads of Indian universities should send their nominations to the University Grants Commission in New Delhi and heads of Bangladeshi universities to the University Grants Commission in Dhaka); the Commonwealth Scholarship agency in the candidate's own country (for addresses, see the entry for the Commonwealth Scholarship and Fellowship Plan); in special cases, the head of an autonomous non-university institution in the Commonwealth, or the vice-chancellor of a UK university. The Fellowship may not be held concurrently with other awards or with paid employment.

CONCORDIA UNIVERSITY

1455 de Maisonneuve Boulevard West, Montreal, PQ, H3G 1M8, Canada
Tel: (1) 514 848 3801
Fax: (1) 514 848 2812
Email: awardsgs@vax2.concordia.ca
www: http://www.concordia.ca/
Contact: Graduate Studies Office

Concordia University is the result of the 1974 merger between Sir George Williams University and Loyola College. The University incorporates superior teaching methods with an inter-disciplinary approach to learning and is dedicated to offering the best possible scholarship to the student body and to promoting research beneficial to society.

Concordia University Graduate Fellowships

Subjects: All subjects.
Eligibility: Open to graduates of any nationality.
Level of Study: Doctorate, Postgraduate.
Type: Fellowship.
No. of awards offered: Varies.
Frequency: Annual.
Value: C$2,900 per term for Master's level; C$3,600 per term for doctoral level.
Length of Study: A maximum of 4 terms at the Master's level and 9 terms at the doctoral level, calculated from the date of entry in the program.
Study Establishment: Concordia University.
Country of Study: Canada.
Application Procedure: Completed application form, three letters of recommendation and official transcripts of all university studies must be received by the closing date.
Closing Date: February 1st.
Additional Information: Academic merit is the prime consideration in the granting of the award. Awarded for full-time graduate studies.

John W O'Brien Graduate Fellowship

Subjects: Arts and humanities, business administration and management, education and teacher training, engineering, fine and applied arts, mass communication and information, mathematics and computer science, natural sciences, religion and theology.
Eligibility: Open to full-time graduate students of any nationality. Candidates must not have completed more than two terms of Master's study or four terms of doctoral study at Concordia, at the time of application.
Level of Study: Doctorate, Postgraduate.
Purpose: Awarded to applicants in full-time study towards a Master's or doctoral degree.
Type: Fellowship.
No. of awards offered: 1.
Frequency: Annual.
Value: C$3,300 per term at the Master's level and C$4,000 per term at the doctoral level.
Length of Study: A maximum of 3 terms.
Study Establishment: Concordia University.

Country of Study: Canada.
Application Procedure: Application form, three letters of recommendation and official transcripts of all university studies must be submitted by the closing date.
Closing Date: February 1st.
Additional Information: Academic merit is the prime consideration in the granting of awards which are for full-time study in a graduate programme leading to a Master's or doctoral degree.

Stanley G French Graduate Fellowship

Subjects: All subjects.
Eligibility: Open to graduates of any nationality. Candidates must not have completed more than two terms of a Master's programme or four terms of a doctoral programme at Concordia, at the time of application.
Level of Study: Doctorate, Postgraduate.
Type: Fellowship.
No. of awards offered: 1.
Frequency: Annual.
Value: C$3,300 per term for Master's level; C$4,000 per term for doctoral level.
Length of Study: A maximum of 3 terms.
Study Establishment: Concordia University.
Country of Study: Canada.
Application Procedure: Completed application form, three letters of recommendation and official transcripts of all university studies must be submitted by the closing date.
Closing Date: February 1st.
Additional Information: Academic merit is the prime consideration in the granting of awards, which are for full-time study in a graduate programme leading to a Master's or doctoral degree.

COOLEY'S ANEMIA FOUNDATION

129-09 26th Avenue
Suite 203, Flushing, NY, 11354, United States of America
Tel: (1) 718 321 2873
Fax: (1) 718 321 3340
Email: ncaf@aol.com
www: http://www.thalassemia.org
Contact: Ms Pia Levasseur, Special Projects

Cooley's Anemia Foundation funds research to cure this fatal blood disease, supports programmes to enhance the life and quality of patients, educates doctors, trait carriers and the public.

Cooley's Anemia Foundation Research Fellowship Grant

Subjects: Haematology.
Eligibility: Open to researchers of any nationality.
Level of Study: Postdoctorate.

Purpose: To promote an increased understanding of Cooley's anemia, develop improved treatment and achieve a final cure for this life threatening genetic blood disorder.
Type: Fellowship.
No. of awards offered: 10.
Frequency: Annual.
Value: US$30,000.
Length of Study: 1 year.
Country of Study: Any country.
Application Procedure: Application must be submitted to the national office.
Closing Date: March 8th.

COUNCIL FOR INTERNATIONAL EXCHANGE OF SCHOLARS (CIES)

3007 Tilden Street NW
Suite 5L, Washington, DC, 20008-3009, United States of America
Tel: (1) 202 686 8664
Fax: (1) 202 362 3442
Email: appreguest@cies.iie.org
www: http://www.cies.org/
Contact: Mr Janel Showalter, Publications Officer

The Council for International Exchange of Scholars (CIES) is a private, non-profit organisation that facilitates international exchanges in higher education. Under a co-operative agreement with the US information agency, it assists in the administration of the Fulbright Scholar Program. CIES is affiliated with the institute of international education.

Fulbright Scholar Awards for Research and Lecturing Abroad

Subjects: All academic disciplines and some professional fields.
Eligibility: Open to US citizens with a PhD or comparable professional qualifications. University or college teaching experience is normally expected for lecturing awards. For selected assignments, proficiency in a foreign language may be required.
Level of Study: Postdoctorate.
Purpose: To increase mutual understanding between the people of the USA and the people of other nations, strengthen the ties that unite the USA with other nations, and promote international co-operation for educational and cultural advancement.
Type: Research and/or lecturing.
No. of awards offered: 700+.
Frequency: Annual.
Value: Varies by country.
Length of Study: From 2 months to 1 academic year.
Country of Study: Any country.
Application Procedure: Applications are available from CIES.
Closing Date: August 1st.
Additional Information: Individual countries' programs are described in the Council's publication.

THE CROSS TRUST

PO Box 17
25 South Methven Street, Perth, PH1 5ES, Scotland
Tel: (44) 1738 620451
Fax: (44) 1738 631155
Contact: Mrs Barbara Anderson, Assistant Secretary

The Cross Trust

Subjects: Any approved subject.
Eligibility: Open to graduates or undergraduates of Scottish universities or of Central Institutions in Scotland and to Scottish secondary school pupils. Applicants must be of Scottish birth or parentage.
Level of Study: Postgraduate, Undergraduate.
Purpose: To enable young Scottish people to extend the boundaries of human life and to allow travel to extend experience, or encourage performance and participation in drama or opera. The Trust may support the pursuit of studies or research.
No. of awards offered: Varies.
Frequency: Varies.
Value: Varies.
Study Establishment: Anywhere as approved.
Country of Study: Any country.
Application Procedure: Application form must be completed.
Closing Date: No closing date.
Additional Information: Awards will only be considered from postgraduate students who have part funding in place from another organisation.

CROUCHER FOUNDATION

Suite 534
Star House
2 Salisbury Road, Kowloon, Hong Kong
Tel: (852) 2736 6337
Fax: (852) 2730 0742
www: http://coms.hkbu.edu.hk/croucher/
Contact: Ms Elaine Sit

Croucher Foundation Fellowships and Scholarships

Subjects: Natural science, medicine or technology.
Eligibility: Open to permanent residents of Hong Kong. Fellowships are intended for those at postdoctoral or equivalent level. Scholarships are intended for holders of a Master's degree or those in the process of completing an MPhil or PhD programme. In exceptional circumstances an undergraduate in the final year of his/her first degree may apply, but if an award is offered it is conditional on the candidate obtaining first class honours in their first degree.
Level of Study: Doctorate, Postdoctorate.

Purpose: To enable selected students of outstanding promise to devote themselves to full-time postgraduate study or research.
Type: Scholarship, Fellowship.
No. of awards offered: Approx. 20-25.
Frequency: Annual.
Value: £13,680 (fellowships) and £7,140 (scholarships) maintenance allowance (if award is tenable in the UK), assistance towards air fare, plus tuition fees for scholars. Married Fellows/Scholars will be given a special spouse allowance of £2,520 per year including assistance towards air fare if he or she is dependant and accompanying the holder of the award. In addition, children allowance (first child: £336 per year; second child: £289 per year) will also be provided if they are residing with the Fellow/Scholar. If the successful applicant is on paid study leave during the tenure of the award the maintenance allowance will not apply. A one-off grant for books/apparatus and clothing will be given during the first year of tenure. A London weighting allowance of £1,500 per year will be given to candidates who are studying in the London area. An allowance of up to £250 for thesis expenses will be given to final year PhD students on application, against receipts. Fellows and Scholars will be expected to devote their whole time to the objects of their award. Fellows and Scholars will not be debarred from holding another position of emolument but if at the date of application they hold or at a later date are appointed to such a position - or receive concurrently any scholarship or award with monetary value - they must notify the Trustees and must obtain prior approval from them, who may at their discretion modify the value of the Fellowship or Scholarship.
Length of Study: 1-2 years fellowships; 1-3 years scholarships.
Country of Study: Hong Kong, Canada, Australia, New Zealand or United Kingdom.
Application Procedure: Application form can be obtained from the Foundation on production of a study/research proposal and academic qualifications in October.
Closing Date: Mid-November.

CYSTIC FIBROSIS FOUNDATION (CFF)

Office of Grants Management
6931 Arlington Road, Bethesda, MD, 20814, United States of America
Tel: (1) 301 951 4422
Fax: (1) 301 951 6378
Email: rfreundlich@cff.org
www: http://www.cff.org
Contact: Ms Kathleen Curley, Grants Manager

CFF Research Programmes in Cystic Fibrosis

Subjects: Cystic fibrosis.
Eligibility: Some programmes have US citizenship or permanent resident status requirements.
Level of Study: Doctorate, Professional development.

Purpose: Competitive awards for research related to cystic fibrosis.
Type: Research Grant.
No. of awards offered: 8 programmes.
Frequency: Annual.
Value: Depending on the award from US$36,000 to US$100,000.
Country of Study: Any country.
Application Procedure: Please write for application form.
Closing Date: Varies with each award.
Additional Information: The names of the awards are as follows: Therapeutics Development Grants, Pilot Feasibility Awards, Research Grants, Leroy Matthews Physician/Scientist Award, Harry Shwachman Clinical Investigator Award, Clinical Research Grants, CFF/NIH Funding Award, Special Research Awards.

CFF Training Programmes in Cystic Fibrosis

Subjects: Cystic Fibrosis research.
Eligibility: Open to US citizens and permanent residents only.
Level of Study: Doctorate, Professional development.
Purpose: To support individuals interested in careers related to cystic fibrosis research and care.
Type: Varies.
No. of awards offered: 4 programmes.
Frequency: Annual.
Value: Depending on the award from US$1,500 to US$45,000.
Country of Study: Any country.
Application Procedure: Please write for application form.
Closing Date: Varies with the award.
Additional Information: The names of the specific awards are: Postdoctoral Research Fellowships, Clinical Fellowships, Student Traineeships, Summer Scholarships in Epidemiology.

CYSTIC FIBROSIS RESEARCH TRUST (CFRT)

11 London Road, Bromley, Kent, BR1 1BY, England
Tel: (44) 181 464 7211
Fax: (44) 181 313 0472
Contact: Mrs Carol M Eagles, Projects Co-ordinator

CFRT Research Grants

Subjects: Medical and scientific research related to cystic fibrosis.
Eligibility: Open to suitably qualified persons from the United Kingdom.
Level of Study: Doctorate, Postgraduate.

Purpose: To find a cure for cystic fibrosis and also to improve the management, care and treatment of those with cystic fibrosis.
Type: Research Grant.
No. of awards offered: Varies.
Frequency: Twice a year.
Value: From a total fund of £1m per year; grants are made to cover such matters as salaries, expenses and equipment.
Length of Study: Up to 3 years, subject to annual renewal.
Country of Study: United Kingdom.
Application Procedure: Application by CF Trust form plus justification of support requested.
Closing Date: Available on application to the Trust.

DATATEL SCHOLARS FOUNDATION

4375 Fair Lakes Court, Fairfax, VA, 22033, United States of America
Tel: (1) 703 968 9000
Fax: (1) 703 968 4573
Email: scholars@datatel.com
Contact: The Awards Committee

Datatel Scholars Foundation Scholarship

Subjects: All subjects.
Eligibility: Open to students attending a higher learning institution selected from Datatel, Inc.'s more than 450 college, university and non-profit client sites. USA or Canadian citizenship is not required.
Level of Study: Doctorate, Postgraduate, Undergraduate.
Purpose: To award scholarships to eligible students to attend a higher learning institution selected from Datatel's college and client sites.
Type: Scholarship.
No. of awards offered: Determined annually.
Frequency: Annual.
Value: US$700 to US$2,000 depending on tuition amount.
Length of Study: 1 year.
Study Establishment: Datatel client site institution.
Country of Study: USA or Canada.
Application Procedure: Applications must be completed and forwarded by the institution's Office of Financial Aid. The Foundation does not accept applications directly from students.
Closing Date: February 15th.
Additional Information: If requesting applications from the Foundation, please mention the name of your college or university so it can determine if the institution qualifies.

DEAFNESS RESEARCH FOUNDATION (DRF)

15 West 39th Street, New York, NY, 10018-3806, United States of America
Tel: (1) 212 768 1181
Fax: (1) 212 768 1782
Email: drf1@village.ios.com
www: http://www.village.ios.com/~drf1
Contact: Ms Rakeela Khan, Grants Officer

Founded in 1958, the DRF is the nation's largest voluntary health organisation primarily committed to public awareness and support of basic and clinical research directed to unexplored areas of hearing loss and other ear disorders.

DRF Otological Research Fellowship

Subjects: Otological research, otorhinolaryngology.
Eligibility: Open to third year medical students sponsored by a Department of Otolaryngology conducting otological research.
Level of Study: Postgraduate.
Purpose: To increase the number of physicians involved in otological research.
Type: Fellowship.
No. of awards offered: Varies.
Frequency: Annual.
Value: US$10,000 (plus up to US$3,500 for animals and consumable supplies).
Length of Study: 1 year.
Country of Study: USA.
Application Procedure: A letter from the Dean and three letters of recommendation are required.
Closing Date: November 1st.
Additional Information: The Fellowship would be scheduled as a one-year block of time at the end of the third year of medical school, thus requiring a one-year leave of absence from the medical school curriculum.

DRF Research Grants

Subjects: Research into the function, physiology, genetics, anatomy or pathology of the ear.
Eligibility: Open to MDs and PhDs in the field of otologic research. Applicants must be US/Canadian citizens.
Level of Study: Doctorate, Postgraduate.
Purpose: To encourage research into the causes, treatment and prevention of hearing loss and related ear disorders.
Type: Research Grant.
No. of awards offered: Varies.
Frequency: Annual.
Value: Up to US$20,000.
Length of Study: 1 year; renewable for 1 or 2 further years.
Country of Study: USA or Canada.
Closing Date: June 1st (new applications); August 1st (renewal applications).

DEBRA

DEBRA House
13 Wellington Business Park
Dukes Ride, Crowthorne, Berkshire, RG45 6LS, England
Tel: (44) 1344 771961
Fax: (44) 1344 762661
www: http://www.debra.org.uk
Contact: Mr John Dart, Director

DEBRA is a voluntary organisation working on behalf of people with Epidermolysis Bullosa (EB). The main activities of the organisation are funding research into EB, and providing services to benefit EB sufferers.

DEBRA Medical Research Grant Scheme

Subjects: Dermatology, treatment techniques, genetics.
Eligibility: Open to qualified researchers who are able to demonstrate the ability to undertake a specific project in EB.
Level of Study: Postdoctorate.
Purpose: To fund research into all aspects of Epidermolysis Bullosa (EB).
Type: Project Grant.
No. of awards offered: Varies.
Frequency: Twice a year.
Value: Approx. £30,000.
Length of Study: Up to 3 years.
Country of Study: Any country.
Application Procedure: Application forms are available from the DEBRA office or can be downloaded from the DEBRA website.
Closing Date: April 1st, October 1st.

DEMOCRATIC NURSING ORGANISATION OF SOUTH AFRICA (DENOSA)

PO Box 1280, Pretoria, 0001, South Africa
Tel: (27) 12 343 2315
Fax: (27) 12 344 0750
Email: denosahq@cis.co.za
Contact: Executive Director

DENOSA is a professional organisation and labour union for nurses in South Africa.

DENOSA Bursaries, Scholarships and Grants

Subjects: Nursing.
Eligibility: Open to members in good standing of the Organisation who hold the required registered nursing qualifications.

Level of Study: Doctorate, Graduate, Postgraduate, Professional development.
Purpose: To encourage post-basic studies at a South African teaching institution.
Type: Bursary.
No. of awards offered: Varies.
Frequency: Annual.
Value: Varies.
Length of Study: Varies.
Study Establishment: A South African teaching institution.
Country of Study: South Africa.
Application Procedure: Application form must be completed.
Closing Date: January 31st.

THE DENMARK-AMERICA FOUNDATION

Fiolstraede 24
3rd Floor, Copenhagen, DK-1171, Denmark
Tel: (45) 33 12 83 23
Fax: (45) 33325323
Email: fulbdk@unidhp.uni-c.dk
Contact: Ms Marie Monsted, Executive Director

The Denmark-America Foundation was founded in 1914 as a private Foundation, and today its work remains based on donations from Danish firms, foundations and individuals. The Foundation offers scholarships for studies in the USA at the graduate and postgraduate university level and has a trainee programme.

Denmark-America Foundation Grants

Subjects: All subjects.
Eligibility: Open to Danes only.
Level of Study: Doctorate, Postdoctorate, Postgraduate, Professional development.
Purpose: To further understanding between Denmark and the USA.
Type: Bursary.
No. of awards offered: Varies.
Frequency: Twice a year.
Value: Varies.
Length of Study: Between 3 months and 1 year.
Country of Study: USA.
Application Procedure: Special application form must be completed - please contact the Secretariat.
Closing Date: To be announced.

DENTISTRY CANADA FUND/FONDS DENTAIRE CANADIEN (DCF)

427 Gilmour Street, Ottawa, ON, K2P 0R5, Canada
Tel: (1) 613 236 4763
Fax: (1) 613 236 3935
Email: information@dcf-fdc.ca
www: http://www.dcf-fdc.ca
Contact: Mr Richard Munro, Executive Director

DCF Biennial Research Award

Subjects: Dentistry.
Eligibility: Open to graduate or postgraduate students who have conducted their research in association with a Canadian Dental faculty.
Level of Study: Graduate, Postgraduate.
Purpose: To encourage research related to dentistry conducted by graduate or postgraduate students in Canada.
Type: Research Grant.
No. of awards offered: 1.
Frequency: Every two years.
Value: C$2,000 plus a commemorative plaque.
Country of Study: Any country.
Application Procedure: Applicants should submit one typewritten, double-spaced copy and four copies of an original research project in the form of a paper. The manuscript should not exceed 25 pages; or, a previously published paper of the applicant's graduate work either currently in press or already published in a scientific journal provided the date of publication is not more than two years from the date of application and provided the applicant is demonstrably the senior author.
Closing Date: December 1st biennially.
Additional Information: Each entry will be reviewed by three referees appointed by the CDA Committee on Dental Materials and Devices. The decision of the Committee is final.

DCF Fellowships for Teacher/Researcher Training

Subjects: Dentistry.
Eligibility: Applicants must be Canadian citizens or permanent residents who have completed an undergraduate course in dentistry, a dental hygiene programme, or a programme in science and who are also eligible for admission to a graduate or other advanced education programme.
Level of Study: Postgraduate.

Purpose: To provide financial assistance to students who wish to pursue a career in dentistry research and/or teaching at graduate level.
Type: Fellowship.
Country of Study: Any country.
Application Procedure: First-time applications must include official transcripts of previous post-secondary education and letters of recommendation from a faculty member of the applicant's post-secondary institution and from the Administrative Head of the Institution and Department where he/she expects to be employed. All applications must include a CV.
Closing Date: March 1st.

DCF/Wrigley Dental Student Research Awards

Subjects: Oral biology.
Eligibility: Open to students enrolled in Canadian dental schools.
Level of Study: Graduate.
Purpose: To enable applicants to undertake research projects in oral biology.
Type: Research Grant.
No. of awards offered: Up to 3.
Frequency: Annual.
Value: C$3,000.
Country of Study: Any country.
Application Procedure: Each application must include the background on the subject matter, the research objectives, the proposed hypothesis, the research approach and the project's timetable and budget.
Closing Date: March 1st.

DEPARTMENT OF EDUCATION & SCIENCE (IRELAND)

Floor 1J
Block 4
Irish Life Centre
Talbot Street, Dublin, 1, Ireland
Tel: (353) 1 873 4700
Fax: (353) 1 872 9293
Contact: Ms Rita Frawley

Department of Education and Science (Ireland) Exchange Scholarships and Postgraduate Scholarships Exchange Scheme

Subjects: All subjects.
Eligibility: Open to Australian, Austrian, Belgian, Chinese, Finnish, German, Greek, Italian, Japanese, Netherlands, Norwegian, Russian Federation, Spanish and Swiss nationals, who are university graduates or advanced undergraduates who have completed at least three years of academic study. A good knowledge of English and/or Irish is necessary, depending on the course taken.
Level of Study: Postgraduate.

Purpose: To assist students to pursue study or research in Ireland.
Type: Scholarship.
No. of awards offered: 30.
Frequency: Annual.
Value: IR£3,144.
Length of Study: 8 months.
Study Establishment: An Irish university: University College Dublin, University College Cork, University College Galway, Trinity College Dublin, Dublin City University, University of Limerick, St Patrick's College Maynooth, or other similar institution of higher learning.
Country of Study: Ireland.
Application Procedure: Candidates should apply to the appropriate institution in their home country, as follows: Austria - the Federal Ministry for Science and Research, Vienna; Australia - the Ministry of Education, Canberra; Belgium - the Ministry of Education for the Flemish Community, Brussels; China - the Ministries of Foreign Affairs and Education, Beijing; Finland - Finnish Centre for International Mobility (CIMO), Helsinki; France - the Foreign Ministry, Paris; Germany - the German Academic Exchange Board (Deutscher Akademischer Austauschdienst-DAAD), Bonn; Greece - the Ministries of Foreign Affairs and Education, Athens; Italy - the Ministry of Foreign Affairs, Rome; Japan - the Ministries of Foreign Affairs and Education, Tokyo; Netherlands - Netherlands Organisation for International Co-operation in Higher Education (NUFFIC), The Hague; Norway - the Ministry of Foreign Affairs, Office of Cultural Relations, Oslo; Russian Federation - the Ministry of Education of the Russian Federation; Spain - the Ministry of Foreign Affairs, Madrid; Switzerland - Swiss University Authorities, Berne. Five scholarships are offered to students from the United Kingdom to pursue postgraduate studies in Ireland. The value of each scholarship is £6,000. Applications should be made to the Irish Embassy, London.
Closing Date: April 30th.

DoE (Ireland) Summer School Exchange Scholarships

Subjects: All subjects.
Eligibility: Open to Belgian, French, Finnish, German, Hungarian, Italian, Netherlands, Russian Federation and Spanish nationals who are university graduates or advanced undergraduates. A good knowledge of English and/or Irish is necessary, depending on the course taken.
Level of Study: Postgraduate.
Purpose: To assist European students to attend a summer school in Ireland.
Type: Scholarship.
No. of awards offered: 33.
Frequency: Annual.
Value: IR£720 Exception - IR£950 for Hungarian and Russian Federation nationals.
Length of Study: From 2 weeks to 1 month.
Study Establishment: Summer schools at University College Dublin, University College Galway or University College Cork.
Country of Study: Ireland.

Application Procedure: Candidates should apply to the appropriate institution in their home country, as follows: Belgium - the Ministry of Education for the Flemish Community, Brussels; France - the Foreign Ministry, Paris; Finland - Finnish Centre for International Mobility (CIMO), Helsinki; Germany - the German Academic Exchange Board (Deutscher Akademischer Austauschdienst-DAAD), Bonn; Hungary - the Ministry of Culture and Education, Budapest; Italy - the Ministry of Foreign Affairs, Rome; Netherlands - Netherlands Organisation for International Co-operation in Higher Education (NUFFIC), The Hague; Russian Federation - the Ministry of Education of the Russian Federation; Spain - the Ministry of Foreign Affairs, Madrid.
Closing Date: April 30th.

Irish Government Scholarship

Subjects: All subjects.
Eligibility: Open to Australian postgraduate students. The scholar is required to return to Australia on the completion of the scholarship programme or on the completion of further studies leading on from the initial scholarship programme.
Level of Study: Postgraduate.
Type: Scholarship.
No. of awards offered: 1.
Frequency: Annual.
Value: IR£3,144 payable in 8 monthly instalments, plus university or college registration and tuition fees.
Length of Study: 1 academic year.
Study Establishment: University or institute of higher learning.
Country of Study: Ireland.
Application Procedure: Please write to the Grants Management Officer at the Embassy for details.
Closing Date: March.

For further information contact:

Embassy of Ireland
20 Arkana Street, Yarralumla, ACT, 2600, Australia
Tel: (61) 6 273 3022
Fax: (61) 6 273 3741

DEPARTMENT OF EMPLOYMENT, EDUCATION, TRAINING & YOUTH AFFAIRS

Research Grants & Training Section
Loc 731
GPO Box 9880, Canberra, ACT, 2601, Australia
Tel: (61) 6 240 8653
Fax: (61) 6 240 9781
Email: rbfellow@deetya.gov.au
www:
http://www.deetya.gov.au/divisions/hed/research/research.htm
Contact: The Director

The Department of Employment, Education, Training and Youth Affairs is a Ministry within the Australian Government, which works together with the Australian Research Council, and other agencies such as the Higher Education Contribution Scheme and the National Board of Employment, Education and Training on providing employment and training schemes.

Overseas Postgraduate Research Scholarships (OPRS)

Subjects: All subjects.
Eligibility: Applicants cannot be considered if they have commenced a course of study at any university at the same level for which the scholarship is oughjt.
Level of Study: Doctorate, Postgraduate.
Purpose: To assist study leading to the degree of PhD or to a masters research degree.
Type: Scholarship.
No. of awards offered: Varies.
Value: The scholarship covers the course fee and is awarded.
Length of Study: 3 years in the first instance.
Country of Study: Australia.
Application Procedure: Please write for details.
Closing Date: August 30th.
Additional Information: Awarded to varying organisations, The Australian National University being one of them.

DEPARTMENT OF NATIONAL HEALTH AND WELFARE

Research and Program Policy Directorate
Promotion & Programs Branch, Ottawa, ON, K1A 1B4, Canada
Tel: (1) 613 954 8549
Fax: (1) 613 954 7363
Email: nhrdpinfo@isdicp3.hwc.ca
www: http://www.hwc.ca/datahpsb/nhrdp/index.html
Contact: Information & Resource Officer

The National Health Research and Development Programme (NHRDP) funds research with scientific merit to support the Federal Department of Health's mission and national health priorities, and researchers whose work will contribute to policy devlopment and strategic planning. In general, the NHRDP funds research that relates to issues of concern to the federal government and to those that may be of concern to provincial and territorial health ministries pertaining to the health system and the promotion of population health.

Personnel Awards

Subjects: The National Health and Research Development Programme (NHRDP) offers awards to students and new researchers in areas that support Health Canada's research priorities and policy leadership role. The priorities are - population health, health impact of public policies, renewal and restructuring of the health system, research on transfer and uptake of knowledge.

Eligibility: Applicants must clearly identify links between the proposed programme and health policy. Programmes must address the research themes identified in the NHRDP toward 2001. Applicants must be Canadian citizens or landed immigrants.

Level of Study: Doctorate, Postdoctorate, Postgraduate.

Purpose: To help develop and enhance individuals' research skills to ensure Canada has a cadre of researchers to meet future health challenges and to strengthen the country's science and technology research capacity.

Frequency: Annual.

Value: Master and PhD C$18,000, Postgraduate C$30,000, Scholar C$50,000.

Length of Study: Master's 2 years, PhD 4 years, Postgraduate 2 years, Scholar 5 years.

Study Establishment: Canadian Centres.

Country of Study: Master's tenable in Canadian Centres. PhD strong justification required for tenure outside Canada. Postdoctoral strong justification required for tenure outside Canada. Scholar tenable in Canadian Centres.

Closing Date: March 1st.

DEUTSCHE FORSCHUNGSGEMEINSCHAFT (DFG)

Kennedyallee 40, Bonn, 53175, Germany
Tel: (49) 228 885 1
Fax: (49) 228 885 2777
Email: postmaster@dfg.d400.de
www: http://www.dfg.de

The Deutsche Forschungsgemeinschaft is the central public funding organisation for academic research in Germany. The DFG's mandate is to serve science and the arts in all fields by supporting research projects carried out in universities and research institutions in Germany, to promote co-operations between scientists, and to forge and support links between German academic science and industry, and with partners in foreign countries. In doing this, the DFG gives special attention to the education and support of young scientists and scholars. Foreign scientists and scholars who wish to obtain a fellowship to work in Germany may turn to the DAAD or to the Alexander von Humboldt Stiftung.

Collaborative Research Grants

Subjects: All subjects.

Eligibility: Promising groups of German nationals and permanent residents in Germany.

Level of Study: Postdoctorate, Research.

Purpose: To promote long term co-operative research in universtites and academic research.

Type: A variable number of Grants.

No. of awards offered: Varies.

Value: Dependent on the requirements of the project.

Length of Study: 3-15 years.

Study Establishment: Universities and academic institutions in Germany.

Country of Study: Germany.

Application Procedure: Applications must be formally filed by the universities. For further information please write or visit the website.

Closing Date: Please write for details.

Additional Information: A list of Collaborative Research Centres is available (in German only) from the DFG.

Emmy Noethen-Programme

Subjects: All subjects.

Eligibility: Promising young postdoctoral scientists up to the age of approximately 30, who are German nationals, or permanent residents of Germany.

Level of Study: Postdoctorate.

Purpose: To give outstanding young scholars the opportunity to obtain the scientific qualifications needed to be appointed as a lecturer within a period of five years after receiving their PhD.

Type: Project Grant.

No. of awards offered: 100.

Frequency: Annual.

Value: For the two years of research spent abroad the candidate is to receive a project grant in keeping with the requirements of the project, including an allowance, for subsistence and travel. For the three years of research spent at a German university or research institution the candidate is to receive a project grant of up to DM400,000 per annum.

Length of Study: 5 years.

Study Establishment: Universities or research institutions worldwide.

Country of Study: Any country.

Application Procedure: For an application form and further information please contact Dr Bruno Zimmerman, or visit the website.

Closing Date: Please write for details.

For further information contact:

Germany
Tel: (49) 288 855 2254
Fax: (49) 288 885 2180
Contact: Dr Bruno Zimmermann

Eugen and Ilse Seibold Prize

Subjects: Arts and humanities.

Eligibility: Outstanding young German or Japanese scholars.

Level of Study: Postdoctorate.

Purpose: To promote outstanding young scientists and scholars who have made significant contributions to the scientific interchange between Japan and Germany.

Type: Award.

No. of awards offered: 2.

Frequency: Every two years (1999, 2001, 2003).

Value: Approx. DM20,000 per prize.

Length of Study: Varies.

Study Establishment: Universities or research institutions.

Country of Study: Germany or Japan.

Application Procedure: Applications are by nomination. For further information please write or visit the website.
Closing Date: Please write for details.

Fellowships

Subjects: All subjects.
Eligibility: Promising young scientists or scholars who are German nationals or permanent residents of Germany.
Level of Study: Postdoctorate.
Purpose: To promote young scientists and scholars qualified with an outstanding PhD degree.
Type: A variable number of Fellowships.
No. of awards offered: Up to 1000.
Frequency: Annual.
Value: Varies.
Length of Study: Varies.
Study Establishment: Universities worldwide.
Country of Study: Any country.
Application Procedure: Please write for details, or visit the website.
Closing Date: Applications accepted at any time.

Gerhard Hess Awards

Subjects: All subjects.
Eligibility: Promising young scientists and scholars, who are German nationals, or permanent residents of Germany.
Level of Study: Postdoctorate, Predoctorate, Research.
Purpose: To promote young scientists and scholars up to the age of 35 years, who show exceptional promise and achievement and are seeking to establish an independent research group in a qualified research environment.
Type: Award.
No. of awards offered: 10.
Frequency: Annual.
Value: Up to DM200,000 per award.
Length of Study: 2 - 5 years.
Study Establishment: German universities and research institutions.
Application Procedure: Application is by nomination.
Closing Date: Please write for details.

Gottfried Wilhelm Leibnitz Research Prize

Subjects: All subjects.
Eligibility: Outstanding scholars in German universities.
Level of Study: Predoctorate, Research.
Purpose: To promote outstanding scientists and scholars in German universities and research institutions.
Type: Research Grant.
No. of awards offered: Varies.
Frequency: Annual.
Value: DM1.5 - 3million per prize for 5 years study.
Length of Study: 5 years.
Study Establishment: German universities or research institutions.
Country of Study: Germany.
Application Procedure: Application is by nomination. Nominations are restricted to selected institutions (DFG member organisations) or individuals (former prize winners,

chairpersons of DFG review committees). For further information please write or visit the website.
Closing Date: Please write for details.
Additional Information: A list of prize winners is available (in German only) from the DFG.

Graduate Colleges

Subjects: All subjects.
Eligibility: Highly qualified graduate and doctoral students of any nationality.
Level of Study: Postgraduate, Predoctorate.
Purpose: To promote high quality graduate studies at doctoral level through participation of graduate students recruited through country wide calls in research programmes.
Type: A variable number of Fellowships.
No. of awards offered: Varies.
Length of Study: Up to 9 years.
Study Establishment: German universities.
Country of Study: Germany.
Application Procedure: Applications should be submitted in response to calls. For further information please visit the website.
Closing Date: Please write for details.
Additional Information: A list of Graduate Colleges presently funded is available (in Germany only) from the DFG.

Guest Professorships

Subjects: All subjects.
Eligibility: Foreign scientists, whose individual research is of special interest to research and teaching in Germany.
Level of Study: Postdoctorate.
Purpose: To support stays of foreign scientists at German universities, if the stay is of special interest to research and teaching in Germany.
Type: A variable number of Fellowships.
No. of awards offered: Varies.
Frequency: Annual.
Value: Dependent on the duration of the stay.
Length of Study: 3 months - 1 year.
Study Establishment: German universities.
Country of Study: Germany.
Application Procedure: Submission of a proposal by the university intending to host the guest Professor.

Hans Maier-Leibnitz Prize

Subjects: All subjects.
Eligibility: Promising young scholars up to the age of 33, who are German nationals or permanent residents of Germany.
Level of Study: Doctorate, Postdoctorate.
Purpose: To promote outstanding young scientists at doctorate level.
Type: Award.
No. of awards offered: 6.
Frequency: Annual.
Value: DM30,000 per prize.
Length of Study: Varies.
Study Establishment: German universities or research institutions.

Country of Study: Germany.
Application Procedure: Application is by nomination. Please write for details or visit the website.
Closing Date: Please write for details.

Heisenberg Programme

Subjects: All subjects.
Eligibility: High calibre young scientists up to the age of 35 years of age, who are German nationals or permanent residents of Germany.
Level of Study: Postdoctorate.
Purpose: To promote outstanding young scientists up to the age of 35 years of age, who are German nationals, or permanent residents of Germany.
Type: Scholarship.
No. of awards offered: Varies.
Frequency: Annual.
Value: Varies.
Length of Study: 5 years.
Study Establishment: German universities or research institutions.
Country of Study: Germany.
Application Procedure: Applicants must submit a research proposal, a detailed curriculum vitae, copies of degree certificates, a copy of the thesis, a letter explaining the choice of host institution, a list of all the candidates previously published material, and a letter outlining the candidates financial requirements in duplicate. For further information please contact DFG.
Closing Date: Applications are accepted at any time.

Individual Grants

Subjects: All subjects.
Eligibility: Promising researchers and scholars, who are German nationals or permanent residents of Germany.
Level of Study: Postdoctorate, Postgraduate, Predoctorate, Research.
Purpose: To foster the proposed research projects of promising academic scientists or scholars.
Type: A variable number of Grants.
No. of awards offered: Varies.
Frequency: Throughout the year.
Value: Dependent on the requirement of the project.
Length of Study: 2 to 3 years initially, with the option of applying for a renewal.
Study Establishment: Universities worldwide.
Country of Study: Any country.
Application Procedure: Submission of a proposal for a research project. Please write for more details or visit the website: http://www.dfg.de/english/internat-coop.html.
Closing Date: Applications accepted at any time.

Joint Research Projects

Subjects: All subjects.
Eligibility: German scholars and scholars from any participating Eastern European country.
Level of Study: Postdoctorate, Research.

Purpose: To foster co-operation between German scientists and scientists in Middle and Eastern European countries and countries of the former Soviet Union.
Type: A variable number of Grants.
No. of awards offered: Varies.
Frequency: Annual.
Value: Dependent on the length of the research project and the number of participants.
Length of Study: Varies.
Study Establishment: Universities in any participating country.
Country of Study: Any country.
Application Procedure: Applications for sponsorship must be submitted by researchers from German research institutes. Please write for details or visit the website http://dfg.de/english/internat_coop.html.
Closing Date: Please write for details.

Priority Programs

Subjects: All subjects.
Eligibility: Interested groups of scientists from Germany or any country participating in the scheme.
Level of Study: Postdoctorate, Research.
Purpose: To promote proposals made by interested groups of scientists in selected fields.
Type: A variable number of Grants.
No. of awards offered: Varies.
Value: The Senate decides on the financial ceiling for each programme.
Length of Study: Up to 6 years.
Study Establishment: Universities or academic establishments in the countries participating in the scheme.
Country of Study: Any country.
Application Procedure: Priority Programmes are operated through calls for proposals, with all applications subject to open panel review, usually after discussion with the applicants. For further information please write or visit the website.
Closing Date: Please write for details.

Research Groups

Subjects: All subjects.
Eligibility: Interested groups of German nationals and permanent residents of Germany.
Level of Study: Postdoctorate, Research.
Purpose: To promote intensive co-operation between highly qualified researches in one or several institutions in fields of high scientific promise.
Type: Research Grant.
No. of awards offered: Varies.
Frequency: Annual.
Value: Dependent on the requirements of the project.
Length of Study: Up to 6 years.
Study Establishment: German universities.
Country of Study: Germany.
Application Procedure: Please submit proposals to the Senate of the DFG. For further information please write or visit the website.
Closing Date: Please write for details.

Additional Information: A list of currently operating Research Groups is available (in German only) from the DFG.

Additional Information: Conditions are advertised in the medical press.

THE DIGESTIVE DISORDERS FOUNDATION

3 St Andrew's Place
Regent's Park, London, NW1 4LB, England
Tel: (44) 171 486 0341
Fax: (44) 171 224 2012
Email: ddf@digestivedisorders.org.uk
www: http://www.digestivedisorders.org.uk
Contact: G F Oliver

The Digestive Disorders Foundation (formerly the British Digestive Foundation) supports research into the cause, prevention and treatment of digestive disorders, including digestive cancers, ulcers, irritable bowel syndrome, inflammatory bowel disease, diverticulitis, liver disease and pancreatitis. The Foundation also provides information for the public explaining the symptoms and treatment of these and other common digestive conditions.

Digestive Disorders Foundation Fellowships and Grants

Subjects: Gastroenterology. Research Fellowships are awarded for basic or applied clinical research into normal and abnormal aspects of the gastrointestinal tract, liver and pancreas. Research Grants are awarded for specific projects in the same field of interest. Travel Grants are awarded to assist researchers by enabling them to visit overseas institutions with the aim of learning new techniques or otherwise advancing their own research.
Eligibility: Applicants must have been resident in the UK for a minimum of five years. Fellowship projects must contain an element of basic science training.
Level of Study: Doctorate, Postgraduate.
Purpose: To provide funding for gastroenterological research into the prevention and treatment of disorders of the gastrointestinal tract, liver and pancreas.
Type: Fellowships, Research and Travel Grants.
No. of awards offered: Approx. 10.
Frequency: Twice a year.
Value: Up to £34,000 per year, paid quarterly in advance for Fellowships. Research Grants up to £10,000. Travel Grants up to £2,000.
Length of Study: 1, 2 or 3 years.
Study Establishment: Recognised and established research centres.
Country of Study: Primarily the United Kingdom, but training grants for overseas study by British residents can be given.
Application Procedure: An application form must be completed for consideration in a research competition. Competitions are advertised in December and June/July each year. Details are available on the Internet.
Closing Date: As advertised in 'Nature', and 'British Medical Journal'.

DR HADWEN TRUST FOR HUMANE RESEARCH

84A Tilehouse Street, Hitchin, Hertfordshire, SG5 2DY, England
Tel: (44) 1462 436819
Fax: (44) 1462 436844
Contact: Dr G Langley

The Dr Hadwen Trust for Humane Research is a registered charity, established in 1970, to promote research into techniques and procedures to replace the use of living animals in biomedical research, testing, and teaching.

Research Assistant or Technician

Subjects: Research projects must be aimed at the development, validation or implementation of a technique or procedure which would replace one currently using living animals.
Eligibility: Applicants must be UK residents.
Purpose: To provide additional scientific or technical support for a research project.
No. of awards offered: Varies.
Value: Salary for research assistant or technician.
Length of Study: 3 years.
Study Establishment: Various.
Country of Study: United Kingdom.
Application Procedure: In the first instance apply in writing to the Scientific Adviser, Dr G Langley. Applications must be made by the Senior Researcher who will oversee the work.

Research Fellowship

Subjects: The research must aim to develop, validate or implement a technique or procedure which could replace one currently using living animals.
Eligibility: Applicants must be resident in the UK.
Level of Study: Postdoctorate.
Purpose: To attract and retain talented young scientists in non-animal research fields. The funds provide personal support and a contribution to direct research costs.
Type: Fellowship.
No. of awards offered: Varies.
Frequency: Dependent on funds available.
Value: Salary on research analoctous salary scale grade 1A, up to spinal point 9, plus London Allowance where appropriate.
Length of Study: 3 years.
Study Establishment: Various.
Country of Study: United Kingdom.
Application Procedure: In the first instance apply in writing to Dr G Langley, Scientific Adviser. Application forms must be submitted by a Senior Researcher who will oversee the work.

Research Plus PhD Studentship

Subjects: Developing alternatives to animal experiments in biomedical fields.
Eligibility: Applicants must be resident in the UK.
Level of Study: Postgraduate.
Purpose: To encourage young graduates with good honours degrees to train in non-animal methods.
Type: Studentship.
No. of awards offered: Varies.
Frequency: Dependent on funds available.
Value: £7,800 per annum (outside London) £9,580 per annum (London).
Length of Study: 3 years.
Study Establishment: UK based research only.
Country of Study: United Kingdom.
Application Procedure: Initial enquiries to the Scientific Adviser, Dr G Langley. Applications must be submitted by the project supervisor.

DUKE UNIVERSITY CENTER

Box 2908, Durham, NC, 27710, United States of America
Tel: (1) 919 681 8777
Fax: (1) 919 681 8744
Email: grm@duke.edu
www: http://www.geri.duke.edu/education/
Contact: Mr Gail R Marsh, Co-ordinator

Duke University Center Postdoctoral Training in Ageing Research

Subjects: Social and behavioural sciences, natural sciences and medical sciences.
Eligibility: Open to US citizens and permanent residents.
Level of Study: Postdoctorate.
Purpose: To train research scientists in the methods used in research on ageing in any scientific field.
Type: Training Award.
No. of awards offered: Approx. 4.
Frequency: Annual.
Value: Depending on experience. From US$26,256 up to US$41,268 reviewed annually.
Length of Study: 2 years.
Study Establishment: Duke University.
Country of Study: USA.
Application Procedure: Applicants should send CV and letter requesting further application materials. Applicant should also supply a project description, three letters of reference, a training plan, a career plan and graduate transcripts. An application form and further information are available from the website.
Closing Date: April 1st.

EAST-WEST CENTER

Award Services
1601 East-West Road, Honolulu, HI, 96848-1601, United States of America
Tel: (1) 808 944 7735
Fax: (1) 808 944 7730
Contact: Fellowships Office

The East-West Center promotes understanding among the governments and peoples of Asia, the Pacific, and the United States of America; through collaborative research and training and through dialogue and cultural interchange. The Center supports degree Fellows from the region in various educational activities, including study at the University of Hawaii.

Graduate Degree Fellowship

Subjects: Agriculture, forestry and fishery, architecture and town planning, arts and humanities, business administration and management, education and teacher training, engineering, fine and applied arts, law, mass communications and information science, mathematics and computer science, medical sciences, natural sciences, recreation, welfare and protective services, and social and behavioural sciences.
Eligibility: Applicants must have obtained a 4 year bachelor's degree or its equivalent, must be a citizen or permanent resident of the United States of America or a citizen of a country in Asia or the Pacific, and must come to the Center on the Exchange Visitor (J-1) Visa.
Level of Study: Doctorate, Postgraduate.
Purpose: To enable degree study at the University of Hawaii and participation in the educational activities of the Center.
Type: Fellowship.
No. of awards offered: Varies.
Frequency: Annual.
Value: May apply for funding for housing, stipend, tuition, health insurance, books, materials, and supplies.
Length of Study: Initially 12 months, with possible renewal.
Study Establishment: University of Hawaii.
Country of Study: USA.
Application Procedure: Applicants must send the completed East-West Center and University of Hawaii application forms to the East-West Center. Applicants must include test information, curriculum vitae, essay and other documents. Applicants must also arrange for the required test scores, official transcripts, and letters of reference to be submitted to the East-West Center.
Closing Date: October 15th.

EASTMAN DENTAL CENTER

University of Rochester
625 Elmwood Avenue, Rochester, NY, 14620, United States
of America
Tel: (1) 716 275 8315
Fax: (1) 716 256 3153
Email: mfoy@edc.rochester.edu
Contact: Registrar

Eastman Dental Center Clinical Fellowships

Subjects: Postdoctoral training in Advanced Education
General Dentistry.
Eligibility: Open to recent dental graduates who have a DDS
degree or equivalent qualification. Candidates from overseas
must show evidence of high academic achievement and of
their intention to follow an academic or research career.
Level of Study: Postdoctorate.
Purpose: To enable suitably qualified dental graduates to
undertake training and/or research at the Center.
Type: Fellowship.
No. of awards offered: Approx. 25.
Frequency: Annual.
Value: International students pay tuition for Peridontics
Prosthodontics and Orthodontics. Scholarships are
sometimes available for General Dentistry.
Length of Study: 1 or 2 year programs (June - June).
Study Establishment: University of Rochester, Eastman
Dental Center.
Country of Study: USA.
Application Procedure: Please submit application form, CV,
dental transcripts, undergraduate transcripts and three letters
of recommendation from dental professors and Dean of
Dental School.
Closing Date: October 31st.

EDUCATIONAL COMMISSION FOR FOREIGN MEDICAL GRADUATES (ECFMG)

2401 Pennsylvania Avenue NW
Suite 475, Washington, DC, 20037, United States of America
Tel: (1) 202 293 9320
Fax: (1) 202 457 0751
www: http://www.ecfmg.org
Contact: Ms Sally F Oesterling, Staff Assistant

ECFMG serves the public interest through a programme of
evaluation of foreign trained physicians. ECFMG also
sponsors foreign national physicians as exchange visitors in
accredited graduate medical education programmes. The
organisation's aims and missions include promoting
excellence in international medical education and contributing
to the exchange of medical knowledge among nations.

International Fellowships in Medical Education

Subjects: Eligible areas of study include - educational
methodology, curriculum design, evaluation systems, medical
school governance, and the development of basic and clinical
science departments.
Eligibility: Open to citizens of all countries except the United
States and Canada. Candidates must document English
language competence, both written and oral. Candidates
must have a graduate or professional degree that relates to
the proposed area of study. They must have three years of
work experience in their chosen field following completion of
their formal academic and clinical training. They must hold an
academic appointment as a faculty member in a school of
medicine or a postgraduate medical education institute. They
must have the endorsement of the home country medical
school or postgraduate medical education institute for the
proposed programme. Countries with which the US does not
have diplomatic relations excepted.
Level of Study: Professional development.
Purpose: To facilitate placement of faculty from foreign
medical schools in US academic institutions able to provide
educational opportunities of high quality; to match
educational opportunities in the USA with the determined
needs of nations abroad; and to provide opportunities for
faculty from schools of medicine outside the United States to
study aspects of medical education in the United States that
have the potential to improve medical education in their home
country institutions and departments.
Type: Fellowship.
No. of awards offered: 15-20.
Frequency: Annual.
Value: US$2,200 monthly stipend, round trip air fare for the
fellow only; health insurance for the fellow and any
accompanying family members.
Length of Study: Minimum of 6 months to a maximum of 12
months.
Study Establishment: US medical institutions.
Country of Study: USA.
Application Procedure: Application forms must be
requested and completed. Two reference reports must also
be submitted. EFCMG screens applications, matches
approved candidates with appropriate US faculty mentors,
and provides formal recognition for the educational
programme upon its completetion.
Closing Date: August 15th.
Additional Information: Candidates must reside and work in
their home countries at the time of application. Under this
programme fellowships are not provided for degree-granting
educational programmes; programmes that require tuition
payments; tuition grants for short-term courses; specialty
training in residency programmes; or solely for training in
clinical procedures.

ELIZABETH GLASER PEDIATRIC AIDS FOUNDATION

2950 31st Street
Suite 125, Santa Monica, CA, 90405, United States of America
Tel: (1) 310 314 1459
Fax: (1) 310 314 1469
Email: research@pedaids.org
www: http://www.pedaids.org
Contact: Ms Chris Hudnall, Resource Co-ordinator

The Foundation funds basic medical research in paediatric HIV and AIDS.

Elizabeth Glaser Scientist Award

Subjects: Pediatric HIV/AIDS research and investigation.
Eligibility: Applicants must have an MD, PhD, DDS or DVM degree and must be at assistant professor level or above.
Purpose: To build a network of scientists focusing on issues of paediatric HIV and AIDS, and create a generation born free of this infection.
Type: Award.
No. of awards offered: Up to 5.
Frequency: Annual.
Value: Provides up to $650,000 in direct costs over a period of 5 years.
Application Procedure: Please write for details.

Paediatric AIDS Foundation Student Intern Awards

Subjects: Medical research, paediatrics.
Eligibility: Open to highly motivated high-school, college, graduate and medical students who have a sponsor recognised for his or her contributions to paediatric AIDS. The programme may be orientated to either fundamental research or clinical research and care.
Level of Study: Doctorate, Postgraduate, Undergraduate.
Purpose: To encourage students to enter clinical and research programs related to paediatric AIDS.
Type: Award.
No. of awards offered: 50.
Frequency: Annual.
Value: US$2,000 for 320 hours work.
Length of Study: 1 year.
Country of Study: Any country.
Application Procedure: The procedure of application depends on the specific programme; please contact Chris Hudnall for additional information.
Closing Date: March 26th.

Research Grants One-Year and Two-Year

Subjects: Paediatrics.
Purpose: To provide initial funding to investigators to enable them to gather preliminary data to answer questions quickly or obtain sufficient results to apply to other granting agencies.
Type: Research Grant.
Value: Provides up to US$80,000 per year in direct costs for a period of performance not to exceed two years. Research using animal models may apply for supplemental funds directly related to the purchase and care of animals, total direct cost is $100,000/year with supplement. Indirect cost allowed is 20% of total direct.
Length of Study: Determination as to the duration of the support will be made by the Scientific Advisory Committee during peer review. Renewals for 1 year are completely reviewed based on progress. 2 year grants are not renewable.
Application Procedure: Please write for details. Requests for applications sent: March.

Scholar Awards

Subjects: Pediatric HIV/AIDS research.
Eligibility: Applicants must have two to three years of postdoctoral experience. Tenured investigators are not eligible. Applicants must work with a qualified sponsor.
Purpose: To encourage young investigators to select paediatric HIV and AIDS as a research focus for their career.
Value: Provides $66,000 indirect costs, for two years salary support ($32,000 year one and $34,000 year two). Renewable for a third year at $36,000.
Length of Study: 2 years, renewable for a third.
Application Procedure: Only one application for any scholar, sponsor or laboratory, or department. Requests for applications should be sent in March.

Short-Term Scientific Awards

Subjects: Research.
Level of Study: Research.
Purpose: To provide funding for travel and short-term study in a US institution, to initiate a critical research project, obtain preliminary data, learn new techniques in an established laboratory, or sponsor an important workshop.
Type: Award.
Value: Provides up to $5,000. Indirect costs are not applicable. Funds are intended for travel, per diem, housing, research supplies or other costs as needed for short-term projects. Renewals are not granted.
Study Establishment: US institution.
Country of Study: USA.
Application Procedure: Requests for applications sent in March.

ENGINEERING AND PHYSICAL SCIENCES RESEARCH COUNCIL (EPSRC)

Polaris House
North Star Avenue, Swindon, Wiltshire, SN2 1ET, England
Tel: (44) 1793 444000
Fax: (44) 1793 444012
www: http://www.epsrc.ac.uk
Contact: Postgraduate Training

EPSRC promotes and supports high quality, basic, strategic and applied research and related postgraduate training in engineering and physical sciences. It aims to advance knowledge and technology by providing trained scientists and engineers, in order to meet the needs of users and beneficiaries, and thereby contribute to economic competitiveness and quality of life.

EPSRC Overseas Travel Grant

Subjects: All subjects.
Purpose: To allow promising scholars to visit recognised centres abroad to study new techniques or to develop collaborations.
Type: Travel Grant.
Value: Varies.
Study Establishment: Recognised centres abroad.
Country of Study: Any country, except UK.
Application Procedure: Submissions of a proposal on the standard EPS (RP) form.
Closing Date: At least 6 weeks before the proposed visit.

EPSRC Visiting Fellowships

Subjects: All subjects.
Purpose: To enable scientists or engineers of acknowledged standing from within the UK or abroad to visit the proposer's institutions to give advice and assistance in research fields in which the visitor is eminent.
Type: Fellowship.
Value: Appropriate salary including travel allowance and subsistence.
Length of Study: Up to 1 year.
Application Procedure: Applications should be made on form EPS (VF).

Fast Stream Grants

Subjects: All subjects.
Eligibility: Applicants must have been appointed to their first university post within the previous 24 months, and apply the the EPSRC as an individual Principal Investigator for the first time.
Type: A variable number of Grants.
Value: Up to £50,000.
Application Procedure: Submission of a grant proposal to the EPSRC. If the grant proposal is commented on favourably by all three referees in the first stage of the review process,

then approval will be given without the proposal having to enter the rank ordering stage conducted at a panel meeting.

Joint Research Equipment Initative

Subjects: All subjects.
Purpose: To enable high-quality research to be conducted between HEIs and external sponsors of research.

LINK

Subjects: All subjects.
Purpose: To encourage collaborative research between the science and engineering base, and the users of research in industry, commerce, the service sector and elsewhere.
Application Procedure: Submission of application in response to calls for proposals.

MOD Joint Grants Scheme

Subjects: All subjects.
Purpose: To support high-quality research which has been successful at Peer Review and has defense relevance.
Type: Grant.
Application Procedure: Please refer to the guidance notes for applicants.

Realising Our Potential Awards

Subjects: All subjects.
Eligibility: Promising researchers in universities and research council institutions, units or establishments, whose proposals can satisfy the criteria of originality and feasibilty.
Level of Study: Research.
Purpose: To reward researchers who receive substantial financial support from industry for basic/strategic research, by providing research grants to support curiosity driven research of their own choosing.
Value: Varies.
Study Establishment: Universities and research council institutes, units or establishments.

EPILEPSY FOUNDATION

4351 Garden City Drive, Landover, MD, 20785, United States of America
Tel: (1) 301 459 3700
Fax: (1) 301 577 2684
www: http://www.efa.org
Contact: Ms Liz Bryson

The Epilepsy Foundation is a national, charitable organisation, founded in 1968 as the Epilepsy Foundation of America. It is the only organisation wholly dedicated to the welfare of people with epilepsy and to working on their behalf through research, education, advocacy and service.

EF Behavioral Sciences Research Training Fellowship

Subjects: Epilepsy research relative to the behavioural sciences, appropriate fields of study include sociology, social work, psychology, anthropology, nursing, political science, and others relevant to epilepsy research and practice.
Eligibility: Open to individuals who have received their doctoral degree in a field of the behavioural sciences by the time the fellowship commences and desire additional postdoctoral research experience in epilepsy. Applications from women and minorities are encouraged.
Level of Study: Postdoctorate.
Purpose: To offer qualified individuals the opportunity to develop expertise in epilepsy research through a training experience or involvement in an epilepsy research project.
Type: Fellowship.
No. of awards offered: 1.
Frequency: Annual.
Value: A stipend of up to US$30,000, depending on the experience and qualifications of the applicant and the scope and duration of the proposed project.
Length of Study: 1 year.
Study Establishment: An approved facility.
Country of Study: USA.
Application Procedure: Application forms and guidelines are available from the Foundation on request.
Closing Date: February 1st.

EF Health Sciences Student Fellowships

Subjects: Medical and health sciences.
Eligibility: A perceptor must accept responsibility for supervision of the student and the project.
Purpose: To award medical and health sciences students to work on an epilepsy study project.
Type: Fellowship.
Value: $2,000.
Length of Study: 3 months.
Study Establishment: A US institution of the students choice where there are ongoing programmes of research, training, or service in epilepsy.
Country of Study: USA.
Application Procedure: Please write for details.
Closing Date: February 1st to be considered for the same year.

EF International Clinical Research Fellowship

Subjects: Epilepsy research.
Eligibility: Applicants must have received their MD (or foreign equivalent) and completed residency training. Either the Fellow or the host institution must be American.
Level of Study: Doctorate, Postgraduate.
Purpose: To provide an individual with the opportunity to develop expertise in clinical epilepsy and research through a one-year training experience to promote the exchange of medical and scientific information and expertise on epilepsy between the USA and other countries.
Type: Fellowship.
No. of awards offered: 1.

Frequency: Annual.
Value: US$40,000 stipend only.
Length of Study: 1 year.
Study Establishment: An approved facility where there is an ongoing epilepsy research program.
Country of Study: Any country.
Application Procedure: Please write for details.
Closing Date: September 1st.

EF International Visiting Professorship

Subjects: Epilepsy research.
Eligibility: Either the visitor or the host institution must be from the USA.
Level of Study: Professional development.
Purpose: To provide an opportunity for a visiting professor to spend time at a host institution to promote the exchange of medical and scientific information and expertise on epilepsy between the USA and other countries.
Type: Visiting Professorship.
No. of awards offered: Up to 10, depending on funds available.
Frequency: Throughout the year.
Value: To cover travel expenses and minor incidental expenses.
Length of Study: 3-6 weeks.
Study Establishment: An approved facility.
Country of Study: Any country.
Application Procedure: Please write for details.
Closing Date: Applications accepted at any time.

EF Junior Investigator Research Grants

Subjects: Basic biomedical, behavioural and social sciences, particular encouragement is given to applications in the behavioural sciences.
Eligibility: Open to US researchers. Priority is given to beginning investigators just entering the field of epilepsy, to new or innovative projects, and to investigators whose research is relevant to developmental or paediatric aspects of epilepsy. Applications from women and minorities are encouraged; applications from established investigators with other sources of support are discouraged, and Research Grants are not intended to provide support for postdoctoral fellows.
Level of Study: Postdoctorate, Postgraduate.
Purpose: To support basic and clinical research which will advance the understanding, treatment and prevention of epilepsy.
Type: Research Grant.
No. of awards offered: Varies.
Frequency: Annual.
Value: Varies; support is limited to US$40,000.
Length of Study: 1 year.
Country of Study: USA.
Application Procedure: Application forms and guidelines are available from the Foundation on request.
Closing Date: September 1st.

EF Research Training Fellowships

Subjects: Basic or clinical epilepsy research, which must address a question of fundamental importance, a clinical training component is not required.
Eligibility: Open to physicians and PhD neuroscientists who desire postdoctoral research experience; preference is given to applicants whose proposals have a paediatric or developmental emphasis. Applications from women and minorities are encouraged.
Level of Study: Postdoctorate.
Purpose: To offer qualified individuals the opportunity to develop expertise in epilepsy research through involvement in an epilepsy research project.
Type: Fellowship.
No. of awards offered: Varies.
Frequency: Annual.
Value: A stipend of US$40,000.
Length of Study: 1 year.
Study Establishment: A facility where there is an ongoing epilepsy research program.
Country of Study: USA or Canada.
Application Procedure: Application forms and guidelines are available from the Foundation upon request.
Closing Date: September 1st.

EF Research/Clinical Training Fellowships

Subjects: Basic or clinical epilepsy research, with an equal emphasis on clinical training and clinical epileptology.
Eligibility: Open to individuals who have received their MD degree and completed residency training. Applications from women and minorities are encouraged.
Level of Study: Postdoctorate, Postgraduate.
Purpose: To offer qualified individuals the opportunity to develop expertise in epilepsy research through a training experience and involvement in an epilepsy research project.
Type: Fellowship.
No. of awards offered: Varies.
Frequency: Annual.
Value: A stipend of US$40,000.
Length of Study: 1 year.
Study Establishment: A facility where there is an ongoing epilepsy research program.
Country of Study: USA.
Application Procedure: Please write for details.
Closing Date: September 1st.
Additional Information: These Fellowships include the Merrit-Putnam Fellowship.

EXETER COLLEGE

Oxford, OX1 3DP, England
Tel: (44) 1865 279 660
Fax: (44) 1865 279 630
www: http://www.exeter.ox.ac.uk
Contact: Tutor for Graduates

Monsanto Senior Research Fellowship

Subjects: Molecular or cellular biology, or biochemistry.
Eligibility: Open to qualified applicants of any nationality.
Level of Study: Postdoctorate.
Purpose: To support research in molecular or cellular biology, or biochemistry.
Type: Fellowship.
No. of awards offered: 1.
Frequency: Every 3-5 years.
Value: Stipend between £13,941 and £19,326 p.a. Entitled to free lunch and dinner, free rooms in college if unmarried, and housing allowance if not resident in college.
Length of Study: 3-5 years.
Study Establishment: Exeter College.
Country of Study: United Kingdom.
Application Procedure: Enquiries should be addressed to the Tutor for Graduates.

Staines Medical Research Fellowship

Subjects: Medical science widely construed.
Eligibility: Applicants should be close to completing doctoral work, or postdoctoral, and must be under 31 at the time of taking up the fellowship.
Level of Study: Doctorate, Postdoctorate.
Purpose: To support research into medical science.
Type: Fellowship.
No. of awards offered: 1.
Frequency: Every 2-3 year.
Value: Stipend between £300 and £9,228 per year. Entitled to free lunch and dinner, free rooms in college if unmarried, and housing allowance if not resident in college.
Length of Study: 2-3 years.
Study Establishment: Exeter College.
Country of Study: United Kingdom.
Application Procedure: Enquiries should be addressed to the Tutor for Graduates.

FEDERAL COMMISSION FOR SCHOLARSHIPS FOR FOREIGN STUDENTS

Route du Jura 1, Fribourg, CH-1700, Switzerland
Tel: (41) 37 26 74 24
Fax: (41) 37 26 74 04
Contact: Grants Management Officer

Swiss Scholarships for Students from Developing Countries

Subjects: All courses or research work offered at Swiss institutions of higher education.
Eligibility: Open to persons who can satisfy the eligibility requirements of the Swiss educational institution. A good knowledge of French or German is essential and a preliminary language examination is given at the Swiss Embassy in the candidate's country (some scholars may be required to take the language course at Fribourg prior to their proposed course of study). Scholarships for basic academic courses will only be granted to candidates coming from countries

which have no university (yet) or where the university education system is in the process of being developed.

Level of Study: Postgraduate, Undergraduate.

Purpose: To enable students from developing countries to further their studies or begin research work at a Swiss institution of higher education.

Type: Scholarship.

No. of awards offered: Varies.

Frequency: Annual.

Value: Students not having obtained a university degree (the BA and BSc degrees are not necessarily recognised as university degrees) CHF1,450 per month; postgraduates CHF1,650 per month; students attending the language course at Fribourg CHF4,050 total for the duration of the course (three months).

Length of Study: 1 academic year.

Study Establishment: At institutions of higher education. Scholarships for postgraduate students may, in principle, be renewed for a second academic year. Only in exceptional cases will candidates be allowed to continue their studies towards a doctorate by means of the Scholarship.

Country of Study: Switzerland.

Application Procedure: Application forms must be completed and submitted along with: copies of secondary school certificates; copies of certificates, diplomas and university degrees with marks; two academic references; plan outlining the programme of study whilst in Switzerland; curriculum vitae; writeen comfirmation from a professor at the chosen instiution that the applicants project is feasible at the institution; medical certificate. The documents must be written in German, French, Italian or English or translated into one of these languages. Art students must submit Photographs of 3 pieces of their work, rough drafts (with indication of the date) for fine arts; very good quality cassette tapes of 3 different styles of music, composers must submit scores, for music.

Closing Date: Usually end of October of the previous year.

Additional Information: The Commission is part of the Federal Department of Home Affairs. The scholarships are offered to foreign governments and only candidates recommended by their home authorities are eligible. Candidates must apply to the international scholarship agency in their own country.

Swiss Scholarships for Students from Industrial Countries

Subjects: All courses or research work offered at Swiss institutions of higher education.

Eligibility: Open to persons who can satisfy the eligibility requirements of the Swiss educational institution. A good knowledge of French or German is essential and a preliminary language examination is given at the Swiss embassy in the candidate's country (some scholars may be required to take the language course at Fribourg prior to their proposed course of study).

Level of Study: Postgraduate.

Purpose: To enable foreign students to further their studies or begin research work at a Swiss institution of higher education.

Type: Scholarship.

No. of awards offered: Varies.

Frequency: Annual.

Value: Scholars are exempt from tuition fees and insured against illness and accidents. The Scholar pays the fare to Switzerland and the Swiss government pays the return fare only for overseas students (Canada, US, Japan, China, Australia, New Zealand, etc.) Monthly allowances are offered as follows: CHF1,450 for students who have not obtained a university degree (foreign BA and BSc degrees are not always recognised); CHF1,650 for postgraduates; CHF1,650 for fine arts and music students; CHF4,050 for the whole of the language course.

Length of Study: 1 academic year.

Study Establishment: At institutions of higher education. Scholarships for postgraduate students can only exceptionally be renewed for a second academic year.

Country of Study: Switzerland.

Application Procedure: Application forms must be completed and submitted along with: copies of secondary school certificates; copies of certificates, diplomas and university degrees with marks; two academic references; plan outlining the programme of study whilst in Switzerland; curriculum vitae; writen comfirmation from a professor at the chosen instiution that the applicants project is feasible at the institution; medical certificate. The documents must be written in German, French, Italian or English or translated into one of these languages. Art students must submit Photographs of 3 pieces of their work, rough drafts (with indication of the date) for fine arts; very good quality cassette tapes of 3 different styles of music, composers must submit scores, for music.

Closing Date: Usually end of October of the previous year.

Additional Information: The Commission is part of the Federal Department of Home Affairs. The Scholarships are offered to foreign governments and only candidates recommended by their home authorities are eligible. Candidates must apply to the international scholarship agency in their own country (US students: Institution of International Education, 809 United Nations Plaza, New York, New York 10017. Canadian students: Association of Universities and Colleges of Canada, 151 Slater Street, Ottawa, Ontario K1P 5N1. UK students: The British Council, 10 Spring Gardens, London SW1A 2BN). The Commission also administers the Postgraduate Scholarships for Nationals of the Council for Cultured Co-operation, Council of Europe. Those who wish to obtain general information on the courses offered at Swiss universities may consult the brochure 'The Swiss Universities' available at Swiss embassies and consulates.

FIGHT FOR SIGHT, INC.

Research Division of Prevent Blindness America
500 East Remington Road, Schaumburg, IL, 06173, United
States of America
Tel: (1) 708 843 2020
Contact: Research Awards Co-ordinator

Fight for Sight Grants-in-Aid

Subjects: Ophthalmology, vision and related sciences.
Eligibility: Applicants must be residents of the US or Canada.
Level of Study: Doctorate.
Purpose: Awards are made to investigators who are
interested in conducting research in vision and vision related
sciences.
Type: Research Grant.
No. of awards offered: Approx. 20.
Frequency: Annual.
Value: By individual assessment, US$1,000-US$12,000
maximum; to help defray the cost of personnel, equipment
and supplies needed for a specific research investigation.
Length of Study: 1 year, support may be renewed.
Study Establishment: Any institution in the USA or Canada
which offers research facilities suitable to the research project
in question.
Country of Study: USA or Canada.
Application Procedure: Please write for an application form
and programme details.
Closing Date: March 1st.
Additional Information: It is the responsibility of candidates
to make arrangements with the institutions of their choice in
the USA or Canada. Applications for support of pilot projects
are welcome.

Fight for Sight Postdoctoral Research Fellowships

Subjects: Ophthalmology, vision and related sciences - basic
or clinical research.
Eligibility: Applicants must be residents of USA or Canada.
Level of Study: Doctorate.
Purpose: Awards are made to support investigators who are
interested in conducting research in vision or vision related
sciences.
Type: Fellowship.
No. of awards offered: Approx. 15.
Frequency: Annual.
Value: US$5,000-US$14,000 per year. Recipients may
supplement this stipend with institutional funds from another
source, not to exceed US$28,000 per year.
Length of Study: 1 year; possibly renewable.
Study Establishment: At any approved institution in the USA
or Canada.
Country of Study: USA or Canada.
Application Procedure: Please write for application.
Closing Date: March 1st.

Additional Information: It is the responsibility of candidates
to make arrangements with the institutions of their choice in
the USA or Canada.

Fight for Sight Student Research Fellowships

Subjects: Ophthalmology, vision and related sciences.
Eligibility: Open to graduate students who are interested in
eye-related clinical or basic research. Student Fellowships are
not offered to Americans who wish to study abroad.
Level of Study: Postgraduate, Undergraduate.
Purpose: Awards are made to support new investigators who
are interested in conducting research in vision and vision
related sciences.
Type: Fellowship.
No. of awards offered: Approx. 20.
Frequency: Annual.
Value: US$500 per month.
Length of Study: 2-3 months, usually during the summer.
Study Establishment: Approved institutions.
Country of Study: USA or Canada.
Application Procedure: Please write for application and
programme details.
Closing Date: March 1st.
Additional Information: It is the responsibility of candidates
to make arrangements with the institutions of their choice in
the USA or Canada.

FLEMISH COMMUNITY

c/o Embassy of Belgium
3330 Garfied Street NW, Washington, DC, 20008, United
States of America
Tel: (1) 202 625 5850
Fax: (1) 202 342 8346
Contact: Flemish Community Fellowships Office

Fellowship of the Flemish Community

Subjects: Art, music, humanities, social and political
sciences, law, economics, sciences and medicine.
Eligibility: Open to US citizens of no more than 35 years of
age, who hold a Bachelor's or Master's degree, and who have
no other Belgian sources of income.
Level of Study: Postgraduate.
Purpose: To assist American college students who wish to
continue their postgraduate education in Flanders, Belgium.
Type: Fellowship.
No. of awards offered: 5.
Frequency: Annual.
Value: A monthly stipend of BEF26,200; tuition fees at a
Flemish institution up to BEF18,500; health insurance and
public liability insurance in accordance with Belgian law.
There is no reimbursement of travel expenses.
Length of Study: 10 months.
Study Establishment: Universities, conservatories of music,
or art academies affiliated with the Flemish Community.
Country of Study: Belgium.

Application Procedure: Application form must be completed and submitted typed, in triplicate with a certified true copy of the applicant's birth certificate; copy of diplomas; summary of the thesis; official transcripts; two recommendations from current teachers or employers; and latest GPA where applicable.
Closing Date: January 15th.
Additional Information: Applicants will be notified of the result of applications no later than the end of July, and the academic year for most institutes of higher learning in Flanders starts at the end of September.

FONDATION PHILIPPE WIENER-MAURICE ANSPACH

39 avenue Franklin D Roosevelt, Brussels, B-1050, Belgium
Contact: Mr M Philippe de Bruycker, Executive Secretary

Postdoctorate Grants

Subjects: All subjects.
Eligibility: Eligible candidates must have done the doctorate at the Universite Libre de Bruxelles having passed with a minimum of grand distinction.
Level of Study: Postdoctorate.
Purpose: For doctors of all disciplines who completed their thesis at the Universite Libre de Bruxelles and want to continue at Oxford or Cambridge.
Type: Grant.
Value: BEF100,000 per month. Fees and lab costs are paid by the Foundation.
Length of Study: A maximum of 1 year.
Study Establishment: Oxford or Cambridge University.
Country of Study: United Kingdom.
Application Procedure: Applicants must: complete an application form which must be obtained from the secretariat; include a full CV and photocopies of certificates; give information on the research planned- a timetable and someone who will supervise the research in the UK; provide a letter of recommendation from an English sponsor; letters of recommendation from 2 members of university staff.
Closing Date: March 25th.

Predoctorate Grants

Subjects: All subjects.
Eligibility: Open to students who have finished the second stage of their predoctoral course at the Universite Libre de Bruxelles and who want to develop their studies or research during an academic year at Oxford or Cambridge. Access to the grants is dependent on their having completed the first stages of study at the Universite Libre de Bruxelles; having passed with a minimum of grand distinction.
Level of Study: Predoctorate.
Purpose: For student at Universite Libre de Bruxelles who want to continue their studies at Oxford or Cambridge.

Type: Grant.
Value: Between £9,250 and £13,758 with the college fees being paid by the foundation.
Study Establishment: Oxford or Cambridge University.
Country of Study: United Kingdom.
Application Procedure: The following information must be submitted: an application form must be completed which can be obtained from the secretariat; a CV and photocopies of certificates; university grades and details of specific project completed so far; information on the type of study or research the applicant wants to do; two letters of academic reference.
Closing Date: December 1st.

FOULKES FOUNDATION FELLOWSHIP

37 Ringwood Avenue, London, N2 9NT, England
Tel: (44) 181 444 2526
Fax: (44) 181 444 2526
www: http://www.cbcu.cam.ac.uk/foulkes/ff.html
Contact: The Registrar

The aim of the Foulkes Foundation Fellowship is to promote medical research by providing financial support for postdoctoral science graduates who need a medical degree before they can undertake medical research, and similarly for medical graduates who need a science degree.

Foulkes Foundation Fellowship

Subjects: All aspects of medical research, especially in the areas of molecular biology and biological sciences.
Eligibility: Open to recently qualified scientists and medical graduates who have a PhD or equivalent degree or proven research ability and who intend to contribute to medical research. The applicant must study in the UK.
Level of Study: Postdoctorate.
Purpose: To promote medical research by providing financial support for science graduates needing a medical degree before they can undertake medical research, or for medical graduates in need of a science PhD degree.
Type: Fellowship.
No. of awards offered: Varies.
Frequency: Annual.
Value: Varies. The amount of the Fellowship depends on individual need, but the scale for the basic SRC Studentship is used as a guideline. Fellowships do not cover fees.
Length of Study: Up to 3 years.
Country of Study: United Kingdom.
Application Procedure: A stamped self-addressed envelope should be sent to the Registrar for additional information and application form.
Closing Date: March 15th.

FOUNDATION FOR CHIROPRACTIC EDUCATION AND RESEARCH (FCER)

1701 Clarendon Boulevard
1st Floor, Arlington, VA, 22209, United States of America
Tel: (1) 703 276 7445
Fax: (1) 703 276 8178
Email: rosnerfcer@aol.com
www: http://www.fcer.org
Contact: Dr Anthony L Rosner, Director of Research and Education

The goal of FCER is to stimulate both basic and applied research to further our understanding of chiropractic, with particular attention to its clinical and cost effectiveness as well as the mechanisms of the principles upon which chiropractic is founded. Included in FCER's means of support are funding of research grants and support for postgraduate research through the provision of fellowship and residency awards.

FCER Fellowships

Subjects: Chiropractic.
Eligibility: Open to nationals of any country.
Level of Study: Doctorate, Postgraduate.
Purpose: Research development for basic/clinical science projects which specifically relate to chiropractic.
Type: Fellowship.
No. of awards offered: 10.
Frequency: Annual.
Value: US$3,000-US$9,000.
Length of Study: 1-3 years.
Study Establishment: College, university or hospital.
Country of Study: Any country.
Application Procedure: Write or fax FCER with request for application materials and information for appropriate programme.
Closing Date: March 1st.

FCER Research Grants

Subjects: Chiropractic.
Eligibility: Open to nationals of any country.
Level of Study: Doctorate.
Purpose: Research development for basic/clinical science projects which relate specifically to chiropractic.
Type: Grant.
No. of awards offered: 10.
Frequency: Twice a year.
Length of Study: 1-3 years.
Study Establishment: College, university or hospital.
Country of Study: Any country.
Application Procedure: Write or fax FCER with request for application materials and information for appropriate programme.
Closing Date: October 1st, March 1st.

FCER Residencies

Subjects: Chiropractic.
Eligibility: Open to nationals of any country.
Level of Study: Doctorate, Postgraduate.
Purpose: Research development for basic/clinical sciences projects which specifically relate to chiropractic.
Type: Residency.
No. of awards offered: 1.
Frequency: Annual.
Value: US$10,000-US$20,000.
Length of Study: 1-3 years.
Study Establishment: College, university or hospital.
Country of Study: Any country.
Application Procedure: Write or fax FCER with request for application materials and information for appropriate programme.
Closing Date: March 1st.

FOUNDATION FOR HIGH BLOOD PRESSURE RESEARCH

c/o Dept of Physiology
Monash University, Clayton, VIC, 3168, Australia
Tel: (61) 3 9905 2555
Fax: (61) 3 9905 2566
Contact: Ms Jan Morrison, Administrative Officer

The Foundation was established to support research into any aspects of blood pressure, hypertension and associated cardiovascular diseases.

Foundation for High Blood Pressure Research Postdoctoral Fellowship

Subjects: Hypertension research or in areas relevant to the understanding of the causes, prevention, treatment or effects of hypertension.
Eligibility: Open to applicants from Australia or New Zealand, who have a degree in medicine or science, with appropriate PhD.
Level of Study: Postdoctorate.
Purpose: To fund an Australian or New Zealand scientist to perform research into the causes or treatment of hypertension. The research must be performed in Australia.
Type: Fellowship.
No. of awards offered: 1.
Frequency: Two out of three years.
Value: Salary and associated costs, plus project maintenance.
Length of Study: 2-3 years.
Study Establishment: An Australian institute, university or hospital.
Country of Study: Australia.
Application Procedure: Application must be submitted with CV and relevant publications.
Closing Date: Usually July 31st.

Additional Information: The award is not offered every year. It is advertised in Australia and overseas. Interested applicants should contact the Honorary Secretary for further information.

ISH Postdoctoral Fellowship

Subjects: Hypertension research or in areas relevant to the understanding of the causes, prevention, treatment or effects of hypertension.
Eligibility: Open to applicants who have a degree in medicine or science, or appropriate PhD.
Level of Study: Postdoctorate.
Purpose: To fund an international scientist to perform research into the causes or treatment of hypertension. The research must be performed in Australia.
Type: Fellowship.
No. of awards offered: 1.
Frequency: Two out of three years.
Value: Salary and associated costs, in addition to project maintenance.
Length of Study: 2 years.
Study Establishment: An Australian institute, university or hospital.
Country of Study: Australia.
Application Procedure: Application must be completed and submitted with CV and relevant publications.
Closing Date: Usually July 31st.
Additional Information: The award is not offered every year. Details are advertised in Australia and overseas. Interested applicants should contact the Honorary Secretary seeking further information.

FOUNDATION FOR PHYSICAL THERAPY

1111 North Fairax Street, Alexandria, VA, 22314, United States of America
Tel: (1) 703 684 5984
Fax: (1) 703 706 8519
Contact: Scientific Program Officer

The Foundation for Physical Therapy is a national, independent, non-profit corporation to support the physical therapy profession's research needs in three areas: scientific research, clinical research and health services research.

New Investigator Fellowships Training Initiative (NIFTI)

Subjects: Physical therapy.
Eligibility: The applicant must possess a licence to practice physical therapy in the USA and must have received the required post-professional doctoral degree no earlier than five years prior to the year of application.
Level of Study: Postdoctorate.

Purpose: To provide support for new investigators to promote development of a research career and to pursue research that demonstrates clinical effectiveness and functional outcomes of physical therapist practice.
Type: Fellowship.
No. of awards offered: Varies.
Frequency: Annual.
Value: US$30,000.
Country of Study: USA.
Application Procedure: Please write for details or email foundation@apta.org.
Closing Date: January 15th.

Promotion of Doctoral Studies (PODS)

Subjects: Physical therapy.
Eligibility: The applicant must possess a licence to practice physical therapy in the US, and must be enrolled as a student, in a regionally accredited post-professional doctoral programme. The content of this programme should have a demonstrated relationship to physical therapy.
Level of Study: Doctorate.
Purpose: To fund doctoral students who, having completed one full year of coursework, wish to continue their coursework or enter the dissertation phase.
Type: Scholarship.
No. of awards offered: Varies.
Frequency: Annual.
Value: Two levels: US$7,500 and US$15,000.
Length of Study: Up to 5 years.
Country of Study: USA.
Application Procedure: Please write for details or email foundation@apta.org.
Closing Date: January 15th.

FOUNDATION FOR SCIENCE AND DISABILITY, INC.

503 NW 89 Street, Gainesville, FL, 32607, United States of America
Tel: (1) 352 374 5774
Fax: (1) 352 374 5781
Email: rmankin@gainesville.usda.ufl.edu
www: http://www.as.wvu.edu~scidis/organizations
Contact: Dr Richard Mankin, Grants Committee Chair

The Foundation for Science and Disability aims to promote the integration of scientists with disabilities into all activities of the scientific community and of society as a whole, and to promote the removal of barriers in order to enable students with disabilities to choose careers in science.

Foundation for Science and Disability Student Grant Fund

Subjects: Engineering, mathematics, medicine and natural sciences.
Eligibility: Open to candidates from all countries.

Level of Study: Doctorate, Postdoctorate, Postgraduate.
Purpose: To increase opportunities in science for physically disabled students at the graduate or professional level.
Type: Grant.
No. of awards offered: 1-3.
Frequency: Annual.
Value: US$1,000.
Length of Study: 1 year.
Country of Study: Any country.
Application Procedure: Please submit a completed application form, copies of official college transcripts, a letter from research or academic supervisor in support of request, and a second letter from another faculty member.
Closing Date: December 1st.
Additional Information: The award may be used for an assistive device or instrument, or as financial support to work with a professor, or on an individual research project, or for some other special need.

FOUNDATION FOR THE STUDY OF INFANT DEATHS (FSID)

14 Halkin Street, London, SW1X 7DP, England
Tel: (44) 171 235 0965
Fax: (44) 171 823 1986
Email: fsid@sids.org.uk
www: http://www.sids.org.uk/fsid/
Contact: Dr S Levene, Secretary, Scientific Advisory Committee

The Foundation for the Study of Infant Deaths, the leading UK Cot Death charity, raises funds for research, supports families whose babies have died, and disseminates information about cot death and infant care to health professionals and the public.

FSID Research Grant Award

Subjects: Paediatrics, including - developmental physiology, pathology, infection, metabolism, statistics, epidemiology, immunology and infant care practices.
Eligibility: Open to any graduate research worker linked to academic/medical institution within the UK.
Level of Study: Unrestricted.
Purpose: To support relevant experimental and clinical research in sudden unexpected death and well-being in infancy.
Type: Research Grant.
No. of awards offered: Varies.
Frequency: Twice a year; dependent on funds available.
Value: There is no fixed upper limit, but applications are unlikely to succeed if recurrent expenditure exceeds £30,000 and total annual expenditure in any one year exceeds £50,000.
Length of Study: For the duration of the project, normally up to a maximum of 3 years.
Study Establishment: Academic/medical institute.
Country of Study: United Kingdom.

Application Procedure: Application form (10 copies) to be completed.
Closing Date: Early January and early July.

FSID Short Term Training Fellowship

Subjects: Paediatrics.
Eligibility: Open to graduate research workers linked to academic or medical institutions within the UK.
Level of Study: Unrestricted.
Purpose: To allow research workers in the field of sudden infant death to visit and work in specialist labs for short periods to acquire new technical skills, apply new methods of data analysis or establish collaborative research.
Type: Fellowship.
No. of awards offered: Varies.
Frequency: Dependent on funds available.
Value: Usually up to £2,500, maximum £5,000.
Length of Study: 6-26 weeks.
Study Establishment: Academic/medical institute.
Country of Study: United Kingdom.
Application Procedure: Application form must be completed.
Closing Date: Applications are accepted at any time.

FOUNDATION OF THE AMERICAN COLLEGE OF HEALTHCARE EXECUTIVES

Suite 1700
One North Franklin Street, Chicago, IL, 60606-3491, United States of America
Tel: (1) 312 424 2800
Fax: (1) 312 424 0023
Email: srauchenecker@ache.org
www: http://www.ache.org/
Contact: Mr Steven M Rauchenecker, Membership Associate Director

Albert W Dent Student Scholarships

Subjects: Healthcare management.
Eligibility: Open to US and Canadian citizens who are Student Associates of the American College of Healthcare Executives in good standing; minority or handicapped undergraduate students who have been accepted for full-time study for the autumn term in a healthcare management graduate programme accredited by the Accrediting Commission on Education for Health Services Administration or who are enrolled full time and in good academic standing in an ACEHSA-accredited graduate programme in healthcare management; and are able to demonstrate financial need. Candidates may not be previous recipients.
Level of Study: Graduate.

Purpose: To provide financial aid and increase the enrolment of minority and handicapped students in healthcare management graduate programmes, and to encourage students (through structured, formalised study) to obtain positions in middle and upper levels of healthcare management.

Type: Scholarship.

No. of awards offered: Varies.

Frequency: Annual.

Value: US$3,500.

Country of Study: Any country.

Application Procedure: Applications are accepted between January 1st and March 31st and candidates are selected by the Foundation's Scholarship Committee shortly after the deadline date. Candidates should request an application from their programme director or from the Foundation.

Closing Date: Applications accepted between January 1st and March 31st.

Foster G McGaw Student Scholarships

Subjects: Healthcare management.

Eligibility: Open to US and Canadian citizens who are Student Associates of the American College of Healthcare Executives in good standing; who are enrolled full time and are in good academic standing in a graduate programme in healthcare management that is accredited by the Accrediting Commission on Education for Health Services Administration; and who can demonstrate financial need. Candidates may not be previous recipients.

Level of Study: Graduate.

Purpose: To assist financially worthy persons to better prepare themselves for healthcare management, thereby contributing to improvements in the field.

Type: Scholarship.

No. of awards offered: Varies.

Frequency: Annual.

Value: US$3,500.

Country of Study: Any country.

Application Procedure: Because the Foundation receives more applications for Scholarships than it can honour, it has instructed the director of each graduate programme to recommend students with the greatest financial need. To apply, candidates should obtain an application from their programme director. The Foundation accepts applications for Scholarships each year between January 1st and March 31st. Students selected to receive Scholarships are announced soon after the deadline date.

Closing Date: Applications accepted between January 1st and March 31st.

FRANK KNOX MEMORIAL FELLOWSHIPS

48 Westminster Palace Gardens
Artillery Row, London, SW1P 1RR, England
Tel: (44) 171 222 1151
Fax: (44) 171 222 5355
Contact: Ms Anna Mason, Secretary

The Frank Knox Memorial Fellowships were established at Harvard University in 1945 by a gift from Mrs Anna Reid Knox, widow of the late Col Frank Knox, to allow students from the United States, Australia, Canada, New Zealand and the United Kingdom to participate in an educational exchange programme.

Frank Knox Fellowships at Harvard University

Subjects: Arts, sciences (including engineering and medical sciences), business administration, design, divinity, education, law, public administration, public health.

Eligibility: Open to UK citizens normally resident in the UK who, at the time of application, have spent at least two of the last four years at a UK university or university college and will have graduated by the start of tenure.

Level of Study: Postgraduate.

Type: Fellowship.

No. of awards offered: 4.

Frequency: Annual.

Value: US$16,000 plus tuition fees. Unmarried Fellows may be accommodated in one of the university dormitories or halls.

Length of Study: 1 academic year. Depending on the availability of sufficient funds the fellowships may be renewed for Fellows registered for a degree programme of more than 1 year's duration.

Study Establishment: Harvard University, Cambridge, Massachusetts.

Country of Study: USA.

Application Procedure: Harvard University will try to arrange a suitable course for each individual. Fellowships are not awarded for postdoctoral study, and no application will be considered from persons already in the USA. Candidates must file an 'Admissions Application' directly with the graduate school of their choice at an early date; admission to a school is a prior condition of the award of a Fellowship. Candidates wishing to study business administration should apply by November 9th. A period of full-time work since graduation is necessary prior to embarking on the MBA programme. Travel grants are not awarded, although in cases of extreme hardship applications can be made to Harvard University for travel cost assistance.

Closing Date: November 1st.

FRAXA RESEARCH FOUNDATION

45 Pleasant Street, Newburyport, MA, 01950, United States
of America
Tel: (1) 978 462 1866
Fax: (1) 978 463 9985
Email: info@fraxa.org
www: http://www.fraxa.org
Contact: Ms Katherine Clapp, President

FRAXA Research Foundation funds postdoctoral fellowships and investigator-initiated grants to support medical research aimed at the treatment of Fragile X Syndrome. FRAXA is particularly interested in preclinical studies of potential pharmacological and genetic treatments, and studies aimed at understanding the function of the FMRI gene.

FRAXA Postdoctoral Fellowship

Subjects: Medical research aimed at the treatment of Fragile X Syndrome. Preclinical studies of potential pharmacological and genetic treatments and studies aimed at understanding the function of the FMRI gene.
Eligibility: There are no eligibility restrictions.
Level of Study: Postdoctorate.
Purpose: To promote research aimed at finding a specific treatment for Fragile X syndrome.
Type: Fellowship, Grant.
No. of awards offered: 8-15.
Frequency: Twice a year.
Value: Up to US$30,000 for postdoctoral fellowships. No limit for investigator-initiated grants.
Length of Study: 1 year; renewable.
Country of Study: Any country.
Application Procedure: Applications are accepted twice each year. An application form is available on the internet at www.fraxa.org/grants.html, or from FRAXA Research Foundation.
Closing Date: May 1st and November 1st every year.
Additional Information: Potential applicants are welcome to submit a one-page initial inquiry letter describing the proposed research, before submitting a full application.

FRIENDS OF ISRAEL EDUCATIONAL TRUST

Academic Study Group
PO Box 7545, London, NW2 2OZ, England
Tel: (44) 171 435 6803
Fax: (44) 171 794 0291
Email: foi_asg@msn.com
Contact: Mr John Levy

The Friends of Israel Educational Trust aim to encourage a critical understanding of developments, and to forge new collaborative links between Israel and the Arab world.

Friends of Israel Educational Trust Academic Study Bursary

Subjects: All subjects.
Eligibility: Open to research or teaching postgraduates. The Academic Study Group will only consider proposals from British academics who have already linked up with professional counterparts in Israel and agreed terms of reference for an initial visit.
Level of Study: Postdoctorate.
Purpose: To provide funding for British academics planning to pay a first research/study visit to Israel.
Type: Bursary.
No. of awards offered: 15.
Frequency: Annual.
Value: £300 per person.
Country of Study: Israel.
Application Procedure: There is no application form.
Closing Date: November 15th and March 15th.

FULBRIGHT SCHOLAR PROGRAM

Suite 5M
3007 Tilden Street NW, Washington, DC, 20008-3009, United
States of America
Tel: (1) 202 686 8664
Fax: (1) 202 362 3442
Email: apprequest@cies.iie.org
www: http://www.cies.org/
Contact: Grants Management Officer

Fulbright Postdoctoral Research and Lecturing Awards for Non-US Citizens

Subjects: All subjects.
Eligibility: Open to nationals of countries and territories having US diplomatic or consular posts, who have a doctoral degree or equivalent qualification. Preference is given to those persons who have not had extensive previous experience in the USA.
Level of Study: Postdoctorate.
Type: Grant.
No. of awards offered: Varies, approx. 700.
Frequency: Annual.
Value: A maintenance allowance and international travel expenses.
Length of Study: From 3 months to 1 academic year.
Country of Study: USA.
Application Procedure: Applications must be made to the binational educational commission or the US embassy or consulate in the candidate's home country.
Closing Date: Varies by country.

GERMAN ACADEMIC EXCHANGE SERVICE (DAAD)

950 Third Avenue
19th Floor, New York, NY, 10022, United States of America
Tel: (1) 212 758 3223
Fax: (1) 212 755 5780
Email: daadny@daad.org
www: http://www.daad.org
Contact: Grants Management Officer

The DAAD is a private, publicly funded, self-governing organisation of higher education institutes in Germany. DAAD promotes international academic relations and co-operation, especially through exchange programmes for students and faculty. The head office of DAAD is in Bonn and there are branch offices in Berlin, Beijing, Cairo, Jakarta, London, Moscow, Nairobi, New Delhi, New York, Paris, Rio de Janeiro, San Jose and Tokyo. The addresses of the branch offices are available on the DAAD website, or from the Bonn office.

Alexander von Humboldt 'Bundeskanzler' Scholarships

Subjects: Unrestricted, but a background in the humanities, social sciences, law or economics is preferred.
Eligibility: Candidates with demonstrated leadership qualities and excellence in their field should be nominated by US university presidents. Nominees must be US citizens and no more than 40 years of age.
Level of Study: Postgraduate.
Purpose: To enable highly qualified young Americans in academia, business or politics to gain substantial insight into German political, economic, social and cultural life in the course of an extended, self-structured stay.
Type: Scholarship.
No. of awards offered: Up to 10.
Frequency: Annual.
Value: Varies.
Study Establishment: German universities or research institutions.
Country of Study: Germany.
Application Procedure: For details and application material please write to the Alexander Von Humboldt Foundation, email: humboldt@umail.umd.edu or refer to the DAAD website.

For further information contact:

Alexander von Humboldt Foundation
 US Liason
1055 Thomas Jefferson Street
NW
Suite 2030, Washington, DC, 20007, United States of America
Tel: (1) 202 296 2990
Fax: (1) 202 833 8514
Contact: Grants Management Officer

Alexander von Humboldt Research Fellowships

Subjects: All subjects.
Eligibility: Open to highly qualified scholars and scientists of any nationality, who hold a PhD or equivalent and are not yet 40 years of age.
Level of Study: Postdoctorate.
Purpose: To promote promising young scholars and scientists of any nationality.
Type: Fellowship.
No. of awards offered: Varies.
Frequency: Annual.
Value: Varies.
Study Establishment: German universities or research institutions.
Country of Study: Germany.
Application Procedure: Please write for details.

For further information contact:

Alexander von Humboldt Foundation US Liason
1055 Thomas Jefferson Street N W
Suite 2030, Washington, DC, 20007, United States of America
Tel: (1) 202 296 2990
Fax: (1) 202 833 8514

DAAD Canadian Government Grants

Subjects: All subjects.
Eligibility: Open to Canadian citizens between 18 and 32 years of age who have a good command of German.
Level of Study: Postgraduate.
Purpose: To promote young scholars from Quebec who wish to pursue research in German studies.
Type: Grant.
No. of awards offered: Varies.
Frequency: Annual.
Value: Varies.
Length of Study: 1 academic year.
Study Establishment: German universities or research institutions.
Country of Study: Germany.
Application Procedure: Forms to be obtained from Canadian universities or directly from the DAAD office in New York.
Closing Date: Please write for details.

For further information contact:

(Residents from Québec only)
Direction de la générale de l'enseignement et de la recherche universitaires
Ministére de l'Enseignement supéet de la Science
1035 rue de la Chevrotière, Québec, G1R 5A5, Canada
Tel: (1) 418 643 2955
Fax: (1) 418 643 0622

DAAD Fulbright Grants

Subjects: All subjects.
Eligibility: Open to US citizens between 18 and 32 years of age who have a good command of German. Applicants must have been enrolled at a US university for at least one year at the time of application.
Level of Study: Postgraduate.
Purpose: This scholarship provides funds for graduate study and/ or research in Germany for one academic year.
Type: Grant.
No. of awards offered: Varies.
Frequency: Annual.
Value: Varies.
Length of Study: 1 academic year.
Country of Study: Germany.
Application Procedure: Forms may be obtained from campus Fulbright advisor.
Closing Date: Please write for details.

For further information contact:

Institute of International Education (IIE)
809 United Nations Plaza, New York, NY, 10017, United States of America
Tel: (1) 212 984 5330
Fax: (1) 212 984 5325
Contact: Grants Management Officer

DAAD Information Visits

Subjects: All subjects.
Eligibility: Applicants must have been enrolled at a US university for at least one year at time of application.
Level of Study: Graduate.
Purpose: To increase knowledge of specific German subjects and institutions within the framework of an academic study tour homogenous group of 15-25 students.
Frequency: Annual.
Length of Study: 7-21 days.
Country of Study: Germany.
Application Procedure: Forms may be obtained from the DAAD New York office or they can be downloaded from the internet.
Closing Date: At least six months before the intended visit.

DAAD Research Grants for Recent PhDs and PhD Candidates

Subjects: All subjects.
Eligibility: Open to recent PhDs (up to two years after the degree) of no more than 35 years of age and PhD candidates of no more than 32 years of age. Applicants must have been enrolled at a US university for at least one year at the time of application.
Level of Study: Doctorate, Postdoctorate.
Purpose: The purpose of this grant is to enable PhD candidates and recent PhDs to carry out dissertation or post-doctoral research at libraries, archives, institutes or laboratories in Germany for a period of one to six months during the calender year.
Type: Grant.

No. of awards offered: Varies.
Frequency: Annual.
Value: A monthly maintenance allowance, international travel subsidy, and health insurance.
Length of Study: 2-6 months.
Country of Study: Germany.
Application Procedure: Request forms from the DAAD or download from the internet.
Closing Date: August 1st for visits during the first half of the year; February 1st for visits during the second half of the year.

DAAD Study Visit Research Grants for Faculty

Subjects: All subjects.
Eligibility: Open to individuals with at least two years of teaching and/or research experience after the PhD or equivalent and a research record in the proposed field.
Level of Study: Faculty.
Purpose: To allow scholars to pursue research at universities and other institutions in Germany for one to three months during the calendar year.
Type: Grant.
No. of awards offered: Varies.
Frequency: Annual.
Value: A monthly maintenance allowance.
Length of Study: 1-3 months.
Country of Study: Germany.
Application Procedure: Forms may be obtained from the New York office or downloaded from the internet.
Closing Date: August 1st for visits during the first half of the year; February 1st for visits during the second half of the year.

DAAD/AICGS Grant

Subjects: Topics dealing with postwar Germany.
Eligibility: Open to PhD candidates, recent PhDs and junior faculty members.
Level of Study: Doctorate, Postdoctorate.
Purpose: This fellowship is available to assist doctoral candidates, recent PhDs and junior faculty working on topics dealing with postwar Germany. The grant provides funds for summer residency at the American Institute for Contemporary German Studies (AICGS).
Type: Fellowship.
No. of awards offered: 1.
Frequency: Annual.
Study Establishment: The American Institute for Contemporary German Studies (AICGS).
Country of Study: USA.
Application Procedure: Please write for details.
Closing Date: April 15th.

For further information contact:

AICGS
1400 16th Street NW
Suite 420, Washington, DC, 20036-2217, United States of America
Tel: (1) 202 332 9312
Fax: (1) 202 265 9531

Learn 'German in Germany' for Faculty

Subjects: All fields but in English and German.
Eligibility: Open to faculty of US universities.
Level of Study: Faculty.
Purpose: To enable recipients to attend intensive language courses at the Goethe Institutes.
Frequency: Annual.
Length of Study: 4 and 8 weeks.
Study Establishment: Goethe Institutes.
Country of Study: Germany.
Application Procedure: Forms may be obtained from the DAAD office in New York or they can be downloaded from the internet.
Closing Date: January 31st.

Summer Language Course at the University of Leipzig

Subjects: All fields, but students in the fields of English, German or any other modern language are not eligible.
Eligibility: Applicants must have been enrolled at a US university for at least one year at time of application.
Level of Study: Graduate, Postgraduate, Undergraduate.
Purpose: To support intensive language course, lectures, discussions on contemporary issues, independent project work, and excursions.
Frequency: Annual.
Length of Study: 8 weeks.
Study Establishment: University of Leipzig.
Country of Study: Germany.
Application Procedure: Forms may be obtained from the DAAD New York office or they can be downloaded from the internet.
Closing Date: January 31st.

Summer Language Courses at Goethe Institutes

Subjects: All fields, but students in the fields of English and German are not eligible.
Eligibility: Applicants must be enrolled at a US university at time of application.
Level of Study: Postgraduate.
Purpose: To offer intensive eight week language courses.
Frequency: Annual.
Length of Study: 8 weeks.
Study Establishment: Goethe Institutes.
Country of Study: Germany.
Application Procedure: Forms may be obtained from the New York office or they can be downloaded from the internet.
Closing Date: January 31st.

GILCHRIST EDUCATIONAL TRUST

Mary Trevelyan Hall
10 York Terrace East, London, NW1 4PT, England
Tel: (44) 171 631 8300 ext 773
Contact: Mrs Everidge, Secretary

GET Grants

Subjects: All subjects.
Eligibility: Open to students in the UK who are within sight of the end of a course and are facing unexpected financial difficulties which may prevent completion of their studies; students in the UK who are required to spend a short period studying abroad as part of their course; recognised British university expeditions; and pioneer educational establishments.
Level of Study: Doctorate, Postgraduate.
Purpose: To promote the advancement of education and learning in every part of the world.
Type: Grant.
No. of awards offered: Varies.
Frequency: Dependent on funds available.
Value: Modest.
Country of Study: United Kingdom, or students studying at a United Kingdom university who are required to spend a short period abroad.
Application Procedure: University expeditions are required to complete an application form. Eligible individuals are sent a list of information required.
Closing Date: For University Expeditions: February 28th. All other categories: at any time.
Additional Information: Individuals entitled to a mandatory grant/loan are not eligible.

Gilchrist Expedition Award

Subjects: All scientific subjects.
Eligibility: Open to teams of not more than ten members, most of them British, with the majority holding established positions in research departments at universities or similar establishments, wishing to undertake a field season of over six weeks in relation to one or more scientific objectives. The proposed research must be original and challenging, achievable within the timetable and preferably of benefit to the host country or region.
Purpose: To fund an intermediate level expedition by established scientists or academics.
Type: Grant.
No. of awards offered: 1.
Frequency: Every two years (even-numbered years).
Value: £10,000.
Country of Study: Any country.
Application Procedure: Please write for details.
Closing Date: March 15th.
Additional Information: The award is competitive.

GLAUCOMA RESEARCH FOUNDATION

200 Pine Street
Suite 200, San Francisco, CA, 94104, United States of America
Tel: (1) 415 986 3162
Fax: (1) 415 986 3763
www: http://www.glaucoma.org
Contact: Ms Mel Garrett, Research Manager

The Glaucoma Research Foundation is a national non-profit organisation working to protect the sight and independence of people with glaucoma, through research and education.

Clinician-Scientist Fellowship

Subjects: Glaucoma.
Eligibility: Opthamologists who are US citizens and who will have completed a clinical glaucoma fellowship prior to Clinician-Scientist Fellowship.
Purpose: To increase the number of opthamologists pursuing academic research into glaucoma.
Type: Fellowship.
No. of awards offered: 1.
Frequency: Annual.
Value: US$75,000, a portion going to host institution to support Fellow's research.
Length of Study: 1 year.
Country of Study: USA.
Application Procedure: Please write, phone or visit our website for details, or email clinician@glaucoma.org.
Closing Date: December 31st.

Pilot Project Grants Program

Subjects: Glaucoma.
Eligibility: A graduate degree.
Level of Study: Doctorate.
Purpose: To provide funds for research into glaucoma.
Type: Research Grant.
No. of awards offered: Varies.
Frequency: Annual.
Value: US$15,000-50,000.
Length of Study: 1 year.
Country of Study: USA.
Application Procedure: Please write, phone, or visit out website for details.
Closing Date: December 1st.

Shaffer International Fellowship Program

Subjects: Glaucoma.
Eligibility: MD opthamologists at the level of assistant professor. Must be fluent in written and spoken English.
Level of Study: Postgraduate.
Purpose: To enhance the glaucoma research training of opthamologists from developing countries.
Type: Fellowship.
No. of awards offered: 3-5.
Frequency: Annual.
Value: US$25,000, plus round trip travel.
Length of Study: 1 year.
Country of Study: USA.
Application Procedure: Please write, phone, or visit our website for details.
Closing Date: July 15th.

GREEK MINISTRY OF EDUCATION

Embassy of Greece
Cultural Department
1a Holland Park, London, W1H 3TP, England
Tel: (44) 171 229 3850
Fax: (44) 171 229 7221
Contact: Dr V Solomonidis, Cultural Attaché

Greek Ministry of Education Scholarships for British Students

Subjects: All subjects.
Eligibility: Open to UK nationals who hold at least a Bachelor's degree. Candidates graduating during the year of application will be considered. Some knowledge of Modern Greek is advisable.
Level of Study: Doctorate, Postdoctorate, Postgraduate, Professional development.
Purpose: To support postgraduate research in any subject.
Type: Scholarship.
No. of awards offered: 10.
Frequency: Annual.
Value: 100,000 drachmas monthly plus 20,000 drachmas to meet expenses on first arrival (or 30,000 for those who will settle out of Athens), plus 30,000 drachmas for scholars requiring to travel within Greece for their research.
Length of Study: 4-10 months.
Study Establishment: At any university or institution of higher education in Greece.
Country of Study: Greece.
Application Procedure: Application forms may be requested from January. These must be submitted with references.
Closing Date: March 15th.

GRIFFITH UNIVERSITY

Office for Research and International Projects, Nathan, QLD,
4111, Australia
Tel: (61) 7 3875 6596
Fax: (61) 7 3875 7994
Email: m.brown@or.gu.edu.au
www: http://www.gu.edu.au
Contact: Ms Maxine Brown, Postgraduate Scholarships
Officer

Griffith University Postgraduate Research Scholarships

Subjects: All subjects.
Eligibility: Open to any person, irrespective of nationality,
holding or expecting to hold an upper second class honours
degree or equivalent from a recognised institution.
Level of Study: Postgraduate.
Purpose: To provide financial support for candidates
undertaking full-time research leading to the award of the
degree of Doctor of Philosophy or Master of Philosophy.
Type: Scholarship.
No. of awards offered: Varies.
Frequency: Annual.
Value: A$16,135 per year (tax exempt), plus a dependant
child allowance of A$1,500 per year (tax exempt) for some
overseas students, limited travel allowance and a thesis
production allowance.
Length of Study: Up to 2 years for Research Master's, and
up to 3 years for PhD (with possible extension of up to 6
months for PhD), subject to satisfactory progress.
Study Establishment: Griffith University.
Country of Study: Australia.
Application Procedure: Application form to be received by
October 30th in the year preceding the commencement of
study.
Closing Date: October 30th for commencement by March
30th the following year.
Additional Information: The Scholarship does not cover the
cost of tuition fees which range between A$12,000 and
A$15,000 per annum. Applicants must demonstrate
proficiency in the English language by scoring an overall
score of 6.5 in an International English Language Testing
System (IELTS) test, or test score of 580 on the Test of
English as a Foreign Language (TOEFL) including the Test of
Written English score of no less than 5.0.

The Sir Allan Sewell Visiting Fellowship

Subjects: Available for all faculties of Griffith University.
Eligibility: Open to researchers of any nationality.
Level of Study: Professional development.
Purpose: To commemorate the distinguished service of Sir
Allan Sewell to Griffith University by offering awards to enable
visits by distinguished scholars engaged in academic work
who can contribute to the research and teaching in one or
more areas of interest to a faculty or college of the university.
Type: Fellowship.
No. of awards offered: 4.

Frequency: Annual.
Value: Up to A$6,000.
Length of Study: A minimum of 8 weeks.
Study Establishment: University.
Country of Study: Australia.
Application Procedure: Fellows must be invited by
faculties/colleges of the University to apply.

THE GRUNDY EDUCATIONAL TRUST

Springhill Cottage
Shirley Holms, Lymington, Hampshire, SO41 8NG, England
Contact: Mr P G Grundy, Secretary to the Trustees

The Grundy Educational Trust

Subjects: Courses leading to degrees in technologically or
scientifically based disciplines in industry commerce or the
professions.
Eligibility: UK citizens not over 30 years of age.
Level of Study: Postgraduate.
Purpose: To assist in covering maintenance costs whilst
obtaining postgraduate or second degrees.
Type: Award.
No. of awards offered: 10-12.
Frequency: Annual.
Value: Up to £3,000.
Length of Study: 1-3 years.
Study Establishment: Birmingham, Loughborough, Imperial
College, Southampton, Surrey, UMIST.
Country of Study: United Kingdom.
Application Procedure: Apply only through the six selected
universities.

THE HASTINGS CENTER

Garrison, NY, 10524, United States of America
Tel: (1) 914 424 4040
Fax: (1) 914 424 4545
Email: visitors@thehastingcenter.org
www: http://www.thehastingscenter.org
Contact: Mr Bruce Jennings, Executive Vice President

This Center is a private research and educational institute that
studies ethical, social, and legal issues in medicine, the life
science, health policy, and environment policy.

Hastings Center Eastern European Program

Subjects: Ethical issues in medicine, the life sciences and the
professions.
Eligibility: Open to Eastern European scholars conducting
significant work in biomedical ethics.
Level of Study: Postgraduate.

Purpose: To support independent research or study by Eastern European scholars.
Type: Stipend.
No. of awards offered: 3.
Frequency: Annual.
Value: US$500-US$2,000 depending on length of stay plus partial reimbursement of expenses.
Length of Study: 4-6 weeks.
Study Establishment: The Hastings Center.
Country of Study: USA.
Application Procedure: Write for application materials.
Closing Date: Four months prior to proposed stay.

Hastings Center International Scholars Program

Subjects: Ethical issues in medicine, the life sciences and the professions.
Eligibility: Open to foreign scholars conducting significant work in biomedical ethics.
Level of Study: Doctorate, Postdoctorate.
Purpose: To support independent research or study by foreign scholars.
Type: Stipend.
No. of awards offered: 5.
Frequency: Annual.
Value: Up to US$500, depending on need.
Length of Study: 2-6 weeks.
Study Establishment: The Hastings Center.
Country of Study: USA.
Application Procedure: Write for application.
Closing Date: Two months prior to proposed stay.

HEALTH CANADA/NATIONAL HEALTH RESEARCH AND DEVELOPMENT PROGRAMME (NHRDP)

Information, Analysis and Connectivity Branch
Strategies and Systems for Health Directorate
Health Canada
15th Floor
Jeanne Mance Building
Tunney's Pasture
Postal Locator 1915A, Ottawa, ON, K1A 1B4, Canada
Tel: (1) 613 954 8549
Fax: (1) 613 954 7363
Email: nhrdpinfo@hc-sc.gc.ca
www: http://www.hc-sc.gc.ca/hppb/nhrdp
Contact: Ms Raymone Sharp, Manager

NHRDP National Health Master's Fellowships

Subjects: From a variety of research fields with a broad health and public policy perspective.
Eligibility: Open to Canadian citizens or legally landed immigrants, who have applied, been accepted or have

enrolled in a Master's programme with a health or health policy research focus.
Level of Study: Postgraduate.
Purpose: To support individuals who wish to undertake full-time training leading to a Master's degree.
Type: Fellowship.
No. of awards offered: Varies.
Frequency: Annual.
Value: C$18,000 per year for a maximum of two years; a maximum of five years of support for both Master's and PhD.
Study Establishment: Universities offering suitable programs.
Country of Study: Canada.
Application Procedure: Prior to completing application form, candidates should obtain a copy of the most recent NHRDP Guide and Personnel Awards Update.
Closing Date: March 1st.

NHRDP National Health PhD Fellowships

Subjects: From a variety of research fields with a broad health and public policy perspective.
Eligibility: Open to Canadian citizens or legally landed immigrants, who have applied, been accepted to or have enrolled in a PhD programme with a health or health policy research focus.
Level of Study: Doctorate.
Purpose: To support individuals who wish to undertake full-time training leading to a PhD degree.
Type: Fellowship.
No. of awards offered: Varies.
Frequency: Annual.
Value: C$18,000 per year for a maximum of four years; a maximum of five years of support for both Master's and PhD.
Study Establishment: Universities offering suitable programs.
Country of Study: Canada; in exceptional cases (for example, if there is no equivalent Canadian program) outside Canada.
Application Procedure: Prior to completing application form, candidates should obtain a copy of the most recent NHRDP Guide and Personnel Awards Update.
Closing Date: March 1st.

NHRDP National Health Post-Doctoral Fellowships

Subjects: From a variety of fields with a broad health and public policy perspective.
Eligibility: Open to Canadian citizens or legally landed immigrants who have completed their doctoral degree no more than two years prior to application.
Level of Study: Postdoctorate.
Purpose: To support individuals who wish to acquire up to two years' supervised research experience in an established health or health policy research setting.
Type: Fellowship.
No. of awards offered: Varies.
Frequency: Annual.
Value: C$30,000 per year for a maximum of two years.

Country of Study: Canada; justification required for tenure outside Canada.
Application Procedure: Prior to completing application form, candidates should obtain a copy of the most recent NHRDP Guide and Personnel Awards Update.
Closing Date: March 1st.

NHRDP National Health Research Scholar Awards

Subjects: From a variety of research fields with a broad health and public policy perspective.
Eligibility: Open to Canadian citizens or legally landed immigrants, who have completed their PhD more than two and less than six years since their last doctoral degree.
Level of Study: Postdoctorate.
Purpose: To facilitate the development of a high level of health and health policy research activity in Canada.
No. of awards offered: Varies.
Frequency: Annual.
Value: C$50,000 per year for a maximum of five years.
Study Establishment: Centres with established health or health policy research facilities.
Country of Study: Canada.
Application Procedure: Prior to completing application form, candidates should obtain a copy of the most recent NHRDP Guide and Personnel Awards Update.
Closing Date: March 1st.

HEALTH RESEARCH BOARD (HRB)

73 Lower Baggot Street, Dublin, 2, Ireland
Tel: (353) 1 6761176
Fax: (353) 1 6611856
Email: hrb@hrb.ie
www: http://www.hrb.ie
Contact: Medical and Health Service Research Manager

The Health Research Board (HRB) is comprised of 16 members appointed by the Minister of Health, with eight of the members being nominated on the co-joint nomination of the Universities and Colleges. The main functions of the HRB are: to promote or commission health research; to promote conduct epidemiological research as may be appropriate at national level; to promote or commission health services research; to liase and co-operate with other research bodies in Ireland and overseas in the promotion of relevant research; to undertake such other cognate functions as the Minister may from time to time determine.

Clinical Research on Cancer

Subjects: Biomedical sciences, haematology, oncology, radiography.
Eligibility: Open to applicants from any health profession, academic discipline or other relevant background.

Purpose: To provide an infrastructure for a mutli-disciplinary, multi-institutional approach to clinical cancer research; to focus clinical research in a way that contributes to the knowledge and treatment of the most common cancers in Ireland; and to assist participation in collaborative clinical research with other countries, and in particular EU countries and co-operative groups.
No. of awards offered: Programme Grant 1, Project Grants 2 or 3.
Value: Programme Grant up to £50,000 per annum, project grant £10,000- £15,000 per annum.
Length of Study: Programme Grant up to 4 years, Project Grants up to 4 years.
Application Procedure: Please write for further details.
Closing Date: September 12th.

Clinical Research Training Fellowships

Subjects: Biomedicine.
Eligibility: Candidates should be graduates in medicine or dentistry from post registration up to and including Senior Registrar or equivalent academic level.
Purpose: To enable medical and dental graduates at any stage in their career, up to and including Senior Registrar, Lecturer or equivalent levels, to gain specialised research training in the biomedical field in Ireland.
No. of awards offered: Up to 6.
Value: Awards will be in the range of £26,000-£35,000 per annum.
Length of Study: Normally 2 years.
Study Establishment: At an appropriate academic department in the Republic of Ireland.
Application Procedure: Application should be made by the prospective fellow with the support of the Head of an appropriate sponsoring laboratory in the Republic of Ireland. Candidates may apply to remain in their current laboratory, to return to one where they have worked before, or to move to a new laboratory. Please write to the Research Grants Section at The Health Research Board for more information.
Closing Date: December 14th.
Additional Information: Proposals may be submitted for specialised research training or for training in a basic subject relevant to a particular clinical interest.

Health Research Board and British Council-Research Visits Scheme

Subjects: Disciplines relevant to medicine and health-biomedical sciences, epidemiology, dentistry, psychology, social sciences and economics.
Eligibility: Full-time research staff although part of the funding may be used to support travel and subsistence of research students. Collaboration must be based on a joint research proposal and achievable objectives. At least one of the collaborating partners must be a member of staff of a higher education institution. The focus of the subvention requested should be on the travel and subsistence necessary for bringing the partners together. Priority will be given to projects which demonstrate clear additional benefits which will arise from support.

Purpose: To facilitate Irish and UK researchers in developing collaborative research projects in the biomedical and health research fields, by supporting travel and subsistence associated with short term research visits. There is particular interest in supporting new research links.
No. of awards offered: 20-30.
Frequency: Annual.
Value: £500-£1,000 to cover travel, subsistence, and in exceptional circumstances consumables.
Length of Study: 6 weeks.
Application Procedure: Please write or phone for an application form.
Closing Date: January 15th.

Health Research Board Grants, Fellowships and Projects

Subjects: Medical, epidemiological, health and health services research.
Eligibility: The general academic requirement for the awarding of any grant is the possession of a medical, science, dental, or related biomedical science degree. There are no requirements regarding citizenship or age. However, grants in general are normally available only to workers carrying out research in the Republic of Ireland, and training grants are confined to recent graduates who are working towards a higher degree.
Level of Study: Postgraduate.
Type: Varies.
Frequency: Annual.
Value: Varies.
Country of Study: Ireland.
Application Procedure: Application form must be completed.
Closing Date: Applications are accepted at any time.

Health Services Research Fellowships

Subjects: May involve clinical, epidemiological, public health, statistics, health economics, social science, operational and mangement disciplines. It is concerned with populations, and with both costs and effectiveness of health care interventions.
Eligibility: Candidates must normally hold a primary degree in a discipline relevant to health services research, have acquired appropriate post-graduate experience in the field of health services and research, have support from an approved academic Department or Centre, have obtained the prior approval of a Head of Department for the research study being proposed, be Irish citizens or graduates from overseas with a permanent Irish resident status.
Purpose: To enable graduates with some appropriate relevant experince to pursue a career in health devices and research in Ireland.
Type: Fellowship.
No. of awards offered: Up to 3.
Value: The stipend offered will be in the range of £25,000-£30,000 per annum according to age and experience. A contribution of £5,000 will be provided towards running costs.
Length of Study: Normally the maximum period of the award will be 3 years, with renewal being subject to appropriate annual review.

Study Establishment: Institutions approved by the Board, such as - teaching hospitals, universities, research institutes, and health boards in Ireland.
Country of Study: Ireland.
Application Procedure: Please write or phone for an application form.
Closing Date: April 3rd.
Additional Information: It is envisaged that Fellows will spend up to 30% of their time in an advisory/resource centre role.

HRB Project Grants-Co-Funded in Health Services Research

Subjects: Any discipline relevant to health services research.
Eligibility: Open to applicants from any of the health professions, academic discipline or other relevant background.
Purpose: To facilitate the development of health services research by providing support for health services research projects and pilot studies which might lead to larger research proposals subsequently.
Value: HRB contibution may be up to £10,000 with a matching contribution from a health board, hospital or health agency being required.
Length of Study: Variable - it is expected that most projects will be completed within 1 year.
Application Procedure: To obtain an application form please write or alternatively visit the website.
Closing Date: March 5th.

HRB Project Grants-General

Subjects: Medicine (including any related science subject), epidemiology, health service research.
Eligibility: The principal must hold a full-time academic post in an Irish academic institution and his/her speciality should be within the range of disciplines stated in the subject index. Applicants must reside in the Republic of Ireland and grants are tenable in this country.
Purpose: To facilitate research in medicine, epidemiology, health service research and health research in Ireland.
No. of awards offered: 59.
Value: £20,000 per annum for a maximum of three years. Each successful applicant is entitled to one grant in any given year. In addition start up costs may be requested on a one off basis. The amount available for these is £10,000 and their purpose is to facilitate the start up of the project in the first year. Requests for such supplementary funding will require separate justification.
Study Establishment: An Irish academic institution.
Country of Study: Ireland.
Application Procedure: To obtain an application form please write or, alternatively visit the website.
Closing Date: February 12th.

HRB Research Project Grants - Inter-Disciplinary

Subjects: Engineering, information technology, humanities, medicine, science and the social sciences.

Eligibility: At least one applicant should hold a full-time academic post in an Irish university or college and be actively engaged in research on a relevant health research topic.
Purpose: To promote inter-discplinary research in addressing research topics directly related to improving human health.
No. of awards offered: 2.
Value: £50,000 per annum to cover salary, equipment and consumable components.
Length of Study: 2 years.
Study Establishment: At recognised academic and health services centres in the Republic of Ireland.
Application Procedure: To obtain an application form please write or alternatively visit the website.
Closing Date: March 5th.

HRB Research Project Grants-North South Co-operation

Subjects: Medical sciences.
Eligibility: Applicants should hold a full-time academic post in an Irish university or college and be actively engaged in medical, epidemiological, health service or health research in Ireland.
Purpose: To stimulate co-operation between research investigators in the Republic of Ireland and in Northern Ireland by making grant support available for joint health research projects of a high quality.
No. of awards offered: Up to 4.
Value: £26,000 per annum and may be used for research scholars, small items of equipment, consumables and travel.
Length of Study: Awards may be sought for 1, 2 or 3 years.
Study Establishment: Recognised academic institutions and health service centres in the Republic of Ireland and Northern Ireland.
Application Procedure: Application in the first instance should be made by an individual or research group placed in the Republic of Ireland. In the application the role of a research partner from Northern Ireland in the proposed research project should be clearly demonstrated. In addition evidence that the Northern Ireland partner has access to matching funds or is likely to obtain some in the foreseeable future should be provided. Application forms are available on the website.
Closing Date: March 5th.

HRB Science Degree Scholarship Scheme for Medical Graduates

Subjects: Medical sciences.
Eligibility: Candidates must hold a primary medical degree; be prepared to undertake the proposed research study within 6 months of completing their internship; normally not hold a tenured or substantive post other than demonstratorship; be Irish citizens or be graduates from overseas with permanent Irish resident status.
Purpose: To enable medical graduates to undertake a full-time academic course leading to a degree qualification during the period immediately following their internship.
Type: Scholarship.
No. of awards offered: Up to 4.

Frequency: Annual.
Value: A stipend of £5,000 payable in three instalments, with any fees to be remitted by the host college/instiution.
Length of Study: Normally for a complete academic year.
Study Establishment: Institutions approved by the Board such as teaching hospitals, universities and research institutes.
Application Procedure: Scholarships are awarded in open competition, on the basis of merit and following an interview by the Board. Please write or visit the website for further details.
Closing Date: March 6th.

HRB Summer Student Grants

Subjects: Medical, dental, health service.
Eligibility: Open to students from medical, dental or health service related disciplines.
Purpose: To develop interest in research and give the student the opportunity to become familiar with research techniques.
Type: Grant.
No. of awards offered: 1 per Director.
Value: £80 per week, in monthly arrears.
Length of Study: 8 weeks.
Application Procedure: Please write or phone for an application form.
Closing Date: March 6th.

New Blood Fellowships in Biomedical Science

Subjects: Biomedicine.
Eligibility: Candidates must be medically or dentally qualified, hold a PhD, or be an experienced veterinary scientist. Independent research must have been carried out for at least 4 years in a biomedical or clinical department and on a biomedical subject either in Ireland or overseas. Candidates must have a sponsoring laboratory which is an academic department in the Republic of Ireland (awards are not tenable in Northern Ireland), be proposing to carry out their research in a biomedical field other than cancer, have the full support of a sponsor who will guarantee space and facilities for the prospective lecturer and have an undertaking that he or she will be granted the status and responsibilities of a lecturer or senior lecturer during the fellowship. Also, they must have practical control, if necessary, of a number of patients for investigative work under appropriate supervision, not be expected to carry out more than six hours a week of routine clinical or teaching duties, have a guarantee from the Head of the Institution, or an individual with full authority to commit the institution, that the individual's personal support will be taken over at the end of the grant and that the balance of the Fellow's salary will be paid in the fourth year of the fellowship.
Purpose: To strengthen biomedical research in the Republic of Ireland by providing funds to help universities make appointment to the permanent academic staff. Support under this scheme will be focused at the first appointment of clinical and non-clinical researchers.
Type: Fellowship.
Value: The Fellow's full salary for 3 years, 50% of the salary in the fourth year and 25% in the fifth - the balance of the Fellow's salary in the fouth and fifth year to be paid by the

host institution. The salary paid will be within the salary scales applicable at the time of the award for lecturers and senior lecturers in the Republic of Ireland. Salary requests at the Consultant level will be considered for fellows in receipt of an Honourary Consultant contract during the fellowship. The direct costs of the research programme and allowances to support attendance at scientific meetings but for the first three years only. Support for appropriate research and technical support staff will be considered but funding will not be provided for studentships. Equipment for the programme of research and to enable start-up in a new laboratory will also be provided.

Application Procedure: Application forms are available by writing to New Blood Fellowships at The Health Research Board or by writing to The Grants Section at The Wellcome Trust.

Closing Date: February 19th.

For further information contact:

The Grants Section (Matching Funding in Ireland)
The Wellcome Trust
183 Euston Road, London, NW1 2BE, England

New Blood Research Fellowships in Medical Science in the Republic of Ireland

Subjects: Biomedical research.
Eligibility: Applicants must normally intend to establish a research career and undertake research in an Irish academic institution, be at the stage of establishing themselves in an independent research career and have recognised postdoctoral achievements, have strong background in biomedical research which is reflected in quality publications, and be nominated by the Head of Department in the Institution where the candidate proposes to work.
Level of Study: Postdoctorate.
Purpose: To encourage young postdoctoral researchers, who are medically or dentally qualified, or science graduates, wishing to establish programmes of research at institutions in Ireland.
Type: Fellowship.
No. of awards offered: Up to 2.
Value: Fellows will be appointed at a salary commensurate with experience which would normally be in the lecturer range of IR£30,000-£36,000. Applicants should discuss appropriate commencing salary with their sponsor for inclusion in the proposed budget on the application form. These awards will normally provide the candidates full salary for the first three years, 50% of the salary for the fourth year and 25% for the fifth year. Expenses may also be requested for a research assistant, equipment and consumables for up to three years.
Length of Study: Normally, maximum period will be 5 years, with annual renewal being dependent on receipt of satisfactory progress reports. A mid term assessment of progress will also be undertaken.
Study Establishment: The fellowships are tenable only in institutions approved of by the Board, such as teaching hospitals or universities in Ireland.

Application Procedure: An application form must be completed.
Closing Date: December 1st.

HEALTH RESEARCH COUNCIL OF NEW ZEALAND

PO Box 5541
Wellesley Street, Auckland, 1000, New Zealand
Tel: (64) 9 379 8227
Fax: (64) 9 377 9988
Email: info@hrc.govt.nz
www: http://www.hrc.govt.nz/hrc

Postdoctoral Fellowship

Subjects: Medical sciences.
Eligibility: Intended for the support of outstanding graduates who have recently completed a degree at doctoral level and who propose to conduct research in scientific fields of relevance to the HRC. Open to suitably qualified individuals from any country. Applicants should not normally have had more than three years postdoctoral experience.
Level of Study: Postdoctorate.
Purpose: To provide support for research workers to gain further experience in their chosen fields and for them to become established as an independent researcher.
Type: Fellowship.
No. of awards offered: No fixed number.
Frequency: Annual.
Value: Stipend is based on the recipient's qualifications and the research experience with regards to funding levels set by the University. HRC may provide an additional allowance of up to NZ$1,750 cover limited working expenses associated with research and to enable the Fellow to travel to one scientific meeting in New Zealand or eastern Australia. In the case of Postdoctoral Fellows appointed from overseas the Council may provide financial assistance for travel to New Zealand if detailed at the time of application and if other possible sources of support have been explored.
Length of Study: Awarded for an initial period of 2 years but fellows are eligible to seek an additional 2 years at the same as another host department or instiution, by making a formal reapplication.
Study Establishment: New Zealand universities, hospitals, or other research institutions approved by council. Awards administered through the host institution.
Country of Study: New Zealand.
Application Procedure: Application forms and guidelines are available in paper and computer disk formats from the HRC Secretariat and the Research Office of Host Institutions. Application information can also be downloaded from the website. Applicants are asked not to send applications via disk or on the Internet. The application should describe the proposed research programme for the full duration of the fellowship period being requested.
Closing Date: Published annually in the HRC calendar.

HEBREW IMMIGRANT AID SOCIETY (HIAS)

333 Seventh Avenue, New York, NY, 10001, United States of America
Tel: (1) 212 613 1351
Email: mbellow@hias.org
Contact: Ms Marina Belotserkousky, Associate Director

HIAS is the international migration agency of the organised Jewish community.

HIAS Scholarship Awards

Subjects: All subjects.
Eligibility: Open to HIAS-assisted refugees and their children who arrived in the USA in 1985 or later. Applicants must have completed one year (two semesters) at a USA high school, college, or graduate school.
Level of Study: Doctorate, Postgraduate, Undergraduate.
Purpose: To assist HIAS-assisted refugees and their children.
Type: One-time grant.
No. of awards offered: 150.
Frequency: Annual.
Value: Average award: US$1,000.
Length of Study: 1 year must be completed.
Country of Study: USA.
Application Procedure: Requests for applications must be in writing and must include a self-addressed stamped envelope. Applications are judged on financial need, academic scholarship and community service. Applications are available starting in February each year.
Closing Date: April 15th.

HEED OPHTHALMIC FOUNDATION

Cleveland Clinic Foundation
Desk A-31
9500 Euclid Avenue, Cleveland, OH, 44195, United States of America
Tel: (1) 216 445 81 45
Fax: (1) 216 444 89 68
Contact: Dr F A Gutman, Executive Secretary

Heed Award

Subjects: Diseases and surgery of the eye and/or research in ophthalmology.
Eligibility: Open to US citizens who are graduates of an institution approved by the AMA.
Level of Study: Postgraduate.
Purpose: To provide assistance to men and women who desire to further their education or to do research in Opthalmology.
Type: Fellowship.
No. of awards offered: Approx. 25.
Frequency: Annual.

Value: US$1,250 per month for up to one year.
Length of Study: 1 year; not renewable.
Study Establishment: US universities or research institutions.
Country of Study: USA.
Application Procedure: Please write for details.
Closing Date: January 15th.

HEWLETT PACKARD COMPANY AND AMERICAN ASSOCIATION OF CRITICAL CARE NURSES

Hewlett Packard Company
3000 Minuteman Road MS210, Andover, MA, 01810, United States of America
Tel: (1) 978 659 4748
Contact: Ms Joan Hodges

HP/AACN Critical Care Nursing Research Grant

Subjects: Nursing.
Eligibility: AACN members may apply (current registered nurse members only). Research must be undertaken in the USA only.
Level of Study: Postgraduate.
Purpose: To support research in critical care nursing. Preferred topics will address information technology requirements of patient management in critical care.
Type: Cash and Equipment.
No. of awards offered: 1.
Frequency: Annual.
Value: US$37,000.
Length of Study: 1 year.
Study Establishment: Hospital.
Country of Study: USA.
Application Procedure: Please write to the Hewlett Packard address for applications.
Additional Information: Questions about suitability of research topics should be addressed to: AACN Research Department, 101 Columbia, Aliso Vicjo, CA 92656, USA. Tel: (1) 800 394 5995.

HILDA MARTINDALE EDUCATIONAL TRUST

c/o Registry
Royal Holloway University of London, Egham, Surrey, TW20 0EX, England
Tel: (44) 1784 434 455
Fax: (44) 1784 437 520
Contact: Miss J L Hurn, Secretary to the Trustees

The Trust was set up by Mrs Hilda Martindale in order to help women of the British Isles with the costs of vocational training for any profession or career likely to be of use or value to the community. Applications are considered annually by six women Trustees.

Hilda Martindale Exhibitions

Subjects: Any vocational training for a profession or career likely to be of value to the community.
Eligibility: Open to women of the British Isles.
Level of Study: Postgraduate, Professional development.
Purpose: To assist with the costs of vocational training.
Type: Grant.
No. of awards offered: 25-35.
Frequency: Annual.
Value: Varies, normally £200-£1,000.
Length of Study: 1 year.
Study Establishment: Any establishment in the UK approved by the trustees.
Country of Study: United Kingdom.
Application Procedure: Application form (two copies) to be obtained from and returned to the Secretary to the Trustees.
Closing Date: March 1st, for the following academic year. Late or retrospective applications will not be considered.
Additional Information: Assistance is not given for short courses, courses abroad, elective studies, intercalated BSc years, access courses, or academic research. Awards are not given to those who are eligible for grants from LEAs, research councils, British Academy or other public sources.

HILGENFELD FOUNDATION FOR MORTUARY EDUCATION

PO Box 4311, Fullerton, CA, 92834, United States of America
Contact: The Secretary

Hilgenfeld Foundation Grant

Subjects: Mortuary science education.
Eligibility: Open only to nationals of the United States.
Level of Study: Postgraduate, Professional development, Undergraduate.
Purpose: To support mortuary science education through scholarships and research.
Type: Research Grant, Research Scholarship.
No. of awards offered: Approx. 20.
Frequency: Annual.
Length of Study: Varies.
Study Establishment: Applicants must be enrolled in a funeral service program, or be employed in the funeral service industry or research related to the funeral service industry.
Country of Study: USA.
Application Procedure: Application to be submitted on forms provided by the Hilgenfeld Foundation.
Closing Date: Applications are accepted at any time.

THE HOSPITAL FOR SICK CHILDREN FOUNDATION

555 University Avenue
Suite 1725, Toronto, ON, M5G 1X8, Canada
Tel: (1) 416 813 6101
Fax: (1) 416 813 5024
Email: gwen.burrows@sickkids.on.ca
www: http://www.sickkids.on.ca
Contact: Ms Gwen Burrows, Grants Program Co-ordinator

The Hospital for Sick Children Foundation is a fundraising and granting organisation, dedicated to the betterment of the health of children. The Foundation is committed to supporting the broader aims of child health in Canada through an annual allocation to the National Grants Programme for paediatric research, health promotion, public education, postgraduate training and innovative community projects.

Duncan L Gordon Fellowships

Subjects: Paediatric health care.
Eligibility: Open to physicians and scientists wishing to obtain postdoctoral training, who are Canadian citizens or landed immigrants, are of outstanding academic achievement, and can provide evidence of special aptitude for teaching and research.
Level of Study: Postdoctorate.
Purpose: To provide postdoctoral training.
Type: Fellowship.
No. of awards offered: Up to 3.
Frequency: Annual.
Value: Up to C$46,844 per year, dependent on the number of years of postdoctoral experience.
Length of Study: 1 or 3 years.
Study Establishment: Any agreed institution.
Country of Study: Any country.
Application Procedure: Candidates should be nominated by the Head of the Department in which they are involved. A project proposal, written by the applicant, and three letters of reference are required.
Closing Date: October 1st.
Additional Information: Please contact the office for current guidelines and application forms. The candidate must supply an outline of the course of study and detailed study plans indicating the location and facilities which will be available and the individual who would supervise his/her study. The candidate must indicate his/her objectives in paediatrics upon completion of the fellowship period.

Hospital for Sick Children Foundation External Grants

Subjects: All areas of child health - research, special programs, and health education programs.
Eligibility: Open to researchers in Canada who are working on projects which have significant potential to impact positively on child health in Canada.
Level of Study: Professional development.

Purpose: To support research and innovative programs in child health across Canada.
Type: Grant.
No. of awards offered: Approx. 20.
Frequency: Twice a year.
Value: From C$1,000 per project; not to exceed C$65,000 per year.
Length of Study: 1-2 years.
Study Establishment: Any agreed Canadian institution.
Country of Study: Canada.
Application Procedure: Applications should be made through the institution or organisation under whose auspices the project will be carried out. There are two stages to the procedure: a letter of intent screening stage, and a full application for those who get past the first stage. Applications for health education funding are processed separately.
Closing Date: There are two cycles: one in the spring and one in the autumn. Please contact the office for exact dates. Health education projects may be submitted at any time.
Additional Information: Grants will not be made to support annual campaigns, operating expenses, operating deficits, general endowment or sustaining funds, projects which might result in gain or profit to the organisation, or building construction or improvement. The grant cycle takes about six months from letter of intent to the final decision.

HUMANE RESEARCH TRUST

Brook House
29 Bramhall Lane South
Bramhall, Stockport, Cheshire, SK7 2DN, England
Tel: (44) 161 439 8041
Fax: (44) 161 439 3713
Contact: Ms Margaret Pritchard, Trust Secretary

The Humane Research Trust is a national charity which funds a range of unique medical research programmes into human illness at hospitals and universities around the country. In keeping with the philosophy of the Trust, none of the research involves animals, and much of it seeks to establish and develop pioneering techniques which will replace animal intensive experiments currently undertaken elsewhere.

Humane Research Trust Grant

Subjects: Humane research.
Eligibility: Open to established scientific workers engaged in productive research. Nationals of any country are considered, but for the sake of overseeing, projects should be undertaken in a UK establishment.
Level of Study: Unrestricted.
Purpose: To encourage scientific programmes where the use of animals is replaced by other methods.
Type: Grant.
No. of awards offered: Varies.
Frequency: Dependent on funds available.
Value: Varies.
Country of Study: United Kingdom.

Application Procedure: Application form must be completed.
Closing Date: Varies; the Trustees meet every three to four months.
Additional Information: The Trust is a registered charity and donations are encouraged.

HUMANITARIAN TRUST

36-38 Westbourne Grove, London, W2 5SH, England
Contact: Mrs M Myers, Secretary of Trustees

Humanitarian Trust Awards

Subjects: Unrestricted, subject to the discretion of the Trustees. Awards are not made for journalism, theatre, music or any arts subjects. All aspects of medical sciences are eligible apart from nursing, medical auxiliaries, midwifery, radiology, treatment techniques, and medical technology. Candidates are only considered when studying academic subjects.
Eligibility: Open to persons already holding an original grant.
Level of Study: Graduate, Postgraduate, Undergraduate.
Purpose: General charitable purposes beneficial to the community.
Type: Award.
No. of awards offered: Approx.15.
Frequency: Twice a year.
Value: Approximately £200.
Length of Study: 1 year; not renewable.
Study Establishment: Any approved institution.
Country of Study: United Kingdom.
Application Procedure: Please write in. Submit two references, preferably from tutors or heads of department, and a breakdown of anticipated income and expenditure.
Additional Information: Awards are not made for travel or overseas courses. They are intended only as supplementary assistance and are to be held concurrently with other awards.

HUNTINGTON'S DISEASE ASSOCIATION

108 Battersea High Street, London, SW11 3HP, England
Tel: (44) 171 223 7000
Fax: (44) 171 223 9489
Email: sue_watkin@hda.org.uk
Contact: Ms Sue Watkin, Chair

Huntingtons Disease Association Research Grant

Subjects: Any medical or social research aimed at furthering our understanding of Huntington's disease, improving it's treatment, or otherwise improving the quality of life of patients and carers.
Eligibility: Open to suitably qualified researchers of any nationality.

Level of Study: Postgraduate.
Type: Project Grant, Studentship.
No. of awards offered: Varies, depending on the annual budget.
Frequency: Annual.
Value: Studentship: up to £12,000 per annum; Project Grants: up to £25,000 for 1-3 years.
Country of Study: United Kingdom.
Application Procedure: An application form must be completed, please write for details.
Closing Date: March 1st.

HUNTINGTON'S DISEASE SOCIETY OF AMERICA (HDSA)

158 West 29th Street
7th Floor, New York, NY, 10001-5300, United States of America
Tel: (1) 212 242 1968 ext 20
Fax: (1) 212 239 3430
Email: jhammel_hdsa@hotmail.com
www: http://www.hdsa.mgh.harvard.edu
Contact: Ms Joyce Hammel, Manager of Medical and Scientific Programs

The Huntington's Disease Society of America (HDSA) is dedicated to the care and cure of families afflicted with Huntington's Disease. HDSA is a not-for-profit volunteer health agency whose mission statement is three-fold: to eradicate Huntington's Disease by promoting and supporting research; to help families cope with the problems presented by the disease; and to educate the public and professionals about it.

HDSA Fellowships

Subjects: Cure and treatment of Huntington's Disease at the basic and clinical level.
Eligibility: Open to MDs or PhDs from accredited medical schools and universities.
Level of Study: Postdoctorate.
Purpose: To help promising young postdoctoral investigators in the early stages of their careers, in support of basic or clinical research related to Huntington's Disease.
Type: Fellowship.
No. of awards offered: Varies.
Frequency: Annual.
Value: Up to US$70,000 over 2 years.
Length of Study: Up to 2 years.
Country of Study: Any country.
Application Procedure: Application form must be completed. Email with a request for application.
Closing Date: January 5th.

HDSA Research Grants

Subjects: Cure and treatment of Huntington's Disease at the basic and clinical level.

Eligibility: Open to MDs or PhDs from accredited medical schools and universities.
Level of Study: Postdoctorate.
Purpose: Provided as seed monies for new or innovative research projects focusing on basic or clinical research relating to Huntington's Disease, in the hope that they will develop sufficiently to attract funding from other sources.
Type: Research Grant.
No. of awards offered: Varies.
Frequency: Annual.
Value: Up to US$100,000 over 2 years.
Length of Study: Up to 2 years.
Country of Study: Any country.
Application Procedure: Application form must be completed. Email with a request for application.
Closing Date: January 5th.

HDSA Research Initiative Grants

Subjects: Cure and treatment of Huntington's Disease at the basic and clinical level.
Eligibility: Open to MDs or PhDs from accredited medical schools and universities.
Level of Study: Postdoctorate.
Purpose: To swiftly investigate a novel idea with very little preliminary data.
Type: Grant.
No. of awards offered: Varies.
Frequency: Annual.
Value: Up to US$20,000 per annum.
Length of Study: 1 year.
Country of Study: Any country.
Application Procedure: Application form must be completed. Email with a request for application.
Closing Date: January 5th.

IAN KARTEN CHARITABLE TRUST

The Mill House
Newark Lane, Ripley, Surrey, GU23 6DP, England
Fax: (44) 1483 222420
Contact: Mr Ian H Karten, Trustee and Administrator

Ian Karten Scholarship

Subjects: Most subjects, with varying levels of priority.
Eligibility: Open to British students of any religion or ethnic background. Jewish students of any nationality, under 30 years of age on October 1st of year for which grant is sought, are also eligible.
Level of Study: Doctorate, Postgraduate.
Purpose: To assist eligible students with the costs of postgraduate programmes of research at universities in the United Kingdom.
Type: Scholarship.
No. of awards offered: 100.
Frequency: Annual.

Value: Varies.
Study Establishment: UK university or conservatoire.
Country of Study: United Kingdom.
Application Procedure: Applicants should apply in writing in February for details of application procedure, giving brief details about themselves and their course, enclosing a SAE.
Closing Date: May 31st.

IMPERIAL CANCER RESEARCH FUND

PO Box 123
Lincoln's Inn Fields, London, WC2A 3PX, England
Tel: (44) 171 269 3328
Fax: (44) 171 269 3585
www: http://www.icnet.uk
Contact: Ms Johanna Higgins, Administration Manager

Imperial Cancer Research Fund Clinical Research Fellowships

Subjects: All areas of cancer research.
Eligibility: Open to medical graduates of registrar or senior registrar status having obtained MRCP, FRCS, or other higher medical qualifications.
Level of Study: Doctorate, Postdoctorate.
Purpose: To enable research training.
Type: Fellowship.
No. of awards offered: Approx. 3.
Frequency: Annual.
Value: Remuneration is based on current NHS salary scales.
Length of Study: Up to 4 years.
Study Establishment: Imperial Cancer Research Fund Laboratories and Clinical Units. Fellows based in the Research Laboratories are expected to register for a PhD degree; fellows based in the Clinical Units will submit their work for either a PhD or MD.
Country of Study: United Kingdom.
Application Procedure: As detailed in advertisements.
Additional Information: Fellowships are advertised in scientific and medical journals.

Imperial Cancer Research Fund Graduate Studentships

Subjects: All areas of cancer research.
Eligibility: Candidates should normally have been resident in the UK for at least three years, and have, or be about to obtain, a first or upper second class degree in science, and not be over 25 years of age. Non-residents are not excluded from consideration.
Level of Study: Doctorate.
Purpose: To enable research training.
Type: Studentship.
No. of awards offered: Approx. 20.
Frequency: Annual.

Value: Approximately £11,358-£12,288 (taxable) per year, depending on location, plus additional allowances in some cases.
Length of Study: 3 years.
Study Establishment: Imperial Cancer Research Fund Laboratories and Clinical Units.
Country of Study: United Kingdom.
Application Procedure: As detailed in advertisements.

Imperial Cancer Research Fund Research Fellowships

Subjects: All areas of cancer research.
Eligibility: Applicants must have been awarded a PhD or equivalent, or show written proof of submission of their thesis.
Level of Study: Postdoctorate.
Purpose: To assist postdoctoral research.
Type: Fellowship.
No. of awards offered: Approx. 30.
Frequency: Annual.
Value: Approximate starting salary of £20,015-£25,376 (inclusive) per year, depending on experience.
Length of Study: Up to 3 years.
Study Establishment: Imperial Cancer Research Fund Laboratories and Clinical Units.
Country of Study: United Kingdom.
Application Procedure: As detailed in advertisements.

THE INSTITUTE OF CANCER RESEARCH (ICR)

E Block
15 Cotswold Road, Sutton, Surrey, SM2 5NG, England
Tel: (44) 181 643 8901 ext 4656
Fax: (44) 181 643 6940
Email: lindy@icr.ac.uk
www: http://www.icr.ac.uk/icrhome.htm
Contact: Ms Renate Divers, Assistant Registrar

Over the past 90 years, the Institute has become one of the largest, most successful and innovative cancer research centres in the world. The Institute and the Royal Marsden NHS Trust exist side by side in Chelsea and on a joint site at Sutton, and this close association allows for maximum interaction between fundamental laboratory work and clinical environment.

ICR Research Studentships

Subjects: Cancer research.
Eligibility: There is a minimum entry requirement of a first or upper second class honours degree, or equivalent in a relevant subject.
Level of Study: Postgraduate.
Purpose: To encourage research into the causes, prevention and treatment of cancer.
Type: Studentship.

No. of awards offered: 15-20.
Frequency: Annual.
Value: Equivalent to MRC Studentship rates.
Length of Study: Up to 3 years.
Study Establishment: The Institute.
Country of Study: United Kingdom.
Application Procedure: Apply on application form; attendance at interview is compulsory.
Additional Information: A limited number of Institute Postdoctoral Fellowships are offered from time to time as vacancies occur.

INSTITUTE OF IRISH STUDIES

Queen's University
8 Fitzwilliam Street, Belfast, BT9 6AW, Northern Ireland
Tel: (44) 1232 273386
Fax: (44) 1232 439238
Email: irish.studies@qub.ac.uk
Contact: Dr B M Walker, Director

The Institute of Irish Studies was established in 1965 to promote and co-ordinate research in those fields of study which have a particular Irish interest. The Institute's primary role is to promote research and to communicate the results of this research through seminars, conferences and publications.

Institute of Irish Studies Research Fellowships

Subjects: Any academic discipline relating to Ireland.
Eligibility: Candidates must hold at least a second class honours degree, have research experience, and have a viable research proposal.
Level of Study: Postdoctorate.
Purpose: To promote research.
Type: Fellowship.
No. of awards offered: Up to 3.
Frequency: Annual.
Value: £12,500.
Length of Study: 1 year.
Study Establishment: The Institute of Irish Studies.
Country of Study: Northern Ireland.
Application Procedure: Applicants mus apply for an application form in writing in November. Awards are usually advertised in December.
Closing Date: January 21st.

Institute of Irish Studies Senior Visiting Research Fellowship

Subjects: Any academic discipline relating to Ireland.
Eligibility: Open to established scholars of senior standing with a strong publication record.
Level of Study: Postdoctorate.
Purpose: To promote research.
Type: Fellowship.
No. of awards offered: Up to 2.
Frequency: Annual.

Value: £16,500.
Length of Study: 1 year.
Study Establishment: The Institute of Irish Studies.
Country of Study: Northern Ireland.
Application Procedure: Applicants must apply for an application form in writing in November. Awards are usually advertised in December.
Closing Date: January 21st.

THE INSTITUTE OF SPORTS MEDICINE

University College London Medical School
Charles Bell House
67-73 Riding House Street, London, W1P 7LD, England
Tel: (44) 171 813 2832
Fax: (44) 171 813 2832
Email: m.hobsley@ucl.ac.uk
Contact: D Meynell, Secretary

The Institute of Sports Medicine is a postgraduate medical institute which was established to develop teaching and treatment in sports medicine. It offers national awards to medical practitioners and runs courses on different aspects of this specialist subject. Now that it is based at UCL the Institute hopes to work closely with the College in the fulfilment of its objectives.

Duke of Edinburgh Prize for Sports Medicine

Subjects: Clinical and/or research work in the field of sports medicine in the community.
Eligibility: Open to medical practitioners in the United Kingdom.
Level of Study: Postgraduate.
Purpose: To promote postgraduate work and to signify standards of excellence amongst medical practitioners in the United Kingdom.
No. of awards offered: 1.
Frequency: Annual.
Value: Varies; a substantial cash prize.
Country of Study: United Kingdom.
Application Procedure: Applicants should write for an entry/nomination form in the first instance.
Closing Date: Varies annually. Specified in conditions of entry.

The Robert Atkins Award

Subjects: Sports medicine.
Eligibility: Open to medical practitioners in the United Kingdom.
Level of Study: Postgraduate.
Purpose: To increase medical support for and active involvement in sports medicine and to recognise a doctor who has provided, for not less than five years, the most consistently valuable medical (clinical/preventive) service to a national sporting organisation or sport in general.

No. of awards offered: 1.
Frequency: Annual.
Value: Varies; a substantial cash prize.
Country of Study: United Kingdom.
Application Procedure: Applicants should write for an entry/nomination form in the first instance.
Closing Date: Varies annually.

INSTITUTO NACIONAL DE CANCEROLOGIA

Calle 1 #9-85 Seccion Educacion Medica, Santafé de Bogota, Cundinamarca, Colombia
Tel: (57) 1 333 6585
Fax: (57) 1 333 6619
Contact: Chief of Medical Education

The Institute offers five residency programs in general surgery, internal medicine, nuclear medicine, pathology and radiotherapy, as well as eighteen fellowship programs in surgical and clinical oncologic fields, that last one and two years.

Instituto Nacional de Cancerologia Postgraduate Training in Oncologic Topics

Subjects: Sub-specialisation is in the following specific areas - neck and head surgery, breast tissue surgery, oncology surgery, gastroenterology surgery, plastic oncology surgery, dermatology oncology, pain and palliative care, hemato-oncology, imagenology oncology, ophthalmology oncology, pathology oncology, rehabilitation oncology, urology oncology, thoracic oncology, oral oncology.
Eligibility: Candidates must be medical doctors with a postgraduate degree.
Level of Study: Postgraduate.
Purpose: To train medical specialists in a sub-specialisation in a specific oncologic topic, such as surgical oncology, gynaecological oncology, or haemato-oncology.
Type: Bursary.
No. of awards offered: 10.
Frequency: Annual.
Value: US$250 per month.
Length of Study: 1-2 years.
Study Establishment: Hospital.
Country of Study: Colombia.
Application Procedure: Candidates must submit a letter requesting the specific area, a letter from the home institution with a guarantee that the candidate will be received when he or she goes back, in addition to attending an interview with the chairman of the program.
Closing Date: October, March.

INTERNATIONAL AGENCY FOR RESEARCH ON CANCER (IARC)

150 cours Albert Thomas, Lyon Cedex 08, F-69372, France
Tel: (33) 4 72 73 84 85
Fax: (33) 4 72 73 83 22
Email: elakroud@iarc.fr
www: http://www.iarc.fr/
Telex: 380 023
Contact: Ms Eve Elakroud, Administrative Assistant IARC Fellowship Programme

The International Agency for Research on Cancer (IARC) is part of the World Health Organisation. IARC's mission is to co-ordinate and conduct research on the causes of human cancer, the mechanisms of carcinogenesis, and to develop scientific strategies for cancer control. The Agency is involved in both epidemiological and laboratory research and disseminates scientific information through publications, meetings, courses and fellowships.

IARC Fellowships for Research Training in Cancer

Subjects: Environmental carcinogenesis - biostatistics and epidemiology of cancer and all aspects of chemical and viral carcinogenesis, cell biology, cell genetics, molecular biology and mechanisms of carcinogenesis. Applications are encouraged from epidemiologists and laboratory scientists for interdisciplinary training that will facilitate the conduct of genetic and molecular epidemiological research. Applicants requiring basic training in cancer epidemiology will also be considered.
Eligibility: Open to persons who have some postdoctoral experience in medicine or the natural sciences. Applications can not be accepted and will not be considered if the applicant is receiving postdoctoral training abroad, or has already started postdoctoral work at the host institute. Preference will be given to applicants who have not previously received a postdoctoral training abroad in cancer research.
Level of Study: Postdoctorate.
Purpose: To provide training in cancer research to junior scientists who are actively engaged in research in medical or allied sciences, and who wish to pursue a career in cancer research.
Type: Fellowship.
No. of awards offered: Approx. 15.
Frequency: Annual.
Value: Travel for the Fellow and for one dependant if accompanying the Fellow for at least eight months. Stipends according to country of tenure. Annual family allowance of US$400 for spouse and US$450 for each child.
Length of Study: 1 year.
Study Establishment: An institution in any country abroad where suitable research facilities and material exist.
Country of Study: Any country abroad.
Application Procedure: Application form must be completed. Applications must be supported by the Director of the applicant's own instiution.

Closing Date: December 31st.
Additional Information: Applicants should provide reasonable assurance that they will return to a post in their own country at the end of the Fellowship. Applicants should have an adequate knowledge, both written and spoken, of English or the language of the country in which their fellowship is tenable.

INTERNATIONAL CENTRE FOR GENETIC ENGINEERING AND BIOTECHNOLOGY (ICGEB)

Padriciano 99, Trieste, 34012, Italy
Tel: (390) 40 37 57 1
Fax: (390) 40 22 65 55
www: http://www.icgeb.trieste.it

The International Centre for Genetic Engineering and Biotechnology (ICGEB) is an organisation devoted to advanced research and training in molecular biology, with special regard to the needs of the developing world. The component host countries are Italy and India. The full members of the ICGEB Signatory Council are the following: Afghanistan, Algeria, Argentina, Armenia, Bangladesh, Bhutan, Brazil, Bulgaria, Chile, China, Colombia, Costa Rica, Croatia, Cuba, Ecuador, Egypt, Federal Republic of Yugoslavia, Hungary, Iraq, Kuwait, Macedonia, Mauritus, Mexico, Morocco, Nigeria, Pakistan, Panama, Peru, Poland, Romania, Russia, Senegal, Slovakia, Slovenia, Sri Lanka, Sudan, Tunisia, Turkey, Uruguay, Venezuela and Vietnam.

Predoctoral Fellowship Programme - ICGEB JNU PhD Course in Molecular Genetics

Subjects: All subjects.
Eligibility: Promising young students, ideally in possession of an MSc from a recognised university, who are nationals of one of the member states.
Level of Study: Postgraduate, Predoctorate.
Purpose: To offer postgraduate training with the aim of obtaining a PhD degree in the field of Molecular Genetics at the Jawaharlal Nehru University in New Delhi, in collaboration with the ICGEB.
Type: Fellowship.
No. of awards offered: 3 or 4.
Frequency: Annual.
Length of Study: 4 to 5 years, depending on the academic qualification the individual student has achieved prior to embarking on the course.
Study Establishment: Jawaharial Nehru University in New Dehli.
Country of Study: India.

Application Procedure: For details of the application process, please contact Ms Susan Vincent, Office of the Director (Fellowship Programmes), ICGEB, tel: 39 40 37 57 30 5, fax: 39 40 22 65 55 5, or contact one of the ICGEB Project Leaders in New Delhi, India. Fax: 91 11 616 23 16.
Closing Date: Please write for details.
Additional Information: For more information on this course please refer to the website: http://www.icgeb.trieste.it/phdjnu.htm.

Predoctoral Fellowship Programme - ICGEB SISSA PhD Course in Molecular Genetics

Subjects: Molecular genetics.
Eligibility: Promising predoctoral students under the age of 30 from any member state of the ICGEB.
Level of Study: Predoctorate.
Purpose: To enable promising young students to attend and complete the PhD courses in molecular genetics at the International School for Advanced Studies (SISSA) organised in collaboration with the ICGEB.
Type: Fellowship.
No. of awards offered: 5.
Frequency: Annual.
Length of Study: 3 - 4 years.
Study Establishment: ICGEB Laboratory in Trieste.
Application Procedure: Preselection: submission of a letter of application to the school together with all requested documents, by April 30th. Alternatively a letter of application should be submitted by the end of September to be able to participate in the entrance examination held at the beginning of October in Trieste. Applications and letter of recommendation should be sent directly to the Director of the School.
Closing Date: April 30th for pre-selection/end of September for the entrance exams in October.
Additional Information: For further information please contact the Student Secretariat at the School, write to the ICGEB at the Trieste address or refer to the website: http://www.icgeb.trieste.it/phdsissa.htm.

INTERNATIONAL COUNCIL FOR CANADIAN STUDIES (ICCS)

325 Dalhousie S 800, Ottawa, ON, K1N 7G2, Canada
Tel: (1) 613 789 7828
Fax: (1) 613 7897830
Email: general@iccs-ciec.ca
www: http://www.iccs-ciec.ca
Contact: Program Officer

Commonwealth Scholarship Plan

Subjects: All subjects.
Eligibility: Open to Canadian citizens, or those permanent residents who are graduates of a Canadian university, who have completed a university degree or expect to graduate

prior to the tenure of the award. No age restriction pertains, but reference will be given to applicants who have obtained a university degree within the last five years.

Level of Study: Doctorate, Graduate, Postgraduate, Research.

Type: Scholarship.

No. of awards offered: Varies.

Frequency: Annual.

Value: Varies.

Country of Study: India, New Zealand, Sri Lanka, Tobago, Uganda or United Kingdom.

Application Procedure: Please write for details or visit our website at http://www.iccs-cies.ca.

Closing Date: Applications for New Zealand, December 31st; Applications for other countries, October 31st.

Additional Information: The Canadian Commonwealth and Fellowship Committee will select nominations to be forwarded to the awarding country. The number of nominations varies, but will be approximately double the number of awards expected to be made. The decision of the Canadian Committee is final and not open to appeal. The actual offer of a Scholarship will be made by the Commonwealth Scholarship Agency in the awarding country. In general, the Agency tries to place selected candidates in the institutions of their choice; however, where this is not possible, an alternative institution offering opportunities for the proposed course of study will be chosen.

Foreign Government Awards

Subjects: Any subject, except medicine or introduction to language.

Eligibility: Open to Canadian citizens with a working knowledge of the host country's language and a Bachelor's degree (or PhD for postdoctoral fellowships), completed before the beginning of the award term.

Level of Study: Doctorate, Graduate, Postdoctorate, Postgraduate, Research.

Purpose: To assist Canadians to study or conduct research abroad at the Master's, doctoral or postdoctoral level.

Type: Scholarship.

No. of awards offered: Varies.

Frequency: Annual.

Value: Generally to cover tuition fees, books, a living allowance, transportation and miscellaneous expenses.

Country of Study: Colombia, Finland, France, or Mexico.

Application Procedure: Applications are initially evaluated by a 'preselection committee' of Canadian academics. The committee submits a list of recommended candidates and alternates to each host country, where award recipients are chosen. A list of participating countries is available on request.

Closing Date: October 30th or January 20th for Colombia.

INTERNATIONAL DEVELOPMENT RESEARCH CENTRE (IDRC)

Centre Training and Awards Unit
250 Albert Street
PO Box 8500, Ottawa, ON, K1G 3H9, Canada
Tel: (1) 613 236 6163
Fax: (1) 613 563 0815
Email: cta@idrc.ca
www: http://www.idrc.ca
Contact: Ms Estelle Laferriere, Program Assistant

Canadian Window on Instrumental Development

Subjects: Proposals must indicate comparative research in Canada and a developing region of the world to better understand the common, interrelated problem or issue identitified for in-depth study.

Eligibility: Successful candidates will propose comparative research requiring data from both Canada and a developing region of the world to better understand the common, interrelated problem or issue identified for in-depth study. Selection will favour those proposals which demonstrate the relevance of the research topic for Canada and for the less developed country or countries being studied, and the close linkage between the international.

Level of Study: Doctorate.

Purpose: In recognition of the challenges posed in defining international development in a world which continues to change drastically, IDRC offers this award for doctoral research that explores the relationship between Canadian aid, trade, immigration and diplomatic policy, and international development and the alleviation of global poverty.

No. of awards offered: 1 or 2.

Frequency: Annual.

Value: Up to C$20,000.

Study Establishment: Canadian universties.

Country of Study: Canada.

Application Procedure: Application forms must be completed, please write for details.

Closing Date: February 1st.

INTERNATIONAL EYE FOUNDATION

Tv 21 No 100-20 Piso 7, Bogota, Colombia
Tel: (57) 1 611 17 11
Fax: (57) 1 256 82 74
Email: earenas@cable.net.co
www: http://www.interaction.org/members/ief.html
Contact: Dr Eduardo Arenas

International Eye Foundation (Colombia) Fellowship

Subjects: Anterior segment surgery.

Eligibility: Open to ophthalmologists from any country.

Level of Study: Postdoctorate.

Purpose: To bring ophthalmologists up to date with advances in procedures of cornea, glaucoma and cataract.
Type: Fellowship.
No. of awards offered: 2.
Frequency: Twice a year.
Value: US$200.
Length of Study: 6 months.
Study Establishment: Santa Fe de Bogota Foundation.
Country of Study: Colombia.
Application Procedure: Please write for details.
Closing Date: June, September.

INTERNATIONAL FEDERATION OF UNIVERSITY WOMEN (IFUW)

8 rue de l'Ancien-Port, Geneva, CH-1201, Switzerland
Tel: (41) 22 731 23 80
Fax: (41) 22 738 04 40
Email: ifuw@iprolink.ch
www: http://www.ifuw.org
Contact: Grants Management Officer

A non-profit, non-governmental organisation comprising of graduate women working locally, nationally and internationally to advocate for the improvement of the status of women and girls at the international level; to promote lifelong education; and to enable graduate women to use their expertise to effect change.

The British Federation Crosby Hall Fellowship

Subjects: All subjects.
Eligibility: Women applicants for all awards must be either a member of one of IFUW's national federations or associations or, in the case of women graduates living in countries where there is not yet a national affiliate, an independent member of IFUW.
Level of Study: Doctorate, Postdoctorate, Postgraduate, Research.
Purpose: To encourage advance scholarship and original research.
Type: Fellowship.
No. of awards offered: 1.
Frequency: Every two years, next one offered for 2000-2001.
Value: £2,500.
Study Establishment: An approved institution of higher education.
Country of Study: United Kingdom.
Application Procedure: Applicants should write for details enclosing a stamped addressed envelope. Applicants must apply through their respective Federation or Association. A list of IFUW national federations can be sent upon request or obtained through the internet.
Closing Date: Early September in the year preceding the competition.

Additional Information: Applicants in the US and the UK should write to the addresses shown for these countries; all others should write to the main address.

For further information contact:

BFWG
4 Mandeville Courtyard
142 Battersea Park Road, London, SW11 4NB, England
Tel: (44) 171 498 8037
Fax: (44) 171 498 8037
or
AAUW/IFUW Liason
1111 Sixteenth Street
NW, Washington, DC, 28036, United States of America
Fax: (1) 202 872 1425

Ida Smedley Maclean, CFUW/A Vibert Douglas, IFUW and Action Fellowship

Subjects: All subjects.
Eligibility: Women applicants for all awards must be either a member of one of IFUW's national federations or associations or, in the case of women graduates living in countries where there is not yet a national affiliate, an independent member of IFUW. Applicants should be well started on a research programme and should have completed at least one year of graduate work.
Level of Study: Doctorate, Postdoctorate, Postgraduate.
Purpose: To encourage advanced scholarship and original research.
Type: Fellowship.
No. of awards offered: 1 of each fellowship.
Frequency: Every two years. Next competition will offer awards for 2000-2001.
Value: Maclean Fellowship: CHF8,000-10,000; Douglas Fellowship: C$6,000; SAAP Fellowship: CHF8,000-10,000.
Length of Study: At least 8 months.
Study Establishment: An approved institution of higher education other than that in which the applicant received her education or habitually resides.
Country of Study: Any country.
Application Procedure: Applicants should write for details enclosing a stamped addressed envelope. Applicants must apply through their respective federation or association. A list of IFUW national federations can be sent upon request or be obtained from the internet.
Closing Date: Early September in the year preceding the competition.
Additional Information: Applicants in the US and the UK should write to the addresses shown for these countries; all others should write to the main address.

For further information contact:

BFWG
4 Mandeville Courtyard
142 Battersea Park Road, London, SW11 4NB, England
Tel: (44) 171 498 8037
Fax: (44) 171 498 8037

or

AAUW/IFUW

1111 Sixteenth Street NW, Washington, DC, 28036, United States of America

Fax: (1) 202 872 1425

Winifred Cullis and Dorothy Leet Grants, NZFUW Grants

Subjects: All subjects.

Eligibility: Women applicants for all awards must be either a member of one of the IFUW's national federations or associations or, in the case of women graduates living in countries where there is not yet a national affiliate, an independent member of IFUW.

Level of Study: Doctorate, Graduate, Postdoctorate, Postgraduate.

Purpose: To enable recipients to carry out research, obtain specialised training essential to research, or training in new techniques.

Type: Grant.

No. of awards offered: Varies.

Frequency: Every two years. Next competition will offer awards for 2000-2001.

Value: Varies; CHF3,000-CHF6,000.

Length of Study: Minimum of 2 months.

Country of Study: Any country.

Application Procedure: Applicants should write for details enclosing a stamped addressed envelope. Applicants must apply through their respective federation or association. A list of IFUW national federations can be sent upon request or obtained from the internet.

Closing Date: Early September in the year preceding the competition.

Additional Information: Applicants in the US and the UK should write to the addresses shown for these countries; all others should write to the main address.

For further information contact:

BFWG

4 Mandeville Courtyard

142 Battersea Park Road, London, SW11 4NB, England

Tel: (44) 171 498 8037

Fax: (44) 171 498 8037

or

AAUW/IFUW Liason

1111 Sixteenth Street

NW, Washington, DC, 28036, United States of America

Fax: (1) 202 872 1425

INTERNATIONAL FOUNDATION FOR ETHICAL RESEARCH (IFER)

53 West Jackson Boulevard

Suite 1552, Chicago, IL, 60604, United States of America

Tel: (1) 312 427 6025

Fax: (1) 312 427 6524

www: http://www.ifer.org

Contact: Mr Peter O'Donovan, Deputy Director

The IFER supports the development and implementation of viable, scientifically valid alternatives to the use of animals in research, product testing, and classroom education. IFER is dedicated to the belief that through new technologies and diligent research, we can find solutions that will create a better world for all, without using non-human animals.

International Foundation for Ethical Research Fellowship in Animal Welfare

Subjects: Tissue cultures, cell cultures, organ cultures, gas chromatography, mathematical and computer models, clinical and epidemiological surveys are examples of some of the research areas previously awarded grants.

Eligibility: Open to qualified educators and/or researchers who seek to provide alternatives to the use of live animals in research, testing and education.

Level of Study: Doctorate, Postgraduate.

Purpose: To develop, validate and disseminate alternatives to the use of live animals in research, education and product testing. Alternatives are defined as methods which replace, refine or reduce the number of animals traditionally used.

Type: Fellowship.

No. of awards offered: 2-3.

Frequency: Annual.

Value: Total amount awarded is approximately US$50,000 - US$75,000 annually among several projects. Each individual fellowship is $15,000 per year; renewable for up to 3 years based on eligibility and funding.

Country of Study: Any country.

Application Procedure: Please write for details or visit the website.

Closing Date: March 1st for pre-proposals.

INTERNATIONAL FOUNDATION OF EMPLOYEE BENEFIT PLANS (IFEBP)

18700 W Bluemound Road
PO Box 69, Brookfield, WI, 53008-0069, United States of America
Tel: (1) 414 786 6700
Fax: (1) 414 786 8670
Email: research@ifebp.org
www: http://www.ifebp.org
Contact: Ms Cindy Kabacinski, Research Secretary

The IFEBP is a non-profit educational and research association dedicated to the exchange of information among those who manage or serve employee benefit plans. Founded in 1954, the IFEBP is consistently recognised as the leading educational institution in the employee benefits field.

IFEBP Grants for Research

Subjects: Original research on employee benefit topics - including health care benefits, retirement and income security, and other aspects of employee benefits systems. Special consideration may be given to proposals on particular topics according to the year of application.
Eligibility: Open to citizens of the United States or Canada who are pursuing a graduate or postgraduate degree from an accredited college or university, or who hold a terminal degree from an accredited institution and are employed by a non-profit educational or research institution. The following academic disciplines are examples of appropriate backgrounds for grant applicants: business and finance, labour and industrial relations, economics, law, social/health sciences.
Level of Study: Graduate, Postdoctorate.
Purpose: To encourage original research on employee benefits-related issues.
Type: Research Grant.
No. of awards offered: Varies.
Frequency: Throughout the year.
Value: Up to US$5,000 (graduate) and US$10,000 (postdoctoral).
Country of Study: Any country.
Application Procedure: Interested individuals may apply by submitting a proposal, most recent (unofficial) transcripts and CV.
Closing Date: Applications are accepted at any time.

INTERNATIONAL HUMAN FRONTIER SCIENCE PROGRAMME ORGANIZATION (HFSP)

Bureaux Europe
20 Place des Halles, Strasbourg, 67080, France
Tel: (33) 3 88 21 51 12
Fax: (33) 88 32 88 97
Email: info@hfsp.org
www: http://www.hfsp.org

The Human Frontier Science Programme (HFSP) promotes basic research into the complex mechanisms underlying the function of living organisms, including humans, by supporting interdisciplinary and international collaboration. The Programme only supports research that transcends national boundaries.

Long Term Fellowships

Subjects: Medical sciences, brain functions, molecular approaches to biological functions.
Eligibility: Promising young scientists at postdoctoral level.
Level of Study: Postdoctorate, Research.
Purpose: To provide a period of postdoctoral training for researchers who are expected to play an important role in originating and pursuing creative research.
Type: A variable number of Fellowships.
No. of awards offered: Varies.
Value: Approx. US$40,000 per annum per fellow.
Length of Study: 2 years.
Study Establishment: Outstanding laboratories in any member country.
Country of Study: Any country.
Application Procedure: Please write for details or visit the website.
Closing Date: Please write for details.

Research Grants

Subjects: Medical sciences, brain functions, molecular approaches to biological functions.
Eligibility: Teams of scientists from different countries who wish to combine their expertise to approach questions that could not be answered by individual laboratories.
Level of Study: Research.
Purpose: To foster international co-operation between the best scientists with different expertise working on the same subject.
Type: A variable number of Grants.
No. of awards offered: Varies.
Frequency: Annual.

Value: Approx. US$230,000 per annum.
Length of Study: Up to 3 years.
Study Establishment: Laboratories worldwide.
Country of Study: Any country.
Application Procedure: Please write for details, or visit the website.
Closing Date: Please write for details.

Short Term Fellowships

Subjects: Medical sciences, brain functions, molecular approaches to biological functions.
Eligibility: Open to promising researchers.
Level of Study: Postdoctorate, Research.
Purpose: To enable researchers to learn state of the art techniques already in use abroad or to establish new research collaborations.
Type: A variable number of Fellowships.
Value: Dependant on the length of time spent abroad.
Length of Study: 2 weeks - 3 months.
Study Establishment: Laboratories in any member country.
Country of Study: Any country.
Application Procedure: Please write for further details, or visit the website.
Closing Date: Please write for details.

INTERNATIONAL PEACE SCHOLARSHIP FUND

c/o PEO
3700 Grand Avenue, Des Moines, IA, 50312, United States of America
Tel: (1) 515 255 3153
Fax: (1) 515 255 3820
Contact: Ms Carolyn J Larson, Project Supervisor

PEO International Peace Scholarship

Subjects: All subjects.
Eligibility: Any nationality may apply apart from candidates from USA or Canada. Eligiblility is based on financial need, nationality, degree, full time status and residence the entire term of study.
Level of Study: Doctorate, Postgraduate.
Purpose: Grant-in-Aid for international women studying graduate degrees (Master's, PhD) in the US or Canada.
Type: Grant-in Aid.
No. of awards offered: Approx. 150.
Frequency: Annual.
Value: US$5,000 maximum per year.
Length of Study: Maximum 3 years.
Country of Study: USA or Canada.
Application Procedure: Eligibility must be established before application material is sent. Write to IPS Office and request eligibility form. If eligibile an application form is sent.

Closing Date: December 15th for receipt of eligibility form, January 31st for receipt of application form.
Additional Information: Scholarships cannot be used for travel, research dissertations, internships or practical training. An applicant must have a contact person who is a citizen of the United States or Canada, and who will act as a non-academic adviser. Applicant must have round trip return travel expense guaranteed at the time of the application. Applicants must return to their own country on completion of their studies.

THE INTERNATIONAL SPINAL RESEARCH TRUST (ISRT)

Unit 8
Bramley Business Centre
Station Road
Bramley, Guildford, Surrey, GU5 0AZ, England
Tel: (44) 1483 898 786
Fax: (44) 1483 898 763
Email: research@isrthq.demon.co.uk
www: http://www.spinal-research.org
Contact: Mr John Cavannagh, Head of Research

Fundraising to support research projects that have the aim of repairing or restoring the loss of function that occurs as a result of injury to the spinal cord. A structured research strategy has been developed to target funds towards relevant research topics.

Nathalie Rose Barr PhD Studentship

Subjects: Topics relevant to ISRT's research strategy (Spinal Cord 34:446-459, 1996). Projects will be between collaborative laboratories involved in spinal cord injury research, based in the UK. Both clinical and basic research projects are considered.
Eligibility: Open to graduates with an upper second or first class degree or recently qualified clinicians from EU countries.
Level of Study: Postgraduate.
Purpose: To support basic and clinical students while working towards a research-based PhD degree.
Type: Studentship.
No. of awards offered: Varies.
Frequency: Annually, dependent on funds available.
Value: In line with the Wellcome Trust.
Length of Study: 4 years - basic research studentship; 3 years - clinical research fellowship.
Study Establishment: UK universities.
Country of Study: United Kingdom.
Application Procedure: Following advertisement, supervisors will submit project proposals on an ISRT application form. Supervisors of successful projects will then advertise for students.
Closing Date: To be advertised.

INTERNATIONAL UNION AGAINST CANCER

Fellowships Department
3 rue de Conseil-Général, Geneva, CH-1205, Switzerland
Fax: (41) 22 809 18 10
Email: bbaker@uicc.ch
www: http://www.uicc.ch/fellows/
Contact: Mr Brita M Baker, Head

The UICC Fellowships Programme provides long, medium and short-term fellowships abroad to qualified investigators, clinicians, and nurses, who are actively involved in cancer research, clinical oncology or oncology nursing.

Asia-Pacific Cancer Society Training Grants (APCASOT)

Subjects: Non-medical aspects of cancer society work, such as fundraising, media relations, organisation and managerial skills, surveilance of cancer statistics, behavioural research, advocacy, non-medical patient services, preventions and early detection education programmes.
Eligibility: Open to staff and accredited volunteers from cancer societies in the Asia-Pacific region.
Level of Study: Unrestricted.
Purpose: To support the training of qualified individuals.
Type: Grant.
No. of awards offered: 5.
Frequency: Annual.
Value: US$1,800 to the least expensive round trip fare or other appropriate form of transport and to the living costs. Extra costs for visa, passports, airport taxes, and insurance, are the responsibility of the grant recipient. No financial support is provided for dependents.
Length of Study: 1-2 weeks.
Study Establishment: Cancer Society.
Country of Study: Any country.
Application Procedure: Please write to the UICC Fellowships Department for an application form or download it from the website.
Closing Date: September 1st for December selection.

International Cancer Research Technology Transfer Project (ICRETT)

Subjects: Cancer control and prevention, epidemiology and cancer registration, public education, and behavioural sciences.
Eligibility: Open to qualified investigators and experienced clinicians.
Level of Study: Professional development.
Purpose: To enable recipients to learn or teach up-to-date research techniques, transfer appropriate technology, or acquire advanced clinical management, diagnostic and therapeutic skills.
Type: Fellowship.
No. of awards offered: 120.
Frequency: Annual.
Value: The average stipend is US$3,000.

Length of Study: 1-3 months (with stipend support for 1 month).
Country of Study: Any country.
Application Procedure: Applications may be submitted at any time. Awards are normally notified within 60 days of registration of a complete application. Applications may be obtained from the Fellowships Department or downloaded from the website.
Closing Date: Applications are accepted at any time.
Additional Information: The Fellowships are funded by: National Cancer Institute, USA; Eurpean Commission Europe Against Cancer Programme; Norwegian Agency for Development (NORAD); Norwegian Cancer Society; Cancer Research Campaign, UK Imperial Cancer Research Fund, UK; Swedish Cancer Society; Nordi Cancer Union; National Cancer Institute of Canada/Cancer Society of Canada; Italian Cancer Research Foundation; Dutch Cnacer Society; French National League Against Cancer; Dr Mildred Scheel Foundation Deutsche Krebshilfe, Germany; Finnish International Development Agency (FINNIDA); Cancer Society of Finland; Australian Cancer Society Inc.; Israel Cancer Association; Cancer Association of South Africa; Assocition of UICC Fellows; UICC Roll of Honour.

International Cancer Technology Transfer Fellowships (ICRETT) for Bilateral Exchanges Between Indonesia and the Netherlands

Subjects: Epidemiology and cancer registration.
Eligibility: The short-term fellowships permit successful candidates to spend up to three months at a suitable host institute in the Netherlands. Qualified cancer investigators should be in the early stages of their careers whilst clinicians should be well established in their oncology practice. Experts from the Netherlands who have been invited to teach these specialised skills at institutes in Indonesia are also eligible to apply.
Level of Study: Professional development.
Purpose: To foster the acquisition of up-to-date clinical management, diagnostic and therapeutic expertise; exchange knowledge and enhance skills in cancer control and prevention; and facilitate rapid transfer of cancer research and technology.
Type: Fellowship.
No. of awards offered: 6-8.
Frequency: Annual.
Value: 1 month stipend and travel of US$3,000, home and or host institutions are expected to cover living costs for any additional periods. UICC also contributes to the least expensive international return air fares or other appropriate form of transport. Travel estimates should not include costs for internal travel within the home and/or host countries. These and extra costs for visa, passports, airport taxes, and insurance, are the responsibility of the Fellow. No allowances are made for accompanying dependents.
Length of Study: Maximum 3 months.
Application Procedure: Application forms are availble from the Fellowships Department or can be downloaed from the website.
Closing Date: Applications may be submitted at any time.

International Fellowships for Beginning Investigators (ACSBI)

Subjects: Epidemiology, prevention, causation, detection, diagnosis, treatment, psycho-oncology.
Eligibility: Candidates should be in the early stages of their careers and applications that are geared to the development of specific cancer control measures in developing and central and east European countries are particularly encouraged. Candidates should holds assistant professorships or similar positions at their home institutes and ordinarily have a minimum of two and a maximum of 10 years postdoctoral experience after obtaining their MD or PhD degrees or equivalents. Awards are conditional on the return of the fellow to the home institute at the end of the fellowship and on the availability of appropriate facilities and resources to apply newly acquired skills. Candidates who are physically present at the proposed host institute whilst their applications are under consideration are not eligible for UICC fellowships.
Level of Study: Professional development.
Purpose: To enable investigators and clinicians, who are in the early stages of their careers to carry out basic, translational, or clinical projects and to develop, acquire and apply advance research procedures and techniques that foster a bi-directional flow of knowledge, experience, expertise and innovation to and from the USA.
Type: Fellowship.
No. of awards offered: 8-10.
Frequency: Annual.
Value: Average value of US$35,000 for travel and stipend support. Calculation of travel and stipend awards are based on the candidate's estimates, which are adjusted, if need be to published fares and UICC scales. Travel awards contribute to least expensive international return air fares or other appropriate form of transport. Travel estimates should not include costs for internal travel within the home and/or host countries. These and extra costs for visa, passports, airport taxes, and insurance, are the responsibility of the Fellow. No allowances are made for accompanying dependents.
Length of Study: 12 months, no extensions are permitted.
Application Procedure: Completed applications with all supporting documentation must reach the UICC by the application closing date. Application forms may be obtained from the Fellowships department or downloaded from the website.
Closing Date: October 1st, selection results notified in mid-April the following year.

International Oncology Nursing Fellowships

Subjects: Cancer nursing training.
Eligibility: Open to English-speaking nurses who are actively engaged in the care of cancer patients in their home institutes and who come from developing or Eastern European countries where specialist cancer nursing training is not yet widely available.
Level of Study: Professional development.
Purpose: To support English-speaking nurses who are actively engaged in the care of cancer patients and who come from developing and East European countries.
Type: Fellowship.

No. of awards offered: 5.
Frequency: Annual.
Value: The average stipend is US$2,800.
Length of Study: 1-3 months (with stipend support for 1 month).
Country of Study: Any country.
Application Procedure: Applications complete with supporting documentation must be received by the UICC Geneva Office by the application closing date. Application forms can be obtained from the Fellowships Department or downloaded from the website.
Closing Date: November 1st for notification mid-February.
Additional Information: The Fellowships are funded by the Oncology Nursing Society and Hoechst Marion Roussel Inc, USA.

Latin America COPES Training and Education Fellowships (LACTEF)

Subjects: Non-medical aspects of cancer society work.
Eligibility: Open to staff and accredited volunteers from cancer societies in the Latin American region.
Level of Study: Unrestricted.
Purpose: To support the training of qualified individuals in non-medical aspects of cancer society work.
Type: Fellowship.
No. of awards offered: 5.
Frequency: Annual.
Value: US$1,800.
Length of Study: 1-2 weeks.
Country of Study: Any country.
Application Procedure: Please write to the UICC Fellowships Department for an application form or it can be downloaded from the website.
Closing Date: May 1st, with selection in mid-August.

Translational Cancer Research Fellowships (TRCF)

Subjects: The bridging of areas that effectively connect the cell and molecular biologists to the patients in the clinic.
Eligibility: The fellowships are subject to the UICC General Conditions for fellowships.
Level of Study: Postdoctorate.
Purpose: To accelerate the translation of basic, experimental, and applied research insights into their clinical applications in the form of new drugs and treatments and of vaccines and effective prevention or intervention strategies.
Type: Fellowship.
No. of awards offered: Varies.
Frequency: Annual.
Value: The average award value is US$55,000.
Length of Study: 12 months.
Country of Study: Any country.
Application Procedure: Application forms may be obtained from the Fellowships Department.
Closing Date: December 1st.

Yamagiwa-Yoshida Memorial International Cancer Study Grants

Subjects: Cancer research.
Eligibility: Open to appropriately qualified investigators from any country who are actively engaged in cancer research. Candidates who are already physically present at the proposed host institute are not eligible.
Level of Study: Professional development.
Purpose: To enable cancer investigators from any country to carry out bilateral research projects which exploit complementary materials or skills, including advanced training in experimental methods or special techiques.
Type: Grant.
No. of awards offered: 15.
Frequency: Twice a year.
Value: The average stipend is US$9,000 (if a Fellows return to home is delayed beyond the extra approved period, 50 per cent of the travel award, the return portion has to be reimbursed to the UICC). Calculation of travel and stipend awards are based on the candidate's estimates, which are adjusted, if need be to published fares and UICC scales. Travel awards contribute to least expensive international return air fares or other appropriate form of transport. Travel estimates should not include costs for internal travel within the home and/or host countries. These and extra costs for visa, passports, airport taxes, and insurance, are the responsibility of the Fellow. No financial support is provided for dependents.
Length of Study: 1-3 months and may be extended at no additional cost to UICC, by their original duration and subject to written approval of the home and host supervisors. Funding for these additional periods may be secured from other funding agencies.
Country of Study: Any country.
Application Procedure: Application forms may be obtained from the Fellowships Department or downloaded from the website.
Closing Date: January 1st for notification by mid-April; July 1st for notification by mid-October.
Additional Information: These grants are funded by the Kyowa Hakko Kogyo Company Ltd, Toray Industries Incorporated, Tokyo, and the Japan National Committee for UICC.

IRIS FUND FOR PREVENTION OF BLINDNESS

York House
199 Westminster Bridge Road, London, SE1 7UT, England
Tel: (44) 171 928 7743
Fax: (44) 171 928 7919
Contact: Mr Stephen D Cochrane, The Executive Director

The Iris Fund supports nationwide research into the prevention and cure of all forms of blindness and serious eye disorders, whether inherited, congenital or acquired. The Fund also focuses on current needs by sponsoring screening programmes and helping ophthalmology departments purchase vital innovative equipment when funds are unavailable from other sources.

Iris Fund Award

Subjects: Ophthalmology.
Eligibility: Open to UK citizens only, under the age of forty.
Level of Study: Professional development.
Purpose: In recognition of distinction either in training or in the chosen area of ophthalmic research.
No. of awards offered: 1.
Frequency: Every two years.
Value: £5,000.
Country of Study: United Kingdom.
Application Procedure: Application form must be completed and submitted with six copies of supporting paperwork.
Closing Date: Please contact the Iris Fund for confirmation.

Iris Fund Grants for Research and Equipment (Ophthalmology)

Subjects: Ophthalmology.
Eligibility: Open to suitably qualified individuals. Applications must be submitted by qualified consultant ophthalmologists or equivalent for research under his/her supervision. Research projects can only take place in the UK.
Level of Study: Unrestricted.
Purpose: To prevent and cure blindness and serious eye disorders.
Type: Grant.
No. of awards offered: Varies.
Frequency: Annual.
Value: As funds become available.
Length of Study: Usually for a maximum of 3 years.
Country of Study: United Kingdom.
Application Procedure: Application form with eight copies, including supporting paperwork, must be submitted to the Iris Fund.
Closing Date: March 31st.

JAMES COOK UNIVERSITY OF NORTH QUEENSLAND

Research Students Office, Townsville, QLD, 4811, Australia
Tel: (61) 77 81 4575
Fax: (61) 77 81 6204
www: http://www.jcu.edu.au
Contact: Research Students Officer

James Cook University Postgraduate Research Scholarship

Subjects: Most subjects offered at the University.
Eligibility: Open to any student who has attained at least a Bachelor's degree at honours level (Class 2A).
Level of Study: Postgraduate.

Purpose: To encourage full-time postgraduate research leading to a Master's or PhD degree.
Type: Scholarship.
No. of awards offered: Up to 4.
Frequency: Annual.
Value: A$15,888 per year. The award does not cover annual tuition fees for overseas students.
Length of Study: 3 years with a possible additional 6 months in exceptional circumstances (PhD); or for 2 years (Master's program).
Study Establishment: James Cook University.
Country of Study: Australia.
Closing Date: October 31st.

JANE COFFIN CHILDS MEMORIAL FUND FOR MEDICAL RESEARCH

333 Cedar Street, New Haven, CT, 06510, United States of America
Tel: (1) 203 785 4612
Fax: (1) 203 785 3301
Contact: Office of the Director

Jane Coffin Childs Memorial Fund for Medical Research Fellowships

Subjects: Medical and related sciences relevant to the causes, origins and treatment of cancer.
Eligibility: Open to persons who possess an MD or PhD degree in the field in which they propose to work.
Level of Study: Postdoctorate.
Type: Fellowship.
No. of awards offered: 25.
Frequency: Annual.
Value: US$28,000 in the first year, US$29,000 in the second year, US$30,000 in the third year; plus dependant child allowance of US$750 each, and usually US$1,500 per year departmental grant.
Length of Study: 2-3 years.
Study Establishment: Laboratories and other institutions where the candidate's proposed research is acceptable and where adequate facilities for work exist.
Country of Study: Any country (US citizens) or USA (non-US citizens).
Application Procedure: Please contact the Fund for further details.
Closing Date: February 1st.

JAPAN SOCIETY FOR THE PROMOTION OF SCIENCE (JSPS)

Jochi Kioizaka Bldg
6-26-3 Kioi-cho
Chiyoda-ku, Tokyo, 102, Japan
Tel: (81) 3 3263 1721
Fax: (81) 3 3263 1854
Contact: Mr Nagahide Onozawa

JSPS Postdoctoral Fellowships for Foreign Researchers

Subjects: Humanities, social sciences, natural sciences, engineering and medicine.
Eligibility: Open to citizens of countries which have diplomatic relations with Japan. Applicants must have a doctorate degree.
Level of Study: Postdoctorate.
Purpose: To assist promising and highly-qualified young foreign researchers wishing to conduct research in Japan.
Type: Fellowship.
No. of awards offered: Varies.
Frequency: Annual.
Value: A round-trip airfare is provided with a monthly maintenance allowance of Y270,000, a settling-in allowance of Y200,000, a monthly housing allowance not to exceed Y100,000, a monthly family allowance of Y50,000 if accompanied by dependants, and accident/sickness insurance coverage for the Fellow only.
Length of Study: 2 years (12 month tenure may be considered).
Study Establishment: Japanese universities and similar institutions.
Country of Study: Japan.
Application Procedure: Please write for details.

JAPANESE GOVERNMENT

Embassy of Japan
112 Empire Circuit, Yarralumla, ACT, 2600, Australia
Tel: (61) 6 273 3244
Fax: (61) 6 273 1848
www: http://www.jwindow.net/GOV/gov.html
Contact: Ms E Prior

Japanese Government (Monbusho) Scholarships Research Category

Subjects: Humanities and social sciences - literature, history, aesthetics, law, politics, economics, commerce, pedagogy, psychology, sociology, music and fine arts. Natural sciences - pure science, engineering, agriculture, fisheries, pharmacology, medicine, dentistry, and home economics.

Eligibility: Open to Australian graduates under 35 years of age and likewise nationals of any country which has diplomatic relations with Japan.
Level of Study: Doctorate, Postgraduate.
Type: Scholarship.
No. of awards offered: Approx. 20.
Frequency: Annual.
Value: Return air fare, plus Y185,500 per month.
Length of Study: 18-24 months.
Study Establishment: A Japanese university.
Country of Study: Japan.
Application Procedure: Application form available.
Closing Date: June.
Additional Information: Applicants must be willing to study the Japanese language.

JEWISH FOUNDATION FOR EDUCATION OF WOMEN

330 West 58th Street
Suite 509, New York, NY, 10019, United States of America
Tel: (1) 212 265 2565
Fax: (1) 212 765 2675
Email: fdnscholar@aol.com
www: http://www.jfew.org
Contact: Ms Marge Goldwater, Executive Director

The Jewish Foundation for Education of Women is a private, non-sectarian organisation. It provides scholarship assistance for higher education to women with financial need within a 50-mile radius of New York City through several specific programmes.

Scholarships for Émigrés in the Health Professions

Subjects: Medicine, dentistry, nursing, pharmacy.
Eligibility: Applicants must be female, émigrés from the former Soviet Union, live within a 50-mile radius of NYC, and demonstrate a financial need.
Level of Study: Graduate, Undergraduate.
Type: Scholarship.
No. of awards offered: Approx. 48.
Value: US$5,000.
Application Procedure: Applications available in late October.

JOHN E FOGARTY INTERNATIONAL CENTER FOR ADVANCED STUDY IN THE HEALTH SCIENCES

Division of International Training and Research
Building 31
Room B2C39
Fogarty International Center
31 Center Drive
MSC 2220, Bethesda, MD, 20892, United States of America
Tel: (1) 301 496 1653
Fax: (1) 301 402 0779
www: http://www.nih.gov/fic
Contact: Grants Management Officer

The John E Fogarty International Center (FIC) for Advanced Study in the Health Sciences, a component of the National Institutes of Health (NIH), promotes international co-operation in the biomedical and behavioural sciences. This is accomplished primarily through long and short-term fellowships, small grants, and training grants. This compendium of international opportunities is prepared by the FIC with the hope that it will stimulate scientists to seek research-enhancing experiences abroad.

AIDS International Training and Research Programme (AITRP)

Subjects: Biomedical and behavourial research related to AIDS.
Eligibility: Decisions about whom to accept for training are made by the programme directors. All current programme directors have developed collaborative activities with specific countries. The relevant US programme director should be contacted for country-specific information, necessary qualifications, eligibility, and application procedures. Scientists from the participating countries are eligible to apply for these training programmes. Scientists from other countries may wish to contact the Fogarty International Center for further information and suggestions as to which programmes may be able to accommodate their interests: AIDS International Training and Research Programs, Division of International Training and Research, Fogarty International Center, National Institutes of Health, Building 31, Room B2C32, 31 Center Drive MSC 2220, Bethesda MD 20892-2220, Fax: 1 301 402-2056, email: Ken_Bridbord@nih.gov.
Level of Study: Research.
Purpose: To enable scientists from developing countries to increase their profiency to undertake biomedical and behavioural research related to AIDS and to develop these acquired skills in clinical trials and prevention and related research.

Type: Research Grant.
No. of awards offered: Varies.
Frequency: Annual.
Application Procedure: Applications are accepted from US institutions in response to a specific request for applications. Individuals who wish to become trainees must apply to the project director of an awarded grant. Application forms are available from the website: http://www.nih.gov/fic/opportunities.

Fogarty International Research Collaboration Award (FIRCA)

Subjects: Biomedical and behavioural sciences.
Eligibility: For the purpose of this programme, eligible countries include those in the following regions: Africa, Asia (except Japan, Singapore, South Korea and Taiwan), Central and Eastern Europe (Hungary, Poland, the Czech and Slovak Republics, Romania, Bulgaria, Albania and the countries of the former Yugoslavia), Russia and the Newly Independent States (NIS) of the FSU, Latin America and the Caribbean, the Middle East, and the Pacific Ocean Islands (except Australia and New Zealand). The US scientist will apply as principal investigator with a colleague from a single laboratory or research site in an eligible country.
Level of Study: Unrestricted.
Purpose: The FIRCA will extend and enhance the research interests of both the US scientist and the collaborating foreign scientist and will help to increase the research capacity of the foreign scientist and institution. These small grants were established, under the auspices of the FIC's Central and Eastern European and Latin American and Caribbean Initiatives, to facilitate collaborative research between US scientists and scientists from Central and Eastern Europe (Bulgaria, the Czech and Slovak Federal Republic, Hungary, Poland, Romania, the USSR, and Yugoslavia), Latin America, and the non-US Caribbean. Eligibility has been expanded to more (developing) countries.
Type: Research Grant.
No. of awards offered: Approx. 35, depending on funds available.
Frequency: Three times each year.
Value: Up to US$32,000 in direct costs per year are available for up to three years. These funds may cover the purchase of supplies for the foreign collaborator's laboratory, a small stipend for the foreign investigator, and travel for the US and foreign collaborators and their research associates, as justified by the needs of the collaborative research.
Length of Study: 1-3 years.
Study Establishment: Awards are made to the US applicant institution to support a collaborative research project that will be carried out mainly at the foreign collaborator's research site.
Country of Study: Developing countries.
Application Procedure: Applications must be submitted on the grant application form PHS 398. Special instructions and conditions apply. Please refer to the website for further information: http://www.nih.gov/fic/opportunities/firca.html.
Closing Date: March 25th, July 25th, November 25th.

HIV-AIDS and Related Illnesses Collaboration Award (AIDS-FIRCA)

Subjects: HIV and AIDS research.
Eligibility: Most countries are eligible for collaboration under the AIDS-FIRCA, consistent with US foreign policy considerations. For the purpose of this programme, developing countries eligible to use AIDS-FIRCA funds for equipment are considered to include those in the following regions: Africa, Asia (except Japan, Singapore, South Korea and Taiwan), Central and Eastern Europe (Hungary, Poland, the Czech and Slovak Republics, Romania, Bulgaria, Albania and the countries of the former Yugoslavia), Russia and independent countries of the former Soviet Union, Latin America, the Middle East, and the Pacific Ocean Islands (except Australia and New Zealand).
Purpose: To foster international research partnerships between NIH supported US scientists and their collaborators through the world in all aspects of HIV-AIDS research and new and resurgent infectious diseases related to HIV infection. The AIDS-FIRCA programme aims to enhance the US investigator's research grant while benefiting the scientific interests of the foreign scientist.
Type: Institution training grant.
Value: US scientists who have an AIDS related NIH grant are eligible to apply. Up to US$32,000 in direct costs per year, for a maximum of three years, is available for US investigators and their foreign collaborators to conduct research, mainly at the foreign site. AIDS-FIRCA grants will provide funds to the foreign collaborator, through the US grantee institution, for a small stipend for the foreign investigator, for supplies at the foreign institution, and for research-related travel and subsistence expenses for both the US and foreign investigators.
Length of Study: Up to 3 years.
Application Procedure: The US scientist will apply as principal investigator with a colleague from a single laboratory or research site in an eligible country. Applications may be submitted by US non-profit organisations, public and private, such as universities, colleges, hospitals and laboratories. Racial/ethnic minority individuals, women, and persons with disabilities are encouraged to apply as principal investigators and collaborators. For further information and application details please refer to the website: http://www.nih.gov/fic/opportunities/.
Closing Date: September 1, January 2, and May 1.

John E Fogarty International Research Fellowship Program

Subjects: Biomedical and behavioural sciences.
Eligibility: Open to foreign scientists who have been selected by the Nominating Committee in their country; have a doctoral degree; have ten years or less of postdoctoral experience; have demonstrated the ability to engage in independent basic or clinical research; have been invited by a scientist employed in a US non-profit institution; have assurance from a non-profit institution in the home country of a position after completion of the Fellowship; and are proficient in spoken and written English.
Level of Study: Postdoctorate.

Purpose: To allow foreign scientists to extend their research experiences in US laboratories.
Type: Fellowship.
No. of awards offered: Approx. 25 depending on funds available.
Frequency: Dependent on funds available.
Value: A stipend of US$20,000-US$33,100 per year (the level is determined by the number of years since receipt of the doctoral degree); and round-trip air travel expenses for the Fellow only. The US host institution receives an allowance to cover mandatory health insurance for the Fellow and accompanying family members, trips to domestic scientific meetings, and incidental research expenses.
Length of Study: 12-24 months.
Country of Study: USA.
Application Procedure: Please write for application form from the nominating committee.
Closing Date: July 1st, October 15th.
Additional Information: More than 60 countries participate in this program. Countries and areas with Nominating Committees are: Argentina, Australia, Austria, Belgium, Bolivia, Brazil, Bulgaria, the Cameroon, Canada, Chile, China, Colombia, Costa Rica, the Czech and Slovak Federal Republics, Denmark, Egypt, Ethiopia, Finland, France, the Federal Republic of Germany, Ghana, Greece, Hong Kong, Hungary, Iceland, India, Ireland, Israel, Italy, Japan, Kenya, the Republic of Korea, Lebanon, Mexico, Mongolia, the Netherlands, New Zealand, Nigeria, Norway, Peru, the Philippines, Poland, Romania, Singapore, Spain, Sudan, Sweden, Switzerland, Tanzania, Thailand, the UK, Uruguay, the former USSR, Venezuela, former Yugoslavia, Zimbabwe, and Taiwan. Regional committees are located in Africa, the Caribbean, and Central/South America. Nominating Committees are being formed in other regions; candidates should enquire if their country of interest is not listed.

John E Fogarty Senior International Fellowship Program

Subjects: Biomedical and behavioural sciences.
Eligibility: Open to scientists who are US citizens or permanent residents invited by foreign host scientists to participate in research projects of mutual interest. Candidates should hold a doctoral degree in one of the biomedical, behavioural, or health sciences; have five years or more of postdoctoral experience; have professional experience in one of the biomedical, behavioural, or health sciences for at least two of the last four years; hold a full-time appointment on the staff of a public or private not-for-profit research, clinical or educational institution; be invited by a not-for-profit foreign institution; and not have received more than one Senior International Fellowship previously.
Level of Study: Postdoctorate.
Purpose: To provide opportunities for research experience and the exchange of information.
Type: Fellowship.
No. of awards offered: Approx. 30, depending on funds available.
Frequency: Dependent on funds available.

Value: A stipend of US$1,250 per month (or a maximum of US$15,000 per year); a foreign living allowance of US$2,000 per month (or a maximum of US$24,000 per year); economy class round-trip air travel for the Fellow only on a US air carrier between the US city and the host city abroad; and a host institutional allowance of up to US$6,000 per year or a pro-rated allowance for a shorter time. (US home institutions use these funds to help defray the costs of research supplies and equipment that are required at the foreign host institutions).
Length of Study: 3-12 months. The award may be divided into as many as 3 terms, utilised over a 3-year period, with a minimum term of 3 months.
Country of Study: Any country.
Application Procedure: Prospective applicants should request the special instructions from the Fogarty International Center. A prospective applicant must: complete the application forms (PHS 416-1, rev. 8/95); describe the benefits of the fellowship to both the fellow and the foreign sponsor and to both the applicant's and the sponsor's institution; carefully justify the benefits of each visit proposed for this fellowship; obtain a letter of invitation and curriculum vitae from the foreign sponsor; the letter should indicate that an understanding has been reached with regard to the plan proposed by the applicant.
Closing Date: April 5th, August 5th, December 5th.
Additional Information: The stipend plus the home institution salary during the tenure of the fellowship cannot exceed the awardee's annual salary. No stipend will be provided if the awardee receives salary from other federal sources. Because fellowships are intended to support an individual's expenses abroad, the foreign host is expected to have the resources to support the research project. Types of activities in which fellows engage include collaboration in basic or clinical research and familiarisation with or utilisation of special techniques and equipment not otherwise available to the applicant. The programs do not provide support for activities which have as their principal purpose conducting brief observational visits; attending scientific meetings or formal training courses; or providing full-time clinical, technical or teaching services.

NIH Visiting Program

Subjects: Biomedical research.
Eligibility: Open to talented foreign scientists throughout the world. An appointment or award to the Visiting Programme must be requested by a senior investigator in an NIH laboratory.
Level of Study: Doctorate, Postdoctorate, Postgraduate.
Purpose: To provide talented foreign scientists throughout the world with the opportunity to share in the varied resources of the NIH. Through this program, scientists at all levels of their careers are invited to the NIH for further experience and to conduct collaborative research in their biomedical specialties.
Type: Fellowship.
Frequency: Dependent on funds available.
Length of Study: Varies, usually 2 years.
Country of Study: USA.

Application Procedure: An award or appointment to the Visiting Programme must be requested by a senior scientist in one of the NIH's intramural laboratories and is offered based on the candidate's qualifications and the research needs of the host laboratory. The NIH senior scientist serves as the participant's sponsor and supervisor during the period of award or appointment. Individuals interested in a Visiting Programme fellowship award or appointment should write to NIH senior scientists working in the same research field, enclosing a resume and brief description of their particular research area.

Additional Information: Each participant works closely with a senior NIH investigator, who serves as a sponsor or supervisor during the period of award or appointment. Anyone interested in a Visiting Programme fellowship appointment or award should send a résumé and brief description of research interests to individual NIH senior staff scientists working in those fields. These investigators are listed in the Scientific Director and Annual Bibliography, which is published each year by the NIH and is available in many libraries throughout the world. Also, the Postdoctoral Research Fellowship Opportunities Catalogue describes research being conducted in laboratories at the NIH and is available on request.

JOSEPH COLLINS FOUNDATION

787-7th Avenue
Rm 3950, New York, NY, 10019-6099, United States of America
Fax: (1) 212 728 8111
Email: apacker@wilkie.com
Contact: Ms Augusta L Packer, Secretary-Treasurer

Joseph Collins Foundation Grants

Subjects: Medicine towards an MD degree.
Eligibility: Open to anyone attending an accredited medical school in the USA, located east of the Mississippi River, who intends to specialise in neurology, psychiatry or general practice. Applicants must have successfully completed their first year at an accredited medical school. No grants are available to students attending medical schools west of the Mississippi River.
Level of Study: Doctorate.
Purpose: To aid needy medical students with broad cultural interests who wish to receive an adequate medical education and obtain an MD degree without sacrificing other interests.
Type: Grant.
No. of awards offered: Varies.
Frequency: Annual.
Value: Varies; up to a maximum of US$10,000 annually, to be applied towards tuition.

Length of Study: 1 year; renewable at the discretion of the Foundation.
Study Establishment: Any accredited medical school, located east of the Mississippi River.
Country of Study: USA.
Application Procedure: Application form must be completed.
Closing Date: March 15th.
Additional Information: Consideration of all applicants will be based on financial need, scholastic record and demonstrated interest in arts and letters or other cultural pursuits or to outside the field of medicine. Preference is given to students who reside within 200 miles of the medical school they attend. Applications should be obtained through medical school authorities. Awards are not made to pre-medical or postgraduate medical students or to chiropracter, osteopathic, or to podiatry students.

KEELE UNIVERSITY

Staffordshire, ST5 5BG, England
Tel: (44) 1782 584002
Fax: (44) 1782 632343
Email: aab01@admin.keele.ac.uk
www: http://www.keele.ac.uk
Contact: Director of Academic Affairs

Keele University Graduate Teaching Assistantships

Subjects: Various subjects from the fields of arts and humanities, business administration and management, education and teacher training, fine and applied arts, law, mathematics and computer science, medical sciences, natural sciences, social and behavioural sciences.
Eligibility: Candidates should hold a good honours degree and are required to register as full-time candidates for a higher degree at the University of Keele.
Level of Study: Postgraduate.
Purpose: To assist research and give teaching experience.
Type: Studentship.
No. of awards offered: 2-3.
Frequency: Annual.
Value: £6,455 per year.
Length of Study: 1 year; may be extended for an unspecified additional period.
Study Establishment: Keele University.
Country of Study: United Kingdom.
Application Procedure: Please contact the admissions office for details.
Closing Date: February 1st.

KENNEDY MEMORIAL TRUST

48 Westminster Palace Gardens
Artillery Row, London, SW1P 1RR, England
Tel: (44) 171 222 1151
Fax: (44) 171 222 5355
Contact: Ms Anna Mason, Secretary

As part of the British National Memorial to President Kennedy, the Trust awards scholarships to British postgraduate students for study at Harvard University or the Massachusetts Institute of Technology. -The awards, which are offered annually following a national competition, cover tuition costs and a stipend to meet living expenses.

Kennedy Scholarships

Subjects: All fields of arts, science, social science and political studies.
Eligibility: Open to UK citizens who are resident in the UK, and who have been wholly or mainly educated in the UK. At the time of application, candidates must have spent at least two of the last five years at a UK university or university college, and must have graduated by the start of tenure in the following year, or have graduated not more than three years prior to the commencement of studies.
Level of Study: Postgraduate.
Purpose: As part of the British National Memorial to President Kennedy to enable students to undertake a course of postgraduate study in the United States.
Type: Scholarship.
No. of awards offered: 12.
Frequency: Annual.
Value: US$16,000 to cover support costs, special equipment and some travel in the USA, plus tuition fees and travelling expenses to and from the USA.
Length of Study: 1 year. In certain circumstances, students who are applying for PhD or 2-year Master's programmes may be considered for extra funding to help support a second year of study.
Study Establishment: Harvard University and the Massachusetts Institute of Technology, Cambridge.
Country of Study: USA.
Application Procedure: Please submit a form, statement of purpose, references, and letter of endorsement from applicant's British university. Applications should come via the applicant's UK university.
Closing Date: November 7th.
Additional Information: No application will be considered from persons already in the USA. Scholarships for the study of business administration and management will only be granted in exceptional circumstances, and candidates must have completed two years' employment in business or public service since graduation. An independent application to Harvard or MIT is necessary. Scholars are not required to study for a degree in the USA but are encouraged to do so if they are eligible and able to complete the requirements for it.

THE KIDNEY FOUNDATION OF CANADA

300-5165 Sherbrooke Street West
Suite 300, Montreal, PQ, H4A 1T6, Canada
Tel: (1) 514 369 4806
Fax: (1) 514 369 2472
Email: research@kidney.ca
www: http://www.kidney.ca
Contact: Ms Jennifer Gee

Kidney Foundation of Canada Allied Health Doctoral Fellowship

Subjects: Nephrology/urology nursing, social work, dietetics.
Eligibility: Open to Canadian citizens who are nephrology/urology nurses and technicians, social workers, dieticians, transplant co-ordinators and other allied health professionals.
Level of Study: Doctorate.
Purpose: To provide for full-time academic and research preparation at the doctoral level; to promote and enhance the development of nephrology/urology allied health investigators.
Type: Fellowship.
Frequency: Annual.
Value: Up to C$31,000.
Length of Study: Up to 4 years.
Country of Study: Any country.
Application Procedure: Application forms and guidelines are available.
Closing Date: October 15th.

The Kidney Foundation of Canada Allied Health Research Grant

Subjects: Social/preventive medicine; dietetics; nephrology; urology; nursing, organ donation.
Eligibility: Open to Canadian citizens.
Level of Study: Professional development, Research.
Purpose: To encourage research relevant to clinical practice in the area of nephrology and urology by allied health professionals.
Type: Grant.
Frequency: Annual.
Value: Up to C$40,000 per year.
Length of Study: Up To 2 years.
Country of Study: Canada.
Application Procedure: Application forms and guidelines are available.
Closing Date: October 15th.

The Kidney Foundation of Canada Allied Health Scholarship

Subjects: Social/preventive medicine; dietetics; nephrology; urology; nursing.

Eligibility: Open to Canadian citizens who are nurses and technicians, social workers, dieticians, transplant co-ordinators, or other allied professionals who demonstrate commitment to the area of nephrology/urology, or organ donation.
Level of Study: Graduate, Postgraduate, Professional development.
Purpose: To assist the student in pursuing education at the Master's, doctoral, or nurse practitioner levels.
Type: Scholarship.
Frequency: Annual.
Value: C$5,000.
Length of Study: 1 year (renewable).
Country of Study: Any country.
Application Procedure: Application forms and guidelines are available.
Closing Date: October 15th.

The Kidney Foundation of Canada Biomedical Fellowship

Subjects: Nephrology; urology.
Eligibility: Open to Canadian citizens and landed immigrant status.
Level of Study: Postdoctorate, Research.
Purpose: To provide for full-time postdoctoral research training in the renal and urinary tract field.
Type: Fellowship.
Frequency: Annual.
Value: Up to C$46,844.
Length of Study: Up to 4 years.
Country of Study: Any country.
Application Procedure: Application forms and guidelines are available.
Closing Date: October 15th.

The Kidney Foundation of Canada Biomedical Research (Operating) Grant

Subjects: Nephrology; urology.
Eligibility: Open to Canadian citizens.
Level of Study: Postdoctorate, Research.
Purpose: To assist in defraying the cost of research. Includes the purchase and maintenance of experimental animals, purchase of materials, supplies and equipment and the payment of laboratory assistants.
Type: Grant.
Frequency: Annual.
Value: Up to C$40,000 per year.
Length of Study: 1 or 2 years.
Country of Study: Canada.
Application Procedure: Application form and guidelines are available.
Closing Date: October 15th.

The Kidney Foundation of Canada Biomedical Scholarship

Subjects: Nephrology; urology.
Eligibility: Open to Canadian citizens.
Level of Study: Postdoctorate.
Purpose: To provide salary support for two years of an initial faculty appointment at the rank of assistant professor or its assistant at an approved medical school.
Type: Scholarship.
Frequency: Annual.
Value: C$45,000 per year.
Length of Study: 2 years.
Study Establishment: An approved medical school.
Country of Study: Canada.
Application Procedure: Application forms and guidelines are available.
Closing Date: October 15th.

THE KIDSACTION RESEARCH

1185 Eglinton Avenue East
Suite 706, North York, ON, M3C 3C6, Canada
Tel: (1) 416 429 1529
Fax: (1) 416 969 9351
Email: amichie@kidsaction.comg
www: http://www.kidsaction.com
Contact: The Administrator

KidsAction Research Fellowships and Grants

Subjects: Treatment techniques.
Eligibility: Funding is limited to Canadian citizens or landed immigrants in the province of Ontario only. If an applicant is temporarily working outside of the country and planning to return to Ontario, funding will be considered.
Level of Study: Doctorate, Postdoctorate, Professional development.
Purpose: To support research, development and professional training concerned with the prevention, treatment and management of physical disabilities in children and young adults in the province of Ontario.
Type: Fellowships; Scholarships; Grants.
No. of awards offered: Varies.
Frequency: Annual.
Value: C$3,000-C$30,000.
Length of Study: 1-2 years.
Country of Study: Canada (if the applicant plans to practise in Canada then there is proviso for them to study in any country).
Application Procedure: Application form must be completed.
Closing Date: March 1st (studentships) and April 15th.
Additional Information: Grants are not made for special projects, operating funds, building funds, emergency funds, conferences and seminars, deficit financing, endowment funds, equipment funds, matching funds, and seed money.

KING EDWARD VII BRITISH-GERMAN FOUNDATION

10 Langton Street, London, SW10 0JH, England
Contact: Secretary

The Foundation provides scholarships to postgraduate students of British nationality under the age of 30 to study in Germany and promote Anglo-German relations and understanding.

King Edward VII Scholarships

Subjects: All subjects.
Eligibility: Open to British nationals who are graduates of British universities, are under 30 years of age, and who wish to study further in Germany.
Level of Study: Postgraduate.
Purpose: To promote Anglo-German relations.
Type: Scholarship.
No. of awards offered: Up to 3.
Frequency: Annual.
Value: DM1200 per month, a book grant of DM150, exemption from tuition fees, plus travelling expenses between a Scholar's home in the UK and his/her place of study in Germany.
Length of Study: 10 months.
Study Establishment: A university or other institution of higher education.
Country of Study: Germany.
Application Procedure: Write for application form, enclosing A5 SAE.
Closing Date: December 31st.

KING FAISAL FOUNDATION

PO Box 22476, Riyadh, 11495, Saudi Arabia
Tel: (966) 1 465 2255
Fax: (966) 1 465 8685
Email: info@kff.com
www: http://www.kff.org
Telex: 401180 FAISAL SJ
Contact: Dr Abd Allah S Al-Uthaimin, Secretary General

King Faisal International Award for Medicine

Subjects: Medicine.
Eligibility: There are no restrictions on eligibility except that applications from political parties will not be accepted.
Level of Study: Unrestricted.
Purpose: To show appreciation to scholars who have made significant breakthrough and advance in medicine.
Type: Prize.
No. of awards offered: 1.
Frequency: Annual.
Value: US$200,000.
Country of Study: Any country.

Application Procedure: Universities, international institutes and scientific organisations are invited to nominate candidates each year.
Closing Date: May 31st for the following year.
Additional Information: In the year 2000 the award will be given in the field of research into ageing.

KOSCIUSZKO FOUNDATION

15 East 65th Street, New York, NY, 10021-6595, United States of America
Tel: (1) 212 734 2130
Fax: (1) 212 628 4552
Email: thekf@pegasusnet.com
www: http://www.kosciuszkofoundation.org/
Contact: Mr Thomas J Pniewski, Director Cultural Affairs

The Kosciuszko Foundation founded in 1925, is dedicated to promoting educational and cultural relations between the United States and Poland, and to increasing American awareness of Polish culture and history. In addition to its grants and scholarships, which total more than $1 million annually, the Foundation presents cultural programmes including lectures, concerts and exhibitions, promoting Polish culture in the United States, and nurturing the spirit of multicultural co-operation.

Kosciuszko Foundation Graduate and Postgraduate Studies and Research in Poland Program

Subjects: All subjects.
Eligibility: Open to US graduate and postgraduate students who wish to pursue a course of graduate or postgraduate study and/or research at institutions of higher learning in Poland. Also eligible are university faculty who wish to spend a sabbatical pursuing research in Poland.
Level of Study: Graduate, Postgraduate.
Purpose: To enable Americans to continue their graduate and postgraduate studies in Poland.
Type: Grant.
No. of awards offered: Varies.
Frequency: Annual.
Value: Tuition and housing, plus a monthly stipend in Polish currency for living expenses.
Country of Study: Poland.
Application Procedure: Please write for details.
Closing Date: January 16th.
Additional Information: Applicants must have a working knowledge of the Polish language and are reviewed based on academic background, motivation for pursuing graduate studies and/or research in Poland, and a proposal of studies and research in Poland.

LA TROBE UNIVERSITY

Bundoora Campus, Melbourne, VIC, 3083, Australia
Tel: (61) 3 9479 2971
Fax: (61) 3 9479 1464
Email: c.cocks@latrobe.edu.au
www: http://www.latrobe.edu.au/www/rgso
Contact: Scholarships and Candidature Co-ordinator

La Trobe University is one of the leading research universities in Australia. The University has internationally regarded strengths across a diverse range of disciplines. It offers a detailed and broad research training programme and provides unique access to technology transfer and collaboration with end users of its research and training via its Research and Development Park.

Australian Postgraduate Awards

Subjects: Health sciences, humanities and social sciences, science technology and engineering, law and management.
Eligibility: Applicants must have completed at least 4 years of tertiary education studies at a high level of achievement (for example, first class honours degree or equivalent) at an Australian university. Applicants must be Australian citizens or have permanent resident status and have lived in Australia continuously for the twelve months prior to the closing date for application. Applicants who have previously held an Australian Government Award (APA, APRA or CPRA) for more than 3 months are not eligible for an APA. Applicants who have previously held an Australian Postgraduate Course Award (APCA) may apply only for an APA to support PhD research.
Level of Study: Doctorate, Postgraduate.
Purpose: To support research leading to Masters or Doctoral degrees.
Type: Award.
No. of awards offered: Varies.
Value: $16,135 per annum full-time (tax exempt plus allowances; $8,734 per annum part-time (taxable) plus allowances.
Length of Study: Master's candidates 2 years, PhD candidates 3 years. Periods of study already undertaken towards the degree will be deducted from the tenure of the award.
Study Establishment: Bundoora Campus, La Trobe University.
Country of Study: Australia.
Application Procedure: Application kits are available from the school in which the candidate wishes to study. Applications must be submitted in duplicate, to the Research and Graduate Studies Office, La Trobe University, Bundoora Campus, Bundoora, Victoria, Australia 3083.
Closing Date: October 31st.
Additional Information: APA holders are required to pay the annual General Service Fee- $320 (Bundoora Campus), $276 (Bendigo Campus). The awards may be held concurrently with other nonAustralian government awards. Paid work may be permitted to a maximum of 8 hours per week (full time award) or 4 hours per week (part time award).

International Postgraduate Research Scholarships (IPRS)

Subjects: Health sciences, humanities and social sciences, science, technology and engineering, law and management.
Eligibility: IPRS are awarded on the basis of academic merit and research capacity to suitably qualified overseas graduates eligible to commence a higher degree (doctoral or Masters) by research. The IPRS may be held concurrently with a university research scholarship and applicants for an IPRS are advised to apply for La Trobe University Postgraduate Research Scholarship (LTUPRS). The scheme is open to citizens of all overseas countries (excluding New Zealand). Successful applicants will research specialisation and, in most instances, will become members of a research team working under the direction of senior researchers. Applicants who have already commenced a Masters or PhD candidature are not eligible to apply for and IPRS to support the degree course for which they have already enrolled. Applicants for Masters Candidature by coursework and minor thesis are not eligible to apply for the IPRS.
Level of Study: Doctorate, Postgraduate.
Purpose: To attract top quqality overseas postgraduate students to areas of research strength in higher education institutions and to support Austrlia's research effort.
Type: Scholarship.
No. of awards offered: Varies.
Value: Tuition fess, basic health care cover.
Length of Study: Masters 2 years, PhD 3 years.
Study Establishment: Bundoora Campus, La Trobe University.
Country of Study: Australia.
Application Procedure: Application forms should be submitted on the application form for international candidates available from the International Programmes Office email: international@latrobe.edu.au.
Additional Information: APA holders are required to pay the annual General Service Fee- $320 (Bundoora Campus), $276 (Bendigo Campus).

La Trobe University Postdoctoral Research Fellowship

Subjects: All subjects.
Eligibility: Open to students who have been awarded their doctorates within the last five years. Applicants must hold a doctoral degree or equivalent at the date of appointment. The university may also take into account the proposed area of research having regard to the university's research promotion and management strategy policies.
Level of Study: Postdoctorate.
Purpose: To advance research activities on the various campuses of the university by bringing to or retaining in Australia promising scholars.
Type: Fellowship.
No. of awards offered: 1.
Frequency: Annual.
Value: A$33,200-A$45,055 per year, plus air fares and a resettlement allowance.
Length of Study: 2 years.
Country of Study: Australia.

Application Procedure: An application form and guidelines will be available either upon request in writing or via email, or they can be downloaded from the University's website. Administrative contact: Ms Jennie Somerville, Grants Administrator, Research & Graduate Studies Office, tel: (61) 3 9479 2049, fax: (61) 3 9479 1464; email: j.somerville@latrobe.edu.au.

Closing Date: September.

Additional Information: A project must be proposed by the applicant in collaboration with a La Trobe University research worker or team. The approved project will be designated in the letter of offer and the major objectives of a Fellow's project shall not be altered without the written approval of the university.

La Trobe University Postgraduate Research Scholarships (LTUPRS)

Subjects: Health sciences, humanities and social sciences, science, technology and engineering, law and management.

Eligibility: Open to citizens of all countries including Australia and New Zealand. Applicants must have completed four years of tertiary education studies at a very high level of achievement (first class honours degree or equivalent at an Australian university or recognised overseas university. Applicants who have previously held an LTUPRS for more than 3 months are not eligible to apply.

Level of Study: Postgraduate.

Purpose: To support research leading to Masters of Doctoral degrees.

Type: Scholarship.

No. of awards offered: Vaies.

Value: A$15,800 per annum full-time (tax exempt plus allowances; A$8,500 per annum part-time (taxable) plus allowances.

Length of Study: Masters 2 years, PhD 3 years. Periods of study already undertaken towards the degree will be deducted from the tenure of the award.

Study Establishment: Bundoora Campus, La Trobe University.

Country of Study: Australia.

Application Procedure: Application kits are available from the school in which the candidate wishes to study. Applications must be submitted in duplicate, to the Research and Graduate Studies Office, La Trobe University, Bundoora Campus, Bundoora, Victoria, Australia 3083.

Additional Information: Paid work may be permitted to a maximum of 8 hours per week.

LADY TATA MEMORIAL TRUST

Academic Dept of Haemotology and Cytogenetics
The Royal Marsden Hospital
Fulham Road, London, SW3 6JJ, England
Tel: (44) 171 352 8171
Fax: (44) 171 351 6420
Contact: Professor D Catovsky, Secretary

Lady Tata Memorial Trust Scholarships

Subjects: Leukaemia.

Eligibility: Open to qualified applicants of any nationality.

Level of Study: Postdoctorate.

Purpose: To encourage study and research in diseases of the blood, with special reference to leukaemias and furthering knowledge in connection with such diseases.

Type: Scholarship.

No. of awards offered: Normally 10.

Frequency: Annual.

Value: Ranging between £10,000-£20,000 per year.

Length of Study: 1-2 years.

Country of Study: Any country.

Application Procedure: Eight copies of the application, including form, summary of proposed research, and two letters of reference, must be submitted.

Closing Date: March 1st.

LANCASTER UNIVERSITY

Student Support Office
University House
Bailrigg, Lancaster, LA1 4YW, England
Tel: (44) 1524 65201
Fax: (44) 1524 594294
www: http://www.lancs.ac.uk
Contact: Ms Lorna M Mullett

Cartmel College Scholarship Fund

Subjects: Any subject offered by the University.

Eligibility: Open to candidates of any nationality, who must have a place at Lancaster University. Priority is given to members of Cartmel College and to new students.

Level of Study: Postgraduate.

Purpose: To assist students unable to obtain adequate grants from other bodies.

Type: Scholarship.

No. of awards offered: Varies.

Frequency: Annual.

Value: £300-£500 not including fees.
Study Establishment: Lancaster University.
Country of Study: United Kingdom.
Application Procedure: Please write to Lorna M Mullet at the Student Support Office for details.
Closing Date: June 1st.

Lancaster University County College Awards

Subjects: Any subject offered by the University.
Eligibility: Open to candidates of any nationality, who must have place at Lancaster University. Candidates must be former members of the County College and must be prepared to reside in the College.
Level of Study: Postgraduate.
Purpose: To assist students whose course of study will lead to financial hardship.
No. of awards offered: Varies.
Frequency: Annual.
Value: Free residence.
Study Establishment: Lancaster University; recipients must reside in County College, and be former members of the College.
Country of Study: United Kingdom.
Application Procedure: Please write to Lorna M Mullett at the Student Support Office.
Closing Date: June 1st.

Lancaster University International Bursaries

Subjects: All subjects.
Eligibility: Open to nationals of India and the People's Republic of China, who have not previously studied at Lancaster University.
Level of Study: Postgraduate.
Purpose: To offer financial support.
Type: Bursary.
No. of awards offered: 6.
Frequency: Annual.
Value: £2,000.
Length of Study: 1 year minimum.
Study Establishment: Lancaster University.
Country of Study: United Kingdom.
Application Procedure: Applications are available on request; please contact the International Office.
Closing Date: June 30th.

Peel Awards

Subjects: Any subject offered by the University.
Eligibility: Open to candidates of any nationality, who must have a place at Lancaster University and must be over 21 years of age.
Level of Study: Postgraduate, Undergraduate.
Purpose: To enable students who are unable to secure finance from other sources to study at Lancaster University.
No. of awards offered: Varies.
Frequency: Annual.
Value: Varies. Awards do not cover fees.
Study Establishment: Lancaster University.
Country of Study: United Kingdom.

Application Procedure: Application form available on request from Lorna M Mullett in the Student Support Office.
Closing Date: June 1st.

LEAGUE FOR THE EXCHANGE OF COMMONWEALTH TEACHERS

Commonwealth House
7 Lion Yard
Tremadoc Road
Clapham, London, SW4 7NF, England
Tel: (44) 171 498 1101
Fax: (44) 171 720 5403
Contact: S Browning, Publicity

LECT's aim is to develop and support a wide range of exchanges for teachers and others in all sectors of the educational profession in the United Kingdom with similarly qualified colleagues in other parts of the Commonwealth for a fixed period, so that shared experiences may be of benefit to students, teachers and their employing institutions.

UK Government Grants

Subjects: All subjects.
Eligibility: Open to teachers (in all types of schools - primary, secondary, special, technical colleges, colleges of education) from the UK who are accepted for exchange with teachers in selected Commonwealth countries. Teachers should be between 25 and 45 years of age and have not less than five years' teaching experience in the UK, with at least two years' under the current employing authority.
Level of Study: Professional development.
Purpose: To facilitate the exchange of British teachers to other Commonwealth countries.
Type: Grant.
No. of awards offered: Approx. 300.
Frequency: Annual.
Value: Return air fare.
Length of Study: 1 academic year.
Study Establishment: Schools or colleges in selected Commonwealth countries.
Country of Study: Australia, Bahamas, Bermuda, Canada, India, Jamaica, Kenya (Nairobi), New Zealand, Sierra Leone or Trinidad.
Application Procedure: Application form must be completed.
Additional Information: There is also a separate programme to support teacher exchanges between different parts of the UK.

LEPRA (THE BRITISH LEPROSY RELIEF ASSOCIATION)

Fairfax House
Causton Road, Colchester, Essex, CO1 1PU, England
Tel: (44) 1206 562286
Fax: (44) 1206 762151
Email: lepra@lepra.org
www: http://www.lepra.org.uk
Contact: Information Officer

LPRA is a secular organisation whose aim is the eradication of leprosy. To that end it undertakes leprosy surveys to find and treat as many cases of leprosy as it can, and also trains staff to ensure the widest possible coverage of leprosy control.

LEPRA Grants

Subjects: Any relevant medical subject.
Level of Study: Postgraduate.
Purpose: To encourage an interest in leprosy among doctors and research workers.
Type: Grant.
No. of awards offered: Varies.
Frequency: Dependent on funds available.
Value: Dependent on funds available and the nature of the research or training.
Study Establishment: As appropriate to the nature of the research or training. Arrangements are made to enable interested medical students to spend their elective period anywhere in the world where a suitable project can be arranged, working on a specific leprosy research project.
Country of Study: Any country.
Application Procedure: For research, the applicant must submit a programme considered useful by the Medical Board; for training, the applicant must submit a course deemed useful by the Board and will be expected to undertake work in leprosy after completion of training.
Closing Date: End of March, August or November.
Additional Information: Annual awards are also given to registered medical students in the UK for the best essay or essays on a specific subject in the field.

LEUKAEMIA RESEARCH FUND

43 Great Ormond Street, London, WC1N 3JJ, England
Tel: (44) 171 405 0101
Fax: (44) 171 242 1488
Email: lrf@leukres.demon.co.uk
www: http://www.phoenix.jrz.ox.ac.uk/lrf/lrfhome.htm
Contact: Dr David Grant

To discover the causes of leukaemia and related diseases, to ensure accurate and early diagnosis, to understand the malignant process and to exploit this knowledge in the development of new therapeutic strategies. The goal is the selective and routine cure of leukaemia and other blood cancers.

Gordon Piller Studentships

Subjects: All life science disciplines. The research topic must be applicable to leukaemia.
Eligibility: Open to graduates of any nationality who work and reside in the UK.
Level of Study: Postgraduate.
Purpose: To train graduates in life sciences in research and allow them to submit for a PhD degree.
Type: Studentship.
No. of awards offered: 4.
Frequency: Annual.
Value: Varies.
Length of Study: 3 years.
Study Establishment: Universities, medical schools and research institutes.
Country of Study: United Kingdom.
Application Procedure: Application form to be completed.
Closing Date: August.

Leukaemia Research Fund Clinical Research Fellowship

Subjects: All life science disciplines. The research topic must be applicable to leukaemia.
Eligibility: Open to researchers of any nationality who work and reside in the UK.
Level of Study: Clinical.
Purpose: To train registrar-grade clinicians in research and allow them to submit for a higher degree (MD or PhD).
Type: Fellowship.
No. of awards offered: 4.
Frequency: Annual.
Value: Varies.
Length of Study: 2 or 3 years.
Study Establishment: Universities, medical schools, research institutes and teaching hospitals.
Country of Study: United Kingdom.
Application Procedure: Application form must be completed.
Closing Date: March.

Leukaemia Research Fund Clinical Training Fellowship

Subjects: Haematology, oncology.
Eligibility: Open to researchers of any nationality who work and reside in the UK.
Level of Study: Clinical.
Purpose: To train registrar-grade clinicians in the care and treatment of patients with a haematological malignancy.
Type: Fellowship.
No. of awards offered: 11.
Frequency: Three times each year.
Value: Varies.
Length of Study: 2 years.
Study Establishment: Any UK centre of excellence for leukaemia medicine.
Country of Study: United Kingdom.

Application Procedure: Application form must be completed.
Closing Date: Available on request.

Leukaemia Research Fund Grant Programme

Subjects: All life science disciplines.
Eligibility: Open to researchers who work and reside in the UK.
Level of Study: Unrestricted.
Purpose: To give long-term support to research groups studying the causes and treatment of haematological malignancies.
Type: Research Grant.
No. of awards offered: Varies.
Frequency: Three times each year.
Value: Varies.
Length of Study: Varies.
Study Establishment: Universities, medical schools, research institutes and teaching hospitals.
Country of Study: United Kingdom.
Application Procedure: Application form to be completed only after discussion with Scientific Director.
Closing Date: Available on request.

Leukaemia Research Fund Grant Project

Subjects: All life science disciplines.
Eligibility: Open to researchers of any nationality who work and reside in the UK.
Level of Study: Postdoctorate, Postgraduate.
Purpose: To support laboratory and clinical based research into the causes and treatment of the haematological malignancies.
Type: Grant.
No. of awards offered: Varies.
Frequency: Three times each year.
Value: Varies.
Length of Study: Varies.
Study Establishment: Universities, medical schools, research institutes and teaching hospitals.
Country of Study: United Kingdom.
Application Procedure: Application form must be completed.
Closing Date: Available on request.

LEUKEMIA RESEARCH FUND OF CANADA

1110 Finch Avenue West
Suite 220, Toronto, ON, M3J 2T2, Canada
Tel: (1) 416 661 9541
Fax: (1) 416 661 7799
Email: leukemia@istar.ca
www: http://www.leukemia.ca
Contact: National Executive Director

LRFC is a volunteer driven organisation with branches across Canada whose goal is to raise money to support Canadian research for the cure of leukemia and related blood diseases.

Leukemia Research Fund Awards

Subjects: Research on leukemia and related blood diseases.
Eligibility: Open to researchers and postdoctoral students engaged in work in Canada in the field of leukaemia and related blood diseases.
Level of Study: Postdoctorate, Research.
Purpose: To provide funds for researchers in the field of leukemia and blood diseases, and to provide a limited number of postdoctoral fellowships in the same field.
Type: Fellowships and studentships.
No. of awards offered: Varies.
Frequency: Annual.
Value: Varies.
Length of Study: 1 year.
Country of Study: Canada.
Application Procedure: All applications must be prepared on the Fund's forms and submitted by the deadline for evaluation, on a merit basis, by the Scientific Review Panel. Applications are available through Deans of Medicine or the LRFC Office.
Closing Date: February 1st.
Additional Information: Special grant available for study of CLL, gene therapy at a maximum of C$50,000 for up to two years. Deadline is March 1st.

LEUKEMIA SOCIETY OF AMERICA

600 Third Avenue
4th Floor, New York, NY, 10016, United States of America
Tel: (1) 212 450 8843
Fax: (1) 212 856 9686
Email: lermandb@leukemia.org
www: http://www.leukemia.org
Contact: Ms Barbara P Lermand, Director of Research Administration

The Leukemia Society of America, Inc is a national voluntary health agency dedicated to the conquest of leukemia, lymphoma and myleloma through research. Through its research programme, the society hopes to encourage an promote research activity of the highest quality. In addition the Society also supports patient aid, public and professional education and community service programmes.

Leukemia Society of America Scholarships, Special Fellowships and Fellowships

Subjects: Leukemia, lymphona, Hodgkins disease and myeloma research.
Eligibility: Applications may be submitted by individuals working in domestic or non-profit organisations, such as universities, hospitals, or unites or state and local governments.
Level of Study: Postdoctorate.
Purpose: To provide support for individuals pursuing careers in basic, clinical or translational research in leukemia, lymphona, Hodgkins disease and myeloma.

Type: Career Development.
No. of awards offered: Varies.
Frequency: Annual.
Value: US$33,250-US$70,000 per year for up to five years, plus 8% institutional overhead.
Length of Study: 3-5 years, based on experience and training.
Study Establishment: Domestic or foreign non-profit organisations.
Country of Study: USA.
Application Procedure: Please contact the Director of Research Administration at the LSA or visit our website for details of the Career Development Award Application Packet.
Closing Date: September 15th for the preliminary (two page) application. October 1st for the complete application.
Additional Information: Plese write for further details.

Leukemia Society of America Translational Research Award

Subjects: Leukemia, lymphona, Hodgkins disease and myeloma research.
Eligibility: Applications may be submitted by individuals working in domestic or foreign non-profit organisations, such as universities, hospitals or units of State and Local Governments.
Level of Study: Postdoctorate.
Purpose: To encourage and provide early stage support for clinical research on leukemia, lymphona, Hodgkins disease and myeloma; emphasising novel approaches and strategies.
Type: Research Grant.
No. of awards offered: Varies.
Frequency: Annual.
Value: Annual maximum of US$100,000 in direct costs plus 8% overhead.
Length of Study: 3 years (with possibly 2 additional years).
Study Establishment: Domestic or foreign non-profit organisations.
Country of Study: USA.
Application Procedure: Please contact the Director of Research Administration at the LSA or visit our website for details of the Translational Research Grant Application Packet.
Closing Date: February 15th for the preliminary (two page) application, and March 15th for the complete application.
Additional Information: Please write to LSA for further details.

THE LINNEAN SOCIETY OF NEW SOUTH WALES

PO Box 457, Milsons Point, NSW, 1565, Australia
Tel: (61) 9 929 0253
Fax: (61) 9 929 0253
www:
http://bioscience.babs.unsw.edu.au/linnsoc/welcome.htm
Contact: Ms Claudia G Ford

The Society is concerned with the publication of original scientific research papers and the encouragement of scientific research through grants and public lectures.

Linnean Macleay Fellowship

Subjects: Animal and plant physiology and pathology, anthropology, biochemistry, botany, comparative anatomy and embryology, general biology, geography, geology, palaeontology and zoology, research.
Eligibility: Candidates must be residents of New South Wales, Australia, and must have taken a degree in science or agricultural science in the University of Sydney, and must be a member of the Linnean Society of New South Wales.
Level of Study: Postgraduate.
Purpose: To encourage the study of natural history in New South Wales.
Type: Fellowship.
No. of awards offered: 1.
Frequency: Annual.
Value: A$3,200.
Length of Study: 1 year.
Study Establishment: University of Sydney or elsewhere, subject to the approval of the Council of the Linnean Society.
Country of Study: Australia.
Closing Date: November 15th.

THE LISTER INSTITUTE OF PREVENTIVE MEDICINE

The White House
70 High Road, Bushey Heath, Hertfordshire, WD2 3JG, England
Tel: (44) 181 421 8808
Fax: (44) 181 421 8818
Email: secretary@lister-institute.org.uk
www: http://www.lister-institute.org.uk
Contact: Mr Keith Cowey, Secretary

Originally founded in 1891, the Lister Institute now operates as a medical research charity whose sole function is to sponsor research fellowships in the area of biomedicine. A rolling portfolio of 25-30 research fellowships, supported by investment income, is maintained within UK universities and research institutions.

Lister Institute Senior Research Fellowships

Subjects: Biomedicine. There are no priority diseases or scientific disciplines, provided that the proposed research has implications for preventive medicine. The research is primarily laboratory based and is targeted at generating understanding and underpinning knowledge through fundamental research.
Eligibility: Open to UK residents with a PhD, DPhil, MD, or MB BCh with membership of the Royal College of Physicians, who must be aged 35 or under for non-clinicians, and 37 or under for clinicians. Applicants must have at least two years' postdoctoral experience. Research must be performed in the UK.
Level of Study: Postdoctorate.
Purpose: To support postdoctoral scientific research into the causes and prevention of disease in man.
Type: Senior Postdoctoral Fellowship.

No. of awards offered: 5.
Frequency: Annual.
Value: Full salary plus employer's superannuation and national insurance costs reimbursed, together with up to £8,500 per year consumables allowance.
Length of Study: 5 years.
Study Establishment: Employing university, research institute or unit, or hospital.
Country of Study: United Kingdom.
Application Procedure: Application form should be submitted along with CV and two letters of reference on approved form.
Closing Date: End of third week in January.
Additional Information: Potential applicants between 35 and 40 years of age for non-clinicians, and between 37 and 40 years of age for clinicians, must request permission to make a full application. In exceptional circumstances fellowships may be extended by 1-3 years. Research topics are of the applicant's own choosing. Projects are assessed on scientific merit and potential. Applicants cannot be permanent employees of research councils or charities.

MARCH OF DIMES BIRTH DEFECTS FOUNDATION

1275 Mamaroneck Avenue, White Plains, NY, 10605, United States of America
Tel: (1) 914 997 4555
Fax: (1) 914 997 4560
Email: research-grants@modimes.org
www: http://www.modimes.org
Contact: Grants Administration

Basil O'Connor Starter Scholar Research Award Program

Subjects: The research interests of the Foundation include the broader aspects of pregnancy outcome, for example factors underlying the birth and survival of a healthy infant, the cognitive development of low birthweight infants, as well as the function of chromosomes, their subunits, genes, supporting structures and the like.
Eligibility: Open to young investigators (MDs or PhDs) who are interested in undertaking independent research after completion of their doctoral and postdoctoral training.
Level of Study: Faculty.
Purpose: To support young scientists at the level of instructor or assistant professor who are just embarking on their independent research careers.
Type: Research Grant.
No. of awards offered: Varies.
Frequency: Annual.
Value: US$50,000.
Study Establishment: An appropriate institution.
Country of Study: Any country.

Application Procedure: Candidates interested in this programme should submit a brief abstract, a copy of their curriculum vitae with a covering letter mentioning the BOC programme and a letter of nomination, written by the Chairman of the Department, Director of the Institute, the Dean, or an equivalent person. The Foundation will respond indicating whether he/she qualifies administratively for this programme, or, if not, whether he/she should apply to one of the Foundation's other research programmes. Please note that BOC applicants may not submit an application simultaneously for another MOD research grant programme. They must also not be the recipient of any other major grants.
Closing Date: Abstract due by January 31st, with application due by May 31st.

MASSEY UNIVERSITY

Academic Section
Private Bag 11-222, Palmerston North, New Zealand
Tel: (64) 6 350 5549
Fax: (64) 6 350 5603
Email: m.e.gilbert@massey.ac.nz
www: http://www.massey.ac.nz
Contact: Ms Margeret E Gilbert, Scholarships Adminstrative Assistant

Massey University has over 30,000 students, 12,000 studying on campus with the remaining 18,000 studying by correspondence. The four colleges - Business, Education, Humanities and Social Sciences, and Sciences - provide a comprehensive range of undergraduate and graduate degrees and diplomas all geared to meeting national and international needs.

Massey Doctoral Scholarship

Subjects: Agriculture, forestry, town planning, arts and humanities, business administration and management, education and teacher training, engineering, commercial law, media studies, mathematics and computer science, nursing, midwifery, natural sciences, social welfare and social work, environmental studies, religious studies, tourism, social and behavioural studies, air transport.
Eligibility: Minimum qualification of a first class honours degree.
Level of Study: Doctorate.
Purpose: For research towards a PhD degree.
Type: Scholarship.
No. of awards offered: 20-30.
Frequency: Annual.
Value: NZ$12,000 per year.
Length of Study: 3 years.
Study Establishment: University.
Country of Study: New Zealand.
Application Procedure: Application form must be completed.
Closing Date: October 1st, July 1st.

THE MATSUMAE INTERNATIONAL FOUNDATION

Room 6-002
New Marunouchi Bldg
1-5-1 Marunouchi
Chiyoda-ku, Tokyo, 100-0005, Japan
Tel: (81) 3 3214 7611
Fax: (81) 3 3214 7613
Contact: Mr S Nakajima

Matsumae International Foundation Research Fellowship

Subjects: Engineering, mathematics, medicine, natural sciences and agriculture.
Eligibility: Open to applicants under 40 years of age, of non-Japanese nationality, who hold a doctorate or have two years' research experience after receipt of a Master's degree, and who have not been in Japan previously.
Level of Study: Postdoctorate, Professional development.
Purpose: To provide the opportunity for foreign scientists to conduct research at Japanese institutions.
Type: Fellowship.
No. of awards offered: 20.
Frequency: Annual.
Value: Covers the cost of an air ticket, personal accident/sickness insurance and research stipend plus 300,00 yen on arrival in addition to 150,000 yen monthly.
Length of Study: 3-6 months.
Study Establishment: Unrestricted.
Country of Study: Japan.
Application Procedure: Applicants should obtain the current issue of the Fellowship announcement from the Foundation.
Closing Date: July 31st.
Additional Information: Priority will be given to fields of science, engineering and medicine.

THE MEDICAL MISSIONARY ASSOCIATION

157 Waterloo Road, London, SE1 8XN, England
Tel: (44) 171 928 4694
Fax: (44) 171 620 2453
Email: 106173.333@compuserve.com
Contact: Dr David Clegg, General Secretary

The Medical Missionary Association is developing a health resource centre to promote Christian medical mission. Other support includes elective days, a refresher course, overseas update publications, and grants.

Medical Missionary Association Grants

Subjects: Medical mission (Church related or Christian Healthcare).

Eligibility: Open to committed Christians (UK based) who have spent at least one tour working in a mission/church-related medical post and who will be going back to continue this work for at least one further tour of three years, and to committed Christian medical students who are going to the Developing World for their elective period in mission or church related medical work.
Level of Study: Postgraduate.
Purpose: To assist doctors and nurses and other paramedicals who have served at least one tour in a mission/church-related medical post in the developing world to gain a postgraduate qualification, or to assist Christian medical students to spend their elective in a mission/church-related hospital in the developing world.
Type: Grant.
Frequency: Varies.
Value: Postgraduate up to £750. Undergraduate up to £250.
Country of Study: United Kingdom or developing world countries.
Application Procedure: Write for application form.
Closing Date: At least six months before the course is due to start.
Additional Information: Each request is discussed on its own merit.

MEDICAL RESEARCH COUNCIL (MRC)

20 Park Crescent, London, W1N 4AL, England
Tel: (44) 171 636 5422
Fax: (44) 171 670 5002
Email: fellows@headoffice.mrc.ac.uk
www: http://www.mrc.ac.uk
Contact: Ms Rosa Parker, Research Career Awards

The Medical Research Council offers support for talented individuals who want to pursue a career in the bio-medical sciences, public health and health services research. It provides its support through a variety of personal award schemes that are aimed at each stage in a clinical or non-clinical research career.

MRC Advanced Course Studentships

Subjects: Any science relevant to medicine.
Eligibility: Candidates should have graduated with a good honours degree. A copy of the regulations governing residence eligibility may be obtained from the Council.
Level of Study: Postgraduate.
Purpose: To enable graduates to take an approved postgraduate course of instruction.
Type: Studentship.
No. of awards offered: 10.
Frequency: Annual.
Value: To include a tax-free maintenance grant depending on location and nature of living accommodation, compulsory university and college fees, certain travel expenses, additional allowances for dependents in certain circumstances. The stipends for 1998/99 are: first year postgraduate students

£7,070 per annum (London £9,400), second year postgraduate students £7,490 per annum (London £9,860) and third year postgraduate students £7,910 per annum (London £10,330) as well as a research Training and Support Grant of £1,000 per annum and a Conference Allowance of £300 per annum.
Length of Study: A period corresponding to the duration of the course.
Study Establishment: A recognised institution.
Country of Study: United Kingdom.
Application Procedure: Applications must be made by Heads of Department on behalf of candidates. Awards are made only in respect of full-time courses. Applications for a quota of awards should be submitted by departments by October 1st.
Closing Date: October 9th.

MRC Career Development Award

Subjects: Biomedical science.
Eligibility: Residence requirements apply. It is normally expected that all applicants will hold a PhD/MPhil in a basic science and will have at least three years postdoctoral research experience.
Level of Study: Postdoctorate.
Purpose: To award outstanding researchers who wish to consolidate and develop their research skills and make the transition from postdoctoral research and training to becoming independent investigators, but who do not hold established positions.
Type: Fellowship.
No. of awards offered: 10.
Frequency: Annual.
Value: Appropriate academic salary plus support for running costs, equipment and research support staff and a travel allowance of £1,000.
Length of Study: Up to 4 years.
Study Establishment: A suitable university department or similar institution.
Country of Study: United Kingdom (including one year in a recognised research establishment overseas or in UK industry).
Application Procedure: Personal application. Forms and further details are available from MRC.
Closing Date: November.

MRC Clinical Scientist Fellowship

Subjects: Biomedical science.
Eligibility: The scheme is open to hospital doctors, dentists, general practitioners, nurses, midwives and members of the Professions Allied to Medicine.
Level of Study: Postdoctorate.
Purpose: To provide an opportunity for outstanding clinical researchers who have already secured a PhD in a basic science subject who wish to consolidate their research skills and make the transition from postdoctoral research and training to becoming independent investigators.
Type: Fellowship.
No. of awards offered: Up to 10.
Frequency: Annual.

Value: Comprises salary at appropriate point on clinical academic scale plus support for technician, consumables, equipment and travel allowance of £1,000.
Length of Study: Up to 4 years.
Study Establishment: A suitable university department or similar institution.
Country of Study: United Kingdom (including one year in a recognised research establishment overseas or in UK industry).
Application Procedure: Personal application. Form and further details can be obtained from MRC.
Closing Date: August.

MRC Clinical Training Fellowships

Subjects: Biomedical sciences.
Eligibility: Residence requirements apply. The scheme is open to hospital doctors, dentists, general practitioners, nurses, midwives and members of the Professions Allied to Medicine (PAMS).
Level of Study: Postgraduate.
Purpose: To provide an opportunity for specialised or further research training in the biomedical sciences within the UK leading to the submission of a PhD/DPhil or MD.
Type: Fellowship.
No. of awards offered: Up to 58.
Frequency: Twice a year.
Value: Appropriate point on current NHS or university lecturer scale, Research Training Support Grant of £4,500 per year and travel allowance of £450.
Length of Study: Up to 3 years.
Study Establishment: A suitable university department or similar institution.
Country of Study: United Kingdom.
Application Procedure: Personal application. Forms and further details are available from MRC.
Closing Date: January, September.
Additional Information: In addition to this scheme, the MRC also offers Joint Training Fellowships with the Royal Colleges of Surgeons of England and Edinburgh, and the Royal College of Obstetricians and Gynecologists. These awards are aimed at individuals whose long-term career aspirations involve undertaking academic clinical research.

MRC NHS Special Fellowships in Health Services Research

Subjects: Health Services.
Eligibility: Hospital doctors, nurses, dentists, midwives, members of the professions allied to medicine interested in specialist training in multi-disciplinary research.
Level of Study: Doctorate, Postdoctorate.
Purpose: To provide hospital doctors, dentists, GPs, nurses, midwives, members of the professions allied to medicine and non-medical graduates an opportunity for specialist training in multi-disciplinary research, addressing problems of direct relevance to the health services within the UK.
Type: A variable number of Fellowships.
Frequency: Annual.
Value: Varies.
Length of Study: Varies.

Study Establishment: Appropriate academic or research institutions in the UK.
Country of Study: United Kingdom.
Application Procedure: For details please contact the Fellowships Section, Research Career Awards of the MRC.
Closing Date: Please write for details.

MRC Research Fellowship

Subjects: Biomedical science.
Eligibility: Residence requirements apply. Applicants would normally be expected to holds a PhD/DPhil in basic science (or expect to receive their doctorate by the time they intend to take up an award). Applicants who hold a research-oriented Master's degree and who have at least three years appropriate postgraduate research experience may, exceptionally be considered for example medical statisticians.
Level of Study: Postdoctorate.
Purpose: To provide an opportunity for high calibre non-clinical postdoctoral scientists, who wish to develop their careers in biomedical and public health research (including related biological sciences and health services research), to gain specialised of further research training.
Type: Fellowship.
No. of awards offered: Up to 20.
Frequency: Annual.
Value: Appropriate academic salary, a Research Training Support Grant of £6,500 and travel allowance of £500.
Length of Study: Up to 3 years.
Study Establishment: A suitable university department or institution.
Country of Study: United Kingdom; but one year may be spent in a recognised research establishment overseas.
Application Procedure: Personal application. Form and further details are available from the MRC.
Closing Date: January.

MRC Research Studentships

Subjects: Any biomedical science.
Eligibility: Candidates should have graduated with a good honours degree. A copy of the regulations governing residence eligibility may be obtained from the Council.
Level of Study: Postgraduate.
Purpose: To enable individuals of special promise to receive full-time training in research methods in a biomedical field under suitable direction.
Type: Research Studentship.
No. of awards offered: Approx. 220.
Frequency: Annual.
Value: To include a tax-free maintenance grant depending on location and nature of living accommodation, compulsory university and college fees, certain travel expenses, additional allowances for dependents in certain circumstances. In addition, a support grant is paid to the university as a contribution towards the incidental departmental costs incurred in the student's training.
Length of Study: Up to 3 years.
Study Establishment: A recognised institution.
Country of Study: United Kingdom.
Application Procedure: Applications must be made by heads of department on behalf of candidates. Applications for a quota of awards should be submitted by departments by the beginning of October. Application forms are available from July.
Closing Date: October 1st.

MRC Royal College of Obstetricians and Gynaecologists Training Fellowship

Subjects: Gynaecology and obstetrics.
Eligibility: Members of the Royal College of Obstetrics and Gynaecology wishing to pursue research at PhD or MD level.
Level of Study: Postdoctorate.
Purpose: To provide members of the Royal College with an opportunity for specialist or further research training in a basic science relevant to obstetrics and gynaecology leading to the submission of a PhD, a DPhil or an MD.
Type: A variable number of Fellowships.
No. of awards offered: Varies.
Frequency: Annual.
Value: Varies.
Length of Study: Varies.
Study Establishment: Royal College of Obstetrics and Gynaecology.
Country of Study: United Kingdom.
Application Procedure: For details please contact the Fellowships Section, Research Career Awards of the MRC.
Closing Date: Please write for details.

MRC Royal College of Surgeons Training Fellowships

Subjects: Medicine and surgery.
Eligibility: Members of the Royal College of Surgeons of England and members of the Royal College of Surgeons of Edinburgh, wishing to pursue research at PhD or MD level.
Level of Study: Postdoctorate.
Purpose: To encourage and promote research of direct relevance to surgery and to provide members of these Royal Colleges with an oppurtunity for specialised or further research training leading to the submission of a PhD, and MPhil or an MD.
Type: A variable number of Fellowships.
No. of awards offered: Varies.
Value: Varies.
Length of Study: Varies.
Study Establishment: Royal College of Surgeons of England and Royal College of Surgeons of Edinburgh.
Country of Study: United Kingdom.
Application Procedure: For details please contact the Fellowships Section, Research Career Awards of the MRC.
Closing Date: Please write for details.

MRC Senior Clinical Fellowship

Subjects: Biomedical science.
Eligibility: Open to nationals of any country. Applicants are expected to have proved themselves to be independent researchers, be well qualified for an academic research career and demonstrate the promise of becoming future research

leaders. The scheme is open to hospital doctors, dentists, general practitioners, nurses, midwives and members of the Professions Allied to Medicine (PAMS).

Level of Study: Postdoctorate.

Purpose: To provide an opportunity for clinical researchers of exceptional ability (who do not have tenured positions) to concentrate on a period of research.

Type: Fellowship.

No. of awards offered: Up to 4.

Frequency: Annual.

Value: Appropriate point of clinical academic scale plus support for postdoctoral/technicians, consumables and some equipment and travel allowance (£1,000).

Length of Study: Up to 5 years, renewable for a further 5 years.

Study Establishment: A suitable university department or similar institution.

Country of Study: United Kingdom.

Application Procedure: Personal application. Forms and further details are available from MRC.

Closing Date: September.

Additional Information: Possibility of a further five years of funding (renewal through open competition).

MRC Senior Non-Clinical Fellowship

Subjects: Biomedical sciences.

Eligibility: Open to nationals of any country. Applicants are expected to have proven themselves to be independent researchers, be well qualified for an academic research career and demonstrate the promise of becoming future research leaders. It is usually expected that all applicants will hold a PhD/DPhil in a basic science project and that they will have at least six years relevant postdoctoral research experience.

Level of Study: Postdoctorate.

Purpose: To provide support for non-clinical scientists of exceptional ability (who do not have tenured positions) to concentrate on a period of research.

Type: Fellowship.

No. of awards offered: Up to 10.

Frequency: Annual.

Value: Appropriate academic salary, support for technician/postdoctoral, consumables and some equipment and a travel allowance of £1,000.

Length of Study: Up to 5 years.

Study Establishment: Suitable university department or similar institution.

Country of Study: United Kingdom.

Application Procedure: Personal application. Forms and further details are available from MRC.

Closing Date: November.

Additional Information: Possibility of a further five years funding (renewal through open competition).

MRC Special Training Fellowship in Bioinformatics

Subjects: Biomedical sciences.

Eligibility: Residence requirements apply. The scheme is aimed at individuals from a variety of backgrounds: non-biological as well as biological, non-clinical as well as clinical, and individuals with PhD's/MD's or with informatics research experience at a predoctoral level.

Level of Study: Postdoctorate.

Purpose: To provide specialist, multidisciplinary research training at doctoral or postdoctoral level. Fellows may undertake a Master's degree during the first part of their fellowship, followed by a period of specialist research training.

Type: Fellowship.

No. of awards offered: Up to 7.

Frequency: Annual.

Value: Appropriate academic salary, a research Training Support Grant of up to £6,500 and travel allowance of £500.

Length of Study: Up to 4 years.

Study Establishment: A suitable university department or similar institution.

Country of Study: United Kingdom (but one year may be spent in a recognised research establishment overseas or in UK industry).

Application Procedure: Personal application. Form and further details are available from MRC.

Closing Date: January.

Additional Information: Award holders are encouraged to apply for a PhD (or MD) if they do not already have one.

MRC/Joint MRC Health Regions Special Training Fellowship in Health Services Research

Subjects: Biomedical sciences.

Eligibility: Residence requirements apply. The scheme is open to non-medical graduates, hospital doctors, dentists, general practitioners, nurses, midwives and members of the Professions Allied to Medicine (PAMS) who are seeking a research career in health services and research.

Level of Study: Postdoctorate.

Purpose: To provide support for researchers wishing to gain further training in multi-disciplinary research to address problems of direct relevance to the health services within the UK.

Type: Fellowship.

No. of awards offered: Up to 15.

Frequency: Annual.

Value: Appropriate academic salary, Research Training Support Grant of £4,500 and travel allowance of £450.

Length of Study: Up to 3 years.

Study Establishment: A suitable university department or similar institution.

Country of Study: United Kingdom; but one year may be spent at a recognised research establishment overseas.

Application Procedure: Personal application. Form and further details are available from MRC.

Closing Date: January.

MEDICAL RESEARCH COUNCIL OF CANADA

Communications Branch
5th Floor
Tower B
1600 Scott Street, Ottawa, ON, K1A 0W9, Canada
Tel: (1) 613 941 2672
Email: mrcinfocrm@hpb.hwc.ca
www: http://www.mrc.gc.ca
Contact: Awards Officer

The Medical Research Council of Canada is the major federal agency responsible for funding biomedical research in Canada. Its role is to promote, assist and undertake basic, applied and clinical research in Canada in the health sciences. MRC does not operate laboratories of its own nor does it employ its own scientists. The research it supports is carried out by scientists in universities, hospitals and research institutions across Canada.

Doctoral Research Awards

Subjects: General medical sciences.
Eligibility: Students engaged in full-time research training in a Canadian graduate school, who have completed at least one year of graduate study at Master's or PhD level but have been registered for no more than two years as a full-time student in a doctoral programme. Candidates must be Canadian citizens or permanent residents of Canada.
Level of Study: Postgraduate, Predoctorate.
Purpose: To provide special recognition and support to students who are pursuing a doctoral degree in the health sciences in Canada.
Type: Award.
No. of awards offered: Varies.
Frequency: Annual.
Value: A stipend of C$17,300 to C$19,000 and a travel allowance of C$500 per annum.
Length of Study: 3 years maximum.
Study Establishment: Canadian universities or research institutions.
Country of Study: Canada.
Application Procedure: Application forms and programme guidelines are available on the MRC website.
Closing Date: October 15th.
Additional Information: For further information please write for details or contact the MRC Awards unit on 613 954 1690.

MD PhD Programme Studentships

Subjects: General Medical Sciences.
Eligibility: Candidates must have been admitted to a combined MD/PhD programme.
Level of Study: Graduate, Postgraduate, Predoctorate.
Purpose: To promote promising students embarking on a combined MD/PhD programme at approved Canadian Universities.

Type: Studentship.
No. of awards offered: Up to 10.
Frequency: The MRC will only provide support for 40 students under this programme, therfore it will only run for four or five years.
Value: A stipend of C$16,300 per annum.
Length of Study: 6 years maximum.
Study Establishment: The universities of British Columbia, Calgary, Dalhousie, McGill, Montreal, Toronto and Western Ontario.
Country of Study: Canada.
Application Procedure: By nomination. Candidates must be endorsed and selected by the director of the MD/PhD programme of each institution.
Closing Date: Please write for details.
Additional Information: For further information please contact the MRC or refer the website. In addition to the combined MD/PhD Studentship Programme, MRC has also established a Master's or PhD Studentship Programme under very similar conditions, details of which are available from the MRC or on the website.

MRC Fellowship Programme

Subjects: Rehabilitive science or veterinary medicine.
Eligibility: Promising postdoctoral scholars, researchers or health professionals, preferbaly holding licensure in Canada. For information on obtaining medical licensure in Canada please contact Director of Credentials and Registration, The Medical Research Council of Canada, 2283 St Laurent Boulevard, PO Box 8234, Station T, Ottawa, Ontario K1G 3H7 Tel: 613 521 6012 Fax: 613 521 9417.
Level of Study: Postdoctorate.
Purpose: To provide support for highly qualified postdoctoral candidates to add to their experience by engaging in research either in Canada or abroad.
Type: A variable number of Fellowships.
No. of awards offered: Varies.
Frequency: Twice a year.
Value: Depending on the experience, stipend of C$26,790 to C$2,585 per annum including a yearly research and travel allowance of C$1,800 in the first year and C$1,300 thereafter.
Length of Study: 5 years maximum.
Study Establishment: Universities or research institutions in Canada (or possibly abroad - if the required nature and calibre of training is not available in Canada).
Country of Study: Canada.
Application Procedure: Candidates must compile the following for a complete application package: training module, CV module for both the candidate and the supervisor(s), official transcripts of the candidates graduate and/or professional training including proof of any degrees completed, proof of Canadian licensure, at least three assessments from persons under whom the candidate has studied and a letter of support from the proposed supervisor of foreign candidates.
Closing Date: April 1st and November 1st.
Additional Information: In addition to this fellowships programme the MRC has established the more long-term and prestigious Centennial Fellowship Programme for candidates of special academic distinction and Awards for Clinical

Scientists, as well as Awards for distinguished Scientists and Senior Scientists and the Michael Smith Award for Research Personnel. For details of these programmes please refer to the website htp://www.mrc.gc.ca/gag/9798/b.

MRC Scholarship Programme

Subjects: General Medcal Sciences.
Eligibility: Promising scholars or researchers who hold a health professional degree or PhD (or the equivalent) and shown promise of attaining competence as independent investigators. Candidates should not be registered for a higher degree at the time of application or undertake such studies during the period of the appointment.
Level of Study: Doctorate, Predoctorate.
Purpose: To enable promising scholars and researchers to develop and demonstrate their ability to initiate and carry out independent health research, unhampered by the necessity of carrying out the full teaching duties expected of a regular member of the university staff.
Type: 1 Scholarship.
No. of awards offered: Varies.
Frequency: Annual.
Value: C$50,000 per annum.
Length of Study: 5 years.
Study Establishment: Candian universities or research institutions.
Country of Study: Canada.
Application Procedure: For details please write to the MRC Awards Unit.
Closing Date: Please write for details.

MRS Wellcome Trust Agreement

Subjects: Biomedical Science.
Eligibility: Biomedical research scientists who are nationals of the UK or Canada or permanent residents of these countries.
Level of Study: Postdoctorate.
Purpose: To promote promising bio-medical research scientists.
Type: Travel Grant.
No. of awards offered: Varies.
Frequency: Annual.
Value: Travel costs, research expenses of up to C$1,000 and a subsistence allowance of C$3,000 for up to 30 days, C$2,410 for 31 to 60 days and C$1,950 thereafter.
Length of Study: Up to 3 months.
Study Establishment: Universities or research institutions in the UK or Canada.
Country of Study: UK or Canada.
Application Procedure: Submission of an application on form MRC 26 (Application for a Visiting Scientist Award) Forms are available from the MRC.
Closing Date: October 1st.
Additional Information: For further please contact The Wellcome Trust, 183 Euston Road, London NW1 2BE, UK. Tel: +44 171 611 8888, Fax: +44 171 611 8545. In addition to this international exchange programme the MRC also has similar agreements with CONCICET (Argentina), CNP(Brazil), NNSFC(China), CNRS (France), INSERM (France), CNR (Italy).

For details about these programmes please refer to the website http://www.mrc.gc.ca/gag/9798/ggise.html.

University Industry Program

Subjects: All medical sciences including dentistry, nursing, pharmacy, optometry and veterinary medicine and other academic departments, as long as the research is relevant to humasn health.
Eligibility: Canadian citizens involved in medical research and citizens of the countries participating in international scientific exchanges such as Argentina, Brazil, the Peoples Republic of China, France and Italy.
Level of Study: Graduate, Postdoctorate, Research.
Purpose: To allow industry to put the the results of university research into practice more speedily and effectively.
Type: A variable number of Grants.
No. of awards offered: Variable, depending on funding available.
Frequency: Annual.
Value: Dependent on the individual or research project requirements.
Length of Study: 1 to 5 years.
Study Establishment: Canadian University.
Country of Study: Canada.
Application Procedure: Submission of applications for funding.
Additional Information: For general enquiries Tel: 613 941 2672. For more information on the MRC and it's progammes write to The Medical Research Council of Canada, Communications Branch, 5th Floor, Towe B, 1600 Scott Street, Ottawa, Ontario K1A 0W9, Canada.

Wyeth Ayerst and MRC PMAC Health Programme Clinical Research Chairs in Women's Health

Subjects: Women's health in the fields of perinatology, reproductive endocriminology, mental health and cardiovascular health.
Eligibility: Promising scholars with a degree in medicine who have completed their training and hold a faculty appointment at the time of taking up the award.
Level of Study: Postdoctorate.
Purpose: To champion women's health as a field of medical research and to promote promising scholars wishing to pursue research in this field.
Type: Award.
No. of awards offered: 4.
Frequency: Annual.
Value: Up to C$120,000 per annum.
Length of Study: Varies.
Study Establishment: Canadian universities or research institutions.
Country of Study: Canada.
Application Procedure: Nomination by the Dean of Faculty or Head of the Institution where the research is to be undertaken. The nomination must be accompanied by a letter of intent which includes the candidate's affiliation, mailing address and contact numbers, the location where the proposed research is to be conducted, a detailed curriculum vitae, an outline of the research programme (two pages

maximum) and a letter of support by the Dean of Faculty or Head of the Institution indicating how the proposal will fit into the Institution's overall research plan.

Closing Date: April 30th.

Additional Information: For further information or to submit a letter of intent please write to Beranard M Leduc, Vice President, Canadian Regional Research, Wyeth Ayerst Canada, Inc, 110 Sheppard Avenue East, North York, Ontario M2N 6R5, Canada or telephone the Project Co-ordinator, Michelle Davies on 416 226 7620 or fax: 416 225 3785.

THE MENTAL HEALTH FOUNDATION

20-21 Cornwall Terrace, London, NW1 4QL, England
Email: mhf@mentalhealth.org.uk
www: http://www.mentalhealth.org.uk
Contact: Ms Kate Rogers, Grants Research Support Officer

The Mental Health Foundation is the leading charity in the UK working for the needs of people with mental health problems and those with learning disabilities. The Foundation's work includes funding research and community projects, promoting the development of good services, and providing easily accessible information to the general public.

Mental Health Foundation Grants in Aid of Travel During Medical Students Elective Periods

Subjects: Psychiatry.
Eligibility: Open to student electives in psychiatry.
Level of Study: Postgraduate.
Type: An unlimited number of grants.
No. of awards offered: Maximum 8 grants per year.
Frequency: Annual.
Value: Up to £400.
Country of Study: United Kingdom.
Application Procedure: Contact the Grants Administrator.
Additional Information: The Foundation makes the awards to each medical school in the UK. Candidates should obtain application forms from their Medical School Office. All grants will be advertised via the Medical School Office.

Mental Health Foundation Research Grant

Subjects: Psychiatry and mental health, nursing, cognitive sciences, psychology, experimental psychology, and educational psychology.
Eligibility: There are no restrictions within the UK. Awards are dependent on quality.
Level of Study: Unrestricted.
Purpose: To further research into the areas of mental health and psychiatry. Also to undertake community or social projects in the area of mental health and learning disabilities.
Type: Research Grant.
No. of awards offered: Varies.
Value: Normally to a maximum of £70,000.
Length of Study: Special projects run for 3-5 years.

Country of Study: United Kingdom.
Application Procedure: Application form and any other documentation deemed a requirement for a specific grant giving round. After a new programme has been announced, application forms are available from the Grants Administrator.
Closing Date: Variable, throughout the financial year.
Additional Information: Information on current programmes of work can be obtained from the Grants Administrator. Current programmes include: community projects and scientific research in the field of dementia; older people with learning disabilities; children and young people's mental health. See website for further details. The majority of funding is allocated in research within themed programmes.

Mental Health Foundation Studentship

Subjects: Psychiatry and mental health, nursing, cognitive sciences, psychology, experimental psychology, and educational psychology.
Eligibility: There are no restrictions within the UK. Awards are dependent on quality.
Level of Study: Doctorate.
Purpose: To further research into the areas of mental health and psychiatry.
Type: Studentship.
Country of Study: United Kingdom.
Application Procedure: Application form and any other documentation deemed a requirement for a specific grant can be obtained from the Grants Administrator.
Closing Date: Variable, throughout the financial year.
Additional Information: Future studentships will be in the field of demention.

MICHIGAN SOCIETY OF FELLOWS

University of Michigan
3030 Rackham Building
915 E Washington Street, Ann Arbor, MI, 48109-1070, United States of America
Tel: (1) 734 763 1259
Fax: (1) 734 763 2447
Email: society.of.fellows@umich.edu
www: http://www.rackham.umich.edu/faculty/society.htm
Contact: Ms Luan McCarthy Briefer, Administration Assistant

The Michigan Society of Fellows provides financial and intellectual support to individuals selected for outstanding achievement, professional promise, and interdisciplinary interests. The Society invite applications from qualified candidates for three year postdoctoral fellowships at the University of Michigan.

Michigan Society of Fellows Postdoctoral Fellowships

Subjects: All subject fields offered by the University of Michigan.

Eligibility: Applicants must have completed the PhD or comparable professional or artistic degree within three years of appointment.
Level of Study: Postdoctorate.
Purpose: To provide financial and intellectual support for individuals selected for outstanding achievement, professional promise, and interdisciplinary interests.
Type: Fellowship.
No. of awards offered: 4.
Frequency: Annual.
Value: Stipend of US$36,000 per year.
Length of Study: 3 years.
Study Establishment: University of Michigan.
Country of Study: USA.
Application Procedure: Application form must be completed; please write to request application materials.
Closing Date: Early October - this date will vary from year to year.

MIGRAINE TRUST

45 Great Ormond Street, London, WC1N 3HZ, England
Tel: (44) 171 278 2676
Fax: (44) 171 831 5174
Email: migrainetrust@compuserve.com
www: http://www.migrainetrust.org/
Contact: Dr Cathy Fernandes

Migraine Trust Grants

Subjects: All aspects of migraine and associated headaches.
Eligibility: Grants are awarded on merit and not according to predetermined criteria.
Level of Study: Doctorate, Postdoctorate, Postgraduate.
Purpose: To fund research into migraine.
Type: Research Grant, Fellowship, Studentship.
No. of awards offered: Varies.
Frequency: Annual.
Value: Varies.
Length of Study: Up to 3 years.
Study Establishment: Approved universities or research institutions.
Country of Study: Unrestricted (except for the studentships which must be United Kingdom only).
Application Procedure: Applicants should write for a grant, fellowship or studentship application form in the first instance. Studentship applications should be made by host institution and not directly by the student.
Closing Date: March 31st.

MINISTÈRE DES AFFAIRES ÉTRANGÈRES

Bureau des Boursiers Français a l'Etranger
244 boulevard Saint-Germain, Paris, F-75303, France
Tel: (33) 1 43 17 72 22
Fax: (33) 1 43 17 97 57
Email: boursiers-francais@diplomatie.fr
Contact: Mr Serge François

Lavoisier Award

Subjects: All subjects.
Eligibility: Applicants must be French and under 40 years of age.
Level of Study: Doctorate, Postdoctorate, Postgraduate.
Purpose: To encourage scientific co-operation abroad.
Type: Scholarship.
No. of awards offered: 350.
Frequency: Dependent on funds available.
Value: Between FF40,000 and FF80,000 per year, depending on the cost of living in the host country.
Length of Study: 1 year.
Study Establishment: Unrestricted.
Country of Study: Any country.
Application Procedure: Please write for application forms between October and February.
Closing Date: March 1st.

MONASH UNIVERSITY

Wellington Road, Clayton, VIC, 3168, Australia
Tel: (61) 3 9905 2009
Fax: (61) 3 9905 5042
Email: research.training.support@adm.monash.edu.au
www: http://www.monash.edu.au
Contact: Manager, Research, Training and Support Branch

Logan Research Fellowships

Subjects: All subjects.
Eligibility: There are no restrictions, other than applicants must hold a PhD and have 2-6 years' postdoctoral research experience.
Level of Study: Postdoctorate.
Purpose: To attract outstanding researchers with 2-6 years' postdoctoral research experience.
Type: Fellowship.
No. of awards offered: 5.
Frequency: Annual.
Value: Salary of research fellowship level B (A$46,269) per year or above, plus research support grants of between A$5,000 and A$20,000 per year depending on the nature of the research. Return air fare provided.

Length of Study: 3 years with the possibility of an additional 3 years.
Study Establishment: Monash University.
Country of Study: Australia.
Application Procedure: Application forms and referees report forms must be submitted.
Closing Date: April 30th.
Additional Information: Electronic lodgement of application is preferred.

Monash Graduate Scholarships

Subjects: All subjects.
Eligibility: Open to graduates or graduands of any Australian or overseas university, who should hold at least a first class honours Bachelor's degree or the equivalent, or should be completing the final year of a course leading to such a degree.
Level of Study: Doctorate, Research.
Purpose: To provide support for supervised full-time research at Master's and doctorate level.
Type: Scholarship.
No. of awards offered: 110.
Frequency: Annual.
Value: A$16,135 stipend plus thesis preparation and other allowances.
Length of Study: Up to 2 years for the Master's degree; up to 3 years with the possibility of an additional 6 month extension for the doctoral degree.
Study Establishment: Monash University.
Country of Study: Australia.
Application Procedure: Application kit available four months before closing date.
Closing Date: October 31st.
Additional Information: International students must meet English language proficiency requirements.

Monash University Partial Tuition Postgraduate Research Scholarship Scheme

Subjects: All subjects.
Eligibility: Open to graduates or graduands of any Australian or overseas university, who should hold at least a first class honours Bachelor's degree or the equivalent, or should be completing the final year of a course leading to such a degree.
Level of Study: Doctorate, Research.
Purpose: To provide support for supervised full-time research at Master's and doctoral level.
Type: Scholarship.
No. of awards offered: 9.
Frequency: Annual.
Value: The award meets two thirds of the tuition fee for international students.
Length of Study: Up to 2 years for the Master's degree; up to 3 years with the possibility of an additional 6 month extension for the doctoral degree.
Study Establishment: Monash University.
Country of Study: Australia.

Application Procedure: Application kit available four months before closing date.
Closing Date: October 31st.

Monash University Silver Jubilee Postgraduate Scholarship

Subjects: 2000 science, 2001 arts and art design, 2002 law or education, or business and economics, 2003 engineering and computing and information technology.
Eligibility: Open to graduates or graduands of any Australian or overseas university, who should hold at least a first class honours Bachelor's degree or the equivalent, or should be completing the final year of a course leading to such a degree.
Level of Study: Doctorate, Research.
Purpose: To provide supervised full-time research at Master's and doctorate level.
Type: Scholarship.
No. of awards offered: 1.
Frequency: Annual.
Value: Stipend: A$20,822 per year plus establishment, relocation, incidentals and thesis allowance.
Length of Study: Up to 2 years for the Master's degree; up to 3 years with the possibility of an additional 6 month extension for the doctoral degree.
Study Establishment: Monash University.
Country of Study: Australia.
Application Procedure: Application kit is available four months before the closing date.
Closing Date: October 31st.
Additional Information: International students must meet English proficiency requirements.

Sir James McNeill Foundation Postgraduate Scholarship

Subjects: Engineering, medicine, music or science.
Eligibility: Open to graduates or graduands of any Australian or overseas university, who should hold a first class honours Bachelor's degree or the equivalent, or should be completing the final year of a course leading to such a degree.
Level of Study: Doctorate.
Purpose: To enable a PhD scholar to pursue a full-time programme of research which is both environmentally responsible and socially beneficial to the community.
Type: Scholarship.
No. of awards offered: 1.
Frequency: Annual.
Value: A$21,322 per year, plus allowances.
Length of Study: Up to 4 years.
Study Establishment: Monash University.
Country of Study: Australia.
Application Procedure: Application kit is available four months before the closing date.
Closing Date: October 31st.
Additional Information: International students must meet English proficiency requirements.

MONTREAL NEUROLOGICAL INSTITUTE

McGill University
3801 University Street, Montreal, PQ, H3A 2B4, Canada
Tel: (1) 514 398 8998
Fax: (1) 514 398 8248
Email: fil@mni.lan.mcgill.ca
www: http://www.mcgill.ca/mni
Contact: Ms Fi L Lumia, Liason Officer

The Montreal Neurological Institute is dedicated to the study of the nervous system and neurological disorders. Its 70 principal researchers hold teaching positions at McGill University. The Institute is characterised by close interaction between basic science researchers and the clinicians at its affiliated hospital.

Jeanne Timmins Costello Fellowships

Subjects: Neurology, neurosurgery or neuroscience - research and study.
Eligibility: Open to candidates of any nationality who have an MD or PhD degree. Those with MD degrees will ordinarily have completed clinical studies in neurology or neurosurgery.
Level of Study: Doctorate, Postgraduate.
Purpose: To support research in neurology, neurosurgery and neuroscience.
Type: Fellowship.
No. of awards offered: 4.
Frequency: Annual.
Value: C$25,000 per year.
Length of Study: 1 year; possibly renewable for 1 further year.
Study Establishment: MNI.
Country of Study: Canada.
Closing Date: October 15th.

Preston Robb Fellowship

Subjects: Neurology, neurosurgery or neuroscience.
Eligibility: Open to researchers of any nationality.
Level of Study: Postdoctorate.
Purpose: To support research.
Type: Fellowship.
No. of awards offered: 1.
Frequency: Annual.
Value: C$25,000.
Length of Study: 1 year.
Country of Study: Canada.
Application Procedure: Please write for details.
Closing Date: October 15th.

MOUNT DESERT ISLAND BIOLOGICAL LABORATORY

PO Box 35
Department NIA
Old Bar Harbor Road, Salsbury Cove, ME, 04672, United States of America
Tel: (1) 207 288 3605
Fax: (1) 207 288 2130
Email: bkb@mdibl.org
www: http://www.mdibl.org
Contact: Dr Barbara Kent, Administrative Director

Mount Desert Island Biological Laboratory is a seasonal marine and biomedical research laboratory which uses unique models such as shark, skate and flounder to solve questions related to human and environmental health.

Mount Desert Island New Investigator Award

Subjects: Biological and life sciences.
Eligibility: Open to US citizens and permanent residents. African Americans, Hispanic, Native American Indian and Native Pacific Islanders are targeted.
Level of Study: Postdoctorate, Professional development.
Purpose: To support independent investigators spending one to two months in the summer doing physiological research on marine animals at MDIBL.
Type: Fellowship.
No. of awards offered: 15-20.
Frequency: Dependent on funds available.
Value: $5,000.
Length of Study: 2-3 months.
Study Establishment: Mount Desert Island Biological Laboratory.
Country of Study: USA.
Application Procedure: The application form can be obtained from MDIBL.
Closing Date: January 15th.

MULTIPLE SCLEROSIS SOCIETY OF CANADA (MSSC)

250 Bloor Street East
Suite 1000, Toronto, ON, M4W 3PG, Canada
Tel: (1) 416 922 6065
Fax: (1) 416 922 7538
www: http://www.mssoc.ca
Contact: Ms Jackie Munroe

MSSC Career Development Award

Subjects: Multiple sclerosis.
Eligibility: Open to individuals holding a doctoratal degree who have recently completed their training in research and are capable of carrying out independent research relevant to MS on a full-time basis.
Level of Study: Postdoctorate.

Purpose: To encourage full-time research.
No. of awards offered: Limited.
Frequency: Annual.
Value: The salary scale, conditions of remuneration and allowable involvement in non-research activities will be similar to Medical Research Council Scholarships.
Length of Study: 3 years initially; with the opportunity for renewal twice.
Study Establishment: A Canadian school of medicine.
Country of Study: Canada.
Closing Date: October 1st.

MSSC Postdoctoral Fellowship

Subjects: Multiple sclerosis and allied diseases.
Eligibility: Open to qualified persons holding an MD or PhD degree and intending to pursue research work relevant to MS and allied diseases. The applicant must be responsible to an appropriate authority in the field he or she wishes to study.
Level of Study: Postdoctorate.
Purpose: To encourage research.
Type: Fellowship.
No. of awards offered: Varies.
Frequency: Annual.
Value: Salary scales follow those suggested by the Medical Research Council for fellowships, plus C$1,000.
Length of Study: 3 years; may be extended for 1 additional year under exceptional circumstances.
Study Establishment: A recognised institution which deals with problems relevant to MS.
Country of Study: Applicants proposing to go abroad are encouraged to seek the advice of the panel members regarding suitable laboratories for advanced training.
Closing Date: October 1st.
Additional Information: Maximum funding three years, but under exceptional circumstances may be extended for one additional year.

MSSC Research Grant

Subjects: Multiple sclerosis.
Eligibility: Open to researchers working in Canada or intending to return to Canada.
Level of Study: Postgraduate.
Purpose: To fund research projects.
Type: Research Grant.
No. of awards offered: Limited.
Frequency: Annual.
Value: Varies.
Length of Study: 1, 2 or 3 years; if further funding is requested reapplication in full must be made.
Study Establishment: An approved institution.
Country of Study: Any country.
Closing Date: October 1st.

MSSC Research Studentship

Subjects: Multiple sclerosis research.
Eligibility: Open to qualified persons holding other than an MD or PhD degree. Applicants directed towards understanding the pathogenesis and potential treatment of MS will receive priority.
Level of Study: Postgraduate.
Purpose: To provide further training in a specialised area related to research in multiple sclerosis and allied diseases.
Type: Studentship.
No. of awards offered: Varies.
Frequency: Annual.
Value: Salary scales for studentships follow those suggested by the Medical Research Council.
Length of Study: 4 years; under exceptional circumstances this may be extended. Renewal must be obtained each year.
Study Establishment: A recognised institution.
Country of Study: Any country.
Closing Date: October 1st.

MULTIPLE SCLEROSIS SOCIETY OF GREAT BRITAIN AND NORTHERN IRELAND

25 Effie Road, London, SW6 1EE, England
Tel: (44) 171 610 7153
Fax: (44) 171 736 9861
Email: ldytrych@mssociety.org.uk
www: http://www.ifmss.org.uk

Multiple Sclerosis Society Research Grants

Subjects: Multiple sclerosis.
Eligibility: Open to nationals of all countries.
Level of Study: Doctorate, Postdoctorate.
Purpose: To promote medical research into the cause and treatment of multiple sclerosis.
Type: Research Grant.
No. of awards offered: Varies.
Frequency: Varies.
Value: Research Grants may be awarded in the form of fellowships and PhD studentships, to provide remuneration for research workers. They may also be awarded for the provision of scientific assistance in connection with some particular aspect of research by a qualified medical or graduate scientist, to meet the entire or part cost of technical laboratory assistance, equipment and materials.
Length of Study: Innovative awards 1 year; PhD and junior fellowships 4years; project grants 2 years; senior fellowships 5 years.
Study Establishment: Suitable institutions.
Country of Study: Any country.

Application Procedure: Application form must be completed.

Closing Date: Contact the Society.

Additional Information: Applications should, where applicable, be sponsored by the Head of the hospital Department or laboratory on which the work is to be carried out.

MUSCULAR DYSTROPHY ASSOCIATION

Research Department
3300 East Sunrise Drive, Tucson, AZ, 85718, United States of America
Tel: (1) 520 529 2000
Fax: (1) 520 529 5300
Email: grants@mdausa.org
www: http://www.mdausa.org
Contact: Ms Karen Mashburn, Grants Manager

MDA supports research into 40 diseases of the neuromuscular system to identify the causes of, and effective treatments for, the muscular dystrophies and related diseases which include spinal muscular atrophies and motor neuron diseases, peripheral neuropathies, inflammatory myopathies, metabolic myopathies and diseases of the neuromuscular junction.

Muscular Dystrophy Association Grant Programs

Subjects: The muscular dystrophies and related diseases which include spinal muscular atrophies and motor neuron diseases, peripheral neuropathies, inflammatory myopathies, metabolic myopathies and diseases of the neuromuscular junction.

Eligibility: Open to persons who are professional or faculty members at appropriate educational, medical, or research institutions and qualified to conduct and supervise programmes of original research; who have access to institutional resources necessary to conduct the proposed research project; and who hold a Doctor of Medicine, Doctor of Philosophy, Doctor of Science or equivalent degree.

Level of Study: Postdoctorate.

Purpose: To support research into 40 diseases of the neuromuscular system to identify the causes of, and effective treatments for, the muscular dystrophies and related diseases.

Type: Grant.

No. of awards offered: Varies.

Frequency: Annual.

Value: Amount not specified; overhead limited to a maximum of 8% of the total amount of the grant requested.

Length of Study: 1 year; renewable for a further 2 or 3 years.

Country of Study: Any country.

Application Procedure: The Request for Research Grant Application must be completed to formally request an application for a grant.

Closing Date: Pre-applications due no later than December 15th nad June 15th.

Additional Information: Proposals from applicants outside the USA will only be considered for projects of highest priority to MDA and when, in addition to the applicants having met the eligibility requirements noted above, one or more of the following conditions exist: the applicant's country of residence has inadequate sources of financial support for biomedical research; collaboration with an MDA-supported US investigator is required to conduct the project; or an invitation to submit an application has been extended by MDA. The research program, under which a full application may be invited, is determined at MDA's sole discretion. Research is sponsored under the following grant programs: Neuromuscular Disease Research; Neuromuscular Disease Research Development; Task Force on Genetics; Neuromuscular Disease Special Grants.

MUSCULAR DYSTROPHY GROUP OF GREAT BRITAIN AND NORTHERN IRELAND

Strangeways Research Laboratory
Wort's Causeway, Cambridge, CB1 4RN, England
Tel: (44) 1223 411706
Fax: (44) 1223 411609
www: http://www.muscular-dystrophy.org
Contact: Dr Sarah Yates, Director of Scientific Affairs

Muscular Dystrophy Programme Grant

Subjects: Biomedicine.

Eligibility: Only awarded in exceptional circumstances - a site visit would be made prior to approval.

Level of Study: Postdoctorate.

Purpose: To provide continuity of funding for high quality research of central importance to the Muscular Dystrophy Group's research objectives.

Type: Programme Grant.

No. of awards offered: Varies.

Frequency: Dependent on funds available.

Value: Salary of research staff, equipment and consumables. Salary of grant holder is not funded.

Length of Study: 5 years.

Study Establishment: University or hospital.

Country of Study: United Kingdom.

Application Procedure: Individual applicants should contact the Director of Scientific Affairs with a summary of proposed research.

Closing Date: To be announced.

Muscular Dystrophy Project Grant

Subjects: Biomedicine. Muscular Dystrophy and allied neuromuscular diseases.

Eligibility: Open to research workers with appropriate qualification and experience. Grant holder must have tenured position. UK nationals (usually restricted).

Level of Study: Postdoctorate.

Purpose: For the advancement of medical research into Muscular Dystrophy and allied neuromuscular conditions.
Type: Project Grant.
No. of awards offered: Varies.
Frequency: Annual.
Value: Salary of research staff, equipment and consumables.
Length of Study: 3 years.
Study Establishment: University or hospital.
Country of Study: Any country.
Application Procedure: Summary of proposal to Director of Scientific Affairs in the first instance.
Closing Date: To be announced.
Additional Information: Grant holder must have tenured position.

Muscular Dystrophy Research Grants

Subjects: Muscular Dystrophy and allied neuro muscular diseases.
Eligibility: Open to UK nationals who have appropriate qualifications and experience.
Level of Study: Postdoctorate.
Purpose: To support research into neuromuscular function in health and in disease, with particular reference to Muscular Dystrophy and related disorders.
Type: Research Grant.
No. of awards offered: Varies.
Frequency: Dependent on funds available.
Value: Varies, according to the nature of the research and the qualifications and experience of the applicant.
Length of Study: 3 years.
Study Establishment: Universities, hospitals and other research institutions.
Country of Study: United Kingdom.
Application Procedure: Send summary of proposal to the Director of Scientific Affairs, in the first instance.
Additional Information: Grant holder must have tenured position.

THE MYASTHENIA GRAVIS FOUNDATION

222 S Riverside Plaza
Suite 1540, Chicago, IL, 60606, United States of America
Tel: (1) 312 258 0522
Fax: (1) 312 258 0461
Email: myastheniagravis@msn.com
www: http://www.myasthenia.org
Contact: Research and Grants Committee

The Foundation was established in order to find a cure for Myasthenia Gravis and related disorders of the neuromuscular junction, and to improve the lives of all people affected, through programs of medical research, patient care, professional education and public information.

Henry R Viets Medical/Graduate Student Research Fellowship

Subjects: Scientific basis of MG or related neuromuscular conditions.
Eligibility: There are no eligibility restrictions.
Level of Study: Doctorate, Postgraduate.
Purpose: To promote research into the cause and cure of myasthenia gravis.
Type: Stipend.
No. of awards offered: 4-8.
Frequency: Annual.
Value: US$3,000.
Length of Study: Short-term.
Country of Study: Any country.
Application Procedure: Briefly describe, in abstract form, the question proposed for study, its association to MG or related neuromuscular conditions, and research methodology. Further information may then be requested by the Foundation.
Closing Date: March 15th.

Myasthenia Gravis Nursing Fellowship

Subjects: Research designed to strengthen the contribution of nursing to the treatment of Myasthenia Gravis.
Eligibility: There are no eligibility restrictions.
Level of Study: Postgraduate.
Purpose: To strengthen the linkages between myasthenia gravis treatment and the nursing profession.
Type: Stipend.
No. of awards offered: 2-3.
Frequency: Annual.
Value: US$1,500-US$2,000.
Length of Study: Short-term.
Country of Study: Any country.
Application Procedure: Please contact the Foundation for further details.
Closing Date: Applications are accepted at any time.

Osserman Research Fellowship

Subjects: Research pertinent to Myasthenia Gravis (MG), concerned with neuromuscular transmission, immunology, molecular cell biology of the neuromuscular synapse, the etiology/pathogenesis, diagnosis or treatment of MG.
Eligibility: There are no eligibility restrictions.
Level of Study: Postdoctorate.
Purpose: To investigate the fundamental nature of myastenia gravis.
Type: Fellowship.
No. of awards offered: 2-4.
Frequency: Annual.
Value: US$30,000.
Length of Study: 1 year.
Country of Study: Any country.
Application Procedure: Application form must be completed.
Closing Date: November 1st.

NANSEN FUND

77 Saddlebrook Lane, Houston, TX, 77024, United States of
America
Tel: (1) 713 686 3963
Fax: (1) 713 680 8255
Contact: Fellowships Office

John Dana Archbold Fellowship

Subjects: All subjects.
Eligibility: Eligibility is limited to those aged between 20 and
35, in good health, of good character, and citizens of the
USA, who are not recent immigrants from Norway.
Level of Study: Postdoctorate, Postgraduate, Professional
development.
Purpose: To support educational exchange between the
United States and Norway.
Type: Fellowship.
No. of awards offered: 1-2.
Frequency: Every two years.
Value: Grants vary, depending on costs and rates of
exchange. The University of Oslo will charge no tuition and
the Nansen Fund will pay up to US$10,000 for supplies,
maintenance and travel. The maintenance stipend is sufficient
to meet expenses in Norway for a single person. Air fare from
the US to Norway is covered.
Length of Study: 1 year.
Study Establishment: University of Oslo.
Country of Study: Norway.
Application Procedure: Application form must be completed
and submitted with references and transcripts.
Closing Date: January 31st.
Additional Information: Every other year the Norway-
America Association, the sister organisation of the Nansen
Fund, offers fellowships for Norwegian citizens wishing to
study at a universityin the USA. For further information please
contact: The Norway - America Association, Drammensveien
20c, Oslo, N0 255, Norway, Tel: +47 224 477 16.

NATIONAL ALLIANCE FOR RESEARCH ON SCHIZOPHRENIA AND DEPRESSION (NARSAD)

Grants Adminstration
60 Cutter Mill Road 404, Great Neck, NY, 11021, United
States of America
Tel: (1) 516 829 0091
Fax: (1) 516 487 6930
www: http://www.mhsource.com/narsad.html
Contact: Ms Brenda Berman, Grants Adminstrator

NARSAD Distinguished Investigator Awards

Subjects: Mental illness.
Eligibility: Open to senior researchers of any nationality who
are of professor status (or equivalent).

Level of Study: Postdoctorate.
Purpose: To encourage experienced scientists to pursue
innovative projects in diverse areas of mental illness research.
Type: Grant.
No. of awards offered: Varies.
Frequency: Annual.
Value: Up to US$100,000.
Country of Study: Any country.
Closing Date: Mid-June.

NARSAD Independent Investigator Award

Subjects: Psychiatry and mental health.
Eligibility: This award is intended for scientists at the
academic level of associate professor or equivalent, who
have won national competitive support as a principal
investigator.
Level of Study: Postdoctorate.
Purpose: To support independent investigation.
Type: Grant.
No. of awards offered: 1.
Frequency: Annual.
Value: Up to US$100,000.
Country of Study: Any country.
Closing Date: February 5th.

NARSAD Young Investigator Awards

Subjects: Mental illness.
Eligibility: Open to investigators of any nationality who have
attained a doctorate or equivalent degree, are affiliated with a
specific research institution and who have a mentor or senior
collaborator who is performing significant research in an area
relevant to schizophrenia, depression or other serious mental
illnesses. Candidates should be at the postdoctoral through
assistant professor level.
Level of Study: Postdoctorate.
Purpose: To encourage basic or clinical investigators in the
beginning phase of a research career.
Type: Grant.
No. of awards offered: Varies.
Frequency: Annual.
Value: US$30,000 for up to two years, (for example, the
investigator may apply for US$60,000 at US$30,000 a year).
Length of Study: Up to 2 years.
Country of Study: Any country.
Closing Date: October 25th.

NATIONAL ASSOCIATION OF DENTAL ASSISTANTS

900 South Washington Street
G-13, Falls Church, VA, 22046, United States of America
Tel: (1) 703 237 8616
Contact: Scholarship Department

National Association of Dental Assistants Annual Scholarship Award

Subjects: Dental assistant certification, recertification, dental training, continuing dental education seminars or any course that is related to or required in the dental degree program. All courses must be approved by the board.
Eligibility: Open to dental assistants who have a minimum of two years' membership in good standing (members only). Applicants may also be a member's dependant, spouse or grandchild.
Level of Study: Unrestricted.
Purpose: To enable dental assistants to further their education.
Type: Scholarship.
No. of awards offered: 1-2.
Frequency: Annual.
Value: US$250.
Study Establishment: appropriate institutions.
Country of Study: Any country.
Application Procedure: Applicants must submit one recommendation from their current or previous employer, one recommendation from someone other than a member (if a member's dependant), such as a school counsellor or another dental assistant, and a completed application form and up-to-date student transcript.
Closing Date: May 31st.

NATIONAL ASTHMA CAMPAIGN

Providence House
Providence Place, London, N1 0NT, England
Tel: (44) 171 226 2260
Fax: (44) 171 704 0740
Contact: Office for Funding

National Asthma Campaign Project Grants

Subjects: The organisation are particularly interested in receiving applications concerned with research into delivery or care, interaction of asthma and environment, evaluation of complementary therpies, genetics, mechanisms of severe asthma and primary prevention.
Eligibility: Tenured individuals working in the UK.
Level of Study: Research.
Purpose: To fund research in applied, basic or clinical research relevant to asthma and/or related allergy.
Type: Project Grant.
Frequency: Annual.
Value: Varies.

Length of Study: 3 years maximum.
Country of Study: Normally UK.
Application Procedure: Application form available on request from research department.
Closing Date: Last Friday in November.

NATIONAL ATAXIA FOUNDATION

2600 Fernbrook Lane
Suite 119, Minneapolis, MN, 55447, United States of America
Tel: (1) 612 553 0020
Fax: (1) 612 553 0167
Email: naf@mr.net
www: http://www.ataxia.org
Contact: Research Director

The National Ataxia Foundation was founded in 1957 to combat the hereditary ataxias through education, service and research programs.

Ataxia Research Grant

Subjects: Neurology and genetics, in relation to the study of ataxia.
Eligibility: There are no eligibility restrictions.
Level of Study: Unrestricted.
Purpose: Proposed research projects should relate to the cause and treatment for the inherited ataxias or closely related disorders of concern to the National Ataxia Foundation.
Type: Research Grant.
No. of awards offered: Approx. 6.
Frequency: Annual.
Value: US$5,000-US$20,000.
Length of Study: 1 year.
Country of Study: USA or Canada.
Application Procedure: Application and guidelines are available upon request.
Closing Date: August 31st.

National Ataxia Foundation Friedreich's Ataxia Research Grant

Subjects: Friedreich's Ataxia is a recessively progressive neurological disorder that often has its onset in young teens. Studies aimed at understanding the basic, underlying cause of Freidreich's in the hope of developing a method of treatment will be supported.
Eligibility: Please write for details.
Purpose: To study the cause of Ataxia and devlop treatment models.
Type: Research Grant.
No. of awards offered: Varies.
Value: $25,000-$200,000.
Country of Study: Any country.
Application Procedure: Contact the national Ataxia Foundation after May 15th for application details.

Closing Date: August 31st.
Additional Information: This award was offered for the first time in 1999.

NATIONAL BACK PAIN ASSOCIATION

16 Elmtree Road, Teddington, Middlesex, TW11 8ST, England
Tel: (44) 181 977 5474
Fax: (44) 181 943 5318
Email: 101540.1065@compuserve.com
www: http://homepages.nildram.co.uk/~backtalk/
Contact: Ms Jane Puzey, Fundraising

National Back Pain Association Research Grants

Subjects: Studies related to back pain - causation and diagnosis of back pain, identification of those most susceptible to back pain, identification of the main environmental and occupational hazards, trials of different methods of treatment to alleviate back pain, methods of preventing back pain, reduction in back pain disability by influencing health education, lifestyles, patient behaviour and clinical practice, social and psychological factors relevant to back pain, back pain and primary care.
Eligibility: Open to appropriately qualified and experienced persons.
Level of Study: Postgraduate.
Purpose: To encourage and support scientific research into the causes, treatment and prevention of back pain. The objective is to reduce the incidence of, and disability from, back pain and improve its treatment by gaining through research a better understanding of its manifestation and causes.
Type: Research Grant.
Value: Varies; dependent on funds available. The association is not a major funding organisation.
Length of Study: Up to 2 years.
Study Establishment: Suitable establishments.
Country of Study: United Kingdom.
Application Procedure: Applicants should write, in the first instance, for a copy of the detailed application procedure, as failure to comply with all conditions may diminish the success of an application.
Closing Date: June 1st, November 1st.
Additional Information: Applicants should first satisfy themselves that their proposed research falls within the remit of the National Back Pain Association as defined in the Grant Policy Statement. The association is unable to fund educational courses, attendance at meetings or conferences, or the purchase of computers.

NATIONAL BLACK MBA ASSOCIATION

180 North Michigan
Suite 1515, Chicago, IL, 60601, United States of America
Tel: (1) 312 236 2622
Fax: (1) 312 236 4131
www: http://www.nbmbaa.org
Contact: Ms Lisa Collins, Program Manager

National Black MBA Association Scholarships

Subjects: An essay topic is selected annually by the Scholarship Committee.
Eligibility: Open to minority full-time students enrolled in an accredited US business programme pursuing an MBA degree.
Level of Study: Doctorate, Postgraduate.
Type: Scholarship, Fellowship.
No. of awards offered: 25 for MBA, 2 for PhD.
Frequency: Annual.
Value: MBA - US$3,000 average; PhD - US$10,000 and US$5,000.
Country of Study: USA.
Application Procedure: Application form must be completed and submitted with official transcripts.
Closing Date: March 31st.

NATIONAL CANCER INSTITUTE OF CANADA (NCIC)

Suite 200
10 Alcorn Avenue, Toronto, ON, M4V 3B1, Canada
Tel: (1) 416 961 7223
Fax: (1) 416 961 4189
Email: ncic@cancer.ca
www: http://www.cancer.ca
Contact: Dr Michael Wosnick, Research Programs Director

The National Cancer Institute of Canada (NCIC) and the Canadian Cancer Society (CCS) are organisations that have evolved from the need for a co-ordinated attack on the problem of cancer in Canada and have formed 50-year partnership. The Terry Fox Foundation has also entered into partnership with the NCIC, which is the sole recipient of funds raised by the Foundation for Cancer Research.

American Cancer Society International Fellowships for Beginning Investigators (ACBSI)

Subjects: Cancer research.
Eligibility: Candidates should be in the early stages of their career. Applications that are geared to the development of cancer control measures in developing central and east European countries are particularly encouraged.
Level of Study: Postgraduate.

Purpose: The NCIC financially supports the International Union Against Cancer (UICC) which administers a number of fellowships to qualified professionals.
Type: Research Grant.
No. of awards offered: 8-10.
Frequency: Annual.
Value: Average value US$30,000 per year.
Length of Study: 12 months.
Country of Study: Any country.
Application Procedure: Please write for details.
Closing Date: October 1st.

For further information contact:

3 rue du Conseil-General, Geneva, 1205, Switzerland
Tel: (41) 22 809 1811
Fax: (41) 22 809 1810
Contact: UICC Fellowships Department

CCS Feasibility Grants

Subjects: Cancer research.
Eligibility: This programme is open to all applicants but priority will be given where it is apparent that no other resouces are available. These grants will not be awarded to support travel to conduct planning meetings. These funds will also not be awarded for conference travel or for the purchase of permanent equipment.
Level of Study: Postgraduate.
Purpose: The NCIC recognises that it is difficult to submit a full application for a research grant without having first conducted preliminary studies.
Type: Grant.
No. of awards offered: Varies.
Frequency: Annual.
Value: Up to a maximum of C$35,000.
Length of Study: 1 year.
Country of Study: Canada.
Application Procedure: Please write for details.

CCS Grants for Molecular Epidemiologic/Clinical Correlative Studies

Subjects: Cancer research.
Eligibility: Please write for details.
Level of Study: Postgraduate.
Purpose: In 1992 the Institute announced a special programme and issued a request for applications. For the current year the Institute has again decided to accept further applications for this special programme, and to incorporate them into the regular grant cycle.
Type: Research Grant.
No. of awards offered: Varies.
Country of Study: Canada.
Application Procedure: Please write for details.

CCS Student Travel Award

Subjects: Medical sciences - oncology (cancer research).

Eligibility: Applicants must be enrolled at a Canadian Institution and be in the final phase of study of a PhD or MD/PhD program.
Level of Study: Doctorate.
Purpose: To provide financial assistance to senior level PhD or MD/PhD students by helping to defray travel costs associated with making a scientific presentation at a conference or symposium.
Type: Travel Grant.
No. of awards offered: 20.
Frequency: Three times each year.
Value: Up to a maximum of C$1,000.
Study Establishment: A Canadian university.
Country of Study: Canada.
Application Procedure: Please write for details or refer to the website.
Closing Date: April 1st, September 1st, December 1st.

CCS Travel Award for Senior Level PhD Students

Subjects: Cancer research.
Eligibility: Please write for details.
Level of Study: Postgraduate.
Purpose: To expand research in the areas of behavioural research and cancer control.
Type: Travel Grant.
No. of awards offered: Varies.
Frequency: Annual.
Value: Varies.
Country of Study: Canada.
Application Procedure: Please write for details.
Closing Date: April 1st, September 1st, December 1st.

International Cancer Technology Transfer (ICRETT) Fellowships

Subjects: Cancer research.
Eligibility: Please write for details.
Level of Study: Postgraduate.
Purpose: The NCIC financially supports the International Union Against Cancer (UICC) which administers a number of fellowships to qualified professionals.
Type: Research Grant.
No. of awards offered: Varies.
Frequency: Annual.
Value: Average value US$3,000.
Country of Study: Any country.
Application Procedure: Please write for details.
Closing Date: Applications are accepted at any time.

NCIC Clinical Research Fellowships

Subjects: Clinical cancer research.
Eligibility: Open to Canadian citizens or residents who are graduates in medicine from an institution recognised by the Institute and licensed to practise in Canada, who have normally qualified for admission to Fellowship of the Royal College of Physicians and Surgeons of Canada.
Level of Study: Postdoctorate, Professional development.

Purpose: To assist outstanding medically qualified individuals who seek specialised training.
Type: Research Fellowship.
No. of awards offered: Varies.
Frequency: Annual.
Value: C$29,200 minimum, to a maximum of C$45,400 per year.
Length of Study: Up to a maximum of 3 years.
Study Establishment: A teaching hospital.
Country of Study: Canada, or outside as approved.
Application Procedure: Please write to the Institute for application information.
Closing Date: February 1st.
Additional Information: Stipends are subject to annual review. Recipients of these fellowships are eligible to apply for a contribution of C$1,000 towards the cost of conference travel per award year. Also available are Terry Fox Clinical Research Fellowships. Apply as above.

NCIC Research Fellowships

Subjects: Cancer research.
Eligibility: Open to Canadian citizens or residents who have graduated from universities approved by the Institute. Candidates must be accepted for postdoctoral training or research towards a PhD degree in a university laboratory or teaching hospital approved by the Institute, and be engaged in the field of cancer research. The supervisor must be affiliated at the institute/university recognised by the Institute.
Level of Study: Postdoctorate.
Purpose: To provide training in cancer research for outstanding candidates who plan a career in Canada.
Type: Research Fellowship.
No. of awards offered: Varies.
Frequency: Annual.
Value: Minimum of C$29,200 per year, to a maximum of C$45,400.
Length of Study: 3 years, no renewal.
Study Establishment: A university laboratory or teaching hospital approved by the Institute.
Country of Study: Any country.
Application Procedure: Please write for details.
Closing Date: February 1st.
Additional Information: A Fellow may apply for a transportation grant to and from the laboratory where the training will take place, and if married, an amount to assist in the expense of moving their family. Research Fellowships are not awarded for the purpose of providing practical clinical training. For further details and conditions of Research Fellowships, consult the manual Support for Research and Training, which is available from the Institute.

NCIC Research Grants to Individuals

Subjects: Cancer research.
Eligibility: Open to persons with research experience and competence, holding appointments at Canadian universities or other institutions.
Level of Study: Postgraduate.

Purpose: Designed to stimulate Canadian investigators in a very broad spectrum of research having relevance to cancer.
Type: Research Grant.
No. of awards offered: Varies.
Frequency: Annual.
Value: To cover the purchase and maintenance of animals, expendable supplies, minor items of equipment, and payment of graduate students, postdoctoral Fellows, and technical and research assistants, but not personal support for the grantee.
Length of Study: 3 years in the first instance; renewable for periods of 1-5 years.
Study Establishment: Universities or other institutions.
Country of Study: Canada.
Application Procedure: Please write for details.
Closing Date: October 15th.
Additional Information: Grants will be awarded to projects deemed worthy of support, provided that the basic equipment and research facilities are available in the institution concerned and that it will provide the necessary administrative services. Grants are made only with the consent and knowledge of the administrative head of the institution at which they are to be held, and applications must be countersigned accordingly. The Institute also makes available to individuals engaged in studies related to cancer research, grants for purchase of permanent equipment, including specialised major equipment. For further information and conditions of application, consult the manual Support for Research and Training which is available from the Institute.

NCIC Research Scientist Awards

Subjects: Cancer research.
Eligibility: Open to trained investigators interested in careers in cancer research who hold a doctorate in medicine or in related science, and have completed three years of postdoctoral training in research, but not more than five, and who intend to remain in Canada. PhD or MD degrees must be from universities recognised by the NCIC, and the proposed lab is also recognised by the NCIC.
Level of Study: Postdoctorate.
Purpose: To develop the abilities and research potential of candidates, and to enable them to work full-time on the research project without involvement in major teaching responsibilities.
Type: Research Grant.
No. of awards offered: Varies.
Frequency: Annual.
Value: Initial salary will depend on the experience and competence of the individual. The university must be willing to provide space and two years salary at the end of the award.
Length of Study: 6 years for the initial appointment.
Study Establishment: A Canadian university or research establishment.
Country of Study: Canada.
Application Procedure: Please contact the Institute for application forms.
Closing Date: February 3rd.

Additional Information: Research scientists should apply to the Institute for funds to carry out the research under the regulations set forth in 'Research Grants to Individuals'. Regarding eligibility, receipt of an NCIC Operating Research Grant is seen as the base line requirement. Candidates may not have more than five years' research experience.

Terry Fox Equipment Grants for New Investigators

Subjects: Cancer research.
Eligibility: Applicants should be new investigators who have no more than two years' experience as an independent investigator as of October 15, 1997.
Level of Study: Postgraduate.
Purpose: The purpose of this programme is to make it possible for new investigators to set up cancer research facilities in Canada.
Type: Grant.
No. of awards offered: Varies.
Frequency: Dependent on funds available.
Value: Applicants may request up to C$75,000 for equipment under this category.
Country of Study: Canada.
Application Procedure: Please write for details.
Closing Date: Please write for details.
Additional Information: It is understood that applicants may submit similar applications to other agencies.

Terry Fox New Frontiers Initiative

Subjects: Discovery research with an orientation towards cancer cure.
Eligibility: Must include at least two scientists with different expertise working toward a common goal, which would be difficult to achieve without the combined strength of approaches. Grants will be awarded for discovery research with an orientation towards cancer cure.
Level of Study: Professional development.
Type: Grant.
No. of awards offered: Varies.
Frequency: Annual.
Value: Between C$150,000 and C$300,000.
Country of Study: Canada.
Application Procedure: Please write for details.
Closing Date: December 1st.

For further information contact:

10 Alcorn Avenue
Suite 200, Toronto, ON, M4V 3B1, United States of America
Contact: Dr Michael A Wosnick, Director Research Programs

Terry Fox Post-PhD and Post-MD Research Fellowships

Subjects: Cancer research.
Eligibility: Please write for details.
Level of Study: Postgraduate.
Purpose: To expand research in the area of behavioural research and cancer control.

Type: Fellowship.
No. of awards offered: Varies.
Frequency: Annual.
Value: Varies.
Study Establishment: A Canadian institute.
Country of Study: Canada.
Application Procedure: Please write for details.
Closing Date: February 3rd.

Terry Fox Research Grants for New Investigators

Subjects: Cancer research.
Eligibility: Applicants should be new investigators who have no more than two years' experience as an independent investigator as of October 15, 1997; and who have not previously received a research grant from the National Cancer Institute of Canada or other comparable agency.
Level of Study: Postgraduate.
Purpose: The purpose of this programme is to facilitate the possibility for new investigators to obtain grant support for cancer research. The award is designed for new investigators, and is not intended for relocation expenses.
Type: Research Grant.
No. of awards offered: Varies.
Frequency: Annual.
Value: Varies.
Study Establishment: A Canadian institute.
Country of Study: Canada.
Application Procedure: Please write for details.
Closing Date: Please write for details.
Additional Information: Grantees are asked to play a direct role in the Institute's efforts to provide more funds for research in the future. Recipients of the award are expected to acknowledge the support of the Institute and its financial partners in all scientific communications and press releases related to the award.

Terry Fox Research Studentships

Subjects: Cancer research, available in two broad categories - biomedical research, and behavioural/psychosocial/cancer control research.
Eligibility: Applicants must be residents of Canada and enrolled in a PhD programme at a Canadian institution at the time of application. In addition, the candidate must have completed at least two years of research training at the graduate level or have equivalent research experience.
Level of Study: Postgraduate.
Purpose: The National Cancer Institute of Canada (NCIC) has initiated a new studentship programme to provide training to PhD students in cancer research. Beginning in 1998 a limited number of studentships will be offered to outstanding individuals who plan a career in cancer research in Canada.
Type: Research Grant.
No. of awards offered: Varies.
Value: The annual stipend will begin at C$18,000 and rise by C$500 for each year of the award up to a maximum of C$19,000. Recipients of this award are also eligible for up to C$1,000 per year towards the cost of conference travel.
Length of Study: Awards will be made up to a maximum of 4 years and will not be renewable.

Study Establishment: A Canadian institution.
Country of Study: Canada.
Application Procedure: For information and application forms, please see the research office of your host institution or contact the NCIC directly.
Closing Date: February 3rd.
Additional Information: We invite all members of the research community to identify and approach qualified individuals, and encourage them to apply.

Yamagiwa-Yoshida Memorial International Cancer Study Grants

Subjects: Cancer research.
Eligibility: Candidates should be qualified and experienced investigators with publications in international peer-reviewed periodicals.
Level of Study: Postgraduate.
Purpose: The NCIC financially supports the International Union Against Cancer (UICC) which administers a number of fellowships to qualified professionals.
Type: Research Grant.
No. of awards offered: 8-10.
Frequency: Annual.
Value: Average value US$9,000.
Length of Study: 3-6 months.
Country of Study: Any country.
Application Procedure: Please write for details.
Closing Date: January 1st, July 1st.

THE NATIONAL CHAPTER OF CANADA IODE

Suite 254
40 Orchard View Boulevard, Toronto, ON, M4R 1B9, Canada
Tel: (1) 416 487 4416
Fax: (1) 416 487 4417
Contact: Grants Management Officer

The mission of IODE, a Canadian women's charitable organisation, is to improve the quality of life for children, youth and those in need, through educational, social service and citizenship programs.

IODE War Memorial Doctoral Scholarship

Subjects: All subjects.
Eligibility: Open to Canadian citizens who hold a first degree from a recognised Canadian university. At the time of applying a candidate must be enrolled in a programme at the doctoral level or equivalent.
Level of Study: Doctorate.
Purpose: To honour the memory of the men and women who gave their lives for Canada in World Wars I and II, this memorial was established to provide scholarships for study at the doctoral level.
Type: Scholarship.
No. of awards offered: 9.

Frequency: Annual.
Value: C$12,000 for study in Canada; C$15,000 for study overseas within the Commonwealth.
Country of Study: Canada or other Commonwealth countries.
Application Procedure: Applications and supporting documents are available in September and must be submitted by December 1st.
Closing Date: December 1st.

THE NATIONAL COLLEGIATE ATHLETIC ASSOCIATION

6201 College Boulevard, Overland Park, KS, 66211-2422,
United States of America
Tel: (1) 913 339 1906
Fax: (1) 913 339 0035
www: http://www.ncaa.org
Contact: Ms Julie M Quickel, Committee and Scholarship Co-ordinator

NCAA Postgraduate Scholarship

Subjects: All subjects.
Eligibility: Minimum GPA of 3.000 on a 4.000 scale or its equivalent; student athlete enrolled at an NCAA member institution must be in last year of intercollegiate competition.
Level of Study: Postgraduate.
Purpose: To honour outstanding student athletes from NCAA member institutions who are also outstanding scholars.
Type: Grant.
No. of awards offered: 174.
Frequency: Annual.
Value: Award (one time grant of US$5,000) is not earmarked for a specific area of postgraduate study but awardee must use as a full time graduate student in a graduate or professional school of an academically accredited institution.
Country of Study: Any country.
Application Procedure: Candidates are nominated by their Faculty Athletics Representative or Director of Athletics.
Closing Date: Three deadlines - may vary slightly each year.

NATIONAL FOUNDATION FOR INFECTIOUS DISEASES (NFID)

4733 Bethesda Avenue
Suite 750, Bethesda, MD, 20814, United States of America
Tel: (1) 301 656 0003
Fax: (1) 301 907 0878
Email: nfid@aol.com
www: http://www.nfid.org
Contact: Grants Management Officer

The National Foundation for Infectious Diseases (NFID) is a not-for-profit, non-governmental organisation whose mission is public and professional education and promotion of research on the causes, treatment, and prevention of infectious diseases.

Colin L Powell Minority Postdoctoral Fellowship in Tropical Disease Research

Subjects: Tropical diseases.
Eligibility: The applicant must hold a doctorate from a recognised university and be a permanent resident or citizen of the United States, or a spouse of a citizen or permanent resident of the United States. Each applicant will be required to have arranged for an American or foreign laboratory in which to conduct his/her research. The laboratory should be supervised by a recognised leader in tropical disease research qualified to oversee the work of the selected fellow. The fellowship may not be awarded if the applicant has received or will receive a major fellowship, research grant, or traineeship from the federal government or another foundation in excess of the total amount of this award (US$30,000).
Purpose: To encourage and assist a qualified minority researcher to become a specialist investigator in the field of tropical diseases.
Value: A stipend of US$30,000 for the year, of which US$3,000 may be used for travel supplies (at investigators discretion). Although it is anticipated that the award will be tax-exempt, no guarantee of IRS rulings can be made. No overhead to the sponsoring institution will be paid. The stipend may be supplemented by other monies up to US$30,000 to achieve salary levels consistent with other fellows within the supporting institution.
Length of Study: 1 year.
Application Procedure: The original application and four copies must be postmarked no later than the deadline and be addressed to the Grants Manager.
Closing Date: Must be postmarked no later than January 11th.
Additional Information: Minority in the context of this fellowship refers to Black, Hispanic, American Indian, or Alaskan Native, and Asian or Pacific Islander (From US Bureau of the Census).

John P Utz Postdoctoral Fellowship in Medical Mycology

Subjects: Medical mycology.
Eligibility: The applicant must be a physician who is a citizen of the United States. He/she must demonstrate aptitude and accomplishment in research, and must confirm arrangements for conduct of the proposed research in a recognised host laboratory. The applicant must be sponsored by a university-affiliated medical centre. The fellowship may not be awarded if the applicant has received or will receive a major fellowship, research grant or traineeship from the Federal government or another foundation in excess of the amount of this award. A letter from the Chairman of the Department of Infectious Diseases expressing a willingness to assume responsibility for training the applicant must accompany the application.
Level of Study: Postdoctorate.

Purpose: To encourage and assist a qualified physician to become a specialist and investigator in medical mycology.
Type: Fellowship.
No. of awards offered: 1.
Frequency: Annual.
Value: A stipend of US$30,000 for the year and an additional US$1,000 for travel and supplies. Although it is anticipated that the award will be tax-exempt, no guarantee of IRS rulings can be made. No overhead will be paid to the sponsoring institution.
Length of Study: 1 year.
Study Establishment: Approved research institutions.
Country of Study: USA.
Application Procedure: Detailed guidelines are available from the NFID.
Closing Date: Postmark January 11th for notification in April.

New Investigator Matching Grants

Subjects: Infectious diseases.
Eligibility: A legal resident or citizen of the United States or Canada with full-time junior faculty (instructor or assistant professor) status at a recognised accredited institution of higher learning in the United States or Canada. Priority will be given to those who do not have research grants and whose studies represent pilot work with a new intent for further research.
Level of Study: Doctorate.
Purpose: To assist new investigators who are beginning their research.
Type: Grant.
No. of awards offered: Varies.
Frequency: Annual.
Value: US$2,000.
Application Procedure: A proposal must be completed and be based on research relevant to infectious diseases, microbiology, clinical medicine, epidemiology, and nursing. The topics included in the top 10 infectious diseases as recognised by NFID will receive highest priority for funding. Those top 10 are as follows: antimicrobial resistance and emerging infections, HIV and AIDS, vaccine and preventable diseases, hospital-aquired and opportunistic infections, gastrointestinal, diarrheal, and foodbourne diseases, viral hepatitis, tuberculosis, sexually transmitted diseases, zoonotic diseases, tropical infectious diseases. Application forms are available on request and applications should be addressed to the Grants Manager at NFID.
Closing Date: February 16th.

NFID Fellowship in Infectious Diseases

Subjects: Infectious diseases.
Eligibility: Open to physicians who are citizens of the USA and have satisfactorily completed three or more years of postgraduate medical training (internal medicine, surgery, paediatrics, epidemiology). The applicant must be sponsored by a university-affiliated medical centre. This fellowship may not be awarded if the applicant has received or will receive a major fellowship, research grant or traineeship in excess of the amount of this award from the Federal government or another foundation. A letter from the Chairman of the

Department of Infectious Diseases expressing a willingness to assume responsibility for training the applicant must accompany the application.

Level of Study: Postdoctorate.

Purpose: To encourage and assist young qualified physicians to become specialists and investigators in the field of infectious diseases.

Type: Fellowship.

No. of awards offered: 1.

Frequency: Annual.

Value: A stipend of US$24,000 for the year and an additional US$1,000 for travel and supplies. Although it is anticipated that the award will be tax-exempt, no guarantee of IRS rulings can be made. No overhead will be paid to the sponsoring institution.

Length of Study: 1 year.

Country of Study: USA.

Application Procedure: Please write for details.

Closing Date: Postmark January 11th for notification in April.

NFID New Investigator Matching Grants

Subjects: The proposal must be based on research relevant to infectious diseases, microbiology, clinical medicine, epidemiology, and nursing. Those topics included in the 'top ten' infectious diseases problems as recognised by the NFID will receive highest priority for funding, as follows, HIV and AIDS, antimicrobial resistance and emerging infections, vaccine preventable diseases, hospital acquired and opportunistic infections, viral hepatitis, gastrointestinal, diarrheal and foodborne diseases, sexually transmitted diseases, tuberculosis, zoonotic diseases and tropical infectious diseases.

Eligibility: Open to young investigators, defined as individuals with full-time junior faculty (Instructor or Assistant Professor) status at a recognised and accredited institution of higher learning. Priority will be given to those who do not have research grants and whose studies represent pilot work with intent to further develop their research.

Level of Study: Postgraduate.

Purpose: To assist new investigators who are beginning their research.

Type: Grant.

No. of awards offered: Varies.

Frequency: Annual.

Value: US$2,000. Each application must be accompanied by an agreement from the applicant's sponsoring institution to match the award with equal funds. No indirect costs may be included.

Country of Study: USA or Canada.

Application Procedure: 4-page application in proposal form is available from the NFID or can be downloaded form HFID's website.

Closing Date: February 16th, awarded in May.

NFID Postdoctoral Fellowship in Emerging Infectious Diseases

Subjects: Epidemiology research.

Eligibility: Open to physicians who are US citizens and have completed an infectious diseases fellowship.

Level of Study: Postdoctorate.

Purpose: To encourage and assist a qualified physician to become a recognised authority on emerging infectious diseases and epidemiology.

Type: Fellowship.

No. of awards offered: 1.

Frequency: Annual.

Value: US$50,000.

Length of Study: 1 year.

Study Establishment: Fellow will be assigned to the National Center for Infectious Diseases, CDC Atlanta, GA.

Country of Study: USA.

Application Procedure: Four copies of application must be submitted, to include CV, letter of recommendation and a signed statement indicating that the applicant will acknowledge support received from this grant in publications associated with or resulting from this grant.

Closing Date: Postmarked no later than January 11th.

NFID Postdoctoral Fellowship in Nosocomial Infection Research and Training

Subjects: Medical research into nosocomial infections.

Eligibility: Open to physicians in training who are citizens of the USA. Applicants must demonstrate aptitude or accomplishments in research, and must confirm arrangements for conduct of the proposed research in a recognised host laboratory. Applicants receiving or to be awarded grants in the same academic year in excess of the amount of this award are not eligible for funding under this proposal. Applicants with no grant support will receive priority consideration.

Level of Study: Postdoctorate.

Purpose: To encourage and assist a qualified physician trainee researcher to become a specialist and investigator in the field of nosocomial infections.

Type: Fellowship.

No. of awards offered: Varies.

Frequency: Annual.

Value: A stipend of US$25,000 for the year, of which US$1,000 may be used for travel and supplies (at investigator's discretion). Although it is anticipated that the award will be tax-exempt, no guarantee of IRS rulings can be made. No overhead to the sponsoring institution will be paid. The stipend may be supplemented by other monies to achieve salary levels consistent with other fellows within the supporting institutions.

Length of Study: 1 year.

Country of Study: USA.

Closing Date: Postmark January 11th for notification in April.

NATIONAL HEADACHE FOUNDATION

428 West Saint James Place
2nd Floor, Chicago, IL, 60614, United States of America
Tel: (1) 773 388 6399
Fax: (1) 773 525 7357
www: http://www.headaches.org
Contact: Ms Suzanne E Simons, Executive Director

The Foundation disseminates information, funds research, sponsors public and professional education programs and has a nationwide network of support groups, with 20,000 members. The Foundation is the recognised authority in headache and head pain, and offers the award-winning newsletter, NHF Head Lines, patient education brochures, audio and video tapes.

National Headache Foundation Research Grant

Subjects: Causes of and treatments for headache.
Eligibility: Open to researchers in neurology and pharmacology departments in US medical schools. Submissions from other departments and individual investigators are also welcome.
Level of Study: Doctorate, Postdoctorate.
Purpose: To encourage better understanding and treatment of headache and head pain.
Type: Research Grant.
No. of awards offered: Varies, depending on funds available and worthy projects submitted.
Frequency: Annual.
Value: Amount is dependent on funds available. Grant covers only direct costs of carrying out research, no overhead or salaries.
Country of Study: USA.
Closing Date: December 1st for notification by the following March.

NATIONAL HEALTH AND MEDICAL RESEARCH COUNCIL (NHMRC)

Research Management Unit
GPO Box 9848, Canberra, ACT, 2601, Australia
Tel: (61) 6 289 7077
Fax: (61) 6 289 8617
www: http://www.health.gov.au/nhmrc
Contact: Ms Ann Donovan, Director

Burnet Fellowships

Subjects: Any field of health and medical sciences.
Eligibility: Open to Australian citizens or permanent residents who are not under bond to any foreign government. Candidates should have a current academic or hospital appointment overseas (for at least seven years) equivalent to an Australian Professor/Associate Professor, and be actively engaged in research and apply in conjunction with a host institution which must undertake to provide infrastructural support and administer the award (normal access procedures for receipt of NHMRC funds will apply).
Level of Study: Professional development.
Purpose: To attract back to Australia health and medical researchers of a high calibre who have spent considerable time overseas (at least seven years) and who have not returned because of the lack of suitable opportunities.
Type: Fellowship.
No. of awards offered: Varies.
Frequency: Dependent on funds available.
Value: A setting up grant of up to A$250,000 per year to cover the senior investigator's salary at the appropriate level on the NHMRC Research Fellowship scales, maintenance/equipment and/or salaries for a limited number of associate investigators who wish to return with the senior investigator, plus appropriate travel/removal allowances.
Length of Study: 5 years.
Study Establishment: Australian research institutions.
Country of Study: Australia.
Application Procedure: There is no application form. Applications should be submitted in writing with CV attached.
Closing Date: Applications are accepted at any time.

For further information contact:

Fellowships Unit - Mail Group 33
GPO Box 9848, Canberra, ACT, 2601, Australia
Tel: (61) 6 289 5034
Fax: (61) 6 289 1329
Contact: Ms H Murray

C J Martin Fellowships

Subjects: Biomedical sciences.
Eligibility: Open to Australian citizens or graduates from overseas with permanent Australian resident status who are not under bond to any foreign government. Candidates should hold a doctorate in a medical, dental or related field of research, be actively engaged in such research in Australia and have no more than two years postdoctoral experience at the time of application.
Level of Study: Postdoctorate.
Purpose: To enable Fellows to develop their research skills and work overseas on specific research projects within the biomedical sciences under nominated advisers.
Type: Fellowship.
No. of awards offered: Varies.
Frequency: Annual.
Value: Varies.
Length of Study: 4 years, the first 2 of which are to be spent overseas and the final 2 in Australia.
Study Establishment: Institutions approved by the NHMRC, such as teaching hospitals, universities and research institutes.
Country of Study: Any country.
Application Procedure: Application form must be completed.
Closing Date: July 31st.

For further information contact:

Training Awards Office
MDP 33
GPO Box 9848, Canberra, ACT, 2601, Australia
Tel: (61) 6 289 5843
Fax: (61) 6 289 1329
Contact: Ms Marian Blake

Dora Lush (Biomedical) and Public Health Postgraduate Scholarships

Subjects: Biomedical sciences.
Eligibility: Open to Australian citizens who have already completed a science degree (or equivalent) at the time of submission of the application, science honours graduates and unregistered medical or dental graduates from overseas, who have permanent resident status and are currently residing in Australia. The scholarship shall be held within Australia.
Level of Study: Postgraduate.
Purpose: The purpose of the scholarship is to encourage science honours or equivalent graduates of outstanding ability to gain full-time medical research experience. All candidates must enrol for a higher degree.
Type: Scholarship.
No. of awards offered: Varies.
Frequency: Annual.
Value: A variable stipend per year, plus an allowance of A$1,500 per year, payable to the department where the scholar is working.
Length of Study: 1 year; renewable for up to 2 further years.
Study Establishment: Institutions of higher learning.
Country of Study: Australia.
Application Procedure: Please write for details.
Closing Date: August 13th.

For further information contact:

Training Awards Office
MDP 33
GPO Box 9848, Canberra, ACT, 2601, Australia
Tel: (61) 6 289 5609
Fax: (61) 6 289 1329
Contact: Ms Christine Chapman

Eccles Awards

Subjects: Any field of the health and medical research; preference will be given to fields recognised as high priority to the health of the nation.
Eligibility: Open to investigators with an outstanding record in research, who have potential for appointment at a level equivalent to Australian Professor/Associate Professor, and who are Australian citizens currently working overseas or have permanent Australian resident status and are not under bond to any foreign government. Applicants must have been working overseas for at least seven years.
Level of Study: Professional development.
Purpose: To assist in the appointment of distinguished and productive expatriate medical and dental researchers, to an academic position in Australia.

Type: Award.
No. of awards offered: Varies.
Frequency: Dependent on funds available.
Value: No more than A$150,000 per year to be used for equipment, maintenance and/or salaries for associate investigators, excluding the salary of the potential appointee. This grant must be matched by the appointing institution in an appropriate and adequate way.
Length of Study: 3 years.
Study Establishment: Australian research institutions.
Country of Study: Australia.
Application Procedure: There is no application form. Applications should be submitted in writing with a full CV attached.
Closing Date: Applications are accepted at any time.

For further information contact:

Fellowships Unit - Mail Group 33
GPO Box 9848, Canberra, ACT, 2601, Australia
Tel: (61) 6 289 5034
Fax: (61) 6 289 1329
Contact: Ms H Murray

Neil Hamilton Fairley Fellowships

Subjects: Scientific research, including the social and behavioural sciences, which can be applied to any area of clinical or community medicine.
Eligibility: Open to Australian citizens or graduates from overseas with permanent Australian resident status who are not under bond to any foreign government. Candidates should hold a doctorate in a health related field of research or have submitted a thesis for such by December of the year of application and be actively engaged in such research in Australia and have no more than two years postdoctoral experience at the time of application.
Level of Study: Postdoctorate.
Purpose: To provide training in scientific research methods.
Type: Fellowship.
No. of awards offered: Varies.
Frequency: Annual.
Value: Varies.
Length of Study: 4 years, the first 2 of which are to be spent overseas and the final 2 in Australia.
Study Establishment: Institutions approved by the NHMRC, such as teaching hospitals, universities and research institutes.
Country of Study: Any country.
Application Procedure: Application form must be completed.
Closing Date: July 31st.

For further information contact:

Training Awards Office
MDP 33
GPO Box 9848, Canberra, ACT, 2601, Australia

Tel: (61) 6 289 5843
Fax: (61) 6 289 1329
Contact: Ms Marion Blake

NHMRC Equipment Grants

Subjects: All fields of medicine and dentistry.
Eligibility: Open to individuals, groups or institutions which are normally eligible for NHMRC support. Grants will be made on the basis of scientific merit, taking into consideration factors including whether the applicant(s) hold NHMRC grants; the institutional ranking of the application; and institutional or regional availability of major equipment.
Level of Study: Unrestricted.
Purpose: To provide funding support for the purchase of items of equipment required for biomedical research costing in excess of A$10,000.
Type: Grant.
No. of awards offered: Varies.
Frequency: Annual.
Value: To cover the cost of equipment in excess of A$10,000.
Country of Study: Australia.
Application Procedure: Application form must be completed.
Closing Date: April 30th.

For further information contact:

Project Grants Office
GPO Box 9848, Canberra, ACT, 2601, Australia
Tel: (61) 6 289 8278
Fax: (61) 6 289 8617
Contact: Ms J Sewell

NHMRC Medical and Dental and Public Health Postgraduate Research Scholarships

Subjects: Medical or dental research.
Eligibility: Open to Australian citizens who are medical or dental graduates registered to practice in Australia, with the proviso that medical graduates can also apply during their intern year, and that Dental Postgraduate Research Scholarships may be awarded prior to graduation provided that the evidence of high quality work is shown. Also open to medical and dental graduates from overseas who hold a qualification that is registered for practice in Australia and who have permanent resident status and are currently residing in Australia. Evidence of residence status must be provided. The scholarship shall be held within Australia.
Level of Study: Postgraduate.
Purpose: To encourage medical and dental graduates to gain full-time research experience. All candidates must enrol for a higher degree.
Type: Scholarship.
No. of awards offered: Varies.
Frequency: Annual.
Value: Stipend varies per year, plus an allowance of A$1,500 per year payable to the department where the scholar is working.
Length of Study: 1 year; renewable for up to 2 further years.
Study Establishment: Institutions of higher learning.

Country of Study: Australia.
Application Procedure: Application form must be completed.
Closing Date: August 13th.

For further information contact:

Training Awards Office
MDP 33
GPO Box 9848, Canberra, ACT, 2601, Australia
Tel: (61) 6 289 5609
Fax: (61) 6 289 1329
Contact: Ms Christine Chapman

NHMRC Research Programme Grants

Subjects: All fields of health and medical research.
Eligibility: Open to research teams that would normally comprise several outstanding established investigators. Essential criteria include evidence of significant and innovating research on a broad central theme over a lengthy period, and evidence of collaboration.
Level of Study: Unrestricted.
Purpose: To provide guaranteed support over five years for a collaborative research team.
Type: Grant.
No. of awards offered: Varies.
Frequency: Annual.
Value: Varies.
Length of Study: 5 years.
Study Establishment: Australian research institutions.
Country of Study: Australia.
Application Procedure: There is a two stage application process. Application forms and information kits are available from Mr T Biden.
Closing Date: August 31st.

For further information contact:

Program Grants Unit
GPO Box 9848, Canberra, ACT, 2601, Australia
Tel: (61) 6 289 5235
Fax: (61) 6 289 1329
Contact: Mr T Biden

NHMRC Research Project Grants

Subjects: All fields of medicine and dentistry.
Eligibility: Open to Australian researchers only.
Level of Study: Unrestricted.
Purpose: To provide support for work on problems which are likely to be capable of solution in a reasonably short period of time.
Type: Grant.
No. of awards offered: Varies.
Frequency: Annual.
Value: To cover salary, equipment, maintenance and other specific expenses.
Country of Study: Australia.
Application Procedure: Application form must be completed.
Closing Date: March 6th.

For further information contact:

Project Grants Office
GPO Box 9848, Canberra, ACT, 2601, Australia
Tel: (61) 6 289 6974
Fax: (61) 6 289 8617
Contact: Ms E Hoole

NHMRC/INSERM Exchange Fellowships

Subjects: Biomedical sciences.
Eligibility: Open to Australian citizens and permanent residents, who are not under bond to any foreign government, who hold a doctorate in a medical, dental or related field of research or have submitted a thesis for such by December in the year of application, are actively engaged in such research in Australia and have no more than two years postdoctoral experience at the time of application.
Level of Study: Postdoctorate.
Purpose: To enable Fellows to work overseas on specific research projects.
Type: Fellowship.
No. of awards offered: 1.
Frequency: Annual.
Value: Varies.
Length of Study: 4 years: the first 2 of which are to be spent in France and the final 2 in Australia.
Study Establishment: Institutions approved by the NHMRC, such as teaching hospitals, universities and research institutes, and INSERM laboratories in France.
Country of Study: France or Australia.
Application Procedure: Application form must be completed.
Closing Date: July 31st.
Additional Information: This Fellowship is awarded in association with l'Institut National de la Santé et de la Recherche Médicale (INSERM), France.

For further information contact:

Training Awards Office
MDP 33
GPO Box 9848, Canberra, ACT, 2601, Australia
Tel: (61) 6 289 8187
Fax: (61) 6 289 6957
Contact: Ms Marian Blake

Peter Doherty Fellowships

Subjects: Biomedical sciences.
Eligibility: Open to Australian citizens or graduates from overseas with permanent Australian resident status who are not under bond to any foreign government. Candidates should hold a doctorate in a medical, dental or related field of research or have submitted a thesis for such by December in

the year of application, be actively engaged in such research in Australia or overseas and have no more than two years' postdoctoral experience at the time of application.
Level of Study: Postdoctorate.
Purpose: To provide a vehicle for training in clinical and basic research in Australia, and to encourage persons of outstanding ability to make medical research a full-time career.
Type: Fellowship.
No. of awards offered: Varies.
Frequency: Annual.
Value: Varies.
Length of Study: 4 years.
Study Establishment: Institutions approved by the NHMRC, such as teaching hospitals, universities and research institutes.
Country of Study: Australia.
Application Procedure: Application form must be completed.
Closing Date: July 31st.

For further information contact:

Training Awards Office
GPO Box 9848, Canberra, ACT, 2601, Australia
Tel: (61) 6 289 5843
Fax: (61) 6 289 1329
Contact: Ms Marian Blake

R Douglas Wright Awards

Subjects: All fields of health and medical research.
Eligibility: Open to applicants who have completed postdoctoral research training or have equivalent experience, and are seeking to establish themselves in a career in medical research in Australia.
Level of Study: Postdoctorate, Professional development.
Purpose: To provide outstanding researchers at an early stage in their career with an opportunity for independent research together with improved security.
Type: Award.
No. of awards offered: Varies.
Frequency: Annual.
Value: Salary in the range of Senior Research Officer Level 1 to Senior Research Officer Level 4, with annual increments, plus an allowance of A$10,000 per year.
Length of Study: 4 years.
Study Establishment: Australian research institutions.
Country of Study: Australia.
Application Procedure: Applications are available from Ms H Murray.
Closing Date: April 30th.

For further information contact:

Fellowships Unit - Mail Drop Point 33
GPO Box 9848, Canberra, ACT, 2601, Australia
Tel: (61) 6 289 5034
Fax: (61) 6 289 1329
Contact: Ms H Murray

NATIONAL HEART FOUNDATION OF AUSTRALIA

PO Box 2, Woden, ACT, 2606, Australia
Tel: (61) 2 6282 2144
Fax: (61) 2 6282 5147
Email: debra.green@heartfoundation.com
www: http://www.heartfoundation.com.au
Contact: Ms Debra Greer, Research Manager

The National Heart Foundation of Australia is a non-government, non-profit health organisation funded mostly by public donation. The Foundation's mission is to prevent early death and disability from heart disease and stroke. The Foundation funds biomedical research, provides clinical leadership and develops health promotion strategies and initiatives.

National Heart Foundation of Australia Overseas Research Fellowships

Subjects: Clinical or basic medical sciences related to cardiovascular problems.
Eligibility: Open to persons normally resident in Australia with at least two years' postgraduate experience and significant achievement in research.
Level of Study: Postgraduate.
Purpose: To allow Fellows to obtain skills in cardiovascular research.
Type: Fellowship.
No. of awards offered: 1-2.
Frequency: Annual.
Value: A$39,335-A$47,780 plus allowances.
Length of Study: 3 years.
Study Establishment: Approved institutions.
Country of Study: Overseas for the first two years and Australia for the third year.
Application Procedure: Please write for details.
Closing Date: May 31st.
Additional Information: Fellowships are awarded on the understanding that the Fellow will return to Australia to continue his or her career upon completion of the Fellowship.

National Heart Foundation of Australia Postgraduate (Non-Medical) Research Scholarship

Subjects: Cardiovascular research.
Eligibility: Open to Australian citizens and permanent residents only.
Level of Study: Postgraduate.
Purpose: To assist non-medical graduates to undertake a period of training in research under the full-time supervision and tuition of a responsible investigator.
Type: Scholarship.
Frequency: Annual.
Value: A$18,135 plus A$1,200 departmental allowance per annum, plus up to A$500 thesis allowance (final year).
Length of Study: Up to 3 years.

Study Establishment: Universities, hospitals, research institutions.
Country of Study: Australia.
Application Procedure: Application submission outlining research proposal stating name of supervisor and host institution. References are also required.
Closing Date: October 31st.

National Heart Foundation of Australia Postgraduate Medical Research Scholarship

Subjects: Cardiovascular research.
Eligibility: Open to Australian citizens and permanent residents only.
Level of Study: Postgraduate.
Purpose: To enable medical graduates to undertake a period of training in research under the full-time supervision and tuition of a responsible investigator.
Type: Scholarship.
No. of awards offered: Varies.
Frequency: Annual.
Value: A$23,997 plus A$1,200 departmental allowance per annum plus up to A$500 thesis allowance (final year).
Length of Study: 3 years.
Study Establishment: University, hospitals, and research institutions.
Country of Study: Australia.
Application Procedure: Application outlining research proposal must be accompanied by supervisor's reference and backing.
Closing Date: May 31st.

National Heart Foundation of Australia Research Grants-in-Aid

Subjects: Cardiovascular research.
Eligibility: Open to Australian citizens only.
Level of Study: Professional development.
Purpose: To support research in the cardiovascular field.
Type: Grant.
No. of awards offered: 50-60.
Frequency: Annual.
Value: Dependent on project and funds available; grants may cover salaries and equipment/supply costs.
Length of Study: Up to 2 years.
Study Establishment: An approved Australian institution.
Country of Study: Australia.
Application Procedure: Application must be submitted outlining research proposal. References are also required.
Closing Date: April 30th.

Warren McDonald International Fellowship

Subjects: Cardiovascular research.
Eligibility: Open to senior research workers of proven ability in the cardiovascular field, whose normal employment is outside Australia.
Level of Study: Professional development.

Purpose: To enable a senior overseas researcher of proven ability in the cardiovascular field to make a significant research contribution to an Australian research group.
Type: Fellowship.
No. of awards offered: 1.
Frequency: Annual.
Value: An appropriate stipend, plus a travel grant to cover the minimum cost return airfare for the Fellow and his/her immediate family dependants (if any) from his/her home to Australia. The Foundation also makes a grant of up to A$4,000 to cover departmental expenses.
Length of Study: Up to 1 year.
Study Establishment: Universities, hospitals or research institutions.
Country of Study: Australia.
Application Procedure: Applicants must be nominated by the head of the host department or institution.
Closing Date: May 31st.

NATIONAL HEART FOUNDATION OF NEW ZEALAND

PO Box 17-160
Greenlane
Newmarket, Auckland, New Zealand
Tel: (64) 9 524 6005
Fax: (64) 9 524 7854
Email: boyds@akl.nhf.org.nz
www: http://www.nhf.org.nz
Contact: Medical Director

The National Heart Foundation of New Zealand aims to promote good health and to reduce suffering and premature death from diseases of the heart and circulation.

National Heart Foundation of New Zealand Fellowships

Subjects: Any aspect of cardiovascular disease including research, rehabilitation and education.
Eligibility: Normally open to New Zealand graduates only.
Level of Study: Postgraduate.
Purpose: To promote the aims of the National Heart Foundation of New Zealand.
Type: Fellowship.
No. of awards offered: Varies.
Frequency: Annual.
Value: Varies, according to the determination of the Scientific Committee and within an annual budget.
Study Establishment: New Zealand institutions.
Country of Study: New Zealand, but Travel Grants and Clinical Training Fellowships may be held abroad.
Application Procedure: Candidates should apply to the Foundation for the publication 'A Guide to Applicants for Research and Other Grants'.
Closing Date: June 1st.

National Heart Foundation of New Zealand Grants-in-Aid

Subjects: Any aspect of cardiovascular disease including research, rehabilitation and education.
Eligibility: Normally open to New Zealand graduates only.
Level of Study: Postgraduate.
Purpose: To promote the aims of the National Heart Foundation of New Zealand.
Type: Grant.
No. of awards offered: Varies.
Frequency: Annual.
Value: Varies, according to the determination of the Scientific Committee and within an annual budget.
Study Establishment: New Zealnd institutions.
Country of Study: New Zealand, but Travel Grants and Clinical Training Fellowships may be held abroad.
Application Procedure: Please write for details.
Closing Date: February 1st, June 1st, October 1st.

National Heart Foundation of New Zealand Project Grants

Subjects: Any aspect of cardiovascular disease including research, rehabilitation and education.
Eligibility: Normally open to New Zealand graduates only.
Level of Study: Postgraduate.
Purpose: To promote the aims of the National Heart Foundation of New Zealand.
Type: Grant.
No. of awards offered: Varies.
Frequency: Annual.
Value: Varies, according to the determination of the Scientific Committee and within an annual budget.
Study Establishment: New Zealand Institutions.
Country of Study: New Zealand, but Travel Grants and Clinical Training Grants may be held abroad.
Application Procedure: Please write for details.
Closing Date: March 1st.

National Heart Foundation of New Zealand Travel Grants

Subjects: Any aspect of cardiovascular disease including research, and education.
Eligibility: Normally open to New Zealand graduates only.
Level of Study: Postgraduate.
Purpose: To promote the aims of the National Heart Foundation of New Zealand.
Type: Grant.
No. of awards offered: Varies.
Frequency: Annual.
Value: Varies, according to the determination of the Scientific Committee and withiin an annual budget.
Study Establishment: New Zealand institutions.
Country of Study: New Zealand, but Travel Grants and Clinical Training Fellowships may be held abroad.
Application Procedure: Please write for details.
Closing Date: February 1st, June 1st, October 1st.

NATIONAL HUMAN GENOME RESEARCH INSTITUTE (NHGRI)

9000 Rockville Pike
Building 38A, Bethesda, MD, 20892, United States of America
Contact: Ms Jean Cahill, Grants Management Officer

The National Human Genome Institute (NHGRI) was originally established in 1989 as the National Center for Human Genome Research (NCHGR). Its mission is to head the Human Genome Project for the National Institutes of Health (NIH). NHGRI is one of 24 institutes, centres, or divisions that make up the NIH, the Federal US Government's primary agent for the support of biomedical research. The collective research components of the NIH make up the largest biomedical research facility in the world. NIH is part of the US Department of Health and Human Services. To carry out these diverse duties, NHGRI is organised into several administrative units.

Ethical, Legal and Social Implications of Human Genome Research - Research

Subjects: All subjects.

Genome Informatics Programme Research Grants

Subjects: All subjects.

Genome Science and Technology Centres Research Grant

Subjects: All subjects.

Pilot Projects or Feasibility Studies for Genomic Mapping, Sequencing and Analysis - Research Grants

Subjects: All subjects.

Small Business Innovation Research Programme - Research Grants

Subjects: All subjects.

Small Business Technology Transfer Programme - Research Grants

Subjects: All subjects.

Technologies for Genomic Mapping, Sequencing and Analysis Research Grants

Subjects: All subjects.

NATIONAL INSTITUTE OF GENERAL MEDICAL SCIENCES (NIGMS)

45 Center Drive
MSC 6200, Bethesda, MD, 20892-6200, United States of America
Tel: (1) 301 496 7301
Fax: (1) 301 402 0224
Email: pub_info@nigms.nih.gov
www: http://www.nih.gov/nigms/
Contact: Office of Communications and Public Liaison

The NIGMS is a component of the National Institutes of Health, the biomedical agency of the US government. NIGMS supports biomedical research that is not targeted to specific diseases, but that increases understanding of life processes and lays the foundation for advances in disease diagnosis, treatment and prevention.

MARC Faculty Predoctoral Fellowships

Subjects: Biomedicine.
Eligibility: Applicants must be full time faculty members in a biomedically related science or mathematics programme for at least three years at the time of submission.
Level of Study: Postgraduate.
Purpose: To provide an opportunity for faculty who lack the PhD degree to obtain the research doctorate.
No. of awards offered: Varies.
Frequency: Annual.
Value: An applicant may request a stipend equal to his or her annual salary, but not to exceed the stipend of a level 1 postdoctoral fellow. The applicant may also request tuition and fees as determined by the training institution as well as an allowance of US$2,000 per year for training related costs.
Study Establishment: A US institution.
Country of Study: USA.
Application Procedure: Please write for details or contact Dr Adolphus Toliver, tel: 1 301 594 3900. Further details are also available from the website: http://www.nih.gov/nigms.

NIGMS Fellowship Awards for Minority Students

Subjects: Biomedicine and the behavioural sciences.
Eligibility: Eligible for this award are highly qualified students who are members of minority groups that are under-represented in the biomedical or behavioural sciences in the United States. These groups include African Americans, Hispanic Americans, Native Americans, and Natives of the Pacific Islands.
Level of Study: Postgraduate, Predoctorate.
Purpose: The intent of this fellowship programme is to encourage students from minority groups who are underrepresented in the biomedical and behavioural sciences to seek graduate degrees, and thus further the goal of increasing the number of minority scientists who are prepared to pursue careers in this field.
No. of awards offered: Varies.
Frequency: Annual.

Value: The fellowship provides an annual stipend of US$14,688; a tuition fee allowance; and an annual institution fee of US$2,000, which may be used for travel to scientific meetings and for laboratory and other training expenses.
Length of Study: Up to 5 years.
Country of Study: USA.
Application Procedure: Please write for details or contact Dr Adolphus Toliver, tel: 1 301 594 3900. Further information is also available from the website: http://www.nih.gov/nigms.

NIGMS Fellowship Awards for Students With Disabilities

Subjects: Biomedicine and the behavioural sciences.
Eligibility: Please write for details.
Level of Study: Postgraduate, Predoctorate.
Purpose: The intent of this fellowship programme is to encourage students with disabilities to seek graduate degrees, and thus further the goal of increasing the number of scientists with disabilities who are prepared to pursue careers in biomedical and behavioural research.
No. of awards offered: Varies.
Frequency: Annual.
Value: The fellowship provides an annual stipend of US$14,668; a tuition fee allowance; and an annual institution fee of US$2,000, which may be used for travel to scientific meetings and for laboratory and other training expenses.
Length of Study: Up to 5 years.
Study Establishment: A US institution.
Country of Study: USA.
Application Procedure: Please write for details or contact Dr Anthony René, tel: 1 301 594 3833.

NIGMS Postdoctoral Awards

Subjects: Biomedicine.
Eligibility: The applicant must have received the doctoral degree (domestic or foreign), and must have had at least seven years of relevant research experience.
Level of Study: Postdoctorate.
Purpose: NIGMS welcomes NRSA applications from eligible individuals who seek postdoctoral biomedical research training in areas related to the scientific programs of the Institute.
No. of awards offered: Varies.
Frequency: Annual.
Value: The stipend awarded a senior fellow may range up to US$41,268 per 12 month period, based on the salary of the applicant at the time of the award.
Study Establishment: The institutional setting may be domestic or foreign, public or private.
Country of Study: Any country.
Application Procedure: Please write for details.

NIGMS Research Project Grants

Subjects: Biomedicine.
Eligibility: A research project grant is awarded to an eligible institution on behalf of a principal investigator.
Level of Study: Postgraduate.

Purpose: To support a discrete project related to the investigator's area of interest and competence.
Type: Research Grant.
No. of awards offered: Varies.
Frequency: Annual.
Value: These grants may provide funds for reasonable costs of the research activity, as well as for salaries, equipment, supplies, travel, and other related expenses.
Country of Study: USA.
Application Procedure: Please write for details, or contact the Office of Extramural Outreach and Information Resources, Office of Extramural Research, NIH, Room 6207, 6701 Rockledge Drive, MSC 7910, Bethesda, MD 20892-7910, tel: 1 301 435 0714, Email grantsinfo@nih.gov.
Additional Information: Research grants may be awarded to nonprofit organisations and institutions, governments and their agencies, and occasionally to individuals who have access to adequate facilities and resources for conducting the research, as well as profit making organisations. Foreign institutions and international organisations are also eligible to apply for these grants.

NIGMS Research Supplements for Underrepresented Minorities

Subjects: Biomedicine.
Eligibility: Please write for details.
Level of Study: Unrestricted.
Purpose: To help minority scientists and students develop their capabilities for independent research careers.
Type: Research Supplements.
No. of awards offered: Varies.
Frequency: Annual.
Value: Varies.
Length of Study: 2 years.
Study Establishment: A US institution.
Country of Study: USA.
Application Procedure: Please write for details or contact Dr Anthony René, tel: 1 3014 594 3833. Further information is available from the website http://www.nih.gov/nigms.

NATIONAL INSTITUTE ON AGING

GW 218, Bethesda, MD, 20892, United States of America
Tel: (1) 301 496 9322
Fax: (1) 301 402 2945
Email: mk46u@nihigov
www: http://www.nih.gov
Contact: Dr Miriam Kelty, Associate Director

The National Institute on Ageing conducts and supports research and research training in all facts of biological ageing, the neuroscience and neuropsychology of ageing, geriatrics, and the social and behavioural sciences of ageing.

NIH Research Grants

Subjects: The biology of ageing neuroscience and neuropsychology of ageing, geriatrics, and social and behavioural sciences of ageing.
Eligibility: Varies, depending on mechanism, but generally open to US citizens only.
Level of Study: Postdoctorate, Professional development.
Purpose: To support research and training in biological, clinical, behavioral and social aspects of ageing mechanisms and processes.
Type: Research Grants, Fellowships, Career Development Awards, Institutional Training Awards.
No. of awards offered: Varies.
Frequency: Annual.
Value: Varies.
Length of Study: 1-5 years.
Country of Study: USA and others depending on mechanism.
Application Procedure: Please write for application form PHS 398 or access it on the WWW.
Closing Date: Staggered, please see form PHS 398.
Additional Information: For further information refer to NIH home page.

NATIONAL KIDNEY FOUNDATION OF SOUTH AFRICA

PO Box 891
Houghton, Johannesburg, 2041, South Africa
Tel: (27) 11 484 7547
Fax: (27) 11 2711 6438777
Email: 014alwyn@cahiron.wits.ac.za
Contact: Secretary

Charlotte Roberts Trust Kidney Research Award

Subjects: Kidney disease.
Eligibility: Open to suitably qualified medical practitioners and allied medical workers registered in South Africa.
Level of Study: Professional development.
Purpose: To sponsor a suitable person on a short-term overseas visit devoted to research or study.
Type: Travel Grant.
No. of awards offered: 1-2.
Frequency: Every two years.
Value: R20,000 (if more then one applicant is successful, the grant money wil be divided between them).
Length of Study: Varies.
Study Establishment: An appropriate research institute or university department.
Country of Study: Any country.
Application Procedure: Applications should include the completed application form, a summary of the proposed study, evidence of suitability to undertake the research

programme, and names and addresses of two referees. Application forms are available from mid-march from the National Kidney Foundation.
Closing Date: July 15th 2000.
Additional Information: In determining the award, the value of the proposed research project to kidney research in South Africa is taken into consideration. The award will not be disbursed until the Foundation is satisfied that the successful applicant has been accepted by an appropriate research institute or university department, and the recipient must undertake to return to South Africa on the termination of the project and to submit a comprehensive report on the research.

NATIONAL KIDNEY RESEARCH FUND

King's Chambers
Priestgate, Peterborough, Cambridgeshire, PE1 1FG, England
Tel: (44) 1733 704650
Fax: (44) 1733 704699
Contact: Mr Sam Badni

The National Kidney Research Fund aims to advance and promote research into kidney and renal disease generally; the acute failure of kidneys and chronic renal failure; and congenital malformations of the kidney and bladder. The Fund's research also incorporates the development of artificial kidney and dialysis machines.

NKRF Research Project Grants

Subjects: Renal research projects.
Eligibility: Open to suitably qualified researchers of any nationality. Work must be carried out in the United Kingdom.
Level of Study: Unrestricted.
Purpose: To support renal research.
No. of awards offered: Varies.
Frequency: Annual.
Value: Up to £75,000.
Length of Study: 1-3 years.
Country of Study: United Kingdom.
Application Procedure: Applications forms are available from Department RG.
Closing Date: Please write for details.

NKRF Senior Fellowships

Subjects: Scientific aspects of renal medicine.
Eligibility: Open to postdoctoral researchers in the biomedical field with evidence of independent research, including two years' postdoctoral research. Applicants may be of any nationality, but project work must be carried out in the UK.
Level of Study: Postdoctorate.
Purpose: To support renal research projects.
Type: Fellowship.
No. of awards offered: Varies.

Frequency: Annual.
Value: Salary will be at Registrar/Senior Registrar level or at the appropriate university scale. An allowance for consumables and minor equipment is available, and technical support.
Length of Study: 3-5 years, subject to review in the third year.
Country of Study: United Kingdom.
Application Procedure: Application forms are available from Department SF.
Closing Date: Please write for details.

NKRF Special Project Grants

Subjects: Renal disease.
Eligibility: Open to suitably qualified researchers of any nationality.
Level of Study: Professional development.
Purpose: To provide support for substantial projects in scientific disciplines related to renal disease and its management.
Type: Grant.
No. of awards offered: Varies.
Frequency: Annual.
Value: Up to £150,000.
Length of Study: 3 years.
Country of Study: United Kingdom.
Application Procedure: Applications forms are available from Department SP.
Closing Date: Please write for details.

NKRF Studentships

Subjects: Renal medicine.
Eligibility: Open to applicants of any nationality. Project work must take place in the United Kingdom.
Level of Study: Postgraduate.
Purpose: To support renal research projects.
Type: Studentship.
No. of awards offered: Varies.
Frequency: Annual.
Value: University fees are met by the NKRF, and a bench fee is available to the host institution. Student stipend of £10,000 per year in London or £9,000 elsewhere.
Length of Study: 3 years, subject to a satisfactory annual report.
Country of Study: United Kingdom.
Application Procedure: Applications are available from Department S.
Closing Date: Please write for details.

NKRF Training Fellowships

Subjects: Renal medicine and related scientific studies.
Eligibility: Open to medical candidates of immediate post-registration to Registrar level and to science candidates with a PhD or DPhil.
Level of Study: Postgraduate.
Purpose: To enable medical or scientific graduates to undertake specialized training in the renal field.
Type: Fellowship.

No. of awards offered: Varies.
Frequency: Annual.
Value: Level of financial support will be based on an appropriate point on current NHS or university pay scales. A training support allowance will be available to the host institution.
Length of Study: 1-3 years, subject to annual review.
Country of Study: United Kingdom.
Application Procedure: Application forms are available from Department TF.
Closing Date: Please write for details.

NATIONAL LIBRARY OF MEDICINE

8600 Rockville Pike
Building 38A, Bethesda, MD, 20894, United States of America
Tel: (1) 301 496 4221
Fax: (1) 301 402 0421
Email: shelley_carow@nlm.nih.gov
www: http://www.nlm.nih.gov
Contact: Ms Shelley Carow, Grants Management Officer

As the nation's premier repository of bio medical information, NLM has a vital interest in information management and in the enormous utility of computers and telecommunications for improving storage, retrieval, access and use of bio medical information. The Library offers support for qualified investigators, be they individuals or institutions, in three separate but related programme areas: medical informatics, biotechnology information and health sciences library and information science.

NLM Fellowship in Applied Informatics

Subjects: Health informatics.
Eligibility: Individuals with a BA/BSc, MA/MSc or PhD in a field related to health, who are US nationals or permanent residents of the US.
Level of Study: Doctorate, Graduate, Postdoctorate, Postgraduate.
Purpose: To improve the American healthcare system by educating health professionals in the technology of health informatics, thus enabling them to help solve biomedical information management problems.
Type: Fellowship.
Frequency: Annual.
Value: Up to US$58,000 per annum, based on the salary or renumeration the individual would have been paid from their home institution.
Length of Study: Varies.
Study Establishment: Universities, colleges, hospitals, laboratories, units of State and certain agencies of the Federal Government in the US.
Country of Study: USA.
Application Procedure: Applications must be submitted by an organisation on behalf of the individual seeking the scholarship, on the standard grant application form PHS 416-

1 (rev 8/95). Application forms are available from Extramural Outreach/ Information Resources, National Institute of Health, 6701 Rockledge Drive, MSC 7910, Bethesda, MD 20892-7910, USA. Tel: 1 301 435 0714, fax: 1 301 480 0525, email: grantsinfo@nih.gov. The completed original and two legible copies, the Personal Data form, the Check list, appendix material, sealed references and other required information must then be sent to: Center for Scientific Review, National Institute of Health, 6701 Rockledge Drive, MSC 7710, Suite 1040, Bethesda, MD 20892-7710, USA (Or Bethesda, MD 20817-7710, USA for express/courier service).

Closing Date: April 5th, August 5th, December 5th.

Additional Information: The NLM encourages potential applicants to clafify any issues or questions. For enquiries regarding programmematic issues, please contact Peter Clepper, Programme Officer, Division of Extramural Programmes, National Library of Medicine, Rockledge One Building, Suite 301, 6705 Rockledge Drive, Bethesda, MD 20892, USA. Tel: 1 301 594 4882, fax: 1 301 402 2952, email: peter_clepper@nlm.nih.gov. For enquiries regarding Division of Nursing programmematic issues, please contact: Division of Nursing, Parklawn Building, Room 9-36, 5600 Fishers Lane, Rockville, MD 20857, USA. Tel: 1 301 443 5786, Fax: 1 301 443 8586. For enquiries regarding fiscal matters, please contact: Ms Shelley Carrow, Grants Management Officer, Division of Extramural Programmes, National Library of Medicine, Tel: 1 301 496 4221, Fax: 1 301 402 0421, email: shelley_carrow@nlm.nih.gov.

NLM Integrated Advanced Information Management System (IAIMS) Apprenticeships

Subjects: Health sciences administration, education, research and/or clinical care.

Eligibility: Promising graduate and doctoral students. Requirements depend on the principle investigator of the IAIMS, but doctoral degrees are usually not mandatory.

Level of Study: Doctorate, Predoctorate.

Purpose: To allow promising graduate and doctoral students to participate in the IAIMS projects. The goal of these projects is to create an organisational mechanism to manage more effectively the knowledge of medicine, and provide for a system of comprehensive and convenient information access.

Type: Apprenticeship.

Value: Up to US$50,000 per annum.

Study Establishment: Established Integrated Advanced Information Management Systems.

Country of Study: USA.

Application Procedure: Details available from Fact Sheets, Office of Public Information, National Library of Medicine, 8600 Rockville Pike, Bethesda, Maryland 20894, USA. Fax: 1 301 496 4450, email: publicinfo@nlm.nih.gov, or on the website: http://www.nlm.nih.gov.

Closing Date: Please write for details.

NLM Investigator Initiated Project Grant

Subjects: Medical informatics, biotechnology information, health sciences library/information science.

Purpose: To support individual investigators and their colleagues to pursue a discreet, circumscribed line of investigation to its logical conclusion.

Type: Project Grant.

Frequency: Three times each year.

Length of Study: Up to 3 years.

Study Establishment: US universities or research institutions.

Country of Study: USA.

Application Procedure: Applications must be submitted on the PHS form 398 (rev 5/95) which is available from Extramural Outreach/Information Resources, National Institute of Health, 6701 Rockledge drive, MSC 7910, Bethesda, MD 20892-7910, USA. Tel: 1 301 435 0714, fax: 1 301 480 0525, email: grantsinfo@nih.gov.

Closing Date: February 1st, June 1st, October 1st.

Additional Information: For further information and assistance, please contact: Peter Clepper, Division of Extramural Programs, National Library of Medicine, Rockledge One Building, 6705 Rockledge Drive, Suite 301, Bethesda, MD 20892, USA. Tel: 1 301 594 4882, fax: 1 301 402 2952, email: peter_clepper@nlm.nih.gov.

NLM Publication Grant Programme

Subjects: Medical and health sciences.

Eligibility: Public or private, non profit institutions and individuals, who are involved in research.

Purpose: To provide assistance for the preparation of book length manuscripts and, in some cases, the publication of important scientific information needed by US health professionals.

Type: Project Grant.

Frequency: Three times each year.

Value: US$35,000 direct costs per annum over a period of 3 years maximum.

Length of Study: 1 to 3 years.

Country of Study: USA.

Application Procedure: Applications must be submittted on the PHS FORM 398 (Rev 5/95) grant application kit, which is available from Extramural Outreach/ Information Resources, National Institutes of Health, 6701 Rockledge Drive, MSC 7910, Bethesda, MD 20892-7910, tel: 1 301 435 0714, fax: 1 480 0525, email: grantsinfo@nih.gov.

Closing Date: February 1st, June 1st, October 1st.

Additional Information: Potential applicants are strongly encouraged to discuss projects early with the Programme staff, who will discuss programme status and experience with them, provide additional information in response to specific application plans and review draft proposals for completeness if desired. For further information please contact Publication Grant Programme, Division of Extramural Programmes, National Library of Medicine, Rockledge One Building, Suite 301, 6705 Rockledge Drive, Bethesda, MD 20892, USA. Tel: 1 301 594 4882, fax: 1 301 402 2952, email: sparks@nlm.nih.gov or refer to the website http://www.nlm.nih.gov/pubs/factssheet/pubgrant.html. For a complete list of NLM Factsheet, please contact Factsheets, Office of Public Information, National Library of Medicine, 8600 Rockville Pike, Bethesda Maryland 20894, USA. Fax: 1 301 496 4450, email: publicinfo@nlm.nih.gov.

THE NATIONAL MULTIPLE SCLEROSIS SOCIETY

733 Third Avenue, New York, NY, 10017, United States of America
Tel: (1) 212 986 3240
Fax: (1) 212 986 7981
Email: nat@nmss.org
www: http://www.nmss.org
Contact: Grants Management Officer

The National Multiple Sclerosis Society is dedicated to ending the devastating effects of multiple sclerosis.

National Multiple Sclerosis Society Junior Faculty Awards

Subjects: Neurosciences related to multiple sclerosis.
Eligibility: Open to US citizens holding a doctoral degree who have had sufficient research training at the pre or postdoctoral levels to be capable of independent research. Individuals who have already carried out independent research for more than five years are not eligible.
Level of Study: Professional development.
Purpose: To enable highly qualified persons who have concluded their research training and have begun academic careers as independent investigators, to undertake independent research.
No. of awards offered: Varies.
Frequency: Annual.
Value: Approximately US$75,000 per year.
Length of Study: 5 years.
Study Establishment: An approved US university, professional or research institute.
Country of Study: USA.
Application Procedure: Application form must be completed.
Closing Date: February 1st for awards to become effective July 1st or September 1st.
Additional Information: The candidate will not be an employee of the society, but rather of the institution. It is expected that the institution will develop plans for continuing the candidate's appointment and for continued salary support beyond the five-year period of the award. Fellows may not supplement their salary through private practice or consultation, nor accept another concurrent award. The grantee institution holds title to all equipment purchased with award funds.

National Multiple Sclerosis Society Pilot Research Grants

Subjects: Multiple sclerosis.
Eligibility: Open to suitably qualified investigators.
Level of Study: Established Investigator.
Purpose: To provide limited short-term support of novel high-risk research.
Type: Research Grant.
No. of awards offered: Varies.
Frequency: Dependent on funds available.

Value: Up to US$25,000 in direct costs may be requested for the one-year period.
Length of Study: 1 year.
Country of Study: Any country.
Application Procedure: Application form must be completed.
Closing Date: Applications are accepted at any time.
Additional Information: Grants are awarded to an institution to support the research of the principal investigator. Progress reports are required.

National Multiple Sclerosis Society Postdoctoral Fellowships

Subjects: Training in research applicable to multiple sclerosis.
Eligibility: Open to unusually promising recipients of MD and/or PhD degrees. The programme of training to be supported by the grant must materially enhance the likelihood of the trainee performing meaningful and independent research on multiple sclerosis, and obtaining a suitable position which will enable him to do so. Foreign nationals are welcome to apply for fellowships in the USA only. Besides its attention to younger researchers, the society will also consider applications from established investigators who seek support to obtain specialised training in some field in which they are not expert, when such training will materially enhance their capacity to conduct more meaningful research on multiple sclerosis. US citizenship is not required for training in US institutions; applicants who plan to train in other countries must be US citizens.
Level of Study: Postdoctorate.
Purpose: To provide postdoctoral training which will enhance the likelihood of performing meaningful and independent research relevant to multiple sclerosis.
Type: Fellowship.
No. of awards offered: Varies.
Frequency: Annual.
Value: Varies according to professional status, previous training, accomplishments in research, and to the pay scale of the institution in which the training is provided. Fellowships may be supplemented by other forms of support, with prior approval.
Length of Study: 1-3 years.
Study Establishment: An institution of the candidate's choice.
Country of Study: USA for foreign postdoctoral applicants.
Application Procedure: Application form must be completed.
Closing Date: February 1st for grants to become effective July 1st or thereafter.
Additional Information: These fellowships are awarded to support training in research and are not awarded to support clinical training directed towards the completion of internship and/or specialty board certification. Similarly, they cannot be used to provide support for individuals whose primary responsibility is teaching and/or service, although fellows are encouraged to spend a reasonable amount of their time (up to 10%) in teaching. Fellows are not considered as employees of the society, but rather of the institution where the training is provided; the fellowship is to be administered in accordance with the prevailing policies of the sponsoring

institution. It is the responsibility of the applicant to make all arrangement for his training with the mentor and institution of his choice.

National Multiple Sclerosis Society Research Grants

Subjects: Multiple sclerosis - cause, prevention, alleviation and cure.
Eligibility: Open to suitably qualified investigators.
Level of Study: Professional development.
Purpose: To stimulate, coordinate and support fundamental or applied, clinical or non-clinical research.
Type: Research Grant.
No. of awards offered: Varies.
Frequency: Twice a year.
Value: Funds may be used to pay in whole or in part the salaries of associated professional personnel, technical assistants and other non-professional personnel in proportion to their time spent directly on the project. Salaries are in accordance with the prevailing policies of the grantee institution. If requested, other expenses, such as travel costs and fringe benefits, may also be paid.
Length of Study: 3 years.
Country of Study: Any country.
Application Procedure: Application form must be completed.
Closing Date: February 1st and August 1st for grants to become effective October 1st and April 1st respectively.
Additional Information: Grants are awarded to an institution to support the research of the principal investigator. Scientific equipment and supplies bought with Grant funds become the property of the grantee institution. Progress reports are required, and appropriate publication is expected.

THE NATIONAL ORGANIZATION FOR RARE DISORDERS

PO Box 8923, New Fairfield, CT, 06812-8923, United States of America
Tel: (1) 203 746 6518
Fax: (1) 203 746 5418
Email: orphan@rarediseases.org
www: http://www.rarediseases.org
Contact: Ms Maria T Hardin, Vice President of Patient Services

NORD is the federation of voluntary health oragnisations dedicated to helping people with rare (orphan) diseases and assisting the organizations that serve them. NORD is committed to the identification, treatment and cure of rare disorders through programs of advocacy, education, research and service.

NORD Clinical Research Grants

Subjects: New treatments for rare diseases - medical research.

Eligibility: Open to American academic scientists.
Level of Study: Doctorate, Postdoctorate, Professional development.
Purpose: To support small clinical trials.
Type: Research Grant.
No. of awards offered: 3-4.
Frequency: Dependent on funds available.
Value: US$20,000 to US$50,000 per year.
Length of Study: Up to 2 years.
Country of Study: USA.
Application Procedure: An application form must be completed.
Closing Date: Inquiries are accepted at any time for future announcements.

NATIONAL RESEARCH COUNCIL OF CANADA

Recruitment Unit
Montreal Road
M58, Ottawa, ON, K1A 0R6, Canada
Tel: (1) 613 998 4126
Fax: (1) 613 990 7669
Email: ra.coordinator@nrc.ca
www: http://www.nrc.ca
Contact: Research Associates Co-ordinator

NRC is a dynamic, nationwide R&D organisation committed to helping Canada realize its potential as an innovative and competitive nation.

Industrial Research Assistance Program

Subjects: All subjects.
Eligibility: Recent college and university graduates who are unemployed or under employed.
Purpose: To help small and medium sized Canadian firms (SMEs) create and adopt innovative technologies that yield new products, create high quality jobs, and make industry more competitive. Another aim is to give recent university and college graduates who are unemployed or underemployed a chance to develop their work skills with SMEs in Canada.
Type: Internship.
No. of awards offered: Up to 1000 internships.
Study Establishment: Small and medium sized businesses in Canada.
Country of Study: Canada.
Application Procedure: Contact the Industrial Research Assistance Programme (IRAP) on the internet: http://pub.irap.nrc.ca/IRAP/web/IRAPcomm.nsf/Home or write to the National Research Council of Canada, Montreal Road, M58, Ottawa, Ontario, K1A OR6.
Additional Information: The programme administers two internship programmes : the Science and Technology Internships Programme and the Science Collaborative Research Internships Programme. Please write for more details or visit the website:http://pub.irap.nrc.ca/IRAP/web/IRAPcomm.nsf/home.

NATIONAL STRENGTH AND CONDITIONING ASSOCIATION

1955 N Union, Colorado Springs, CO, 80909-2229, United States of America
Tel: (1) 719 632 6722
Fax: (1) 719 632 6367
Email: nsca@usa.net
www: http://www.nsca-lift.org/
Contact: Ms Karri Todd Baker, Member Relations Co-ordinator

The National Strength and Conditioning Association is a non-profit, educational organisation dedicated to strength and conditioning for improved physical performance. Now in its 20th year of operation, the NSCA is regarded as the world-wide authority on strength and conditioning.

NSCA Challenge Scholarship

Subjects: A strength and conditioning related field.
Eligibility: Applicants must be NSCA members for at least one year from the application deadline. Must be seeking either an undergraduate or graduate degree in a strength and conditioning-related field.
Level of Study: Postgraduate, Undergraduate.
Purpose: To financially assist members in their pursuit of a career in strength and conditioning.
Type: Scholarship.
No. of awards offered: 1-5 dependent on applications.
Frequency: Annual.
Value: US$1,000.
Study Establishment: Unrestricted.
Country of Study: Any country.
Application Procedure: Applicants must submit: a current resume, cover letter of application, and three current letters of recommendation; an original copy of an authorised transcript from all post-secondary schools attended; an essay of no more than 500 words describing course of study, career goals and need. All material must be mailed together and postmarked by March 1st.
Closing Date: March 1st.

NSCA Student Grant Research Grant

Subjects: Strength and conditioning.
Eligibility: NSCA members who have been members for at least one year from the application deadline. Graduate students, who are members, and are studying in the field of strength and conditioning are invited to apply. A graduate faculty member is required to serve as co-investigator in the study.
Level of Study: Postgraduate.
Purpose: To fund graduate student research in strength and conditioning that is directed by a graduate faculty member.
Type: Grant.
No. of awards offered: Varies, dependent on number of applications.
Frequency: Annual.

Value: Up toUS$2,500.
Length of Study: 1 year.
Study Establishment: Unrestricted.
Country of Study: Any country.
Application Procedure: A grant application submission to the NSCA Student Grant Programme should contain the following sections, not to exceed 10 single-spaced pages. Project title, student investigator with NSCA membership number, proof of enrollement, institution, address, phone, fax and email, abstract, brief review of literature, importance of project to the field, limited bibliography, methods, statistical analysis, itemised budget, "Human Subjects Consent Form" and proof of institutional review board approval, proposed time schedule, abbreviated (3 pages) curriculum vitae of faculty co-investigator.
Closing Date: Letter of intent February 3rd; grant application March 17th.
Additional Information: Application form can be accessed via our website or call 719 632 6722.

NATIONAL UNIVERSITY OF SINGAPORE

Registrar's Office
10 Kent Ridge Crescent, 119074, Singapore
Tel: (65) 874 6576
Fax: (65) 773 1462
Email: reggen42@nus.edu.sg
www: http://www.nus.edu.sg
Contact: Grants Management Officer

ASEAN Graduate Scholarships

Subjects: Graduate studies by coursework leading to the following degrees - MA in English studies, Chinese studies, Southeast Asian studies, urban design, Master of social sciences in economics, applied psychology, social work, applied sociology, Master in public policy, Master of architecture, Master of business administration (English and Chinese medium), Master of dental surgery in oral and maxillofacial surgery, endodontics, orthodontics and prosthodontics, Master of laws, Master of comparative law, Master of clinical embryology, Master of medicine in anaesthesiology, diagnostic radiology, internal medicine, obstetrics & gynaecology, occupational medicine, ophthalmology, paediatric, public health, psychiatry, surgery, Master of science in project management, building science, real estate, management of technology, chemical engineering, civil engineering, electrical engineering, environmental engineering, industrial & systems engineering, material science & engineering, mechanical engineering, safety, health & environmental technology, transportation systems & management, computer & information sciences, Asia-Pacific human resource management, mathematics.
Eligibility: Open to citizens of ASEAN member countries (except Singapore).
Level of Study: Postgraduate.

Purpose: To provide outstanding candidates, from member countries of the Association of Southeast Asian Nations (ASEAN), an opportunity to pursue postgraduate studies at the National University of Singapore.
Type: Scholarship.
No. of awards offered: 10.
Frequency: Annual.
Value: Stipend of S$1,350 each month, a once-only book allowance of S$500, approved fees and expenses, etc.
Study Establishment: National University of Singapore.
Country of Study: Singapore.
Application Procedure: Application forms for the designated degrees must be completed and submitted with supporting documents to the respective Faculties/Graduate Schools.
Closing Date: Concurrent with the closing date of graduate courses of the respective Faculties/Graduate Schools.
Additional Information: ASEAN is the abbreviation for the Association of South East Asian Nation and it comprises the following 9 nations in South East Asia- Brunei, Indonesia, Laos, Malaysia, Myanmar, Philippines, Singapore, Thailand and Vietnam, as on November 1998.

Lee Foundation and Tan Sri Dr Runme Shaw Foundation Fellowships in Orthopaedic Surgery

Subjects: Orthopaedic surgery, hand and reconstructive microsurgery.
Eligibility: Open to doctors from developing countries who have a first medical degree with a minimum of four years' postgraduate experience, of which at least two years must have been in orthopaedic surgery or at least one year must have been in orthopaedic surgery after the completion of basic surgical training. Applicants must be fluent in English. The applicant to be selected for hand and reconstructive microsurgery should have completed his basic orthopaedic training in his own country.
Level of Study: Postgraduate.
Purpose: To offer the opportunity for clinical hospital attachment.
Type: Fellowship.
No. of awards offered: 4 of each fellowship.
Frequency: Annual.
Value: Approximately S$1,200 monthly.
Length of Study: 6 months.
Study Establishment: National University Hospital or at Singapore General Hospital.
Country of Study: Singapore.
Application Procedure: Applicants should write for application form and return it to the Graduate School for Medical Studies , National University of Singapore, Lower Kent Ridge Road, Singapore, 119074.
Closing Date: July 29th.

Mobil-NUS Postgraduate Medical Research Scholarship

Subjects: Anaesthesiology, community, occupational and family medicine, diagnostic radiology, internal medicine, obstetrics and gynaecology, opthamology, orthapaedic surgery, otolaryngology, paediatric medicine, pathology, psychological medicine, surgery.
Eligibility: Applicants must have an MBBS degree or its equivalent, at least three years of post-registration clinical experience in the relevant speciality, an outstanding academic record, and a good command of the English language (determined by a pass of at least 580 marks in TOEFL/a minimal band of 7 and above in IELTS).
Level of Study: Postgraduate.
Purpose: To provide the opportunity for postgraduate medical research in various clinical disciplines.
Type: Scholarship.
No. of awards offered: 20.
Frequency: Twice a year.
Value: Aprox. S$2,000 monthly.
Length of Study: 2 years.
Study Establishment: National University of Singapore.
Country of Study: Singapore.
Application Procedure: Applicants should write for an application form to the Graduate School of Medical Studies, National University of Singapore, Lower Kent Ridge Road, Singapore, 119074, fax (65) 773 1462.
Closing Date: March 1st.

National University of Singapore Postgraduate Research Scholarship

Subjects: Science, humanities, business.
Eligibility: Open to graduates with at least an Honours Class II Upper Bachelor's degree, or equivalent.
Level of Study: Doctorate, Postgraduate.
Purpose: To encourage qualified candidates to pursue postgraduate research in their fields of interest in NUS.
Type: Scholarship.
No. of awards offered: 410.
Frequency: Annual.
Value: S$1,200 - S$1,400 plus full fee subsidy over 2-3 years.
Length of Study: 2 or 3 years.
Study Establishment: NUS.
Country of Study: Singapore.
Application Procedure: Application form must be completed.
Closing Date: Usually mid-May and mid-December.

NATIVE AMERICAN SCHOLARSHIP FUND, INC.

8200 Mountain Road NE
Suite 203, Albuquerque, NM, 87110, United States of America
Tel: (1) 505 262 2351
Fax: (1) 505 262 0534
Email: nasf@nasf.com
www: http://nasf.com/
Contact: Ms Lucille Kelley, Director of Recruitment

NASF offers 2 scholarship programmes. The math, education, science, business, engineering and computer science (MESBEC) provides scholarships to native Americans studying in these fields. The Native American Leadership in Education (NALE) is for Native Americans who are para-professionals in the schools. It helps them to complete their college degrees and earn teaching credentials, administrative certification, and counsellor certification. NASF fund Indian students in other fields such as humanities, fine arts, and social science. Students must be a quarter or more American Indian and enrolled with their tribe.

Native American Scholarship Program

Subjects: All subjects.
Eligibility: Restricted to US citizens of Native American Indian and Alaskan Native ancestry.
Level of Study: Unrestricted.
Purpose: To provide scholarships to high-potential Native American students in the fields that are critical for the political, economic, social and business development of American Indian tribes.
Type: Scholarship.
No. of awards offered: 190.
Frequency: Annual.
Value: US$500 - US$2,500 per academic year.
Length of Study: 4 years.
Study Establishment: An accredited college or university.
Country of Study: USA.
Application Procedure: Please write to reques for application forms.
Closing Date: September 15th for spring, April 15th for fall, and March 15th for summer.

NATURAL SCIENCES AND ENGINEERING RESEARCH COUNCIL (NSERC)

350 Albert Street, Ottawa, ON, K1A 1H5, Canada
Tel: (1) 613 996 3769
Fax: (1) 613 996 2589
Email: schol@nserc.ca
www: http://www.nserc.ca
Contact: Scholarships and Fellowships Branch

The Natural Sciences and Engineering Research Council of Canada (NSERC) is the national instrument for making strategic investments in Canada's capability in science and technology. NSERC supports both basic university research through research grants and project grants and project research through partnerships of universities with industry, as well as advanced training of high qualified people in both areas.

NSERC New Faculty Support Grants

Subjects: All subjects.
Eligibility: The proposed position must be the candidate's first tenured or tenure track appointment in a Canadian university. The candidate should have obtained their PhD in the last five years (not counting period of leave taken to bring up children) and must be qualified for appointment at assistant appointment level, or higher, in a tenured, or tenure track position.
Level of Study: Postdoctorate, Research.
Purpose: To assist universities, jointly with industry, to recruit and place highly qualified persons in junior level faculty positions in research areas of interest to industry.
Type: A variable number of Grants.
No. of awards offered: Varies.
Frequency: Annual, if funds are available.
Value: NSERC provides a grant equivalent to a cash contribution from the industrial sector. The minimum cash contribution from the industrial sector is C$25,000 per annum. The maximum grant available from NSERC is C$75,000 per annum.
Length of Study: Varies.
Study Establishment: Any Canadian university.
Country of Study: Canada.
Application Procedure: There is no application form, but the proposal must contain a Personal Data Form (Form 100) for the candidate; at least three letters of recommendation to support the nomination of the candidate, which should include letters from supervisors of the candidate's doctoral and postdoctoral research; a letter from the candidate indicating their interest in the position and the reasons for wishing to take up the appointment; a statement from an appropriate authority at the university indicating how the candidate fits within the university's recruitment plans and its research strategy, priorities and strengths. Confirmation of the intent to appoint the candidate in a tenured or tenure track position must be included; confirmation from the university of space and basic research facilities for the new appointee; a statement of commitment from the sponsoring corporation including its level of financial support, the reasons it has chosen to sponsor the candidate, and the benefits the corporation expects to accrue from its participation; and a three year budget summary outlining how the contributions of the NSERC, the company and the university will be dispersed.
Closing Date: Proposals may be submitted at any time.

NETHERLANDS GOVERNMENT

Royal Netherlands Embassy
120 Empire Circuit, Yarralumla, ACT, 2600, Australia
Tel: (61) 6 273 3111
Fax: (61) 6 273 3206
Email: nlgovcan@ozemail.com.au
Contact: Grants Management Officer

Huygens Programme

Subjects: All subjects.
Eligibility: Students who have completed or are near completion of a higher education programme, and who hold or are about to be awarded a higher education degree or diploma. Applicants must be no older than 35; have a good command of Dutch or English; have graduated no longer than two years previously, unless the application is for PhD

research; be able to stay in the Netherlands for at least three months; have an admission letter of the host institute indicating how prospective study falls within the framework of institutional co-operation; and be an Australian citizen.

Level of Study: Postgraduate.

Purpose: The Huygens Programme aims to promote the influx of talented foreign students from countries with which the Netherlands has concluded a cultural agreement; and from countries which the Dutch Ministry of Education, Culture and Science has concluded agreements on the award of the scholarships.

Type: Scholarship.

No. of awards offered: 500 worldwide.

Frequency: Annual.

Value: The scholarship includes: a monthly allowance of f1545 for board, lodging and books. This allowance is sufficient for one person only; travel costs from and to your country (up to f500 for EU countries, f1000 for Central and Eastern European countries and f2,500 for other countries); reimbursement of necessary travel expenses in the Netherlands (second-class rail); exemtion from the statutory tuition fees at Dutch institutes of higher education; medical insurance (not including dental treatment); costs of application for permission to stay in the Netherlands.

Length of Study: 3-12 months.

Study Establishment: A university, art academy, school of music or other institute of tertiary education.

Country of Study: Netherlands.

Application Procedure: Applicants are required to submit the following documents in fourfold: a completed application form, with annexes; photocopies of degrees diplomas and academic records; results of English language tests (TOEFL/IELTS) (if English is not their native language); curriculum vitate; motivation for applying for scholarship; two refernce letters from academic supervisors; admisssion letter from the Dutch host institution; a copy of their passport (only for countries where authorization is required for temorary stay); if necessary, a letter stating that, if the institution fee is higher than the statuatory fee for the academic year for which they are applying, they are willing to pay the extra fee themselves. All the documents have to be in English or Dutch (original or translation). Artists are required to include some photographs of their work, and musicians a tape of their performance.

Closing Date: Febrary 1st.

NETHERLANDS ORGANIZATION FOR INTERNATIONAL CO-OPERATION IN HIGHER EDUCATION

NUFFIC
PO Box 29777, The Hague, NL-2502 LT, Netherlands
Tel: (31) 70 4260 260
Fax: (31) 70 4260 229
Email: nuffic@nuffics.nl
www: http://www.nufficcs.nl
Contact: Information Department

Since its founding in 1952, NUFFIC has been an independent non-profit organisation. Its mission is to foster international co-operation in higher education. Special attention is given to development co-operation.

European Development Fund Awards for Citizens of ACP Countries

Subjects: All subjects.

Eligibility: Open to citizens of the African, Caribbean and Pacific countries associated with the European Union.

Level of Study: Unrestricted.

No. of awards offered: Varies.

Value: Course fees, books and field trips, international travel expenses, insurance, monthly allowance and stipend to cover the initial expenseof getting established.

Length of Study: For the duration of the course.

Country of Study: Countries associated with the European Union, ACP countries.

Application Procedure: Information and application forms can be obtained from the Netherlands Embassy in the candidate's country and the EU Delegations and offices of the Commission. The application is submitted through the candidate's employer and government. Delegations of the Commission can be found (usually in the capital cities) in the following countries: Angola, Barbados and the Eastern Caribbean, Benin, Botswana, Burkina Faso, Burundi, Cameroon, Cape Verde, Central African Republic, Chad, Congo (Democratic Republic), Congo (Republic), Cote d'Ivoire, Djibouti, Dominican Republic, Eritrea, Ethiopia, Gabon, Gambia, Ghana, Guinea,Guinea Bissau, Guyana, Haiti, Jamaica, Kenya, Lesotho, Liberia, Madagascar, Malawi, Mali, Mauritania, Mauritius, Mozambique, Namibia, Niger, Nigeria, Papua New Guinea, Rwanda, Senegal, Sierra Leone, Solomon Islands, Somalia, Sudan, Suriname, Swaziland, Tanzania, Togo, Trinidad and Tobago, Uganda, Zambia and Zimbabwe. Offices of the Commission can be found in the following countries: Antigua and Barbuda, Bahamas, Belize, Comoros, Equatorial Guinea, Netherlands Antilles and Aruba, New Caledonia, Samoa, Sao Tome and Principe, Seychelles, Tonga and Vanuatu.

Closing Date: Please contact the Commission for details.

Additional Information: NUFFIC does not administer these awards and will not accept applications.

NFP Netherlands Fellowships Programme of Development Co-operation

Subjects: Most of the courses offered by the Institutes for International Education in the Netherlands.

Eligibility: Open to candidates who have the education and work experience required for the course, as well as an adequate command of the language in which it is conducted (usually English, sometimes French). The age limit is 40 for men and 45 for women. It is intended that candidates, upon completion of training, return to their home countries and resume their jobs. When several candidates with comparable qualifications apply, priority will be given to women. Candidates for a fellowship must be nominated by their employer, and formal employment should be continued during the fellowship period. As a rule the candidate's government is required to state its formal support, except in the case of certain development-oriented non-government organisations.

Level of Study: Postgraduate.

Purpose: To develop human potential through education and training mainly in the Netherlands with a view to diminish qualitative and quantitative deficiencies in the availability of trained manpower in developing countries.

Type: Fellowship.

No. of awards offered: Varies.

Value: Normal living expenses, fees and health insurances. International travel expenses are provided only when the course lasts three months or longer.

Length of Study: For the duration of the course in question.

Country of Study: NFP fellowships are used mainly in the Netherlands.

Application Procedure: For information on the nationality eligibility for these fellowships and on the application procedure, candidates should contact the Netherlands Embassy in their own country. Information on the courses for which the Scholarships are available can be obtained from NUFFIC.

Closing Date: Please write for details.

THE NETHERLANDS ORGANIZATION FOR SCIENTIFIC RESEARCH (NWO)

Lann van Nieuw Oost Indie 131
PO Box 93138, The Hague, AC 2509, Netherlands
Tel: (31) 70 344 0640
Fax: (31) 70 385 0971
Email: nwo@nwo.nl
www: http://www.now.nl
Contact: Ms Consolini, Grants Division

The Netherlands Organisation for Scientific Research (NWO) is the central Dutch organisation in the field of fundamental and strategic scientific research. NWO encompasses all fields of scholarships and consequently plays a key role in the development of science, technology and culture in the Netherlands. NWO is an independent organisation which acts as the national research council in the Netherlands. NWO is the largest national sponsor of fundamental scientific research undertaken in the thirteen Dutch universities and provides many types of funding for research driven by intellectual curiousity.

NWO PIONIER Programme

Subjects: All subjects.

Eligibility: Promising Dutch researchers under the age of 40, who wish to explore a new line of research, in an area of study of great national and international importance.

Purpose: To enable brilliant researchers below the age of 40 to set up their own team in order to explore a new line of research, in an area of study of great national and international importance.

Type: A variable number of Grants.

No. of awards offered: Up to 50.

Frequency: Annual.

Value: 200,000 to 400,000 Dutch Guilders per annum per team. The annual budget for the PIONIER programme is 12 million Dutch Guilders.

Length of Study: Up to 5 years.

Study Establishment: Universities or research institutions in the Netherlands.

Country of Study: Netherlands.

Application Procedure: For details and appication forms please contact Ms Consolini at the grants division, tel: 70 344 06 30.

Closing Date: Please write for details.

NWO SPINOZA Programme

Subjects: All subjects.

Eligibility: Dutch scientists under the age of 55, who are internationally recognised leaders in their field of research.

Level of Study: Postdoctorate, Research.
Purpose: To promote excellent research by identifying and rewarding a limited number of scientists with a large grant, thus enabling them to do high profile and prestigious research.
Type: A variable number of Grants.
No. of awards offered: 3-4.
Frequency: Annual.
Value: 2 to 4 million Dutch Guilders per award recipient.
Length of Study: Varies.
Study Establishment: Research schools in the Netherlands.
Country of Study: Netherlands.
Application Procedure: By nomination.
Closing Date: Please write for details.
Additional Information: Further information and application forms are available from: Ms. Consolini at the Grants Division.

TALENT Programme

Subjects: All subjects.
Eligibility: Highly qualified, young post doctoral students who are Dutch nationals or permanent residents of the Netherlands.
Level of Study: Postdoctorate.
Purpose: To promote highly qualified young postdoctoral students who wish to conduct research at a reputable research institute outside the Netherlands. The programme is designed to make a major contribution to the market value of the recipients of TALENT scholarships.
Type: Scholarship.
No. of awards offered: Varies.
Frequency: Annual.
Length of Study: 1 year maximum.
Study Establishment: University or research institute outside the Netherlands.
Country of Study: Any country.
Application Procedure: For details please contact Ms. Consolini at the grants division. Tel: +31 70 344 06 30.
Closing Date: Please write for details.

NETHERLANDS-SOUTH AFRICA ASSOCIATION

Studiefonds voor Zuidafrikanse Studenten NZAV
Keizersgradet 141, Amsterdam, 1015 CK, Netherlands
Tel: (31) 20 624 9318
Fax: (31) 20 638 2596
Email: nzav@pi.net
Contact: Dr S B I Veltanys-Visser, Secretary

Netherlands-South Africa Study Fund

Subjects: All subjects.
Eligibility: Open to nationals of South Africa.
Level of Study: Postgraduate.
Purpose: To support postgraduate study in Holland.
No. of awards offered: 5-10.
Frequency: Twice a year.

Value: 1,100 Dutch Guilders per month.
Length of Study: Up to 1 year.
Country of Study: Netherlands.
Application Procedure: Please write for details.
Closing Date: May 15th and December 15th.

NEW SOUTH WALES CANCER COUNCIL

PO Box 572, Kings Cross, NSW, 2011, Australia
Tel: (61) 2 9334 1944
Fax: (61) 2 9358 1452
Email: indah@nswcc.org.au
www: http://www.nswcc.org.au
Contact: Ms Cathy O'Callaghan, Research Administration Officer

New South Wales Cancer Council Research Programme Grant

Subjects: Cancer research.
Eligibility: Open to investigators with a sufficient record of research achievement in any field of cancer research.
Level of Study: Postdoctorate.
Purpose: To provide relatively long-term, flexible support for cancer researchers.
Type: Research Grant.
No. of awards offered: Varies.
Frequency: Varies, depending on other priorities.
Value: To cover salaries, consumables and equipment.
Length of Study: 3-5 years; potentially renewable based on results.
Study Establishment: An approved institution in New South Wales.
Country of Study: Australia.
Closing Date: To be advised.

New South Wales Cancer Council Research Project Grants

Subjects: Research projects in all aspects of cancer which elucidate its origin, cause and control at a fundamental and applied level.
Eligibility: Open to Australian residents from NSW who are health care professionals. Recipients of tobacco sponsorship are ineligible.
Level of Study: Unrestricted.
Type: Research Grant.
No. of awards offered: Varies.
Frequency: Annual.
Value: Varies depending on requirements.
Length of Study: 1-3 years.
Study Establishment: An approved institution in New South Wales.
Country of Study: Australia.
Application Procedure: Application forms are available on request.
Closing Date: Mid-June.

NEW ZEALAND COMMONWEALTH SCHOLARSHIPS AND FELLOWSHIPS COMMITTEE

PO Box 11-915, Wellington, New Zealand
Tel: (64) 4 381 8510
Fax: (64) 4 381 8501
Email: schols@nzvcc.ac.nz
www: http://www.nzvcc.ac.nz
Contact: The Scholarships Officer

The New Zealand Commonwealth Scholarships and Fellowships Committee is a secretariat which provides administrative policy services to the seven vice-chancellors of the New Zealand Universities.

New Zealand Commonwealth Scholarships

Subjects: All subjects.
Eligibility: Open to graduates who are citizens of a Commonwealth country and who have graduated within the last five years.
Level of Study: Postgraduate.
Purpose: To enable persons of high intellectual promise to study in New Zealand in the expectation that they will make a significant contribution to life in their own countries on their return.
Type: Scholarship.
No. of awards offered: Approx. 10.
Frequency: Annual.
Value: NZ$1,000 per month, plus travel and allowances.
Length of Study: Up to 3 years.
Country of Study: New Zealand.
Application Procedure: Nominations should be sent to the appropriate agency in the home country.
Closing Date: Differs from country to country. Applications close in New Zealand on August 1st.
Additional Information: Scholarships are provided by the New Zealand government and fall within the framework of the Commonwealth Scholarship and Fellowship Plan.

NEW ZEALAND VICE-CHANCELLORS COMMITTEE

PO Box 11-915, Wellington, New Zealand
Tel: (64) 4 801 5091
Fax: (64) 4 801 5089
www: http://www.nzvcc.ac.nz
Contact: The Scholarships Officer

Claude McCarthy Fellowships

Subjects: Literature, science, medicine.
Eligibility: Open to any graduate of a New Zealand university.
Level of Study: Postgraduate.

Purpose: To enable graduates of New Zealand universities to undertake original work or research.
Type: Fellowship.
No. of awards offered: Varies, depending upon funds available, usually 12-15.
Frequency: Annual.
Value: Varies, according to country of residence during tenure, and the project itself. Assistance for expenses incurred in travel, employment of technical staff, special equipment, etc. may be provided.
Length of Study: Normally for not more than 1 year.
Country of Study: Any country.
Closing Date: August 1st.

L B Wood Travelling Scholarship

Subjects: All subjects.
Eligibility: Open to all holders of postgraduate scholarships from any faculty of any university in New Zealand, provided that application is made within three years of the date of graduation.
Level of Study: Doctorate.
Purpose: To assist graduates of New Zealand universities to undertake doctoral studies in the UK.
Type: Scholarship.
No. of awards offered: 2.
Frequency: Annual.
Value: NZ$3,000 per year, as a supplement to another postgraduate scholarship.
Length of Study: Up to 3 years.
Study Establishment: University or institution of university rank.
Country of Study: United Kingdom.
Closing Date: October 1st.

William Georgetti Scholarships

Subjects: All subjects.
Eligibility: Candidates must be New Zealand citizens or permanent residents. Open to graduates who have been resident in New Zealand for five years immediately before application and who are aged between 21 and 28 years of age.
Level of Study: Postgraduate.
Purpose: To encourage postgraduate study and research in a field which is important to the social, cultural or economic development of New Zealand.
Type: Scholarship.
No. of awards offered: Varies.
Frequency: Annual.
Value: Up to NZ$5,100 for study in New Zealand; up to NZ$10,000 for study overseas.
Study Establishment: Universities in New Zealand or overseas.
Country of Study: Any country.
Closing Date: October 1st.
Additional Information: Age eligibility is recently undergoing a change. Application is currently being made to the New Zealand High Court to make the age restriction open.

THE NEWBERRY LIBRARY

60 West Walton Street, Chicago, IL, 60610, United States of America
Tel: (1) 312 255 3666
Fax: (1) 312 255 3513
Email: research@newberry.org
www: http://www.newberry.org
Contact: Committee on Awards

The Newberry Library, open to the public without charge, is an independent research library and educational institution dedicated to the expansion and dissemination of knowledge in the humanities. With a broad range of books and manuscripts relating to the civilisations of Western Europe and the Americas, the Library's mission is to acquire and preserve research collections of such material, and to provide for and promote their effective use by a diverse community of users.

Hermon Dunlap Smith Center for the History of Cartography Fellowships

Subjects: The history of cartography.
Eligibility: Open to established scholars of any nationality.
Level of Study: Postgraduate.
Type: A variable number of Fellowships.
Value: US$800 per month (maximum stipend of US$30,000).
Study Establishment: In residence, for periods not exceeding 3 months (short-term); or for 6-12 months (long-term).
Country of Study: USA.
Closing Date: March 1st, October 15th (short-term); March 1st (long-term).

For further information contact:

60 West Walton Street, Chicago, IL, 60610, United States of America
Tel: (1) 312 943 9090
Contact: Committee on Awards

NEWBY TRUST LTD

Hill Farm
Froxfield, Petersfield, Hampshire, GU32 1BQ, England
Tel: (44) 1730 827557
Fax: (44) 1730 827557
Contact: Miss W Gillam, Company Secretary

Newby Trust Awards

Subjects: All subjects.
Eligibility: Open to students of any nationality. Students not already in the UK are rarely considered. Foreign students must already be studying in the UK.

Level of Study: Doctorate, Postgraduate, Professional development.
Purpose: General educational purposes among others.
Type: Grant.
No. of awards offered: Varies.
Frequency: Annual.
Value: Up to £1,000 for fees or maintenance.
Study Establishment: University.
Country of Study: United Kingdom, unless there are strong reasons for studying elsewhere.
Application Procedure: Personal letter with CV, two letters of reference, statement of income and expenditure (including fees), and self stamped addressed must be submitted. Application forms are not supplied..
Closing Date: None, but applications in September/October are rarely considered.
Additional Information: Funding is not available for the following- CPS law exam; BSC intercalculated with a medical degree; postgraduate medical/veterinary degrees in the first or second years.

NORTH DAKOTA UNIVERSITY SYSTEM

600 East Boulevard, Bismarck, ND, 58505, United States of America
Tel: (1) 701 328 2960
www: http://www.ndus.nodak.edu
Contact: Ms Rhonda Shaver

North Dakota Indian Scholarship

Subjects: All subjects.
Eligibility: Must be a resident of North Dakota with 1/4 degree Indian Blood. Must be accepted for admission at an institute of higher learning or state vocational programme. Recipients must be enrolled full-time and have a grade point average above 2.00.
Level of Study: Doctorate, Postgraduate.
Purpose: To assist Native American students in obtaining a basic college education.
Type: Scholarship.
No. of awards offered: 140.
Frequency: Annual.
Value: US$700.
Country of Study: USA.
Application Procedure: Send completed forms to: North Dakota Indian Scholarship Program, North Dakota University System, 10th Floor State Capitol, 600 E Boulevard Avenue, Bismarck, ND 58505-0230.
Closing Date: July 15th.

NORWEGIAN INFORMATION SERVICE IN THE UNITED STATES

825 Third Avenue
38th Floor, New York, NY, 10022-7584, United States of America
Tel: (1) 212 421 7333
Fax: (1) 212 754 0583
Email: norcons@interport.net
www: http://www.norway.org
Contact: Grants & Scholarships Department

America-Norway Heritage Fund

Subjects: All subjects.
Eligibility: Candidates must be American of Norwegian descent who have made significant contributions to American culture.
Level of Study: Professional development.
Purpose: To award special grants to Americans of Norwegian descent who have made significant contributions to American culture, enabling them to visit Norway to share the results of their work with the people of Norway.
Type: Travel Grant.
No. of awards offered: Varies.
Frequency: Annual.
Value: Recipients will recieve a grant covering travel expenses as well as an honorarium.
Length of Study: 1-2 weeks. Activities should be planned between October - April.
Country of Study: Norway.
Application Procedure: Applications for the grant are no longer accepted. Candidates will be selected by the Board of Directors of the fund in co-operation with its connections in the United States. However, the Board of Directors of the Fund will appreciate receiving proposals for the possible candidates. Suggestions may be sent to: Nordmanns-Forbundet, Rådhusgt. 23B, N-0158 Oslo, Norway, or Norge-Amerika Foreningen, Drammensveien 20 C, N-0255 Oslo, Norway. For further information please contact these addresses.

American-Scandinavian Foundation

Subjects: All subjects.
Eligibility: Awards are open to US citizens or permanent residents who will have complete their undergraduate education at the the time their overseas programme begins. Proposals from all fields are accepted.
Level of Study: Postgraduate.
Purpose: To encourage advanced study and research in the Scandinavian countries.
Type: Fellowship.
No. of awards offered: Varies.
Frequency: Annual.

Value: Grants normally US$2,500; Fellowships up to US$15,000, not both.
Country of Study: Scandinavian countries.
Application Procedure: All applications must be on ASF application forms, available on request from the ASF.
Closing Date: November 1st.
Additional Information: For further information please contact the ASF.

For further information contact:

15 E 65 Street, New York, NY, 10021, United States of America
Tel: (1) 212 879 9779
Fax: (1) 212 249 3444
Contact: Grants Management Officer

John Dana Archbold Fellowship Program

Subjects: All subjects.
Eligibility: Eligibility is restricted to persons 20 to 35 years old, in good health and good character and citizens of Norway or the USA. Qualified applicants must show evidence of real ability in their chosen field, indicate seriousness of purpose, and have a record of social adaptability. There is ordinarily no language requirement. Undergraduate applicants must have a BA or BSc degree (or equivalent) before their departure date.
Level of Study: Postgraduate.
Purpose: To increase understanding between scholars from one country and their colleagues in the other. Americans go to Norway in even numbered years and Norwegians go to the USA in odd numbered years.
Type: Fellowship.
No. of awards offered: Varies.
Frequency: Annual.
Value: Individual grants vary, depending on projected costs, but generally do not exceed US$10,000. The maintenance stipend is sufficient to meet expenses for a single person. The travel allowance covers return air fare to Oslo.
Study Establishment: Institutions in Norway (not the University of Oslo).
Country of Study: Norway or USA.
Application Procedure: Please write to the Nansen Fund, Inc. for an application form.
Closing Date: January 15th.
Additional Information: The University of Oslo International Summer School offers orientation and Norwegian languages courses six weeks before the start of the regular academic year. For Americans, tuition is paid. Attendance is required. For further information please contact the Nansen Fund, Inc.

For further information contact:

The Nansen Fund, Inc.
77 Saddlebrook Lane, Houston, TX, United States of America
Tel: (1) 713 680 8255
Fax: (1) 713 686 3963

NOVARTIS FOUNDATION

41 Portland Place, London, W1N 4BN, England
Tel: (44) 171 636 9456
Fax: (44) 171 436 2840
Email: jdempster@novartisfound.org.uk
www: http://www.novartisfound.demon.co.uk
Contact: Dr C Langley, Head of Information Services

A scientific and educational charity, Novartis was established in 1997 as the direct successor to the Ciba Foundation which was created in 1947 by Ciba of Basle. There are three functions: the organisation of scientific meetings; the operation of a library and an information service; and the provision of accommodation for overseas visitors.

Novartis Foundation Symposium Bursaries

Subjects: Biomedicine, chemistry and related topics.
Eligibility: Open to applicants (of any nationality), aged between 23 and 35 on the closing date for application, and actively engaged in research on the topic covered by the symposium of their choice.
Level of Study: Doctorate, Postdoctorate.
Purpose: To enable young scientists to attend Novartis Foundation symposia and immediately following the meeting, spend time in the laboratory of one of the symposium participants.
Type: Symposium bursary.
No. of awards offered: Approx. 8.
Frequency: Twice a year.
Value: Covers travel expenses, by the most economical means, bed and breakfast during the symposium, and board and lodging while in the host's laboratory.
Length of Study: Up to a 3-month period, which includes travel, attendance at a Novartis Foundation symposium and up to 12 weeks in the participant's laboratory or institution.
Country of Study: Any country.
Application Procedure: Send full CV and statement of current research, stating symposium of choice (from current advertisements).
Closing Date: Please refer to advertisements.
Additional Information: The availability of the awards is advertised by circular to overseas members of the Novartis Foundation's Scientific Advisory Panel and invited symposiasts, and by an advertisement in 'Nature', or other journal if more appropriate. Awards are advertised every 3-6 months, and at least six months before the date of the relevant meetings. The awardee is selected by the senior staff of the Foundation, usually at least four months before the symposium. Offers to host an awardee are sought from symposiasts at the time of the invitation to the symposium. The successful awardee is asked to select three names from the membership list of the symposium and every effort is made by the Novartis Foundation to accommodate the awardee's choice. Successful candidates are expected to submit a short report following their return home.

NURSES' EDUCATIONAL FUNDS, INC.

555 West 57th Street
Suite 1327, New York, NY, 10019, United States of America
Tel: (1) 212 399 1428
Fax: (1) 212 581 2368
Email: bbnef@aol.com
www: http://www.n-e-f.org
Contact: Ms Barbara Butler, Scholarship Co-ordinator

Nurses' Educational Funds, Inc, is a non-profit corporation awarding scholarships to nurses for graduate education, Master's and doctoral degrees.

Nurses' Educational Funds Fellowships and Scholarships

Subjects: Administration, supervision, education, clinical specialisation and research.
Eligibility: Open to full-time Master's degree students or full or part-time doctoral students who are US citizens or have officially declared the intention of becoming US citizens. Applicants must be members of a professional nursing association.
Level of Study: Doctorate, Postgraduate.
Purpose: To provide the opportunity to registered nurses who seek to qualify through advanced study in a degree programme (Master's and doctoral).
Type: Fellowship.
No. of awards offered: Varies.
Frequency: Annual.
Value: US$2,500-US$10,000.
Length of Study: 1 year.
Study Establishment: Any college or university offering Master's programs in nursing accredited by the National League for Nursing (NLN), or at an accredited University doctoral degree program.
Country of Study: USA.
Application Procedure: To receive an application kit, please send a US$10 cheque to cover postage and handling. Completed applications must be accompanied by official transcripts of academic records, GRE or MAT scores, references, proof of membership in a professional nursing association, and proof of admission to an academic program.
Closing Date: March 1st preceding the academic year for which funds are sought. Applications are not mailed out after February 1st.
Additional Information: Application forms are available from the Fund from August 1st to February 1st. Fellowships and Scholarships administered by the NEF include those donated by: American Journal of Nursing Company, Mead Johnson, F A Davis Company, BOC Group Award, Nurses' Scholarship and Fellowship Fund, National Student Nurses' Association, Edith M Pritchard Award, Isabel Hampton Robb Award, Leisel M Hiemenz Award, Bernhard J Springer Award, Isabel McIsaac Award, Lucy C Perry Award, Elizabeth Carnegie Award, Margaret G Tyson Award, Estelle Massey Osborne

Award, the Judith Whitaker Scholarship and others. Applicants are advised to apply to the school of nursing of their choice concerning fellowships and scholarships available there.

ONTARIO MINISTRY OF EDUCATION AND TRAINING

PO Box 4500
189 Red River Road
4th Floor, Thunder Bay, ON, P7B 6G9, Canada
Tel: (1) 800 465 3957
Fax: (1) 807 343 7278
www: http://edu.gov.on.ca
Contact: G Vibert, OGS Officer

Ontario Graduate Scholarship Programme

Subjects: All subjects.
Eligibility: Open to Canadian residents with an overall A average or equivalent during the previous two years of study. Sixty awards may be allocated to students holding a student authorisation.
Level of Study: Doctorate, Postgraduate.
Purpose: To encourage excellence in graduate studies.
Type: Scholarship.
No. of awards offered: 1,300.
Frequency: Annual.
Value: Approximately C$3,953 per term.
Length of Study: 2 or 3 consecutive terms of full-time graduate study; students must reapply each year and may receive a maximum of 4 awards.
Study Establishment: An Ontario university.
Country of Study: Canada.
Application Procedure: Candidates currently registered in a university in Ontario must submit their applications and supporting documentation through that institution.
Closing Date: November 15th.
Additional Information: Students may hold another award up to C$5,000 and may accept research assistantships or part-time teaching or demonstrating appointments, providing that the total amount paid to the Scholars within the period of the award shall not interfere with their status as full-time graduate students. The total time spent by the student in connection with such an appointment, including preparation, marking examinations, etc., must not exceed an average of ten hours per week.

OPEN SOCIETY FOUNDATION - SOFIA

1 Balsha Street
Block 9, Sofia, 1408, Bulgaria
Tel: (359) 2 919 329
Fax: (359) 2 951 6348
Email: osfinfo@osf.bg
www: http://www.osf.bg
Contact: Ms Illiana Gyulcheva, Education Consultant

Oxford Colleges Hospitality Scheme for East European Scholars

Subjects: All subjects offered by the University of Oxford.
Eligibility: Open to scholars from eastern and central Europe, who have a good knowledge of English and who are in the process of completing work for an advanced degree, or who are working on a book, or a new course of lectures.
Level of Study: Professional development.
Purpose: To enable scholars from eastern and central Europe to work in Oxford libraries or consult Oxford specialists in their subjects.
Type: Scholarship.
No. of awards offered: Up to 6.
Frequency: Annual.
Length of Study: 1-3 months.
Study Establishment: University of Oxford.
Country of Study: United Kingdom.
Application Procedure: Applicants must submit a completed application form, CV, list of publications, and two recommendation letters.
Closing Date: December.

Salzburg Seminars for Physicians

Subjects: Medicine and surgery.
Eligibility: Open to English-speaking Bulgarian medical doctors under the age of 40.
Level of Study: Professional development.
Purpose: Exchange of ideas between physicians from Eastern Europe ans USA.
No. of awards offered: Varies.
Frequency: Annual.
Length of Study: 1 week.
Study Establishment: Salzberg Seminars- Leopoldskron Salzberg, Austria.
Country of Study: Austria.
Application Procedure: Applicants must submit a CV, higher education diploma, and diploma for acknowledged medical speciality.
Closing Date: Varies.

Soros/FCO Chevening Scholarships

Subjects: All subjects offered at Oxford University.
Eligibility: Open to Bulgarian nationals, who have completed five years of university study, who are not older than 28, and who have an excellent knowledge of English.
Level of Study: Postgraduate, Professional development.
Purpose: To support young scholars who wish to use the experience gained from studying in Britain to benefit higher education, research, or public life in their home country.
Type: Scholarship.
No. of awards offered: Up to 6.
Frequency: Annual.
Length of Study: 1 academic year.
Study Establishment: Oxford University.
Country of Study: United Kingdom.
Application Procedure: Applicants must submit a completed application form, a copy of their official diploma, a summary of their dissertation, two confidential evaluation forms, proof of English proficiency, and a list of publications (if any).
Closing Date: January.

University of Warwick Scholarships for East Europe

Subjects: All subjects offered by the University of Warwick.
Eligibility: Open to Bulgarian nationals who have already completed an undergraduate degree. Applicants must have a good command of English and must be under 35 years of age.
Level of Study: Postgraduate.
Purpose: To support postgraduate study.
Type: Scholarship.
No. of awards offered: Up to 4.
Frequency: Annual.
Length of Study: 1 year.
Study Establishment: University of Warwick.
Country of Study: United Kingdom.
Application Procedure: Application form must be completed and submitted with two letters of recommendation, and evidence of English proficiency.
Closing Date: February.

ORENTREICH FOUNDATION FOR THE ADVANCEMENT OF SCIENCE, INC (OFAS)

855 Route 301
Box 375, Cold Spring, NY, 10516-9802, United States of America
Tel: (1) 914 265 4200
Fax: (1) 914 265 4210
Contact: Dr Rozlyn A Krajcik, Assistant Director - Scientific Affairs

OFAS is an operating private Foundation that performs its own research and collaborates on projects of mutual interest.

OFAS Grants

Subjects: Areas of interest to the Foundation including - ageing, dermatology, endocrinology, and serum markers for human diseases.
Eligibility: Applicants must be at or above the postgraduate level in science or medicine at accredited research institutions in the USA. There are, however, no citizenship restrictions.
Level of Study: Postgraduate.
Purpose: To conduct collaborative biomedical research, or research at the Foundation.
Type: Grant.
Frequency: Ussually initiated by OFAS.
Value: Amounts vary depending on the needs, nature, and level of OFAS interest in the project.
Country of Study: USA.
Application Procedure: OFAS is usually the initiator of joint projects. Submit an outline of proposed joint or collaborative research, including, as a minimum, a brief overview of the current research in the field of interest, a statement of scientific objectives, a protocol summary, curriculum vitae of principal investigator, needed funding, and total estimated project funding. Confirming applications are reviewed at least quarterly.
Closing Date: Applications for collaborative research projects may be submitted at any time.
Additional Information: If you have a research question relating to a human disease or disease prevention factor for which there is adequate scientific evidence of a serum marker to justify use of a Serum Treasury, please submit your proposal for consideration to the above address.

ORTHOPAEDIC RESEARCH AND EDUCATION FOUNDATION (OREF)

6300 N River Road
Suite 700, Rosemont, IL, 60018-4261, United States of America
Tel: (1) 847 698 9980
Fax: (1) 847 698 9767
Email: mcguire@oref.org
www: http://www.oref.org
Contact: Mrs Jean Mcguire, Vice President Grants

AAOS/OREF Fellowship in Health Services Research

Subjects: Orthopaedics.
Eligibility: Applicants must be orthopaedic surgeons in either Canada or USA.
Level of Study: Postdoctorate.
Purpose: To develop orthopaedic surgeons with research skills to manage health services and outcomes research.
Type: Fellowship.
No. of awards offered: 1.
Frequency: Annual.
Value: US$70,000 per year, for up to two years.

Length of Study: 2 years.
Study Establishment: At participating institutions.
Country of Study: USA.
Application Procedure: A formal application is required.
Closing Date: August 1st.

Bristol-Myers Squibb/Zimmer Research Grant for Excellence in Orthapedaedic Treatment

Subjects: Treatment techniques, orthopaedics.
Eligibility: PI must be affiliated with a department or division of orthopaedic surgery with strong institutional commitment and competence in orthopaedic research. Applicants must hold either MD, PhD or DVM.
Level of Study: Doctorate, Postdoctorate.
Purpose: To support research which positively affects treatment of orthopaedic diseases leading to improved patient care.
Type: Research Grant.
No. of awards offered: 1.
Frequency: Annual.
Value: US$50,000 per year for up to five years.
Length of Study: 5 years.
Country of Study: USA.
Application Procedure: A formal application is required.
Closing Date: August 1st.

OREF Career Development Award

Subjects: Orthopaedic surgery.
Eligibility: Applicants must be orthopaedic surgeons; not eligible if holders of NIH ROI award.
Level of Study: Professional development.
Purpose: To encourage a commitment to scientific research in orthopaedic surgery.
Type: Basic/clinical research.
No. of awards offered: 1-3.
Frequency: Annual.
Value: Up to US$75,000 per year.
Length of Study: 3 years.
Country of Study: USA or Canada.
Application Procedure: A formal application is required with letters of recommendation.
Closing Date: August 1st.

OREF Clinical Research Award

Subjects: Orthopaedics.
Eligibility: Restricted to members of: American Academy of Orthopaedic Surgeons, Orthopaedic Research Society (ORS), Canadian Orthopaedic Association, Canadian ORS. Alternatively, candidates may be sponsored by a member.
Level of Study: Professional development.
Purpose: To recognise outstanding clinical research related to musculoskeletal disease or injury.
Type: Clinical.
No. of awards offered: 1.
Frequency: Annual.
Value: US$20,000.
Length of Study: 1 year.

Country of Study: USA or Canada.
Application Procedure: Original manuscript must be submitted.
Closing Date: July 1st.

OREF Prospective Clinical Research

Subjects: Orthopaedics.
Eligibility: Applicant must be an orthopaedic surgeon.
Level of Study: Professional development.
Purpose: To provide funding for promising prospective clinical proposals in orthopaedics.
Type: Clinical.
No. of awards offered: 1-3.
Frequency: Annual.
Value: Up to US$50,000 per year.
Length of Study: 3 years.
Study Establishment: Medical center.
Country of Study: USA.
Application Procedure: A formal application is required.
Closing Date: August 1st.

OREF Research Grants

Subjects: Sports medicine, surgery, rheumatology and treatment techniques.
Eligibility: Orthopaedic surgeon must be PI or co PI; PI cannot have NIH ROI award.
Level of Study: Postdoctorate.
Purpose: To encourage new investigators by providing seed money and start-up funding.
Type: Research Grant.
No. of awards offered: 8-12.
Frequency: Annual.
Value: Up to US$50,000 per year.
Length of Study: 2 years.
Study Establishment: A medical center.
Country of Study: USA.
Application Procedure: A formal application is required.
Closing Date: August 1st.

OREF Resident Research Award

Subjects: Orthopaedic research.
Eligibility: Applicants must be orthopaedic surgeon residents or fellows in an approved residency programme in the US.
Level of Study: Professional development.
Purpose: To encourage the development of research interests for residents and Fellows.
Type: Basic research training.
No. of awards offered: Up to 10.
Frequency: Annual.
Value: US$15,000.
Length of Study: 1 year.
Study Establishment: Medical center.
Country of Study: USA.
Application Procedure: A formal application is required.
Closing Date: August 1st.

OSTEOGENESIS IMPERFECTA FOUNDATION, INC.

804 W Diamond Avenue
Suite 210, Gaithersburg, MD, 20878, United States of America
Tel: (1) 301 947 0083
Fax: (1) 301 947 0456
Email: bonelink@aol.com
www: http://www.oif.org
Contact: Ms Ellen Dollar, Director of Public Relations

The Osteogenesis Imperfecta Foundation works to improve the quality of life for individuals affected by OI, through research to find a cure, awareness, education, and mutual support.

Michael Geisman Memorial Fellowship Fund

Subjects: Osteogenesis Imperfecta.
Eligibility: Open to suitably qualified investigators.
Level of Study: Postdoctorate.
Purpose: To encourage research scientists to study Osteogenesis Imperfecta.
Type: Fellowship.
No. of awards offered: 2-3.
Frequency: Annual.
Value: US$25,000 per year salary, plus US$10,000 per year for supplies.
Length of Study: 2 years.
Country of Study: Any country.
Application Procedure: Please write for details.
Closing Date: RFPs distributed in August with November deadline.

Osteogenesis Imperfecta Foundation Seed Research Grant

Subjects: Basic research or clinical studies on Osteogenesis Imperfecta to investigate causes, treatment or cure.
Eligibility: Open to qualified researchers in the field of OI.
Level of Study: Postdoctorate.
Purpose: To fund seed projects which can then be submitted to larger funding bodies.
Type: Research Grant.
No. of awards offered: 1-2.
Frequency: Annual.
Value: Up to US$40,000 (indirect costs and salaries will not be covered).
Length of Study: 1 year.
Country of Study: Any country.
Application Procedure: Please write for details.
Closing Date: RFPs are released in August, with deadline in November.
Additional Information: No PI salaries are allowed; no indirect cost allowed.

PARALYZED VETERANS OF AMERICA, SPINAL CORD RESEARCH FOUNDATION

801 18th Street NW, Washington, DC, 20006, United States of America
Tel: (1) 202 416 7659
Fax: (1) 202 416 7641
Email: scrf@pua.org
www: http://www.pua.org
Contact: Ms Aimee Schimmel, Program Manager

The Spinal Cord Research Foundation was established in 1976 by the Paralyzed Veterans of America for the purpose of supporting research directed to spinal cord injury and disease.

Paralyzed Veterans of America Research Grants

Subjects: Laboratory research in the basic sciences related to spinal cord injury or disease, clinical and functional studies of the medical, psychological, and economic effects of spinal cord injury or disease, as well as interventions proposed to alleviate these effects, design and development of new and improved rehabilitative and assistive devices for individuals with spinal dysfunction. Fellowships for postdoctoral scientists, clinicians, or engineers designed to encourage the training and specialisation of these individuals in the field of spinal dysfunctional research, conferences and symposia that provide opportunities for interactions among scientists, health science providers, and other professionals involved in paralysis.
Eligibility: Open to suitably qualified individuals who are seeking funds to develop a project in the field of spinal cord injury.
Level of Study: Postdoctorate.
Purpose: To improve the quality of life for individuals with spinal cord injuries, and to hasten the discovery of a cure of spinal cord injury.
Type: Research Grant and Fellowship.
No. of awards offered: Approx. 30.
Frequency: Twice a year.
Value: Up to US$75,000 per year.
Length of Study: From 1 to 3 years.
Application Procedure: A brochure, Guidelines and Applications for Grant Request, is available from the foundation.
Closing Date: June 1st, December 1st.
Additional Information: All grant recipients must submit biannual and annual progress reports and an article in layman's language for publications in PVA's monthly publication, Paraplegia News.

PARKER B FRANCIS FELLOWSHIP PROGRAM

Physiology Program
Harvard School of Public Health
Room 1411 Building 1
665 Huntington Ave, Boston, MA, 02115, United States of
America
Tel: (1) 617 432 4099
Fax: (1) 617 277 2382
Email: akirsch@sph.harvard.edu
www:
http://www.usalert.com/htdoc/usoa/fnd/any/any/proc/any/fff0
8199801.htm
Contact: Dr Joseph Brain, Director

Parker B Francis Fellowship Program

Subjects: Pulmonary research.
Eligibility: The director of any training programme, pulmonary
division, or research laboratory may apply on behalf of a
candidate for fellowship. Awards are limited to institutions
located in the USA and Canada. Each department may
submit only one application annually and is limited to a
maximum of two active fellowships at any one time. Parker B
Francis Fellowship grants are awarded to institutions for the
purpose of providing stipends and modest travel expenses in
support of qualified postdoctoral candidates who will devote
the major part of their professional effort to research related
to pulmonary disease. Candidates may hold either an MD,
PhD or other doctoral degree. It is essential there is evidence
of aptitude and proficiency in research. Sponsorship of the
Fellow by an established investigator is required. Open to US
or Canadian citizens, or foreign nationals who are in the
process of becoming permanent residents of the USA or
Canada. The ideal candidate is one who shows evidence of
strong aptitude in the field and is in transition from
postdoctoral trainee to independent investigator and junior
faculty member.
Level of Study: Postdoctorate.
Purpose: To support the development of outstanding
investigators who plan careers in pulmonary research.
Type: Fellowship.
No. of awards offered: 15.
Frequency: Annual.
Value: The total budget is limited to US$38,000 for the first,
US$40,000 for the second, and US$42,000 for the third years.
These totals are to include stipend plus fringe benefits and
may include travel to a maximum of US$1,500. Direct
research project costs and indirect costs are not allowed.
These expenses ought to be supported by research project
grants which are an essential part of the application in
documenting the availability of sufficient research project
support to make possible fulfilment of the Fellow's research
aims.
Length of Study: 3 years.
Country of Study: USA or Canada.

Application Procedure: Application packet with copies of
any applicable publications. Full application details are
available on request. Please email requests to:
brain@hsph.harvard.edu.
Closing Date: Mid-October.
Additional Information: It is permissible, indeed encouraged,
for a grant to span a period during which the awardee
graduates from fellowship to faculty status. Awards are made
to institutions on behalf of the fellows and can be transferred
to other institutions only under special circumstances with
prior approval. Fellows supported by the Fellowships must be
assured of at least 75% of their time available for research.

PARKINSON'S DISEASE SOCIETY OF THE UNITED KINGDOM

215 Vauxhall Bridge Road, London, SW1V 1EJ, England
Tel: (44) 171 931 8080
Fax: (44) 171 233 9908
Email: research@pdsuk.demon.co.uk
Contact: Research Co-ordinator

Parkinson's Disease Society Medical Research Project Grant

Subjects: Medical sciences, neurology, neurosciences,
biochemistry, toxicology, pathology, genetics, geriatrics,
pharmacy.
Eligibility: Restricted to UK residency. The principal applicant
must hold a tenured position for the duration of the award
and hold suitable qualifications.
Level of Study: Postdoctorate, Professional development.
Purpose: To find the cause and cure for Parkinson's Disease.
Type: Project Grant.
No. of awards offered: Varies.
Frequency: Annual.
Value: To include at least one salary plus consumables and
equipment.
Length of Study: Up to 3 years.
Study Establishment: A recognised UK research institution,
university or hospital.
Country of Study: United Kingdom.
Application Procedure: Please write for application form. 20
copies must be completed.
Closing Date: November 29th.
Additional Information: The awards are advertised annually
in Nature, Lancet, BMJ and the PDS newsletter. We do not
fund students.

Parkinson's Disease Society Welfare Research Project Grant

Subjects: Rehabilitation medicine and therapy; nursing;
physiotherapy; speech therapy; occupational therapy; and
cognitive sciences.
Eligibility: Restricted to UK residents with suitable
qualifications and a salaried position for the duration of the
award.

Level of Study: Doctorate.
Purpose: To improve the quality of life of those with Parkinson's Disease and their carers.
Type: Project Grant.
No. of awards offered: Varies.
Frequency: Annual.
Value: From £5,000 over one year to £25,000 over three years.
Length of Study: Up to 3 years.
Study Establishment: A recognised UK teaching, research or clinical institution.
Country of Study: United Kingdom.
Application Procedure: Please write for application form.
Closing Date: Mid-March.
Additional Information: The Society's Welfare Research Committee specifies the research topics for each year. The call for proposals will be advertised in appropriate journals in December of the previous year.

PATERSON INSTITUTE FOR CANCER RESEARCH

Christie Hospital NHS Trust, Manchester, M20 4BX, England
Tel: (44) 161 446 3136
Fax: (44) 161 446 3109
Email: gcowling@picr.man.ac.uk
www: http://christie.man.ac.uk
Contact: Dr G J Cowling, Scientific Administrator

The Patterson Institute is the research arm of a major specialist cancer hospital, the Christie Hospital NHS Trust. It carries out cancer research and oncology education in a large number of areas and has 10 research groups, over 60 research teams and around 250 scientists.

CRC Studentship

Subjects: Role and structure of heparan sulphate in the mediation of basic and acidic FGF responses, the role of 5T4 antigen in developing normal and cancerous epithelia.
Eligibility: Candidates must have a first or upper second class Bachelor of Science degree.
Level of Study: Postgraduate.
Purpose: To support the study of PhD by research, University of Manchester.
Type: Studentship.
No. of awards offered: 2.
Frequency: Annual.
Value: £8,500 per annum stipend and university fees, bench fees.
Length of Study: 3 years.
Country of Study: United Kingdom.
Application Procedure: Adverts in Nature. Reply to cancer research campaign or direct application for further details.
Closing Date: Usually before February 28th.
Additional Information: We often have 2-3 studentships from other sources which are advertised in New Scientists. All positions are advertised on our website. Self funded student accepted, subject to qualifications and 3 year funding.

PETERHOUSE

Peterhouse, Cambridge, CB2 1RD, England
Tel: (44) 1223 338200
Fax: (44) 1223 337578
Contact: The Senior Tutor

Peterhouse Research Fellowship

Subjects: All subjects.
Eligibility: Applicants must hold, or be studying for, a degree from Cambridge or Oxford universities.
Level of Study: Postdoctorate.
Purpose: To support a young scholar in postdoctoral research at Peterhouse.
Type: Fellowship.
No. of awards offered: 2-3.
Frequency: Annual.
Value: Maintenance and allowances.
Length of Study: 3 years.
Study Establishment: For study at Peterhouse only.
Country of Study: United Kingdom.
Application Procedure: Application form must be completed.
Closing Date: Early February.

Peterhouse Research Studentship

Subjects: All subjects.
Eligibility: Applicants should be under 25 years of age on December 1st in the year in which they hope to come into residence.
Level of Study: Postgraduate.
Purpose: To study for a PhD at Peterhouse.
Type: Studentship.
No. of awards offered: 2-3.
Frequency: Annual.
Value: Full fees and maintenance subject to deduction of the emoluments.
Length of Study: 3 years.
Study Establishment: For study at Peterhouse only.
Country of Study: United Kingdom.
Application Procedure: Application form, CV and references must be submitted.
Closing Date: April 1st.

THE PEW CHARITABLE TRUSTS

3333 Califronia Street
Suite 410, San Francisco, CA, 94118, United States of America
Tel: (1) 415 476 8181
Fax: (1) 415 476 4113
www: http://futurehealth.ucsf.edu/pewlatin.html
Contact: The Awards Committee

Pew Latin American Fellows Program

Subjects: Biomedical research in human disease.

Eligibility: Open to postdoctoral level students from any Central or South American country or Mexico. Candidates must have received their MD/PhD degree within the last five years.
Level of Study: Postdoctorate.
Purpose: To serve as a nucleus of scientific exchange and collaboration between investigators in the USA and Latin America.
No. of awards offered: 10.
Frequency: Annual.
Value: US$80,000.
Length of Study: 2 years.
Country of Study: USA.
Application Procedure: Applications are available from the Regional Committee Chairman or the Programme office.
Closing Date: October.

Pew Scholars Programme in the Biomedical Sciences

Subjects: Medical sciences.
Eligibility: Open to qualified candidates of any nationality.
Level of Study: Assistant Professor level or equivalent.
Purpose: To support young investigators of outstanding promise in basic and clinical sciences relevant to the advancement of human health.
Type: Research Grant.
No. of awards offered: 20.
Frequency: Annual.
Value: US$200,000 in total over four years.
Country of Study: USA.
Application Procedure: Applicants must be nominated by one of the invited US institutions.
Closing Date: November 1st.

POLISH EMBASSY

47 Portland Place, London, W1N 3AG, England
Tel: (44) 171 636 6032
Fax: (44) 171 637 2190
Email: pci-lond@pcidir.demon.co.uk
Contact: Ms Marian Dabrouski, Councillor, Science and Education

The Polish Embassy offers grants within the framework of the British-Polish Joint Research Collaboration Programme 1999, which is designed to support joint scientific research.

Polish Embassy Short-Term Bursaries

Subjects: All subjects.
Eligibility: Candidates must be British citizens with a university degree or equivalent qualification, who have some postgraduate research or lecturing experience; preference is given to those undertaking doctoral or postdoctoral work. Married candidates must indicate whether they are prepared to go unaccompanied. Candidates wishing to study Polish philology, Slavonic languages and the history and the geography of Poland must be conversant with Polish or the appropriate Slavonic language.
Level of Study: Doctorate, Postdoctorate, Postgraduate, Professional development.
Purpose: To provide financial support for British students wishing to study in Poland.
Type: Bursary.
No. of awards offered: 40.
Frequency: Annual.
Value: A monthly allowance, free accommodation in student hostels (or possibly in hotels) or a monthly allowance towards accommodation found privately, free meals in a student canteen or a monthly allowance in lieu, a modest book grant, exemption from tuition fees, and free medical care. The Polish authorities will pay for necessary travel expenses within Poland from one academic centre to another; recipients will be required to pay their own fares to and from Poland.
Length of Study: 3-9 months.
Study Establishment: Universities and other institutions of higher education and research.
Country of Study: Poland.
Application Procedure: Please submit completed application form, CV, copy of diploma, research proposal, medical statement, and two letters of recommendation.
Closing Date: March 15th.
Additional Information: The scheme is new under agreement between Poland and the UK on exchanges in the fields of science, humanities and arts. Bursaries cannot normally be taken up during the university summer, except for the summer vacation courses 'Polonicum' and 'Polish Language'.

Polish Government Postgraduate Scholarships Scheme

Subjects: Unrestricted. The following subjects in particular are taught to a high standard in Polish universities - sociology, mathematics, geography and geology, history of Polish architecture, music (performance and composition), the arts and scientific topics.
Eligibility: Candidates must be British citizens with a university degree or equivalent qualification; priority is given to candidates who hold an honours degree and have had some experience of research, laboratory techniques or teaching since graduation. Married candidates must indicate whether they are prepared to go unaccompanied. Candidates wishing to study Polish philology, Slavonic languages and the history and the geography of Poland must be conversant with Polish or the appropriate Slavonic language. Applicants should be under 35 years of age.
Level of Study: Postgraduate, Professional development.
Purpose: To provide financial support for British students wishing to study in Poland.
Type: Scholarship.
Frequency: Annual.
Value: A monthly allowance, free accommodation in student hostels or a monthly allowance towards accommodation found privately, free meals in a student canteen or a monthly allowance in lieu, a modest book grant, exemption from tuition fees, and free medical care.

Length of Study: Periods of up to 10 months. Though applications for shorter periods of study may be considered, preference will be given to those wishing to study for periods of more than 6 months.

Study Establishment: Universities and other institutions of higher education and research.

Country of Study: Poland.

Application Procedure: Completed application form, CV, copy of diploma, research proposal, medical statement, and two letters of recommendation must be submitted. Application forms are obtainable from the Education Officer and should be returned to the Embassy by March 15th.

Closing Date: March 15th.

Additional Information: The scheme is run under agreement between Poland and the UK on exchange in the fields of science, humanities and arts.

THE POPULATION COUNCIL

Policy Research Division
One Dag Hammarskjold Plaza, New York, NY, 10017, United States of America
Tel: (1) 212 339 0671
Fax: (1) 212 755 6052
Email: ssfellowship@popcouncil.org
www: http://www.popcouncil.org
Telex: 9102900660 POPCO
Contact: Ms Jude H Lam, Fellowship Co-ordinator

The Population Council is an independent, non-profit organisation, established in 1952. It conducts multi-disciplinary research and provides technical and professional services in the broad field of population development, population policies, and human productive issues. It also evaluates programs to provide birth planning services and information.

Population Council Fellowships in Population and Social Sciences

Subjects: Economics, demography, sociology, public health, anthropology, biostatistics, epidemiology and women's studies.

Eligibility: Predoctoral: open to applicants who have completed all coursework requirements toward the PhD or an equivalent degree in one of the social sciences in combination with population studies. Applications requesting support for either the dissertation fieldwork or the dissertation writing period will be considered. Postdoctoral: open to persons having a PhD or equivalent degree who wish to undertake postdoctoral training and research at an institution other than the one at which they received their PhD degree. Mid-career: open to persons with a minimum of five years of professional experience in the population field. Mid-career academic awards are open to scholars with a PhD or equivalent degree wishing to undertake specific study in connection with a research institution. Mid-career

professional awards are open to population or development professionals with a keen interest in enhancing and strengthening their professional skills by participating in a one-year diploma, certificate, or Master's degree programme (no MPH candidates will be considered). Awards are open to all qualified persons, but strong preference will be given to applicants from developing countries who have a firm commitment to return home upon completion of their training programmes. Applications by women are particularly encouraged.

Level of Study: Doctorate, postdoctorate, professional development.

Purpose: The Council seeks to make a significant contribution to the advanced training of professionals in the broad field of population studies through the awarding of fellowships on a competitive basis, with particular emphasis on the training of nationals from developing countries.

Type: Fellowship.

No. of awards offered: 20-25.

Frequency: Annual.

Value: Predocoral: US$24,000; postdoctoral: US$32,000; mid-career: varies. A monthly stipend (based on type of fellowship and place of study), tuition payments and related fees, transportation expenses (for fellow only), and health insurance. Some research-related costs may also be part of the award. Tuition at the postdoctoral and mid-career academic levels is not included in the award.

Length of Study: Up to 1 year.

Study Establishment: A training or research institution with a strong programme in population studies, regardless of geographic location.

Country of Study: Any country.

Application Procedure: Applicants must submit application and supporting documents in English. Application forms can be obtained from our homepage.

Closing Date: January 2nd of each year for notification in March.

Additional Information: Selection will be based on the recommendation of the Fellowship Committee, which consists of three distinguished scholars in the field of population. Selection criteria will stress academic excellence and prospective contribution to the population field. Application for independent research funds or for fieldwork not related to a dissertation will not be considered. Requests for application forms should include a brief description of candidates' academic and professional qualifications and a short statement about their research or study plans for the proposed Fellowship period. The Bernard Berelson fellowships are for training at the Population Council of New York office. Prior to submitting a formal application to the Fellowship Office for consideration, the Berelson applicants are required to seek sponsorship from at least one Council staff member from the New York Office. There are two types of Bernard Berelson fellowships: (1) Postdoctoral Berelson is a two year fellowship at the Council, New York. (2) Midcareer academic Berelson is a one year fellowship at the Council, New York.

THE QUEEN'S UNIVERSITY OF BELFAST

Belfast, BT7 1NN, Northern Ireland
Tel: (44) 1232 245133
Fax: (44) 1232 313537
Email: academic.council@qub.ac.uk
www: http://www.qub.ac.uk
Contact: Secretary to Academic Council

Queen's University is over 150 years old and offers degree programmes in all major subject areas, organised for teaching and research purposes into five colleges. The University is located just south of Belfast City Centre, although it has opened an outreach campus in Armagh. Queen's employs over 1,000 academic staff, and 20,000 students attend full and part-time courses.

Musgrave Research Studentships

Subjects: Biology, chemistry, pathology, physics, physiology.
Eligibility: Open only to British subjects who are graduates, with preference being given to graduates of universities in the UK, a UK colony, protectorate, trust or mandated territory or any territory within or associated with the Commonwealth or Republic of Ireland. Candidates must be engaged in or show marked capacity for research in biology, chemistry, pathology, physics, or physiology.
Level of Study: Doctorate, Postgraduate.
Purpose: For personal research.
Type: Studentship.
No. of awards offered: 3-4.
Frequency: Annual.
Value: Dependent upon trust income.
Length of Study: 1 year; may be renewed for 1 or 2 further years.
Study Establishment: Queen's University of Belfast.
Country of Study: United Kingdom.
Application Procedure: Application form must be completed.
Closing Date: June 1st.
Additional Information: The selection panel will take into account other sources of funding for the research.

Queen's University of Belfast Visiting Fellowships

Subjects: Arts and sciences. These fellowships are alternated on an annual basis between the arts-based and science-based areas (before 1997, they were offered on a university-wide basis). This alternating policy will be reviewed but it is likely to continue.
Eligibility: Candidates should be of doctoral degree standing or have undertaken research to an equivalent standard.
Level of Study: Postdoctorate, Professional development.
Purpose: Awarded for personal research.
Type: Fellowship.
No. of awards offered: 2.
Frequency: Annual.
Value: Salary within the first 5 points on the Lecturer's scale.
Length of Study: 1 year.

Study Establishment: Queen's University of Belfast.
Country of Study: United Kingdom.
Application Procedure: Application form must be completed.
Closing Date: December 1st.
Additional Information: Two references are also required at a later stage in the application. We would expect a research proposal which would mean some sort of realistic achievement/results within a one year period.

Queen's University of Belfast Visiting Studentships

Subjects: Arts and sciences. The studentships are currently alternated annually between the arts-based and science-based areas. This policy will be reviewed but will probably continue for the next competition (1999-2000), when visiting studentships will be offered in the science-based areas.
Eligibility: Open only to persons holding at least an upper second class honours degree or equivalent from another university. Candidates must show aptitude for research or other original work.
Level of Study: Doctorate.
Purpose: For original research.
Type: Studentship.
No. of awards offered: 3.
Frequency: Annual.
Value: Currently £5,295 plus fees.
Length of Study: 2 years; renewable for 1 further year.
Study Establishment: Queen's University of Belfast.
Country of Study: United Kingdom.
Application Procedure: Application form must be completed and two references submitted.
Closing Date: December 1st.
Additional Information: Two independent references must be submitted to arrive separately by the closing date.

QUEENSLAND UNIVERSITY OF TECHNOLOGY (QUT)

Office of Research
GPO Box 2434, Brisbane, QLD, 4001, Australia
Tel: (61) 7 3864 1844
Fax: (61) 7 3864 1304
www: http://www.qut.edu.au/draa/or/
Contact: Grants Management Officer

Queensland University of Technology Postdoctoral Research Fellowship

Subjects: All disciplines supported by research centres at QUT.
Eligibility: Open to holders of the PhD who have less than five years' full-time postdoctoral experience and have submitted their thesis for examination prior to closing date.
Level of Study: Postdoctorate.

Purpose: The fellowships serve both as a mechanism for fostering effective and productive interdisciplinary group research and for encouraging excellence in individual research.
Type: Fellowship.
No. of awards offered: Minimum of 2.
Frequency: Annual.
Value: A$38,000-A$41,000.
Length of Study: Up to 2 years.
Study Establishment: Queensland University of Technology in a specified centre or area of research concentration.
Country of Study: Australia.
Application Procedure: Information and application forms are available from the QUT website http://www.qut.edu.au/draa/or/fellow.html.
Closing Date: August 30th.
Additional Information: Referee reports will be called only for applicants supported by QUT research centres.

THE REID TRUST FOR THE HIGHER EDUCATION OF WOMEN

53 Thornton Hill, Exeter, Devon, EX4 4NR, England
Contact: Mrs H M Harvey, Honorary Treasurer

The Reid Trust was founded in 1868 in connection with Bedford College for Women, for the promotion and improvement of women's education. It is administered by a small committee of voluntary trustees.

Reid Trust Awards

Subjects: All subjects.
Eligibility: Open to women educated in the UK who have appropriate academic qualifications and who wish to undertake further training or research.
Level of Study: Unrestricted.
Purpose: To assist in the higher education of women.
No. of awards offered: Usually 6-10.
Frequency: Annual.
Value: £50-£750.
Country of Study: United Kingdom.
Application Procedure: Requests for application forms must be accompanied by an SAE.
Closing Date: May 31st.
Additional Information: This award is for women only.

The Reid Trust For the Higher Education of Women

Subjects: All subjects.
Eligibility: Open to women educated in Britain who have the appropriate academic qualifications, and who wish to undertake further study or research.
Level of Study: Unrestricted.
Purpose: To promote the education of women.
Type: Grant.

No. of awards offered: Usually 10-12.
Frequency: Annual.
Value: £50-£750 each.
Length of Study: Unrestricted.
Country of Study: United Kingdom.
Application Procedure: Please send a stamped self-addressed envelope for an application form.
Closing Date: May 31st.

REMEDI

The Old Rectory
Stanton Prior, Bath, BA2 9HT, England
Tel: (44) 1761 472662
Fax: (44) 1761 472662
Contact: Lt Colonel P D Mesquita OBE, Director

REMEDI, founded in 1973, supports pioneering research into all aspects of disability in the widest sense of the word, with special emphasis on handicap and the way in which it limits the activities and lifestyle of all ages.

REMEDI Research Grants

Subjects: Arthritis, meningitism osteoporosis, Parkinson's Disease, prostatic disease, rehabilitation of the elderly, speech therapy, stroke.
Eligibility: Open to English-speaking applicants living and working in the United Kingdom.
Level of Study: Unrestricted.
Purpose: To support pioneering research into all aspects of disability, in the widest sense of the word, with special emphasis on handicap and the way in which it limits the activities and lifestyle of people of all ages. The Trustees are particularly interested in funding or part-funding initial grants where applicants find it difficult to obtain funding through larger organisations.
Type: Research Grant.
No. of awards offered: Varies.
Frequency: Dependent on funds available.
Value: Varies.
Length of Study: 1-3 years.
Study Establishment: A hospital or university.
Country of Study: United Kingdom.
Application Procedure: Applicants are invited to write to the Director with a summary including costs and start date on one side of A4. If the Chairman considers the research project is of interest, the Director will send the applicant a full application form to complete. Applications are sent out to independent referees for peer review. The Trustees normally make awards bi-annually in June and December.
Closing Date: Applications are accepted at any time.
Additional Information: Grants will not be awarded for course fees, administration and university overheads. Cancer and cancer realted diseases are not normally supported.

THE RESEARCH COUNCIL OF NORWAY

Stensberggata 26
PO Box 2700
St Hanshaugen, Oslo, N-0131, Norway
Tel: (47) 22 03 70 00
Fax: (47) 22 03 70 01
Email: info@forskningsradet.no
www: http://www.sn.no/forskningsradet/
Contact: Grants Management Officer

The Research Council of Norway is a strategic body for Norwegian research and a central advisory body to the government on issues concerning general research policy as well as the development of science and technology. The Council bears overall responsibility for national research strategy and manages nearly one third of the public sector research funding. One of the principal tasks of the Research Council is to promote co-operation and co-ordination among Norwegian academic institutions. Other important objectives include raising the general level of knowledge in society and encouraging innovation in industry and the public sector. The Research Council identifies important fields of research, allocates funds and evaluates R&D.

Bilateral Scholarship Agreements

Subjects: All subjects.
Eligibility: Open to citizens of countries with which Norway has a cultural agreement or a scholarship agreement.
Type: Scholarship.
Application Procedure: Candidates are nominated by the sending country. They must therefore contact relevant authorities in their own country, usually the Ministry of Foreign affairs for further details on application procedures and deadlines.
Additional Information: For details of the courses offered in Norway, admission requirements and application deadlines, please contact the universities directly (attn. Foreign Student Advisor). For further information please contact the International Scholarships Agreements, Norway, telephone or fax as above.

Norwegian Government Scholarship for Foreign Students

Subjects: All subjects.
Eligibility: Open to advanced students from countries with which Norway has cultural agreements and other reciprocal scholarship agreements (most of the European countries and China, Egypt, India, Israel, Japan, and Mexico).
Level of Study: Postgraduate.
Purpose: To establish contacts between Norwegian and foreign students and universities.
Type: Scholarship.
No. of awards offered: Varies, according to each cultural agreement.
Frequency: Annual.

Value: The current rates are NOK25,000 for each of the first two months and NOK10,000 for each succeeding month. Funds to cover travel can be made available.
Length of Study: 1 academic year.
Study Establishment: Norwegian universities, research institutes and other institutions at university level.
Country of Study: Norway.
Application Procedure: Students must apply through the relevant authorities in their home country, usually the Ministry of Foreign Affairs.
Closing Date: June 15th.
Additional Information: It should be noted that lectures are usually given in Norwegian.

Research Programmes of the European Union - Postdoctoral Fellowships

Subjects: All subjects.
Purpose: Under the forth Framework Programme of the European Union (1995-1998), the Programme for Training and Mobility of Researchers (TMR) offers two-year fellowships, preferably at postdoctoral level.
Additional Information: The information package of The TMR is available from Brussels, fax 00 32 2 29 62136, 62133, 56995 or 63270, or on the internet http://www.cordis.lu, or alternatively contact The Research Council of Norway, EU & RD Information Centre on telephone 00 47 22 037163, fax 00 47 22 037001, or email eufi@nfr.no.

RESEARCH INTO AGEING

Baird House
15/17 St Cross Street, London, EC1N 8UW, England
Tel: (44) 171 404 6878
Fax: (44) 171 404 6816
Email: ria@ageing.co.uk
Contact: Dr Gemma Borg, Research Administrator

Research Into Ageing raises funds for research into the causes and incidence of morbidity in old age, and into the ageing process itself. It also aims to encourage able young researchers to enter the fields of ageing research and geriatric medicine.

Queen Elizabeth the Queen Mother Fellowship Award

Subjects: Anaesthesiology, epidemiology, gastroenterology, geriatrics, neurology, ophthalmology, psychiatry and mental health, urology, biochemistry, neurosciences, pharmacology, physiology.
Eligibility: Applicants must be able to speak English. Award is only tenable at UK institutions.
Level of Study: Postdoctorate.
Purpose: To enable outstanding postdoctoral graduates to receive support to develop an independent research career whilst furthering research into the diseases and conditions which most affect the elderly.
Type: Fellowship.

No. of awards offered: 1-2.
Frequency: Annual.
Value: Up to £140,000.
Length of Study: 3 years.
Study Establishment: UK institution.
Country of Study: United Kingdom.
Application Procedure: Application forms can be requested from Research into Ageing. Shortlisted applicants will be invited to interview by the Research Advisory Council.
Closing Date: During December (check exact date with Research Administrator).
Additional Information: Applicants should normally have a maximum of ten years' postdoctoral research experience.

Research into Ageing Prize Studentships

Subjects: Geriatric medicine, gerontology and related disciplines.
Eligibility: Open to potential supervisors wishing to enable a postgraduate to obtain a further degree, usually to PhD standard, through work on a topic connected with age related illness or the ageing process. Applicants must be able to speak English and must be employed by a UK institution.
Level of Study: Postgraduate.
Purpose: To improve the health and quality of life of the elderly, through the initiation, funding and support of medical research relevant to the conditions that affect them.
Type: Studentship.
No. of awards offered: 1-2.
Frequency: Annual.
Value: Varies.
Length of Study: 3 years.
Study Establishment: Suitable UK establishments.
Country of Study: United Kingdom.
Application Procedure: Initially a one page summary of proposed project should be sent in. Application form will then be sent if appropriate.
Closing Date: Mid-September for consideration at November selection meeting. Candidates should apply to Administrator for further details.
Additional Information: Awards should be applied for by supervisors.

Research into Ageing Research Grants

Subjects: Geriatric medicine, gerontology and related disciplines.
Eligibility: Open to suitably qualified clinical or scientific workers who wish to undertake a project studying any aspect of age-related illness or infirmity, or fundamental research into the ageing process. Applicants must speak English.
Level of Study: Postdoctorate.
Purpose: To improve the health and quality of life of the elderly; through the initiation, funding and support of medical research relevant to the conditions that affect them.
Type: Research Grant.

No. of awards offered: Dependent on funds available.
Frequency: Twice a year.
Value: Maximum grant in the region of £90,000 over three years except in exceptional circumstances.
Length of Study: Varies, but usually 1-3 years.
Study Establishment: UK universities, medical colleges, hospitals and general practices.
Country of Study: United Kingdom.
Application Procedure: Initially a one page summary of proposed project should be submitted. Application form will be then be sent if appropriate.
Closing Date: Twice yearly to coincide with the charity's selection meetings. Candidates should apply to Administrator for further details.

REUTER FOUNDATION

85 Fleet Street, London, EC4P 4AJ, England
Tel: (44) 171 542 7015
Fax: (44) 171 542 8599
Email: rtrfoundation@easynet.co.uk
www: http://www.foundation.reuters.com
Contact: Ms Orla Morris

This is an educational and humanitarian trust funded by the Reuters Group, the international news and information organisation. Its first purpose, when it was established in 1982, was to promote high standards in journalism through study and training programs. It now also supports other educational and humanitarian projects.

Reuter Foundation Fellowships in Medical Journalism

Subjects: Medical sciences.
Eligibility: Open to specialist medical writers and broadcasters with at least five years reporting experience.
Level of Study: Professional development.
Purpose: To enable journalists who report on medical issues to research and study at the University of Oxford, England, and Columbia University, New York.
Type: Fellowship.
No. of awards offered: 2.
Frequency: Annual.
Value: The awards cover necessary travel expenses, tuition fees and a cost of living stipend.
Length of Study: 1 term.
Study Establishment: Green College, Oxford University, and Columbia University, New York.
Country of Study: United Kingdom or USA.
Application Procedure: Application form must be completed. Please write for details.
Closing Date: October 30th.

ROCHE RESEARCH FOUNDATION

F Hoffmann-La Roche Ltd, Basel, CH-4070, Switzerland
Tel: (41) 61 688 5227
Fax: (41) 61 688 1460
Email: research.foundation@roche.com
www: http://www.research-foundation.org
Contact: Professor Albert Fischli, Executive Director

Roche Research Foundation

Subjects: Biology, medicine, chemistry.
Eligibility: Open to all qualified researchers for fellowships at Swiss universities or hospitals; and to qualified Swiss students for fellowships abroad.
Level of Study: Doctorate, Postdoctorate, Postgraduate.
Purpose: To promote scientific research at Swiss universities and hospitals in the biomedical field; and to sponsor experimental research of Swiss fellows in biology, chemistry and medicine working at universities and laboratories abroad.
Type: Fellowship.
No. of awards offered: 100.
Frequency: Quarterly.
Value: Living and travelling costs.
Country of Study: Any country.
Application Procedure: An application form must be completed.
Closing Date: January 15th, April 15th, July 15th, October 15th.

THE ROEHER INSTITUTE

Kinsmen Building
4700 Keele Street, North York, ON, M3J 1P3, Canada
Tel: (1) 416 661 9611
Fax: (1) 416 661 5701
www: http://indie.ca/roeher
Contact: Ms Roslyn Ward, Information Officer

Roeher Institute Major Research Grants

Subjects: A broad range of academic disciplines where the study itself has implications for the field of intellectual impairment, including Alzheimer's Disease.
Eligibility: Open to Canadian citizens or landed immigrants who hold a postgraduate degree in a field related to the proposed research. Applicants must have their research projects approved by a Canadian academic or research institute.
Level of Study: Postdoctorate.
Type: Research Grant.
No. of awards offered: Varies.
Frequency: Annual.
Value: Up to C$35,000.
Length of Study: 1-3 years; renewal is contingent on a progress report of the work and research results.
Country of Study: Canada.

Application Procedure: Please contact the Institute for details.
Closing Date: April 30th.

Roeher Institute Research Grants

Subjects: A broad range of fields relating to human services and intellectual impairment.
Eligibility: Open to Canadian citizens or landed immigrants who are graduate students enrolled in graduate programmes at Canadian universities.
Level of Study: Graduate.
Purpose: To enable researchers to examine issues affecting people with an intellectual impairment and other disabilities.
Type: Research Grant.
No. of awards offered: Varies.
Frequency: Annual.
Value: Up to C$10,000.
Length of Study: 1 year; renewable if research project shows results and can be published in related journals.
Study Establishment: An approved university.
Country of Study: Canada.
Application Procedure: Please contact the Institute for details.
Closing Date: April 30th.
Additional Information: Candidates must state intent to pursue a career in Canada and must have definite research projects supported by an academic advisor or an Institute associate or consultant. Applicants must be prepared to forward progress reports and/or publish their results. Research Grants are also offered to associates, associations and agencies.

ROTARY FOUNDATION

One Rotary Center
1560 Sherman Avenue, Evanston, IL, 60201-3698, United States of America
Tel: (1) 847 866 3320
Fax: (1) 847 328 8554
www: http://www.rotary.org
Contact: Resource Development Supervisor/Scholarships

Through the Ambassadorial Scholarships Programme of the Rotary Foundation, Rotarians worldwide strive to promote international understanding and relations between peoples of different nations.

Rotary Foundation Academic Year Ambassadorial Scholarships

Subjects: All subjects.
Eligibility: Open to undergraduates, graduates and those wishing to undertake vocational study. Applicants must have completed two years of university work or appropriate professional experience before starting scholarship studies.

Scholarships are available to individuals of all ages. Spouses or descendants of Rotarians may not apply. Applicants must be citizens of countries in which there are Rotary clubs. Must be proficient in the language of the proposed host country.
Level of Study: Unrestricted.
Purpose: To further international understanding and friendly relations among people of different countries.
Type: Scholarship.
No. of awards offered: Varies.
Frequency: Annually, dependent on funds available.
Value: Funding to cover tuition, fees, room and board, and round-trip transportation, and some educational supplies not to exceed a maximum amount of US$23,000. Funding covers these specific expenses only.
Length of Study: 1 academic year.
Study Establishment: A study institution assigned by the Trustees of the Rotary Foundation.
Country of Study: Any country other than that in which the Scholar resides, providing there are Rotary clubs there.
Application Procedure: Applicants must submit a completed application form, two recommendations, college transcripts, an autobiographical essay, statement of purpose, and a language ability form verifying applicant's background in the language of the proposed host country, if different from his/her native language.
Closing Date: Varies according to local Rotary club, but between March and July, (applicants must apply over a year in advance). Contact a local Rotary club for details.
Additional Information: Scholars will not be assigned to study in areas of a country where they have previously lived or studied for more than six months. During the study year, scholars are expected to be outstanding ambassadors of goodwill through appearances before Rotary clubs, schools, civic organisations and other forums. Upon completion of the scholarship, scholars are expected to share the experiences of understanding acquired during the study year with the people of their home countries. Candidates should contact local Rotary clubs for information on the availability of particular scholarships. Not all Rotary districts are able to offer scholarships. Further details are available from the website.

Rotary Foundation Multi-Year Ambassadorial Scholarships

Subjects: All subjects.
Eligibility: Open to undergraduates and graduates who have completed two years of university work or appropriate professional experience before starting scholarship studies. Scholarships are available to individuals of all ages. Spouses or descendants of Rotarians may not apply. Applicants must be citizens of countries in which there are Rotary clubs.
Level of Study: Unrestricted.
Purpose: To further international understanding and friendly relations among people of different countries and help defray the cost of pursuing a degree.
Type: Scholarship.
No. of awards offered: Varies.
Frequency: Annually, dependent on funds available.

Value: The award provides a flat grant of US$11,000 per year to be applied towards the cost of a degree programme. All additional costs must be absorbed by scholars.
Length of Study: 2 or 3 years.
Study Establishment: A foreign study institution approved by the trustees of The Rotary Foundation.
Country of Study: Any country other than that in which the Scholar resides, providing there are Rotary clubs there.
Application Procedure: Applicants must submit a completed application form, two recommendations, college transcripts, an autobiographical essay and a statement of purpose.
Closing Date: Varies according to local Rotary club, but between March and July (applicants must apply over a year in advance). Contact a local Rotary club for details.
Additional Information: Scholars will not be assigned to study in areas of a country where they have previously lived or studied for more than six months. During the study year, scholars are expected to be outstanding ambassadors of goodwill through appearances before Rotary clubs, schools, civic organisations and other forums. Upon completion of the scholarship, scholars are expected to share the experiences of understanding acquired during the study year with the people of their home countries. Candidates should contact local Rotary clubs for information on the availability of particular scholarships. Not all Rotary districts are able to offer scholarships. Further details are available from the website.

Rotary Grants for University Teachers to Serve in Developing Countries

Subjects: Fields taught must have practical use to the host country.
Eligibility: Applicants must hold a college or university appointment for three or more years, and must be proficient in the language of their prospective host country.
Level of Study: Professional development.
Purpose: To build international understanding while strengthening higher education in low-income countries.
Type: Grant.
No. of awards offered: Set.
Frequency: Dependent on funds available.
Value: Grants are available for a period of either three to five months (receiving US$10,000) or six to ten months (receiving US$20,000), to subsidise expenses of higher education faculty to teach at a college or university in a low-income country.
Length of Study: 3-10 months.
Country of Study: Countries with a per capita GNP of US$6,000 or less in which there are Rotary clubs.
Application Procedure: Teachers must apply through a local Rotary club. Applications should include a completed application form, current CV, statement of intent and two letters of recommendation. Prospective candidates must contact a local Rotary club to confirm the availability of awards, to obtain application materials, and to enquire about the local deadline.
Closing Date: Varies according to local Rotary club, but between March and July (applicants must apply over a year in advance). Please contact a local Rotary club for details.

Additional Information: Grant recipients are expected to be outstanding ambassadors of goodwill to the people of their host and home countries through appearances to Rotary clubs. Not all Rotary districts are able to offer scholarships. Further details are available from the website.

ROYAL ANTHROPOLOGICAL INSTITUTE

50 Fitzroy Street, London, W1P 5HS, England
Tel: (44) 171 387 0455
Fax: (44) 171 383 4235
www: http://lucy.ukc.ac.uk/rai
Contact: Director of Grants

Emslie Horniman Anthropological Scholarship Fund

Subjects: Anthropology.
Eligibility: Open to citizens of the UK, Commonwealth or Irish Republic who are university graduates or who can satisfy the Trustees of their suitability for the study proposed. Preference is given to applicants whose proposals include field work outside the UK. Graduates who already hold a doctorate in anthropology are not eligible. Open to individuals only, no grants are given to expeditions or teams.
Level of Study: Postgraduate.
Purpose: Pre-doctoral grants for fieldwork in anthropology with preference for research outside the United Kingdom.
Type: Scholarship.
No. of awards offered: Approx. 10.
Frequency: Annual.
Value: £500 to £4,000.
Country of Study: Any country.
Application Procedure: Ask for application form.
Closing Date: March 31st.
Additional Information: No grants for library research, university fees, or subsistence in the UK.

ROYAL COLLEGE OF OBSTETRICIANS AND GYNAECOLOGISTS (RCOG)

27 Sussex Place
Regent's Park, London, NW1 4RG, England
Tel: (44) 171 262 5425
Fax: (44) 171 723 0575
www: http://www.rcog.org.uk
Contact: The College Secretary

Bernhard Baron Travelling Scholarships

Subjects: Obstetrics and gynaecology.
Eligibility: Open to Fellows and Members of the College.
Level of Study: Postgraduate.

Purpose: To expand the recipient's knowledge in areas in which he or she already has some experience.
Type: 1 Scholarship.
No. of awards offered: 1.
Frequency: Every two years.
Value: Up to £6,000.
Country of Study: Any country.
Application Procedure: Please contact the College Secretary for further details.
Closing Date: July 31st.

Eden Travelling Fellowship

Subjects: Obstetrics and gynaecology.
Eligibility: Open to medical graduates of not less than two years' standing from any approved university in the UK or Commonwealth.
Level of Study: Postgraduate.
Purpose: To enable the recipient to gain additional knowledge and experience in the pursuit of a specific research project in which he or she is currently engaged.
Type: Fellowship.
No. of awards offered: 1.
Frequency: Annual.
Value: Up to £4,000 according to the project undertaken.
Length of Study: For a specified period of time.
Study Establishment: At another department of obstetrics and gynaecology or of closely related disciplines.
Country of Study: Any country.
Application Procedure: Applications should include information on qualifications; areas of interest and/or publications in a specified area; centre(s) to be visited, with confirmation of arrangements from the head of that centre; estimated costs; and names of two referees.
Closing Date: July 31st.
Additional Information: For more information please contact the College Secretary.

For further information contact:

27 Sussex Place
Regent's Park, London, NW1 4RG, England
Tel: (44) 171 262 5425
Fax: (44) 171 723 0575
Contact: The College Secretary

Edgar Gentilli Prize

Subjects: Gynaecology and obstetrics.
Eligibility: Unrestricted.
Purpose: Awarded to those presenting results of their research in the form of an essay or article on original work done on the cause, nature, recognition and treatment of any form of cancer of the female genital tract.
Type: Prize.
No. of awards offered: 1.
Frequency: Annual.
Value: £500 and book tokens to the value of £100.
Application Procedure: Please contact the Award Secretary at the main address for more information.
Closing Date: July 31st.

Edgar Research Fellowship

Subjects: Obstetrics and gynaecology.
Eligibility: Open to candidates of high academic standing either in obstetrics and gynaecology, or related fields.
Level of Study: Postgraduate.
Purpose: To encourage research, especially into chorion carcinoma or other forms of malignant disease.
Type: Fellowship.
No. of awards offered: 2.
Frequency: Annual.
Value: Up to a maximum of £35,000.
Length of Study: Initially for 1 year's research but a further year's funding may be offered.
Country of Study: Any country.
Application Procedure: Please contact the Research Administrator at the WellBeing address.
Closing Date: First Monday in December.
Additional Information: In making the award the Council of the College will bear in mind the original intention of the Fellowship, which was to encourage research into chorion carcinoma or other forms of malignant disease. Where applications of equal merit are received, priority will be given to the project most closely related to this condition. Fellows are required to submit a report on the work carried out as soon as the tenure of the Fellowship is completed.

For further information contact:

WellBeing
27 Sussex Place
Regent's Park, London, NW1 4SP, England
Tel: (44) 171 772 6338
Fax: (44) 171 724 7725
Contact: The Research Administrator

Ethicon Foundation Fund Travel

Subjects: Obstetrics and gynaecology.
Eligibility: RCOG members, and exceptionally fellows.
Level of Study: Postgraduate.
Purpose: To attend postgraduate training courses and visit research centres.
Type: Travel Grant.
No. of awards offered: Up to 15.
Frequency: Every two years.
Value: Up to a maximum of £750.
Application Procedure: For further information please contact the awards secretary at the main address.
Closing Date: January 31st; July 31st.

Florence and William Blair-Bell Memorial Fellowship

Subjects: Gynaecology and obstetrics.
Eligibility: Fellows or members.
Purpose: To bridge the gap between scientific research and clinical practice.
Type: Fellowship.
No. of awards offered: 1.
Frequency: Annual.
Value: Up to £30,000.

Application Procedure: Please contact The Reseach Administrator at the WellBeing address.
Closing Date: First Monday in December.

For further information contact:

WellBeing
27 Sussex Place
Regent's Park, London, NW1 4SP, England
Tel: (44) 171 772 6338
Fax: (44) 171 724 7725
Contact: The Research Administrator

Green-Armytage and Spackman Travelling Scholarship

Subjects: Obstetrics and gynaecology.
Eligibility: Open to Fellows and Members of the College.
Level of Study: Postgraduate.
Purpose: To visit centres where similar work is carried out to that of the applicants.
Type: Scholarship.
No. of awards offered: 1.
Frequency: Every three years.
Value: Up to £4,000.
Study Establishment: At centre(s) where similar work is being carried out.
Country of Study: Any country.
Application Procedure: Applications should include information on qualifications; area of interest and/or publications in a specified area; centre(s) to be visited, with confirmation of arrangements from the head of that centre; estimated costs; and names of two referees. Applicants should have shown a special interest in some particular aspect of obstetrical or gynaecological practice. The College also offers the Harold Malkin Prize, the Edgar Gentilli Prize and the William Blair-Bell Memorial Lectureships.
Closing Date: July 31st.
Additional Information: For further information please contact the College Secretary.

Green-Armytage Anglo American Lectureship

Subjects: Sterility or sub-fertility.
Eligibility: RCOG Fellows and Members absed in the British Isles (by application) USA lecture (by invitation.
Purpose: To assist RCOG Fellows and Members with travel to the lectureship.
Type: Lectureship.
No. of awards offered: 1.
Frequency: Biennial, rotates between UK and USA.
Value: Under discussion.
Application Procedure: Please contact the Awards Secretary at the main address for information.
Closing Date: July 31st.

Harold Malkin Prize

Subjects: Gynaecology and obstetrics.
Eligibility: RCOG Members or Membership candidates.
Level of Study: Professional development.

Purpose: Awarded to those undertaking best original work whilst holding a Specialist Registrar post in a hospital in the United Kingdom or the Republic of Ireland.
Type: Prize.
No. of awards offered: 1.
Frequency: Annual.
Value: £200.
Application Procedure: Please contact the Award Secretary at the main address for more information.
Closing Date: July 31st.

Medical Student Prizes

Subjects: Obstetrics and gynaecology.
Eligibility: Open to medical students.
Purpose: Awarded to those students showing the greatest understanding of a clinical problem in obstetrics and gynaecology.
Type: Prize.
No. of awards offered: First Prize 1, Second Prize 1, Third Prize 4.
Frequency: Annual.
Value: 1st Prize £500; 2nd Prize £300; 3rd Prize £50.
Application Procedure: Please contact the Award Secretary at the main address for more information.
Closing Date: January 31st.

Menopause Travel Award

Subjects: Menopause.
Eligibility: Open to those holding, or training for, MRCOG in R/SR posts with a special interest in menopause.
Level of Study: Postgraduate.
Purpose: To study advances in clinical practice in the area of the menopause.
Type: Travel award.
No. of awards offered: up to 6.
Frequency: Annual.
Value: Up to £2,500.
Country of Study: Any country.
Application Procedure: For further information please contact the College Secretary.
Closing Date: August.
Additional Information: The award is available to attend UK, Irish or international symposia or to visit institutions to advance clinical practice.

For further information contact:

27 Sussex Place
Regent's Park, London, NW1 4RG, England
Tel: (44) 171 262 5425
Fax: (44) 171 723 0575
Contact: College Secretary

Overseas Fund (Founded by the Aileen Dickens Bequest)

Subjects: Obstetrics and gynaecology.
Eligibility: RCOG Members of equivalent working in obstetrics and gynaecology overseas.

Level of Study: Professional development.
Purpose: To travel to the British Isles for further training.
Type: Travel Grant.
No. of awards offered: Up to 6.
Frequency: Annual.
Value: Up to a maximum of £2,000.
Application Procedure: Please contact the Award Secretary at the main address for further information.
Closing Date: December 1st.

RCOG/Wyeth Historical Lecture

Subjects: Obstetrics and gynaecology with a strong historical content.
Eligibility: RCOG Fellows and Members.
Purpose: To attend a lecture on a current development in obstetrics and gynaecology with a strong historical content.
Type: lecture.
No. of awards offered: 1.
Frequency: Annual.
Value: Honorarium of £100.
Application Procedure: Please contact the Award Secretary at the main address for details.
Closing Date: August 31st.

Research Training Fellowships

Subjects: Gynaecology and obstetrics.
Eligibility: Candidates will have had their basic training in obstetrics and gynaecology, preferably having passed their MRCOG. Candidates will be expected to enrol for a higher degree.
Purpose: To further the training of a young medical graduate in research techniques and methodology in a subject in a subject of direct or indirect relevance to obstetrics and gynaecology.
Type: Fellowship.
No. of awards offered: Varies.
Frequency: Annual.
Value: Up to a maximum of three years salary.
Length of Study: Up to 3 years.
Application Procedure: Enquiries about this award should be directed to The Research Administrator, WellBeing.
Closing Date: First Friday in October.

For further information contact:

WellBeing
27 Sussex Place
Regent's Park, London, NW1 4SP, England
Tel: (44) 171 772 6338
Fax: (44) 171 724 7725
Contact: The Research Administrator

USA/British Isles Visiting Fellowship

Subjects: Gynaecology and obstetrics.
Eligibility: Specialist Registrars in the British Isles or Junior Fellows or those in residency programmes in obstetrics and gynaecology in the United states of America.
Level of Study: Professional development.

Purpose: To visit a specific centre offering new techniques or methods of practice.
Type: Fellowship.
No. of awards offered: 1.
Frequency: Annual.
Value: Up to a maximum of £1,000.
Application Procedure: Please contact the Award Registrar at the main address.
Closing Date: July 31st.

WellBeing Grants

Subjects: Gynaecology and obstetrics.
Eligibility: Specialists in any obstetrics and gynaecology inter-related field.
Level of Study: Professional development.
Purpose: Research into all aspects of Obstetrics and Gynaecology with emphasis on increasing safety of childbirth for mother and baby and prevention of handicap.
Type: Grant.
No. of awards offered: Varies depending on the amount of disposable income.
Frequency: Annual.
Value: Up to a maximum of £80,000 over three years, with not more than £45,000 in the first year.
Application Procedure: Please write to the WellBeing address for more information.

For further information contact:

WellBeing
27 Sussex Place
Regent's Park, London, NW1 4SP, England
Tel: (44) 171 772 6338
Fax: (44) 171 724 7725
Contact: The Research Administrator

Young Obstetrician/Gynaecologist Fellowship

Subjects: Gynaecology and obstetrics.
Eligibility: Young (up to 35 years) obstetricians/gynaecologists from the developing world.
Level of Study: Professional development.
Purpose: To attend a centre in the UK to further their training prior to attendance at the FIGO Congress.
Type: Fellowship.
No. of awards offered: 1.
Frequency: Every three years, 2000 onwards.
Value: Up to a maximum of £4,000.
Country of Study: United Kingdom.
Application Procedure: Please contact the Award Secretary at the main address.
Closing Date: Varies as the award is linked to the FIGO Congress.

ROYAL COLLEGE OF PAEDIATRICS AND CHILD HEALTH

50 Hallam Street, London, WIN 6DE, England
Tel: (44) 171 307 5650
Fax: (44) 171 307 5652
Email: aambalu@rcpch.ac.uk
Contact: Miss Amanda Ambalu, Fellowship Administrator

Royal College of Paediatrics and Child Health works to advance the art and science of Paediatrics; to raise the standard of medical care provided to children; to educate and examine those concerned with health of children; to advance the education of the public - and in particular medical practitioners - in child health.

Heinz Fellowships (Types A and C)

Subjects: Paediatrics.
Eligibility: Type A fellowships are open to paediatricians from any part of the Commonwealth who will benefit from meeting UK paediatricians and seeing something of their work; preference is given in general to applicants from developing countries who are not otherwise likely to visit the UK. Type C fellowships are open to UK paediatricians in the early years of professional life.
Level of Study: Professional development.
Purpose: To enable paediatricians from any part of the Commonwealth overseas to spend up to 12 weeks in the UK and to attend the Spring meeting of the College (Type A) or to enable British paeditriacians in the early years of professional life to spend up to 3 months in a developing country.
Type: Fellowship.
No. of awards offered: Varies.
Frequency: Annual.
Value: To cover the cost of air fares and living expenses.
Length of Study: Up to 12 weeks (Type A); or for a short working visit to a centre for up to 3 months, teaching or conducting research that will benefit the Fellow and hosts (Type C).
Country of Study: United Kingdom (Type A) or a developing country (Type C).
Application Procedure: Application forms are available from Amanda Amabalu. Application form to be completed and submitted with CV and a letter of support from the applicant's Head of Department.
Closing Date: Please write for details.

ROYAL COLLEGE OF SURGEONS OF ENGLAND

35-43 Lincoln's Inn Fields, London, WC2A 3PN, England
Tel: (44) 171 405 3474 ext 4005
Fax: (44) 171 831 9438
Email: msorensen@rcseng.ac.uk
www: http://www.rcseng.ac.uk
Contact: Ms Maura Sorensen, Lectureships and Scholar Administrative Secretary

Ethicon Foundation Fund

Subjects: Surgery.
Eligibility: Open to Fellows of the Royal College of Surgeons of England, preferably surgeons in training or within one year from their appointment as Consultant.
Level of Study: Professional development.
Purpose: To promote international goodwill in surgery and to assist Fellows travelling abroad for research or training purposes.
Type: Grant.
No. of awards offered: 1.
Frequency: Twice a year.
Value: Varies according to number of awards and travel costs.
Length of Study: Varies.
Country of Study: Any country.
Application Procedure: Applications (10 copies) should be addressed to the Secretary and must include the following: a letter of application, to include details of the nature, purpose and date of the proposed visit; a CV, including a list of publications; a letter of support from the Head of Department, or Consultant, under whom the applicant is currently working; a letter of support from another, independent, referee; a financial statement showing expenses to be incurred, with special reference to the cost of personal travel, financial resources already available, and other grants or fellowships being sought. All expenses should be given in sterling.
Closing Date: February 19th and August 20th.

Lionel Colledge Memorial Fellowship in Otolaryngology

Subjects: Head and neck surgery, with an emphasis on laryngology, rhinology or otology.
Eligibility: Open to candidates who are Fellows of the Royal College of Surgeons and between 25 and 35 years of age. Candidates must be senior trainees or recently appointed Consultants, or of similar status, in otolaryngology, rhinology, or otology.
Level of Study: Professional development.
Purpose: To encourage research in the area of head and neck surgery with an emphasis on laryngology, rhinology or otology.
Type: Fellowship.
No. of awards offered: 1.
Frequency: Annual.
Value: Up to £3,000.
Length of Study: Varies.

Study Establishment: Appropriate research institutions outside the UK.
Country of Study: Any country.
Application Procedure: Applications (8 copies) should be addressed to the Secretary and must include the following: name, qualifications and brief CV, including present appointment; proposals for the tour, or visit, to be made during the tenure of the fellowship; letters of support from the applicant's present Consultant (or if already a Consultant, the name of an independent referee in the UK) and from the Head(s) of the Department(s) to be visited; a statement of the expenses to be incurred, and of available financial resources.
Closing Date: April 30th.

Norman Capener Travelling Fellowships

Subjects: Surgery.
Eligibility: Open to medical practitioners. Preference is given to candidates enrolled for Higher Surgical Training or those who have recently completed a course in orthopaedic or hand surgery.
Level of Study: Professional development.
Purpose: To provide travel expenses to and from the UK for the study of orthopaedic surgery and surgery of the hand.
Type: Fellowship.
No. of awards offered: Varies.
Frequency: Every two years.
Value: Varies according to travel costs; paid in one lump sum.
Country of Study: Any country.
Application Procedure: Applications should be submitted to the Secretary of the College and should include the following: a brief CV; an account of the proposed research project and where it is to be carried out; a letter of support from the Consultant under whom the applicant is currently working, or, in the case of the applicant being a Consultant, a letter of support from an independent referee; a statement of the estimated costs to be incurred, including details of stipend, or other resources available, or applied for.
Closing Date: June 31st.

ROYAL IRISH ACADEMY

19 Dawson Street, Dublin, 2, Ireland
Tel: (353) 1 676 2570
Fax: (353) 1 676 2346
Email: admin@ria.ie
www: http://www.ria.ie
Contact: Ms Veronica Barker, Assistant Executive Secretary

The Royal Irish Academy was established in 1875 and is the senior learned institution in Ireland for both the sciences and humanities. It publishes a number of learned journals and monographs. It is Ireland's national representative to a large number of international unions, and through its national committees, runs conferences, lectures and workshops. It also manages a number of scholarly, long-term research projects.

Royal Irish Academy National Committee for Nutritional Sciences Award

Subjects: Dietetics, microbiology.
Eligibility: Open to people who are resident in either Northern or Southern Ireland. Only applicants less than 45 years of age on January 1st of the year of the award are eligible.
Level of Study: Postdoctorate, Professional development.
Purpose: To recognise research contributions in nutritional sciences in referred international journals.
No. of awards offered: 1.
Frequency: Every 2-4 years.
Value: Silver medal.
Country of Study: Ireland.
Application Procedure: Nomination must be made independently by two scientists who are familiar with the work of the nominee. Open to nutritional science and some aspects of microbiology.
Closing Date: Applications are accepted at any time.
Additional Information: A silver medal will be awarded and the recipient will deliver a review lecture at the Royal Irish Academy. A copy of the lecture must be deposited in the Academy's library.

THE ROYAL SOCIETY

6 Carlton House Terrace, London, SW1Y 5AG, England
Tel: (44) 171 451 2516
Fax: (44) 171 930 2170
www: http://www.royalsoc.ac.uk
Contact: Mr Carl Smith, Press Officer

Royal Society Research Grants

Subjects: Any scientific or technological discipline within the remit of the Royal Society, i.e. the natural sciences, including mathematics, engineering science, agricultural and medical research, the scientific aspects of archaeology, geography, experimental psychology and the history of science.
Eligibility: Applicants should normally either be holding or have been appointed to permanent posts in institutions recognised by the Royal Society, or hold or have been appointed to limited-tenure postdoctoral research posts, obtained in open competition, and held in such establishments. Applications from retired scientists may also be accepted where the individual conducts his/her research in, or directly associated with, an eligible organisation. Non-tenured researchers working in association with an eligible institution may apply for support for research in the history of science. No age restriction or preference applies.
Level of Study: Postdoctorate.
Purpose: To meet certain specified costs entailed in undertaking a research project in which the applicant is personally engaged. Such costs are envisaged as normally arising through an applicant initiating or developing specific investigations, entering a promising new or modified field of research, or taking advantage of developments in apparatus offering improved techniques in a promising line of research.
Type: Research Grant.

No. of awards offered: Varies.
Frequency: Twice a year.
Value: Up to £10,000.
Country of Study: United Kingdom, except field research, research at sea, research at a marine biological laboratory or research in the history of science.
Application Procedure: Application form to be completed.
Closing Date: November 1st, April 1st.
Additional Information: Grants are for one or more specific items of expenditure in a given 12-month period. Provision is intended to complement that provided by the host department/institution where an individual's research capacity can be significantly enhanced by such provision. Grants will be made through host institutions. Academic workers in UK universities, or other institutions of higher education or in certain associated, independent non-governmental, non-commercial research institutions recognised by the Royal Society are eligible.

THE ROYAL SOCIETY OF EDINBURGH

22-26 George Street, Edinburgh, EH2 2PQ, Scotland
Tel: (44) 131 225 5000
Fax: (44) 131 220 5024
Email: resfells@rse.org.uk
www: http://www.ma.hw.ac.uk/rse/
Contact: The Research Fellowships Secretary

The Royal Society of Edinburgh is Scotland's National Academy. It is an independent body, founded in 1783 by Royal Charter for 'The Advancement of Learning and Useful Knowledge' and governed by an elected council of Fellows.

Auber Bequest

Subjects: All subjects.
Eligibility: Open to naturalised British citizens or individuals wishing to acquire British nationality who are over 60 years of age, resident in Scotland or England and are bona fide scholars engaged in academic (but not industrial) research.
Level of Study: Unrestricted.
Purpose: To provide assistance for the furtherance of academic research in any of its branches.
No. of awards offered: Varies.
Frequency: Every two years.
Value: Varies; not normally exceeding £3,000.
Length of Study: Up to 2 years.
Country of Study: Scotland or England.
Application Procedure: Application forms are available from the Research Fellowships Secretary.
Closing Date: October 31st.
Additional Information: Applicants should not at birth have been British nationals nor held dual British nationality. Applicants must have acquired British nationality.

CRF/RSE Personal Research Fellowships

Subjects: Biological, biochemical, physical and clinical sciences.
Eligibility: Open to students of all nationalities, who have a PhD and are aged 32 or under on the date of appointment, or who have between 2-6 years' postdoctoral experience.
Level of Study: Postdoctorate.
Purpose: To aid independent research in the biomedical sciences.
Type: Fellowship.
No. of awards offered: Varies.
Frequency: Annual.
Value: Salary according to age, qualifications and experience. Salaries within the scales RGIA-2 for research staff in Higher Education Institutions (£15,986-£24,132). Financial support towards expenses involved in carrying out the research is available, including a start-up grant of £1,000 in the first year only. Fellows receive £1,000 for travel and subsistence each year and are also eligible to make bids annually for equipment and consumables, usually up to a value of £5,000, from a research support pool.
Length of Study: Up to 3 years.
Study Establishment: Any Higher Education Institution in Scotland.
Country of Study: Scotland.
Application Procedure: Application forms are available from the Caledonian Research Foundation. Candidates must negotiate directly with the relevant Head of Department of the proposed host institution.
Closing Date: Mid-March.
Additional Information: The Fellowships are administered by the Caledonian Research Foundation (CRF). Fellows will be expected to devote their full time to research and will not be allowed to hold other paid appointments without the express permission of the Council of the RSE.

For further information contact:

The Caledonian Research Foundation
39 Castle Street, Edinburgh, EH2 3BH, Scotland
Contact: Grants Management Officer

CRF/RSE Support Research Fellowship

Subjects: Biology, biochemical, physical and clinical sciences related to medicine.
Eligibility: Open to existing members of academic staff (aged 40 or under on date of appointment and employed on the lecturer scale) who have held a permanent appointment for at least five years in any Scottish Higher Education Institution.
Level of Study: Professional development.
Purpose: To enable support fellows to take study leave, either in their own institution or elsewhere, whilst remaining in continuous employment with their present employer.
Type: Fellowship.
No. of awards offered: 1.
Frequency: Annual.
Value: The actual cost for non-clinical staff will be reimbursed according to the lecturer 'A' scale (maximum RGI-3) with the placement determined by the employer. If clinically qualified, salary will be within clinical senior lecturer grade. Provision of

£1,000 is made for a start-up grant. There is also a grant of £1,000 for travel and subsistence. Fellows are also eligible to make a bid for equipment and consumables, usually up to a value of £2,000, from a research support pool.
Length of Study: 1 year.
Study Establishment: Any Higher Education Institution in Scotland.
Country of Study: Scotland.
Application Procedure: Application forms are available from the Caledonian Research Foundation.
Closing Date: Mid-March.
Additional Information: This award is administered by the Caledonian Research Foundation.

For further information contact:

The Caledonian Research Foundation
39 Castle Street, Edinburgh, EH2 3BH, Scotland
Contact: Grants Management Officer

Henry Dryerre Scholarship

Subjects: Medical or veterinary physiology.
Eligibility: Open to EC citizens holding a first class honours degree from a Scottish university.
Level of Study: Postgraduate.
Purpose: To support postgraduate research.
Type: Scholarship.
No. of awards offered: 1.
Frequency: Every four years.
Value: Covers the cost of fees; provides for research costs and travel expenses up to £850 per year and a maintenance grant of £5,956 if living away from home.
Length of Study: 3 years full-time research.
Study Establishment: A Scottish institution.
Country of Study: Scotland.
Application Procedure: Applicants must be nominated by a professor, reader or lecturer in a Scottish university.
Closing Date: March 15th.
Additional Information: The Scholarships are administered by the Carnegie Trust for the Universities of Scotland.

For further information contact:

Carnegie Trust for the Universities of Scotland
Cameron House
Abbey Park Place, Dunfermline, Fife, KY12 7PZ, Scotland
Tel: (44) 1383 622148
Fax: (44) 1383 622149
Contact: Professor J T Coppock
or
22-26 George Street, Edinburgh, EH2 2PQ, Scotland
Tel: (44) 131 240 5000
Fax: (44) 131 240 5024
Contact: Ms Anne D G Ferguson, Research Fellowships Secretary

SOEID Personal Research Fellowships

Subjects: All subjects. A proportion of the Fellowships are awarded in fields likely to enhance the development of industry and encourage better uses of resources in Scotland.

Eligibility: Open to persons of all nationalities who have a PhD or equivalent qualification. Candidates must be aged 32 or under on the date of appointment (October 1st) or have between 2-6 years' postdoctoral experience, and must show they have a capacity for innovative research and have a substantial volume of published work relevant to their proposed field of study.

Level of Study: Postdoctorate.

Purpose: To encourage independent research in any discipline.

Type: Fellowship.

No. of awards offered: 2.

Frequency: Annual.

Value: Annual stipends are within the scales RGIA-2 for reseach and analogous staff in Higher Education Institutions (£16,366-£25,092 as at April 1st 1998) with annual increments and superannuation benefits. Expenses to a maximum of £2,500 in year one; £1,000 in years two and three, for travel and attendance at meetings or incidentals may be reimbursed. No support payments are available to the institution but Fellows may seek support for their research from other sources.

Length of Study: Up to 3 years full-time research.

Study Establishment: Any Higher Education Institution, research institution or industrial laboratory approved for the purpose by the Council of the Society.

Country of Study: Scotland.

Application Procedure: Candidates should negotiate directly with the proposed host institution. The Fellowships are offered with the support of the Scottish Office Education and Industry Department (SOEID). Application forms are available from the Research Fellowships Secretary.

Closing Date: Mid-March.

Additional Information: Fellows may not hold other paid appointments without the express permission of the Council, but teaching or seminar work appropriate to their special knowledge may be acceptable.

SOEID/RSE Support Research Fellowships

Subjects: All subjects. A proportion of the fellowships are awarded in fields of research likely to enhance the development of industry and encourage better use of resources in Scotland.

Eligibility: Candidates must be existing members of staff who have held a permanent appointment for not less than five years in any Higher Education Institution in Scotland. Applicants should normally be aged under 40 on the date of appointment (October 1st) and employed on the lecturer (or equivalent) grade.

Level of Study: Professional development.

Purpose: To enable support fellows to take study leave, either in their own institution or elsewhere, whilst remaining in continuous employment with their present employer.

Type: Fellowship.

No. of awards offered: 2.

Frequency: Annual.

Value: The actual cost of replacement staff will be reimbursed according to the Lecturer A scale (maximum RGI-3) with the placement determined by the employer. Superannuation

costs and employer's NI contributions will also be reimbursed.

Length of Study: Up to 12 months full-time research.

Study Establishment: Any Higher Education Institution, research institution or industrial laboratory in Scotland approved for the purpose by the Council of the Society.

Country of Study: Scotland.

Application Procedure: Application forms are available from the Research Fellowships Secretary. Candidates should negotiate directly with the proposed host institution. The Fellowships are offered with the support of the Scottish Office Education and Industry Department (SOEID).

Closing Date: Mid-March.

Additional Information: Awards will take the form of funding for the appointment of a temporary replacement to enable fellows to take study leave. There is provision for reimbursement of approved expenses for support fellows to a maximum of £500 per annum, in respect of actual expenses associated with the research, including travel and attendance at meetings.

THE ROYAL SOCIETY OF MEDICINE

1 Wimpole Street, London, W1M 8AE, England
Tel: (44) 171 290 2900
Fax: (44) 171 290 2909
Email: louisa.bendela@roysocmed.ac.uk
Contact: Ms Louisa Bendela

The Royal Society of Medicine provides academic services and club facilities for its members as well as publishing a monthly journal and a quarterly bulletin, and providing over three hundred educational conferences and meetings per annum.

Colyer Prize

Subjects: Odontology.

Eligibility: Open to dental surgeons educated at a UK dental school who have not been qualified more than 10 years.

Level of Study: Postdoctorate.

Purpose: Awarded for the best original work in dental science completed during the previous five years.

Type: Research Prize.

No. of awards offered: 1.

Frequency: Every three years.

Value: Varies; at least £100.

Country of Study: United Kingdom.

Application Procedure: Candidates should submit a general brief account of their research of not more than 800 words.

Closing Date: March 31st.

John of Arderne Medal

Subjects: Coloproctology.

Eligibility: Open to applicants of any nationality.

Level of Study: Professional development.

Purpose: To award the presenter of the best paper presented at the short papers meeting of the section of Coloproctology. Applicants have to submit an abstract for presentation at the meeting.
Type: Medal and Travelling Fellowship.
No. of awards offered: 1.
Frequency: Annual.
Value: Variable.
Study Establishment: Variable.
Country of Study: Any country.
Application Procedure: Please write for details.
Closing Date: September and November.

Karl Storz Travelling Scholarship

Subjects: Laryngology/rhinology.
Eligibility: Open to senior registrars or consultants of not more than two years standing, who must be members of the section of Laryngology & Rhinology of the RSM.
Level of Study: Postdoctorate.
Purpose: To assist with the cost of travel to overseas centres.
Type: Scholarship.
No. of awards offered: 1.
Frequency: Annual.
Value: £1,000.
Country of Study: Any country.
Application Procedure: The Scholarship is awarded for a paper to be submitted to the RSM Section of Laryngology and Rhinology.
Closing Date: January 31st.
Additional Information: A report is required of the recipient within three months of his/her return to the UK.

Medical Insurance Agency Prize

Subjects: Surgery.
Eligibility: Open to surgeons in training, holding the post of up to the grade of registrar or senior registrar.
Level of Study: Professional development.
Purpose: To enable the recipient to travel to a recognised institution (in the UK or overseas) to further his or her knowledge of surgery, or to attend an overseas conference in the speciality.
Type: Prize.
No. of awards offered: 1.
Frequency: Annual.
Value: £500.
Study Establishment: A recognised institution in the UK or overseas.
Country of Study: Any country.
Application Procedure: Please write for details.
Additional Information: The winner will be required to submit a brief report on the visit, within three months of his or her return.

Mental Health Foundation Essay Prize

Subjects: Psychiatry.
Eligibility: Open to candidates practising medicine in the UK or the Republic of Ireland who are in training at any grade from senior house officer to senior registrar or equivalent.

Level of Study: Unrestricted.
Type: Essay Prize.
No. of awards offered: 1.
Frequency: Annual.
Value: Varies: £500, but depends on available finance. Also, subscription to RSM (if funds available).
Country of Study: United Kingdom.
Application Procedure: Applicants need not be members of RSM. The prize is awarded for an essay on psychiatry, submitted to the RSM Section of Psychiatry (in triplicate).
Closing Date: March 31st.
Additional Information: The subject is left to the candidate. Essays should be approximately 5,000 words in length.

Nichols Fellowship

Subjects: Obstetrics and gynaecology.
Eligibility: Open to suitably qualified UK citizens.
Level of Study: Postdoctorate.
Purpose: To encourage research to advance knowledge in obstetrics and gynaecology.
Type: Fellowship.
No. of awards offered: 1.
Frequency: Every three years (1999).
Value: £500 per year for 2 years (the second year being at the discretion of the Section Council).
Length of Study: 2 years.
Country of Study: Any country.
Application Procedure: Please write for details.

Norman Gamble Fund and Research Prize

Subjects: Otology.
Eligibility: Open to British nationals.
Level of Study: Unrestricted.
Purpose: To support specific research projects in otology.
Type: Prize.
No. of awards offered: 1.
Frequency: Every four years (next 2000).
Value: £300 for research prize; £1,000 for grant-in-aid.
Country of Study: Any country.
Application Procedure: Please write for details.
Closing Date: May 31st.

Norman Tanner Medal and Prize

Subjects: Surgery.
Eligibility: Open to applicants of any nationality.
Level of Study: Professional development.
Purpose: To enable the recipient to travel to a recognised institution (in the UK or overseas) to further his or her knowledge of surgery, or to attend an overseas conference in the speciality.
Type: Medal and Travel Grant.
No. of awards offered: 1.
Frequency: Annual.
Value: £500.
Country of Study: Any country.
Application Procedure: Papers must be presented at a meeting.

Ophthalmology Travelling Fellowship

Subjects: Ophthalmology.
Eligibility: Open to ophthalmologists in the British Isles of any nationality who have not attained an official consultant appointment, nor undertaken professional clinical work or equivalent responsibility for any substantial period before or during the execution of original work.
Level of Study: Professional development.
Type: Fellowship.
No. of awards offered: Varies.
Frequency: Twice a year.
Value: Varies.
Study Establishment: Variable.
Country of Study: Any country.
Application Procedure: Please apply to the Academic Administrator at the RSM.
Closing Date: Entries are evaluated in December and May.

Royal Society of Medicine President's Prize

Subjects: Neurology.
Eligibility: Open to applicants of any nationality.
Level of Study: Professional development.
Purpose: Summaries of cases for clinical presentation.
Type: Prize.
No. of awards offered: 1.
Frequency: Annual.
Value: £100.
Country of Study: Any country.
Application Procedure: Please write for details.
Closing Date: January.
Additional Information: Presentations take place in April.

Royal Society of Medicine Travelling Fellowship

Subjects: Urology.
Eligibility: Open to members of the section of Urology of the Royal Society of Medicine, who should be in urological training or within three years of a consultant appointment.
Level of Study: Professional development.
Purpose: To enable the holder to enhance his or her knowledge and experience by visiting an overseas unit.
Type: Travelling Fellowship.
No. of awards offered: Varies.
Frequency: Annual.
Value: £1,000.
Country of Study: Any country.
Application Procedure: Please write for details.
Closing Date: October 9th.

Sylvia Lawler Prize

Subjects: Oncology.
Eligibility: The awards are intended to go to medically qualified or scientifically qualified trainees.
Level of Study: Postgraduate.
Purpose: To provide two prizes annually in the field of oncology intended to go to medically qualified or scientifically qualified trainees.
Type: Prize.

No. of awards offered: 2.
Frequency: Annual.
Value: £500 for each of the two prize winners. The prize winners may also be reimbursed travel expenses up to the value of £100.
Country of Study: United Kingdom.
Application Procedure: Applicants are invited to submit an abstract of 1 side of A4 to the annually held Sylvia Lawler prize meeting. Abstract forms are available from Louisa Bendela.

RUTH ESTRIN GOLDBERG MEMORIAL FOR CANCER RESEARCH

885 Gloucester Road, Union, NJ, 07083, United States of America
Tel: (1) 908 688 1725
Contact: Ms Myra Abramson

Ruth Estrin Goldberg Memorial for Cancer Research

Subjects: Cancer research.
Eligibility: Open to candidates from Eastern USA: preferably New York, New Jersey, Pennsylvania, Connecticut, Massachusetts, Delaware or Maryland.
Level of Study: Unrestricted.
Purpose: To support cancer research.
No. of awards offered: 2.
Frequency: Annual.
Value: US$10,000 to US$15,000.
Country of Study: USA.
Application Procedure: Please write for application and guidelines.
Closing Date: February 28th.
Additional Information: The Ruth Estrin Goldberg Memorial for Cancer Research is a volunteer organisation.

SAVOY FOUNDATION

PO Box 69
230 Foch, St Jean Sur Richelieu, PQ, J3B 6Z1, Canada
Tel: (1) 450 358 9779
Fax: (1) 450 346 1045
Email: epilepsy@savoy-foundation.ca
www: http://www.savoy-foundation.ca
Contact: Ms Caroline Savoy, Secretary

The Savoy Foundation's main activity is to support and encourage research into epilepsy.

Savoy Foundation Post Doctoral and Clinical Research Fellowships

Subjects: Medical and behavioural science, as they relate to epilepsy.
Eligibility: Candidates must be scientists or medical specialists with a PhD or MD.
Level of Study: Postdoctorate.
Purpose: To support a full-time research project in the field of epilepsy.
Type: Research Grant.
No. of awards offered: Varies.
Frequency: Annual.
Value: C$25,000.
Length of Study: 1 year, in the first instance, but will be renewable once and exceptionally twice, upon request.
Country of Study: Canada.
Application Procedure: For application forms and further information contact the Foundation.
Closing Date: January 15th.
Additional Information: The period of support may begin at any time between May and October.

Savoy Foundation Research Grants

Subjects: Medical and behavioural science, as they relate to epilepsy.
Eligibility: The research grant is intended for launching a project; pre-research; pursuit or completion of a project. It is only available to clinicians and established scientists.
Level of Study: Postdoctorate.
Purpose: To support further research into epilepsy.
Type: Research Grant.
No. of awards offered: Varies.
Frequency: Annual.
Value: Up to C$25,000.
Country of Study: Canada.
Application Procedure: Contact the Foundation for an application form and further information.
Closing Date: January 15th.
Additional Information: The grant is only available to Canadian citizens or for projects conducted in Canada.

Savoy Foundation Studentships

Subjects: Biomedicine, neurology.
Eligibility: The candidate must have a good university record (Bsc, MD or equivalent diploma) and have ensured that a qualified researcher affiliated to a university or hospital will supervise his or her work. Concomitant registration in a graduate programme is encouraged. The awards are available to Canadian citizens or for projects conducted in Canada.
Level of Study: Doctorate, Postgraduate.
Purpose: To support training and research in a biomedical discipline, the health sciences or social sciences related to epilepsy.
Type: Studentship.
No. of awards offered: Varies.
Frequency: Annual.
Value: The stipend will be C$12,000 for the first year, with a C$1,000 increase for each year of renewal. An annual sum of C$1,000 will be allocated to the laboratory or institution as additional support for the research project.
Length of Study: 1-4 years.
Country of Study: Canada.
Application Procedure: For application forms and further information contact the Savoy Foundation.
Closing Date: January 15th.
Additional Information: The studentship is available to Canadian citizens or for projects conducted in Canada.

SCHOLARSHIP FOUNDATION OF THE LEAGUE OF FINNISH-AMERICAN SOCIETIES

Mechelininkatu 10, Helsinki, SF-0010, Finland
Tel: (358) 9 41 333 700
Fax: (358) 9 408 794
Email: sayl@sayl.fi
www: http://www.sayl.fi
Contact: Ms Sisko Rauhala, Culture and Youth Programmes

Scholarship Foundation of the League for Finnish-American Societies

Subjects: All subjects.
Eligibility: Open to Finns only.
Level of Study: Doctorate, Postdoctorate, Postgraduate.
Purpose: To enable Finns to study in the United States.
Type: Scholarship.
No. of awards offered: 2-3.
Frequency: Annual.
Value: US$3,000-US$5,000.
Length of Study: 1 academic year.
Study Establishment: University.
Country of Study: USA.
Application Procedure: Application form and references must be submitted.
Closing Date: First Monday in October.
Additional Information: The Scholarship Foundation also handles awards given to Finns by the American-Scandinavian Foundation and Thanks to Scandinavia Inc, both based in New York.

SIDNEY SUSSEX COLLEGE, CAMBRIDGE

Cambridge, CB2 3HU, England
Tel: (44) 1223 338800
Fax: (44) 1223 338884
Email: aga22@cam.ac.uk
www: http://www.sid.com.ac.uk
Contact: Tutor for Graduate Students

Founded in 1596, Sidney Sussex College admits men and women as undergraduates and graduates. The college presently has 150 graduate students, including 75 working for the PhD degree. The college has excellent sporting, dramatic, and musical facilities, and can house the majority of its graduate students in college rooms.

Sidney Sussex College Research Studentship

Subjects: All subjects.
Eligibility: Applicants must also apply for a postgraduate place at the University of Cambridge. Preference is for candidates under 26 years of age. Candidates must be or must become members of Sidney Sussex College.
Level of Study: Doctorate.
Purpose: To provide full support for one student to do three years of research leading to the degree of PhD at the University of Cambridge.
Type: Studentship.
No. of awards offered: 1.
Frequency: Every two years.
Value: £5,455 maintenance per year plus fees.
Length of Study: 3 years.
Study Establishment: University of Cambridge.
Country of Study: United Kingdom.
Application Procedure: Application form is available from the tutor for graduate studies.
Closing Date: March 1st.

SIGMA THETA TAU INTERNATIONAL

550 West North Street, Indianapolis, IN, 46202, United States of America
Tel: (1) 317 634 8171
Contact: Grants Management Officer

Sigma Theta Tau International exists to promote the development, dissemination and utilisation of nursing knowledge. It is committed to improving the health of people worldwide through increasing the scientific base of nursing practice.

Rosemary Berkel Crisp Research Award

Subjects: Women's health, oncology, and infant/child care.
Eligibility: Applicants must be a registered nurse with a current license, have a Master's or higher degree (those with baccalaureate degrees may be co-investigators), have submitted a complete research application package, be ready to initiate the research project, and be a member of the Sigma Theta Tau International. Submissions should include a completed Sigma Theta Tau research application and research agreement.
Level of Study: Postgraduate.
Purpose: To support nursing research in the critical areas of women's health, oncology, and infant and child care.
Type: Award.
No. of awards offered: 1.
Frequency: Annual.

Value: US$3,000.
Application Procedure: Please write to Sigma Theta Tau International for an application form and details.
Closing Date: March 1st.
Additional Information: Some preference is given to applicants residing in Illinois, Missouri, Arkansas, Kentucky and Tennessee.

Sigma Theta Tau International American Association of Critical Care Nurses

Subjects: Critical care nursing practice.
Eligibility: Applicants must be a registered nurse with a current licence; must have received a Master's degree; and grant proposals must be relevant to critical care nursing practice. Research must be related to critical care nursing practice.
Level of Study: Postgraduate.
Purpose: To encourage qualified nurses to contribute to the advancement of nursing through critical care nursing research.
Type: Research Grant.
No. of awards offered: 1.
Frequency: Annual.
Value: Up to US$10,000.
Study Establishment: Unrestricted.
Country of Study: USA.
Application Procedure: Applications must be sent to AACN. Please write for an information booklet and application form.
Closing Date: October 1st.
Additional Information: Funding date is January 1st.

For further information contact:

American Association of Critical Care Nurses
Department of Research
101 Columbia, Aliso Viejo, CA, 92656-1491, United States of America
Tel: (1) 714 362 2000
Fax: (1) 714 362 2020

Sigma Theta Tau International American Association of Diabetes Educators Grant

Subjects: Research relating to diabetes education and care.
Eligibility: Applicants must be a registered nurse with a current licence, must have received a Master's degree, must have submitted an application package, must be ready to start the research, and must have signed a Sigma Theta Tau research agreement.
Level of Study: Postgraduate.
Purpose: To encourage qualified nurses to contribute to the enhancement of quality and increase the availability of diabetes education and care research.
Type: Research Grant.
No. of awards offered: 1.
Frequency: Annual.
Value: Up to US$6,000.
Country of Study: USA.

Application Procedure: Please write for an information booklet and an application form. Preference will be give to Sigma Theta Tau members, other qualifications being equal.
Closing Date: October 1st.
Additional Information: January 1st is the funding date.

For further information contact:

AADE Foundation Awards
c/o Glenwood Associates
24 Old Georgetown Road, Princeton, NJ, 08540, United States of America
Tel: (1) 732 821 5522
Fax: (1) 732 821 5955

Sigma Theta Tau International American Nephrology Nurses Association Grant

Subjects: Nephrology nursing.
Eligibility: The research topic must be related to nephrology nursing care. Applicants must be a registered nurse with a current licence, must have received a Master's degree, must have submitted an application package, must be ready to start the research project, and must have signed a Sigma Theta Tau research agreement.
Level of Study: Postgraduate.
Purpose: To encourage research related to nephrology nursing practice.
Type: Research Grant.
No. of awards offered: 1.
Frequency: Annual.
Value: Up to US$6,000.
Study Establishment: Unrestricted.
Country of Study: USA.
Application Procedure: Application forms should be sent to the American Nephrology Nurses Association. Please write for an information booklet and application form.
Closing Date: November 1st.
Additional Information: April 1st is the funding date.

For further information contact:

American Nephrology Nurses' Association
East Holly Avenue
PO Box 56, Pitman, NJ, 08071-0056, United States of America
Tel: (1) 609 256 2320
Fax: (1) 609 589 7463

Sigma Theta Tau International American Nurses Foundation Grant

Subjects: Any clinical topic.
Eligibility: Applicants must be a registered nurse with a current licence, must have received a Master's degree, must be ready to start the research project, must have submitted an application package, and must have signed a Sigma Theta Tau research agreement.
Level of Study: Postgraduate.
Purpose: To encourage the research career development of nurses through support of research conducted by beginning

nurse researchers or experienced nurse researchers who are entering a new field of study.
Type: Grant.
No. of awards offered: 1.
Frequency: Annual.
Value: Up to US$6,000.
Study Establishment: Unrestricted.
Country of Study: USA.
Application Procedure: Please write for an information booklet and application form. The selection process is managed jointly - please send proposals to the Sigma Theta Tau International headquarters in even numbered years (use ANF application), and to the American Nurses Foundation in odd numbered years (use STTI) application.
Closing Date: May 1st.
Additional Information: October 1st is the funding date. Preference will be given to Sigma Theta Tau members, other qualifications being equal. Allocation of funds is based on the quality of the proposed research, the future promise of the applicant, and the applicant's research budget.

For further information contact:

American Nurses Foundation
600 Maryland Avenue SW
Suite 100, West Washington, DC, 20024-2571, United States of America
Tel: (1) 202 651 7227
Fax: (1) 202 651 7001

Sigma Theta Tau International Association of Operating Room Nurses Foundation Grant

Subjects: Perioperative nursing science. All relevant topics will be considered although priority will be given to research studies that relate to the AORN research priorities - the relationship of nursing interventions to quality and cost-effective outcomes - prevention of wound infections, protection from injury (thermal, electric, laser, chemical, physical), maintenance of skin integrity, patient satisfaction with care (nursing care, pain management, anxiety management), and patient and family satisfaction with communication and teaching, the relationship of staff mix, cost, and length of stay to quality outcomes, the impact of technology on patient outcomes, the conduct and utilisation of research related to AORN's standards, recommendation and practice guidelines, and ethical issues related to patient outcomes.
Eligibility: The principal investigator is required to be a registered nurse (with a current license) in the perioperative setting, or a registered nurse who demonstrates interest in or significant contributions to nursing practice. The principal investigator must have, as a minimum, a Master's degree in nursing. Applicants must submit a completed AORN research application. Membership of either organisation is acceptable, but not required.
Level of Study: Postgraduate.
Purpose: To encourage qualified nurses to conduct research related to perioperative nursing practice and contribute to the development of perioperative nursing science.
Type: Grant.

Frequency: Annual.
Value: Varies. Allocation of funds is based on the quality of the research, the future promise of the applicant, and the applicant's research budget.
Application Procedure: Please write to the AORN for an application form and general instructions.
Closing Date: April 1st.

For further information contact:

Association of Operating Room Nurses
2170 South Parker Road
Suite 300, Denver, CO, 8023-5711, United States of America
Tel: (1) 800 755 2676 ext 8219
Fax: (1) 303 750 2927
Contact: Ms Mary H Lopez

Sigma Theta Tau International Emergency Nursing Foundation Grant

Subjects: Emergency nursing. All relevant topics will be considered, although priority will be given to studies which relate to ENA Research Initiatives. These are included, but not limited to - mechanisms to assure effective, efficient and quality emergency nursing care delivery systems, factors effecting health care cost, productivity, and market forces to emergency services, ways to enhance health promotion and injury prevention and mechanisms to assure quality and cost effective educational programmes for emergency nursing.
Eligibility: The research must be related to the specialised practice of emergency nursing. Applicants must be a registered nurse with a current licence, must have received a Master's degree, must have submitted an application package, must be ready to start the research project, and must have signed a Sigma Theta Tau research agreement.
Level of Study: Postgraduate.
Purpose: To provide money for research which will advance the specialised practice of emergency nursing.
Type: Research Grant.
No. of awards offered: 1.
Frequency: Annual.
Value: Up to US$6,000.
Study Establishment: Unrestricted.
Country of Study: USA.
Application Procedure: Please write for an information booklet and application form.
Closing Date: May 1st.
Additional Information: October 1st is the funding date.

For further information contact:

ENA Foundation
216 Higgins Road, Park Ridge, IL, 60068 5736, United States of America
Tel: (1) 847 698 9400
Fax: (1) 847 698 9406

Sigma Theta Tau International Glaxo Wellcome New Investigator Mentor Grant

Subjects: Nursing issues related to medication and medication administration. Possible topics include, but are not limited to compliance issues with patients who have asthma or HIV/AIDS, medication management problems in home health care, interventions to increase or enhance the appropriate use of metered dose inhalers by adolescents, or administration of IV medications in nursing homes and training of personnel administering IV medications.
Eligibility: The grant will be given to a novice investigator and an experienced researcher practicing full-time in an adult clinical setting focussing on nursing issues related to medication and medication administration, and is designed to facilitate collaboration between these. Applicants must be a registered nurse with a current licence, must have received a Master's degree, must have submitted an application package, and must have signed a Sigma Theta Tau research agreement.
Level of Study: Postgraduate.
Purpose: To enable research focusing on nursing issues related to medication and medication administration.
Type: Research Grant.
No. of awards offered: 1.
Frequency: Annual.
Value: US$5,500.
Country of Study: Any country.
Application Procedure: Please write for an information booklet and application form.
Closing Date: October 1st.
Additional Information: Preference will be given to Sigma Theta Tau members, other qualifications being equal. Allocation of funds is based on the quality of the proposed research, the future promise of the applicant, and the applicant's research budget.

Sigma Theta Tau International Glaxo Wellcome Prescriptive Practice Grant

Subjects: Practice nursing. Topics may include, but are not limited to - current status of prescriptive privileges by state, nurses or clients' satisfaction with prescriptive authority, barriers and constraints on nursing practice related to prescribing privileges, health policy and delivery system issues in nurses prescribing, needs of specific populations and client outcomes related to nurse prescribers.
Eligibility: The recipient must be dedicated to the prescribing practices of advanced practice nurses. Applicants must be a registered nurse with a current licence, must have received a Master's degree, must have submitted an application package, must be ready to start the research project, and must have signed a Sigma Theta Tau research agreement.
Level of Study: Postgraduate, Professional development.
Purpose: To support research relating to prescribing practices of advanced practice nurses.

Type: Research Grant.
No. of awards offered: 1.
Frequency: Annual.
Value: Up to US$5,000.
Study Establishment: Unrestricted.
Country of Study: Any country.
Application Procedure: Please write for an information booklet and application form. Preference will be given to Sigma Theta Tau members, other qualifications being equal. Allocation of funds is based on the quality of the proposed research, the future promise of the applicant, and the applicant's research budget.
Closing Date: October 1st.
Additional Information: Preference will be given to Sigma Theta Tau members, other qualifications being equal. Allocation of funds is based on the quality of the proposed research, the future promise of the applicant, and the applicant's research budget.

Sigma Theta Tau International Mead Johnson Nutritionals Perinatal Grant

Subjects: Perinatal issues spanning the prenatal period through the first year of life.
Eligibility: Research must be related to prenatal issues spanning the prenatal period through the first year of life. This may include, but is not limited to low and high risk maternal and neonatal care practices and innovative patient care delivery systems. The grant is restricted to the support of Master's or doctorally prepared nurses conducting prenatal research. Applicants must be a registered nurse with a current licence, must have received a Master's degree, must have submitted an application package, must be ready to start the research project, and must have signed a Sigma Theta Tau research agreement.
Level of Study: Postgraduate.
Purpose: To encourage qualified nurses to contribute to the advancement of nursing through research.
Type: Research Grant.
No. of awards offered: 1.
Frequency: Annual.
Value: Up to US$10,000.
Study Establishment: Unrestricted.
Country of Study: USA.
Application Procedure: Please write for an information booklet and application form.
Closing Date: June 1st.
Additional Information: Funding date is September 1st. Preference will be given to Sigma Theta Tau members, other qualifications being equal. Allocation of funds is based on the quality of the proposed research, the future promise of the applicant, and the applicant's research budget.

Sigma Theta Tau International Oncology Nursing Society Grant

Subjects: Clinical oncology.
Eligibility: The research topic must be oncology clinically orientated. Applicants must be a registered nurse with a current licence, must have received a Master's degree, must have submitted an application package, must be ready to start the research project, and must have signed a Sigma Theta Tau research agreement.
Level of Study: Postgraduate.
Purpose: To encourage the research career development of nurses through support of oncology clinically oriented diseases.
Type: Research Grant.
No. of awards offered: 1.
Frequency: Annual.
Value: Up to US$10,000.
Study Establishment: Unrestricted.
Country of Study: USA.
Application Procedure: Proposals for this grant must be sent to the Oncology Nursing Society. Please write for an information booklet and application form.
Closing Date: November 1st.
Additional Information: Funding date is May 1st.

For further information contact:

Oncology Nursing Foundation
501 Holiday Drive, Pittsburgh, PA, 15220-2749, United States of America
Tel: (1) 412 921 7373
Fax: (1) 412 921 6565

Sigma Theta Tau International Rehabilitation Nursing Foundation Grant

Subjects: Rehabilitation nursing.
Eligibility: The research topic must be related to rehabilitation nursing. The principal investigator must be a registered nurse in rehabilitation or a registered nurse who demonstrates interest in and significant contributions to rehabilitation nursing. Proposals that address the clinical practice, educational, or administrative dimensions of rehabilitation nursing are requested. Quantitative and qualitative research projects will be accepted for review. The research project must be completed within 2 years of initial funding. The principal investigator must have a Master's degree in nursing.
Purpose: To encourage research related to rehabilitation nursing.
Type: Grant.
No. of awards offered: 1.
Frequency: Annual.
Value: Up to US$6,000.
Country of Study: USA.
Application Procedure: Please write for details.
Closing Date: April 1st.
Additional Information: The funding date is the following January.

For further information contact:

Rehabilitation Nursing Foudation
4700 West Lake Avenue, Glenview, IL, 60025, United States
of America
Tel: (1) 800 229 7530
Fax: (1) 847 375 4710

Sigma Theta Tau International Research Grant Opportunities

Subjects: Nursing.
Eligibility: Applicants must be a registered nurse with a
current licence, must have received a Master's degree, must
have submitted an application package, must be ready to
start the research project, and must have signed a Sigma
Theta Tau research agreement. Allocation of funds is based
on the quality of the proposed research, the future promise of
the applicant, and the applicant's research budget. Applicants
from novice researchers who have received no other national
research funds are encouraged and will receive preference for
funding, other aspects being equal.
Level of Study: Postgraduate.
Purpose: To encourage qualified nurses to contribute to the
advancement of nursing through research. Multidisciplinary
and international research is encouraged.
Type: Research Grant.
No. of awards offered: 10-15.
Frequency: Annual.
Value: Up to US$5,000.
Study Establishment: Unrestricted.
Country of Study: Any country.
Application Procedure: Write for information booklet and
application form.
Closing Date: March 1st.
Additional Information: Preference is given to Sigma Theta
Tau International Members. Funding date is July 1st.

Virginia Henderson/Sigma Theta Tau International Clinical Research Grant

Subjects: Clinical research.
Eligibility: Applicants must be a registered nurse actively
involved in some aspect of health care delivery, education or
research in a clinical setting; must hold a Master's degree in
nursing; must be a member of Sigma Theta Tau International.
Allocation of funds is based on a research project ready for
implementation, the quality of the proposed research, the
future of potential of the applicant, appropriateness of the
research budget and feasibility of the time frame.
Level of Study: Postgraduate.
Purpose: To encourage the research career development of
clinically based nurses through support of clinically-orientated
research.
Type: Research Grant.
No. of awards offered: 1.
Frequency: Every two years.
Value: US$5,000.
Application Procedure: Please complete a Sigma Theta Tau
International research grant application.
Closing Date: April 15th.

For further information contact:

Virginia Henderson Research Grant
Sigma Theta Tau International
550 West North Street, Indianapolis, IN, 46202, United States
of America

SIR ERNEST CASSEL EDUCATIONAL TRUST

8 Malvern Terrace
Islington, London, N1 1HR, England
Tel: (44) 171 607 7879
Contact: Secretary

The Trust awards overseas research grants -through the
British Academy - in the language, literature, or civilisation of
any country. The Trust also awards the Mountbatten Memorial
Grants to commonwealth students in their final years of study
in the United Kingdom.

Mountbatten Memorial Grants to Commonwealth Students

Subjects: All subjects.
Eligibility: Open to Commonwealth students who are
pursuing a course of study at undergraduate or postgraduate
level at universities or other recognised institutions of higher
education in the UK.
Level of Study: Postgraduate, Undergraduate.
Purpose: To assist overseas students from the
Commonwealth who encounter unforeseen financial
difficulties in their final year of study.
Type: Grant.
No. of awards offered: Varies.
Frequency: Annual.
Value: Up to £500.
Country of Study: United Kingdom.
Application Procedure: Applications in writing, including
brief CV.
Additional Information: Grants are administered and
awarded, on the Trust's behalf, by a number of universities
and other institutions of higher education. Applicants should
consult their university or college student welfare officer for
further information. The Trust does not sponsor or award
scholarships, or pay fees. There are no grants for one-year
courses.

SIR HALLEY STEWART TRUST

88 Long Lane
Willingham, Cambridge, CB4 5LD, England
Tel: (44) 1954 260707
Contact: Mrs Fawcitt

Sir Halley Stewart Trust Grants

Subjects: Medical, social or religious research.
Eligibility: There are no eligibility restrictions.

Level of Study: Unrestricted.
Purpose: To assist pioneering research in medical, social, educational and religious fields.
Type: Research Grant.
Frequency: Dependent on funds available.
Value: Salaries and relevant costs for young research students from PhD level to about £12,000 per year.
Length of Study: Limited to 2 or 3 years.
Study Establishment: Under the auspices of a charitable institution, for example a hospital, laboratory, university department or charitable organisation.
Country of Study: Any country.
Application Procedure: There is no application form. Please contact the Trust for further details.
Closing Date: Applications are accepted at any time.

SIR RICHARD STAPLEY EDUCATIONAL TRUST

PO Box 57, Tonbridge, Kent, TN9 1ZT, England
Contact: The Secretary

The Sir Richard Stapley Educational Trust awards grants to postgraduate students studying for higher degrees, or degrees in medicine, veterinary science or dentistry.

Sir Richard Stapley Educational Trust Grants

Subjects: Medical, dental, or veterinary science.
Eligibility: Open to graduates holding a first or upper second class honours degree who are over the age of 24 on October 1st of the proposed academic year. Students in receipt of a substantial award from local authorities, Research Councils, the British Academy or other similar public bodies will not normally receive a grant from the Trust. Courses which are not eligible include: electives, diplomas, professional training, and intercalated degrees. Council do not normally support students for full-time PhD studies beyond a third year.
Level of Study: Postgraduate.
Purpose: To support postgraduate study for higher degrees and degrees in medicine, veterinary science or dentistry.
Type: Grant.
No. of awards offered: N/A - dependent on funds available each year.
Frequency: Annual.
Value: £250, £500, £800. £1,000+.
Length of Study: Not defined but PhD studies not beyond 3 years. Grants are awarded for 1 full academic year in the first instance.
Study Establishment: A university in the UK.
Country of Study: United Kingdom.
Application Procedure: Enquiries should include a large stamped addressed envelope, or international reply coupons. Application forms will be sent and should be received between March 1st and March 31st, complete with two academic references in sealed envelopes. Applicants will be notified in May.
Closing Date: March 31st.

Additional Information: Grants are paid upon receipt of official confirmation of participation in the course. All matters concerning application are by correspondence only, through the PO Box address shown.

SIR ROBERT MENZIES CENTRE FOR AUSTRALIAN STUDIES

28 Russell Square, London, WC1B 5DS, England
Tel: (44) 171 862 8854
Fax: (44) 171 580 9627
Email: k.mcintyre@sas.ac.uk
Contact: Ms Kirsten McIntyre

The Sir Robert Menzies Centre for Australian Studies is at the Institute of Commonwealth Studies, University of London. There are six broad areas of activity which form the core of the Centre's operations - teaching, postgraduate seminars, public lectures, conferences, research and external lecturing, and its scholarships and fellowships programmes.

Australian Bicentennial Scholarships and Fellowships

Subjects: All subjects.
Eligibility: The scholarship is open to candidates registered as a postgraduate student at a British tertiary institution or eligible for registration at an Australian tertiary institution and usually resident in the UK. The fellowship is open to holders of a good postgraduate degree or relevant experience who are seeking to further their education or professional experience but not through taking a further degree.
Level of Study: Postdoctorate, Postgraduate.
Purpose: To promote scholarship, intellectual links, mutual awareness and understanding between the UK and Australia and to enable UK graduates to study in approved courses or undertake approved research in Australia and to enable Australian graduates to study in approved courses to undertake approved research in the UK. To make allowance for disadvantaged persons.
Type: Scholarship and fellowship.
No. of awards offered: 1-4.
Frequency: Annual.
Value: Up to £4,000.
Study Establishment: Any approved Australian tertiary institution (UK applicants) or in any approved UK tertiary institution (Australian applicants).
Country of Study: Australia or United Kingdom.
Application Procedure: Application form and three references must be submitted plus a letter of acceptance from the proposed host institution.
Closing Date: June 7th for UK applicants; October 29th for Australian applicants.

Northcote Graduate Scholarship

Subjects: All subjects.
Eligibility: Open to applicants resident in the UK who are under 30 years old.
Level of Study: Postgraduate.
Purpose: To enable students to undertake a higher degree at an Australian University.
Type: Scholarship.
No. of awards offered: Up to 2.
Frequency: Annual.
Value: Allowance of A$17,427 per year, plus return economy air fare and payment of compulsory fees.
Length of Study: Up to 3 years.
Study Establishment: Any approved Australian tertiary institution.
Country of Study: Australia.
Application Procedure: Application form, two references, and letter of acceptance from Australian university must be submitted.
Closing Date: August 30th.

SIR ROBERT MENZIES MEMORIAL FOUNDATION

210 Clarendon Street, East Melbourne, Australia
Tel: (61) 3 9419 5699
Fax: (61) 3 9417 7049
Email: menzies@vicnet.net.au
www: http://www.vicnet.net.au/~menzies
Contact: Ms S K Mackenzie, Administration Officer

The Sir Robert Menzies Memorial Research Scholarships in the Allied Health Sciences

Subjects: Occupational therapy, speech pathology, physiotherapy, psychology, nursing, optometry and physical education.
Eligibility: Open to Australian citizens of at least five years standing. Applicants will generally have completed the first year of their PhD project.
Level of Study: Doctorate, Postgraduate.
Purpose: To support an outstanding applicant to carry out doctoral research work likely to improve the health of Australians.
Type: Scholarship.
No. of awards offered: 1.
Frequency: Annual.
Value: A$24,000 free of income tax.
Length of Study: 2 years.
Study Establishment: Australian tertiary institute with appropriate facilities.
Country of Study: Australia.
Application Procedure: Application form must be completed and submitted with academic transcripts and other documents.
Closing Date: June 30th.

Additional Information: Prospectus and application form can be downloaded and completed from the Menzies Foundation website.

THE SMITH AND NEPHEW FOUNDATION

2 Temple Place
Victoria Embankment, London, WC2R 3BP, England
Tel: (44) 171 836 7922
Fax: (44) 171 632 0202
Email: brigitte.swanton@smith-nephew.com
Contact: Foundation Administrator

To improve health care in the United Kingdom by offering awards to individuals in the medical and nursing professions undertaking educational or research projects.

Smith and Nephew Foundation Medical Research Fellowships

Subjects: Orthopaedics, wound management, and endoscopy.
Eligibility: Open to candidates resident in the UK, wishing to undertake one year's postgraduate research the United Kingdom, who have received their medical training and qualifications here and have not yet reached Consultant status. Applicants will be expected to have at least three years clinical experience since qualification.
Level of Study: Postdoctorate, Professional development.
Purpose: To assist those wishing to undertake one year's postgraduate medical research.
Type: Fellowship.
No. of awards offered: Varies.
Frequency: Annual.
Value: Up to £30,000.
Length of Study: 1 year.
Country of Study: United Kingdom.
Application Procedure: Advertised in the relevant medical journals; applications invited.
Closing Date: Varies.
Additional Information: Conditions of Fellowships may change from year to year.

Smith and Nephew Nursing Research Fellowships and Scholarships

Subjects: Postgraduate education and research in nursing. Preference is given to individuals working in wound management, orthopaedics and endoscopy.
Eligibility: Open to nurses, midwives and health visitors, aspiring to leadership positions in clinical, management or education spheres in the nursing professions.
Level of Study: Postgraduate.
Purpose: To enhance the evidence base in relation to clinical practice; to improve patient outcomes.
Type: Fellowship, Scholarship.
No. of awards offered: Varies.

Frequency: Annual.
Value: Varies.
Country of Study: Any country.
Application Procedure: Advertised in the relevant nursing journals.
Closing Date: Varies.
Additional Information: These awards are currently under review; announcements will be made in the near future.

SMITHKLINE BEECHAM PHARMACEUTICALS

New Frontiers Science Park (North)
Third Avenue, Harlow, Essex, CM19 5AW, England
Fax: (44) 1279 622749
Email: beatrice_leigh@sbphrd.com
www: http://www.sb.com
Contact: Ms Beatrice Leigh, Assistant Director - Worldwide Academic Liason

SmithKline Beecham is a major pharmaceutical and health care company. The focus of the company is health care: the treatment, prevention and diagnosis of disease including the concept of proactive health living. SmithKline Beecham is comprised of three integrated businesses: pharmaceuticals, consumer health care and clinical diagnostic services.

Collaborative Research Projects

Subjects: Pharmaceuticals, consumer health care and clinical diagnostic services.
Eligibility: Open to groups whose research activities fit into the company's own programme. Speculative approaches are also welcome from the academic sector.
Level of Study: Doctorate.
Purpose: To target people whose research activities fit into the company's own research programme.
Type: Studentship.
No. of awards offered: 160.
Frequency: Annual.
Country of Study: Any country.
Application Procedure: Please write for details.
Additional Information: It also operates a scheme whereby postdoctoral workers are employed by SB on a contract basis for two years.

Services to Academia

Subjects: Pharmacology, chemistry, biotechnology and toxicology.
Eligibility: Open to candidates working in the listed subject areas.
Level of Study: Professional development.
Purpose: A number of schemes exist to award candidates which are relevant to the subjects listed.
Type: Prizes, sponsored lectures, scholarships.
No. of awards offered: Varies.
Value: Varies.

Country of Study: Any country.
Application Procedure: Details will be advertised locally by the university or instiution concerned.

SMOKELESS TOBACCO RESEARCH COUNCIL

420 Lexington Ave, New York, NY, 10170, United States of America
Tel: (1) 212 697 3485
Fax: (1) 212 986 8631
Email: strc@mindspring.com
Contact: Grant Program

The objective of the Smokeless Tobacco Research Council, Inc, is to continue support through a programme of grants-in-aid of independent research into questions regarding smokeless tobacco and health.

Grants-in-Aid

Subjects: Independent research into smokeless tobacco and health.
Eligibility: N/A.
Level of Study: Doctorate, Postdoctorate.
Purpose: To provide research support.
Type: Grants-in-Aid.
No. of awards offered: Varies, depending on funds available.
Frequency: Twice a year.
Value: Approx. $85,000 annually.
Length of Study: 1-3 years.
Study Establishment: Universites and research organisations.
Country of Study: Any country.
Application Procedure: Application form must be completed.
Closing Date: December 31st for July 1st funding; June 30th for January 1st funding.

SOCIAL SCIENCE RESEARCH COUNCIL (SSRC)

810 Seventh Avenue, New York, NY, 10019, United States of America
Tel: (1) 212 377 2700
Fax: (1) 212 377 2727
Email: lastname@ssrc.org
www: http://www.ssrc.org
Contact: The Awards Committee

The SSRC Soviet Union and Successor States Graduate Training Fellowships

Subjects: Eurasia area studies.

Eligibility: US citizens enrolled in accredited graduate programmes in any discipline of the social sciences or humanities.
Level of Study: Postgraduate.
Purpose: To support training in Eurasia Area Studies.
Type: Fellowship.
Frequency: Annual.
Value: Up to US$15,000.
Length of Study: 2 years.
Country of Study: Any country.
Application Procedure: Application forms; three letters of recommendation; one official copy of all relevant post-secondary study; language self evauation; description of programme of study.
Closing Date: February 3rd.

THE SOCIETY FOR THE SCIENTIFIC STUDY OF SEXUALITY (SSSS)

PO Box 208, Mount Vernon, IA, 52314-0208, United States of America
Tel: (1) 319 895 8407
Fax: (1) 319 895 6203
Email: thesociety@worldnet.att.net
www: http://www.ssc.wisc.edu/ssss
Contact: Mr Howard J Ruppel, Executive Director

The Society for the Scientific Study of Sexuality is an international organisation dedicated to the advancement of knowledge about sexuality. The Society brings together an interdisciplinary group of professionals who believe in the importance of both production of quality research and the clinical, educational, and social applications of research related to all aspects of sexuality.

SSSS Student Research Grant Award

Subjects: Related to the field of human sexuality from any discipline - psychology, anthropology, social work, biology, theology, medical research, etc.
Eligibility: Open to students of any nationality who are enrolled in a degree granting programme.
Level of Study: Unrestricted.
Purpose: To support research in the field of human sexuality.
Type: Grant.
No. of awards offered: 3.
Frequency: Twice a year.
Value: US$750.
Study Establishment: An appropriate institution.
Country of Study: Any country.
Application Procedure: Please send SASE for further details and application packet.
Closing Date: February 1st, September 1st.
Additional Information: The purpose of the research can be a Master's thesis or doctoral dissertation, but this is not a requirement. Funds to support these grants are provided by the Foundation for the Scientific Study of Sexuality.

SOCIETY OF APOTHECARIES OF LONDON

Black Friars Lane, London, EC4V 6EJ, England
Tel: (44) 171 236 1180
Fax: (44) 171 329 3177
Contact: R J Stainger, The Clerk

Gillson Scholarship in Pathology

Subjects: Pathology.
Eligibility: Open to candidates under 35 years of age who are either Licenciates or Freemen of the Society, or who obtain the Licence or the Freedom within six months of election to the Scholarship.
Level of Study: Postgraduate.
Purpose: To encourage original research in any branch of pathology.
Type: Scholarship.
No. of awards offered: 1.
Frequency: Every three years.
Value: £1,800 (£600 per year). Payments are made twice annually for the duration of the Scholarship.
Length of Study: 3 years; renewable for a second term of 3 years.
Country of Study: Any country.
Application Procedure: Candidates should submit two testimonials and present evidence of their attainments and capabilities as shown by any papers already published, and/or a detailed record of any pathological work already done. Candidates should also state where the research will be undertaken.
Closing Date: December 1st.
Additional Information: Preference is given to the candidate who is engaged in the teaching of medical science or in its research. Scholars are required to submit an interim report at the end of the first six months of tenure, and a complete report one month prior to the end of the third year. Any published results should also be submitted to the Society.

SOROPTIMIST INTERNATIONAL OF GREAT BRITAIN AND IRELAND

127 Wellington Road South, Stockport, Cheshire, SK1 3TS, England
Tel: (44) 161 480 7686
Fax: (44) 161 477 6152
www: http://titan.glo.be/~bea/sieorg.htm
Contact: The Chairman

Soroptomist International of Great Britain and Ireland Golden Jubilee Fellowship

Subjects: Any subject, but preference is given to women seeking to train or retrain for a business or profession as mature students. However all applications will be considered by the Committee.

Eligibility: Open to women residing within the boundaries of Soroptimist International of Great Britain and Ireland, who need not be Soroptimists. The countries are Anguilla, Antigua and Barbuda, Bangladesh, Barbados, British Virgin Islands, Cameroon, Gambia, Grenada, Guernsey, India, Isle of Man, Jamaica, Jersey, Republic of Ireland, Malawi, Malta, Mauritius, Nigeria, Pakistan, Seychelles, Sierra Leone, South Africa, Sri Lanka, St Vincent and the Grenadines, Thailand, Trinidad and Tobago, Turks and Caicos Islands, Uganda, United Kingdom, and Zimbabwe.

Level of Study: Unrestricted.

Type: Fellowship.

No. of awards offered: Approx. 40.

Frequency: Annual.

Value: Normally within range £100-£500 per year, from a fund of £6,000.

Study Establishment: Any agreed institution, providing the residential stipulation is met.

Country of Study: Any country.

Application Procedure: Please enclose SAE or IRCs for details.

Closing Date: April 30th for the academic year beginning the following autumn.

SOROS FOUNDATION - LATVIA

Raina bulv 19
Room 243, Riga, LV-1586, Latvia
Tel: (371) 782 0385
Fax: (371) 782 0385
Email: dvisnola@lanet.la
Contact: Mr Dace Sinkevica, Director of EAC

The Soros Foundation was created by George Soros with a view to building and supporting free and open societies. The Foundation hopes to achieve its aim by supporting a wide range of programs in education; media and communications; civil society; science and medicine; arts and culture; economic restructuring; and legal reform.

Soros Foundation (Latvia) Support Programme for Studies Abroad

Subjects: All subjects.

Eligibility: Open to Latvian nationals and residents only.

Level of Study: Doctorate, Postgraduate.

Purpose: To support Latvian students who are studying abroad.

Type: Grant.

No. of awards offered: 20.

Frequency: Annual.

Value: An average of US$1,000, with a maximum of US$3,000.

Length of Study: A minimum of 1semester.

Study Establishment: Any university.

Country of Study: Outside Latvia.

Application Procedure: Application package consists of application forms, description of the study programme, CV and other documentation. Please write for further details.

Closing Date: July 1st, November 1st.

Additional Information: The awards are not to be used to cover study fees, accommodation or living expenses.

SOUTH AFRICAN ASSOCIATION OF UNIVERSITY WOMEN

PO Box 642, Parklands, 2121, South Africa
Tel: (27) 11 836 2027
Fax: (27) 11 784 1338
Email: bell@newaa.co.sa
Contact: Mrs J A Bell, National President

Edna Machanick Award

Subjects: All subjects.

Eligibility: Open to South African women of all races who have successfully completed one year of a course of study and are in need of financial assistance to complete their studies towards a non-degree qualification (diploma or certificate) at the tertiary education level.

Level of Study: Postgraduate.

Purpose: To provide assistance to women at tertiary institutions, other than a university.

Type: Award.

No. of awards offered: 3-4.

Frequency: Annual.

Value: R500 per year.

Study Establishment: Any institution of tertiary education.

Country of Study: Any country.

Application Procedure: Write for application forms.

Closing Date: October 31st.

Additional Information: The awards are generally made by the institutions concerned. SAAUW provides the funding.

Isie Smuts Research Award

Subjects: All subjects.

Eligibility: Open to members of the South African Association of University Women.

Level of Study: Postgraduate.

Purpose: To assist postgraduate women in research.

Type: Award.

No. of awards offered: 1.

Frequency: Annual.

Value: R1,000.

Study Establishment: Any South African university.

Country of Study: South Africa.

Application Procedure: Write for application to Miss V Henley at the main address.

Closing Date: October 31st.

SAAUW International Fellowship

Subjects: Any subject - postgraduate research.
Eligibility: Open to members of the International Federation of University Women.
Level of Study: Postgraduate.
Purpose: To assist members of the International Federation of University Women, who wish to study in South Africa.
Type: Fellowship.
No. of awards offered: 1.
Frequency: Annual.
Value: R1,000.
Length of Study: Not less than 6 months.
Country of Study: South Africa.
Application Procedure: Write for application forms to the address below.
Closing Date: August 31st.
Additional Information: The award is made when a suitable applicant applies.

For further information contact:

21 Templeton Drive, Grahamstown, 6140, South Africa
Contact: Miss V Henley

SOUTH AFRICAN COUNCIL FOR THE AGED

23rd Floor
Golden Acke
Adderley Street, Cape Town, Western Cape, 8000, South Africa
Tel: (27) 21 418 2145
Fax: (27) 21 419 5831
Email: saca@iafrica.com
Contact: Mrs W J M Bryan, Deputy Director

Zerilda Steyn Memorial Trust

Subjects: Needs and care of the aged.
Eligibility: Open to researchers in all disciplines caring for the aged.
Level of Study: Postgraduate.
Purpose: To advance postgraduate research in South Africa.
Type: Project Grant.
No. of awards offered: Several grants are made for a variety of small and large projects.
Frequency: Annual.
Value: R1,500 per year.
Length of Study: 1 year; renewable only in exceptional cases.
Study Establishment: Universities.
Country of Study: South Africa.
Application Procedure: Application form must be submitted to the trustees. A six monthly progress report is required.
Closing Date: January 30th.
Additional Information: In exceptional cases a second grant can be awarded, but this would require substantial motivation.

SOUTH AFRICAN DENTAL ASSOCIATION

Private Bag 1
Houghton, Johannesburg, 2041, South Africa
Tel: (27) 11 484 5288
Fax: (27) 11 642 5718
Email: rswanepoel@sada.co.za
www: http://www.sadanet.co.za
Contact: Ms Rita Swanepoel

The Association's main objective is to promote the interests of its members in order to promote optimal oral health for all.

Lever Pond's Postgraduate Fellowship

Subjects: Any biological field related to dentistry.
Eligibility: Open to residents of South Africa, who are either dentists registered with the South African Medical and Dental Council wishing to qualify themselves further or to equip themselves for research by taking an additional degree, or who are suitably qualified persons wishing to concentrate on dental research.
Level of Study: Postgraduate.
Purpose: To promote dental research and ensure its continuation in South Africa.
Type: Fellowship.
No. of awards offered: 1.
Frequency: Annual.
Value: Up to R20,000.
Length of Study: 1 year; renewable in special circumstances.
Country of Study: South Africa unless facilities are not available.
Application Procedure: Applications must be made on an official application form and must be supported by and submitted through a university or other such institution. An award may be made for research overseas, provided that the application is accompanied by a statement from the sponsoring institution that the proposed project can best be carried out in another country.
Closing Date: October 31st.
Additional Information: A Fellow working overseas must undertake to return to South Africa for a minimum period of two years after completing the project under the award, or refund to the Fellowship Fund any money he/she has received.

SOUTH AFRICAN MEDICAL RESEARCH COUNCIL

Research Grants Administration
PO Box 19070, Tygerberg, 7505, South Africa
Tel: (27) 21 938 0227
Fax: (27) 21 938 0368
Email: mjenkins@mrc.ac.za
www: http://www.mrc.ac.za
Contact: Mrs M Jenkins, Research Grants Administration

The South African Medical Research Council's brief is to undertake excellent research which can be implemented to improve the health of all South Africans. Research priorities are regularly established through broad consultation. The MRC's mission is to improve the health status and quality of life of the nation through excellence in scientific research.

South Africa MRC Grants for Research Units and Centres

Subjects: General medical sciences.
Eligibility: Productive reseacrh teams made up from South African scientists.
Level of Study: Research.
Purpose: To create units or centres at universities or similar institutions under the leadership of a Director who enjoys national and international recognition.
Type: A variable number of grants.
No. of awards offered: Varies.
Frequency: Annual.
Value: Varies.
Length of Study: Initial 5 years, with the option of an extension for a further 5 years.
Study Establishment: South African universities or similar institutions where well qualified and productive research teams and the necessary laboratory and clinical facilities already exist.
Country of Study: South Africa.
Closing Date: March 31st.

South African MRC Dentistry Scholarships

Subjects: Dentistry.
Eligibility: Open to persons who have just obtained their Bachelor's degree in dentistry and have registered with the South African Medical and Dental Council.
Level of Study: Postgraduate.
Purpose: To assist the recipient to undertake research training.
Type: Scholarship.
No. of awards offered: Varies.
Frequency: Annual.
Value: To be determined by the MRC from time to time.
Length of Study: 1 year.
Study Establishment: An approved institution.
Country of Study: South Africa.
Application Procedure: There is no prescribed application form. Applications, in writing, must be directed to the administrative head of the institution where the research will be undertaken, for submission to the MRC. The applicant's study record, proposed research programme and the name of the person under whose supervision the research will be undertaken must be furnished.
Closing Date: April 30th.

South African MRC Distinguished Visiting Scientists Awards

Subjects: Health sciences.
Eligibility: Open to distinguished foreign scientists of any nationality.
Level of Study: Postgraduate.

Purpose: To provide funds to support distinguished scientists from abroad to visit local researchers.
No. of awards offered: Varies.
Frequency: Annual.
Value: Varies; including funds for travel and a daily allowance.
Length of Study: From 2 weeks up to a maximum of 3 months.
Country of Study: South Africa.
Application Procedure: Applications for support must be made by local scientists, in writing, providing the following information: a complete curriculum vitae of the visitor; his work programme; duration of the visit; and funds required for travel.
Closing Date: August 31st.

South African MRC Grants for Research Abroad during Sabbatical Leave

Subjects: General medical sciences.
Eligibility: Established South African researchers.
Level of Study: Research.
Purpose: To provide financial support for established researchers undertaking research at approved institutiuons abroad during their sabbatical leave.
Type: A variable number of Grants.
No. of awards offered: Varies.
Frequency: Varies.
Value: Varies.
Study Establishment: Approved foreign academic institutions.
Country of Study: Any country.
Application Procedure: Submission of application to the MRC.
Closing Date: Applications are accepted at any time.

South African MRC Grants for Research Groups

Subjects: Health Sciences.
Eligibility: Open to South African Scientists.
Purpose: To establish Research groups around an excellent leader who has the potential for developing an international reputation. Research groups are expected to engage in capacity development especially at historically black universities where partnership with white universities may facilitate research development.
Type: Research Grant.
No. of awards offered: Varies.
Frequency: Annual.
Value: Varies.
Length of Study: 5 to 10 years dependent on performance.
Study Establishment: Historically black universities in South Africa.
Country of Study: South Africa.
Closing Date: March 31st.

South African MRC Grants for Research Training Posts

Subjects: General medical sciences.
Eligibility: Medical registrars (clinical assistants) ion their final year of training in a specialist field and medical specialists under the age of 40.
Level of Study: Professional development.
Purpose: To create oppurtunites to stimulate interest, training and experience in research.
Type: Research training posts.
No. of awards offered: Varies.
Frequency: Annual.
Value: Market-related renumeration packet.
Length of Study: Varies.
Study Establishment: South African universities and research institutions.
Country of Study: South Africa.
Closing Date: September 30th.

South African MRC Grants for Self-initiated Research

Subjects: Health Services.
Eligibility: Open to South African Scientists.
Level of Study: Postgraduate.
Purpose: To enable entry level and established researchers to undertake research in the health sciences.
Type: Research Grant.
No. of awards offered: Up to 300.
Frequency: Annual.
Value: Varies.
Length of Study: Up to 3 years.
Study Establishment: Approved research and eduacational institutions.
Country of Study: South Africa.
Application Procedure: Applicants must furnish a proposed research programme and a budget for the full duration of the project.
Closing Date: May 15th.
Additional Information: Please refer to the website http://www.mrc.ac.za/funding/unifund.htm.

South African MRC Post-Intern Scholarships

Subjects: Health sciences.
Eligibility: Open to persons who have obtained a Bachelor's degree in medicine and have just completed their internship.
Level of Study: Doctorate, Postgraduate.
Purpose: To create the opportunity for recently qualified medical doctors to train as researchers.
Type: Scholarship.
No. of awards offered: Varies.
Frequency: Annual.
Value: To be determined by the MRC from time to time.
Length of Study: 1 year.
Study Establishment: Approved institutions.
Country of Study: South Africa.
Application Procedure: There is no prescribed application form. Applications, in writing, must be directed to the administrative head of the institution where the research will

be undertaken, for submission to the MRC. The applicant's study record, proposed research programme and the name of the person under whose supervision the research will be undertaken must be furnished.
Closing Date: June 30th.

South African MRC Research Development Planning Grants

Subjects: General medical sciences.
Purpose: To provide financial support for universities selected by the Group Executive of Research Capacity Development.
Type: Grant.
No. of awards offered: Varies.
Study Establishment: South African universities or research institutions.
Country of Study: South Africa.
Application Procedure: This category of support is purely on invitation after the Group Executive of Research Capacity has visited the university concerned. Please contact Dr R Maharaj, The Manager of Research Capacity Development for further information.

South African MRC Research Supplements for Disadvantaged Students

Subjects: Biomedicine.
Eligibility: South African postgraduate and predocturate students from disadvantaged backgrounds.
Level of Study: Doctorate, Postgraduate, Predoctorate.
Purpose: To provide support for graduate research assistantships at Master's and PhD level for disadvantaged students who wish to develop research skills in biomedical research.
Type: A variable number of Grants.
No. of awards offered: Varies.
Frequency: Annual.
Value: Up to R5,000 toward tuituion fees, a subsistence allowance of up to R12,000 per annum and up to R1,500 for conference attendence.
Length of Study: Varies.
Study Establishment: South African universities, especially historiacally black universities (HBUs).
Country of Study: South Africa.
Application Procedure: Please write for details.
Closing Date: Please write for details.
Additional Information: Before submitting an application for a research supplement, grant applicants should contact Dr R Maharaj, The Manager of the MRC Capacity Development Programme to discuss the application. Tel: +21 938 0436, fax: +1 938 0377. Email; rmaharaj@mrc.ac.za. Or refer to the website http://www.mrc.ac.za/funding/capdev.htm.

South African MRC Scholarships for Post-doctoral Study in South Africa

Subjects: Health sciences.
Eligibility: Open to candidates in the faculties of medicine, dentistry and engineering who hold a PhD degree. Applicants must be South African citizens or in receipt of a permanent

residence permit issued by the state department concerned before the Scholarship, if granted becomes operative.
Level of Study: Postgraduate.
Purpose: To enable researchers in possession of a Doctorate in Health Sciences to undertake research in South Africa. Priority will be given to research projects which would contribute towards improving the health status of the nation.
Type: Scholarship.
No. of awards offered: Varies.
Frequency: Annual.
Value: To be determined by the MRC from time to time.
Study Establishment: An appropriate institution.
Country of Study: South Africa.
Application Procedure: Please write for details.
Closing Date: August 31st.

South African MRC Scholarships for Research and Study Overseas

Subjects: Health sciences.
Eligibility: Open to South African scientists under 50 years of age and holding at least a Master's degree.
Level of Study: Postgraduate.
Purpose: To support research where facilities are not available or are inadequate in South Africa.
Type: Scholarship.
No. of awards offered: Varies.
Frequency: Annual.
Value: To be determined by the MRC from time to time.
Length of Study: 2 years.
Study Establishment: Approved institutions.
Country of Study: Europe, United Kingdom, North America or Canada.
Closing Date: June 30th.
Additional Information: Holders of MRC grants must sign an undertaking that they will return to South Africa for at least three years for every year of support or for five years for two years of support.

South African MRC Scholarships for Study in South Africa

Subjects: Health sciences.
Eligibility: Open to candidates in the faculties of medicine, dentistry and engineering who hold a PhD degree. Applicants must be South African citizens or in receipt of a permanent residence permit issued by the state department concerned before the Scholarship, if granted, becomes operative. For the purposes of this condition, citizens of TVBC states and self governing states within the Republic of South Africa are deemed to be Citizens of the Republic of South Africa.
Level of Study: Postgraduate.
Purpose: To assist students who have obtained an honours degree and wish to obtain a research degree at MSc or PhD Level.
Type: Scholarship.
No. of awards offered: Varies.
Frequency: Annual.
Value: To be determined by the MRC from time to time.
Study Establishment: An appropriate institution.

Country of Study: South Africa.
Application Procedure: Please write for details.
Closing Date: September 30th.

South African MRC Short-Term Research Grants

Subjects: Health sciences.
Eligibility: Open to South African scientists.
Level of Study: Postgraduate.
Purpose: To enable entry level and established researchers to undertake research in the health sciences.
Type: Research Grant.
No. of awards offered: Varies.
Frequency: Annual.
Value: Varies.
Length of Study: Up to 3 years.
Study Establishment: Approved research and educational institutions.
Country of Study: South Africa.
Closing Date: May 15th.

South African MRC Staff Development and Credentialling Grants

Subjects: Health sciences.
Eligibility: Junior academic staff at HBUs, wishing to obtain an MA/PhD.
Level of Study: Graduate, Postdoctorate.
Purpose: To assist junior academic staff at HBUs in improving their credentials. To this end staff are encouraged to take leave to continue their study towards an MD or PhD, with a specific focus on research development.
Type: A variable number of Grants.
No. of awards offered: Varies.
Frequency: Annual.
Length of Study: Varies.
Study Establishment: HBUs in South Africa.
Country of Study: South Africa.
Application Procedure: For information on the application procedure and information on the programme please contact Dr R Maharaj, Tel; +21 938 0436, Fax: +21 938 0377, email: rmaharaj@mrc.ac.za.
Additional Information: For further information please contact Dr R Maharaj or refer to the website http://www.mrc.ac.za/funding/capdev.htm.

South African MRC Technical Assistance Grants to HBUs

Subjects: General medical sciences.
Eligibility: Staf from HBUs who wish to submit research proposals to the MRC.
Level of Study: Research.
Purpose: To enable researchers from other institutions to provide assistance to staff from HBUs who wish to submit proposals to the MRC.
Type: Travel Grant.
No. of awards offered: Varies.
Frequency: Throughout the year.
Value: R10,000 maximum.

Length of Study: Varies.
Study Establishment: South African universities.
Country of Study: South Africa.
Application Procedure: For details about the application procedure and further information about the programme please contact Dr R Maharaj, The Manager of Research Capacity Development of the MRC Tel; +21 938 0436, Fax: +21 938 0377, email; rmaharaj@mrc.ac.za, or refer to the website http://www.mrc.ac.za/funding/capdev.htm.
Closing Date: Please write for details.

South African MRC Travel Grants to International Scientific Meetings

Subjects: General medical sciences.
Eligibility: South African researchers who receive less than R10,000 operating fund per annum.
Level of Study: Research.
Purpose: To give financial support to researchers who are to present a paper or other scientific contribution at an international meeting.
Type: Travel Grant.
No. of awards offered: Varies.
Frequency: Four times per year.
Value: 50% of the estimated travel and subsistance costs, provided that at least 30% of the costs are borne by the researcher's institutions.
Length of Study: Varies.
Study Establishment: International scientific meetings.
Country of Study: Any country.
Application Procedure: Submission of application to the MRC.
Closing Date: February 15th, May 15th, August 15th, October 15th.

South African MRC Travel Grants to Local Scientific Meetings

Subjects: General Medical sciences.
Eligibility: South African researchers who receive less than R10,000 for operating funds.
Level of Study: Research.
Purpose: To give researchers the financial support which enables them to attend local scientific meetings, attend courses or visit laboratories in order to solve problems regarding existing research.
Type: Travel Grant.
No. of awards offered: Varies.
Frequency: Throughout the year.
Value: Varies.
Length of Study: Varies.
Study Establishment: Local scientific meetings, universities or laboratories.
Country of Study: South Africa.
Application Procedure: Submission of applications to the MRC.
Closing Date: At least two months before the meeting/intended visit.

ST ANDREW'S SOCIETY OF THE STATE OF NEW YORK

3 West 51st Street, New York, NY, 10019, United States of America
Tel: (1) 212 397 4849
Fax: (1) 212 397 4846
Email: standrewsny@msn.com
Contact: The Executive Director

St Andrew's Society of the State of New Yorks' constitution states -'For the relief of natives of Scotland and their descendants who might be in want or distress and to promote social intercourse among its members'.

St Andrew's Society of the State of New York Scholarship

Subjects: General, no field of endeavour requirement.
Eligibility: Students who have graduated from an American university, of Scottish-American descent, and New York area address (within a 250 mile radius).
Level of Study: Postgraduate.
Purpose: To promote cultural and intellectual interchange and goodwill between Scotland and the USA.
Type: Scholarship.
No. of awards offered: 2.
Frequency: Annual.
Value: US$10,000.
Length of Study: 1 year.
Study Establishment: Any university in Scotland.
Country of Study: Scotland.
Application Procedure: Application form, documentation of transcripts, and letters of recommendation; the President of each college or university must recommend one student only from that institution.
Closing Date: December 15th.

ST ANDREW'S SOCIETY OF THE STATE OF NEW YORK

42 St Andrew Square, Edinburgh, EH2 2YE, Scotland
Tel: (44) 131 523 2049
Fax: (44) 131 557 9178
Telex: 72230 RBSCOT
Contact: Mr Tony Smith, Executive Assistant

St Andrew's Society of the State of New York Scholarship Fund

Subjects: All subjects.
Eligibility: Open to newly qualified graduates or undergraduates of a Scottish university or of Oxford or Cambridge. Candidates are required to have a Scottish background. The possession of an honours degree is not essential. Personality and other qualities will influence the selection.

Level of Study: Postgraduate.
Purpose: To support advanced study exchanges between the USA and Scotland by individuals with Scottish backgrounds.
Type: Scholarship.
No. of awards offered: 2.
Frequency: Annual.
Value: US$15,000 to cover university tuition fees, room and board, and transportation expenses.
Length of Study: 1 academic year.
Study Establishment: A University in the USA, restricted to a radius of 250 miles from New York City and only if there is an unusual reason and justification will the Society consider other locations for students who cannot find courses for their specialities within the boundaries outlined: thereafter, the scholar is expected to spend a little time travelling in America before returning to Scotland.
Country of Study: USA; restricted to a radius of 250 miles from New York City.
Application Procedure: Please write for further details.
Closing Date: Early January.
Additional Information: Each Scottish University will vet its own applicants and nominate one candidate to go forward to the Final Selection Committee to be held in Edinburgh in early March. Oxford and Cambridge applicants should apply directly to the Society.

STATE SCHOLARSHIPS FOUNDATION

Greek Embassy
Cultural Department
1a Holland Park, London, W11 3TP, England
Tel: (44) 171 229 3850
Fax: (44) 171 229 7221
Contact: Dr Victoria Solomonidis, Cultural Attache

Scholarships for Postgraduate Studies in Greece

Subjects: All subjects.
Eligibility: Open to nationals of countries which are part of the Council of Europe who hold a graduate degree from a foreign university, have a good knowledge of English or French and are not more than 35 years of age.
Level of Study: Doctorate, Postdoctorate, Postgraduate.
Purpose: To fund postgraduate studies.
Type: Scholarship.
No. of awards offered: 10.
Frequency: Annual.
Value: 70,000 drachmas monthly plus 50,000 drachmas for initial expenses; up to 60,000 drachmas for typing of PhD dissertation, up to 60,000 drachmas to cover mandatory laboratory expenses; exemption from tuition fees; free medical care in case of emergency.
Length of Study: 1 academic year; renewable for 2 further years.
Study Establishment: Any university or institution of higher education.

Country of Study: Greece.
Application Procedure: Application forms may be requested from January.
Closing Date: March 31st.
Additional Information: Scholars are strongly recommended to acquire at least an elementary knowledge of Modern Greek.

STIFTELSEN LARS HIERTAS MINNE

Eriksbergsg 3
2tr, Stockholm, S-11430, Sweden
Tel: (46) 8 611 6401
Contact: Ms Elisabeth Norlander

Stiftelsen Lars Hiertas Minne Scientific Research Award

Subjects: Any scientific field.
Eligibility: Open to all nationalities.
Level of Study: Doctorate, Postdoctorate, Postgraduate.
Purpose: To support scientific research.
No. of awards offered: Varies.
Frequency: Annual.
Value: 10-35000 Swedish Crowns.
Study Establishment: Any institution.
Country of Study: Sweden.
Application Procedure: Application form must be completed (the form is in Swedish).
Closing Date: October 1st.
Additional Information: Foreigners must conduct their research in Sweden.

SUSAN G KOMEN BREAST CANCER FOUNDATION

5005 LBJ Freeway
Suite 370, Dallas, TX, 75244, United States of America
Tel: (1) 972 855 4316
Fax: (1) 972 855 1640
Email: mburwell@komen.org
www: http://www.komen.org
Contact: Ms Margaret Burwell, Grants Administrator

Basic Clinical and Translational Breast Cancer Research

Subjects: Studies may be clinical, basic or translational design. The Foundation does not target funding to any specific area of breast cancer study, geographic area or instiution.
Purpose: This programme is intended to foster investigations into the cause, treatment, prevention and cure of breast cancers.

Type: Research Grant.
No. of awards offered: Dependant on funding per project.
Frequency: Annual.
Value: $250,000 (combined direct and indirect costs) over a two year period.
Length of Study: 2 years.
Country of Study: USA.
Application Procedure: Applicants must register before submitting an application. Registration is available on the website. Please contact Elda Railey, Director of National Grants and Sponsored Programs at the main address for more information.
Closing Date: Applications must be received by 5pm CST April 1st.

Dissertation Research Award

Subjects: Particular emphasis will be given to projects offering an indication of the potential to help the Foundation meet its mission to eradicate breast cancer as a life-threatening disease.
Level of Study: Doctorate.
Purpose: Funding is available for doctoral candidates in the fields of health and social sciences to conduct dissertation research on breast health and breast cancer.
Type: Award.
No. of awards offered: Varies.
Frequency: Annual.
Value: US$20,000-US$30,000 over a two year period.
Length of Study: 2 years.
Country of Study: USA.
Application Procedure: Applicants must register before submitting an application. Registration is available on the website. Please contact Elda Railey, Director of National Grants and Sponsored Programs at the main address for more information.
Closing Date: Applications must be received by 5pm CST April 1st.

Imaging Technology

Subjects: To explore and devlop new methods utilising advanced imaging technology to improve diagnostic methods.
Eligibility: Applicants from any country may apply.
Purpose: To fund research and develop methods for early detection and diagnosis of breast cancer.
Type: Research Grant.
No. of awards offered: 4 or 5.
Frequency: Annual.
Value: US$125,000 per year.
Length of Study: 2 years.
Country of Study: USA.
Application Procedure: Applicants must reigister before submitting an application. Registration is available on the website. Please contact Elda Railey, Director of National

Grants and Sponsored Programs, for more information at the main address.
Closing Date: Applications must be received by 5pm CST April 1st.

Population Specfic Research Project

Subjects: The focus of the programme is to identify unique needs, trends and barriers to breast health care among populations such as African American, Asian/Pacific Islander, Hispanic, Native American, lesbian, low literacy and other defined communities.
Eligibility: Applicants from any country may apply.
Level of Study: Unrestricted.
Purpose: For innovative projects addressing breast cancer and epidemiology within specific populations at risk for disease.
Type: Research Grant.
No. of awards offered: Varies.
Frequency: Annual.
Value: US$75,000 per year.
Length of Study: 2 years.
Country of Study: USA.
Application Procedure: Applicants must register before submitting an application. Registration is available on the website. Please contact Elda Railey, Director of National Grants and Sponsored Programs, for more information at the main address.
Closing Date: Applications must be received by 5pm CST April 1st.

Postdoctoral Fellowship in Breast Cancer Research, Public Health or Epidemiology

Subjects: Particular emphasis will be given to projects that are innovative, non-duplicative of other efforts and have the potential to lay the ground work for continuing study.
Eligibility: Applicants from any country may apply.
Level of Study: Postdoctorate.
Purpose: To encourage young scientists to begin a career in breast cancer research or to support continued research continued independent investigations in breast health and breast cancer.
Type: Fellowship.
No. of awards offered: Varies.
Frequency: Annual.
Value: US$35,000.
Length of Study: 3 years.
Country of Study: USA.
Application Procedure: Applicants must register before submitting an application. Registration is available on our website at http://www.komen.org. Please contact Elda Railey, Director of National Grants and Sponsored Programs at the main address for more information.
Closing Date: Applications must be received by 5pm CST April 1st.

SWISS NATIONAL SCIENCE FOUNDATION (SNSF)

Wildhainweg 20
PO Box 3001, Berne, Switzerland
Tel: (41) 31 308 22 22
Fax: (41) 31 301 30 09
www: http://www.snf.ch
Contact: Dr Benno G Frey, Office for Fellowship and Exchange Program

The Swiss National Foundation (SNSF) support scientific research at Swiss universities and other scientific institutions and award fellowships to scientists. The SNSF was established in 1952 as a private Foundation entrusted with the promotion of basic non-commercial research. While the SNSF supports research through grants given to established or promising researchers, it does not maintain its own research institutions. The main objectives of the SNSF are to support basic research in all areas of academic research and to support young scientists and researchers, with the intent of ensuring the continuing high quality of teaching and research in Swiss higher education. In addition to the general research funding, the SNSF is responsible for the National Research Programmes (NRP) and for four of the federal government's Swiss Priority Programmes (SPPs).

Fellowships for Advanced Researchers

Subjects: All subjects.
Eligibility: Postdoctoral (and possibly predoctorate) students under the age of 35, who have at least two years experience in active research and are Swiss nationals or permanent residents in Switzerland. An exception to the age restriction can be made for candidates who have interrupted their scientific career due to family obligations.
Level of Study: Predoctorate.
Purpose: To promote postdoctoral or postgraduate students who have at least two years experience in active research and are Swiss nationals or permanent residents in Switzerland.
Type: A variable number of Fellowships.
No. of awards offered: Varies.
Frequency: Annual.
Value: Varies.
Length of Study: Varies.
Study Establishment: Universities or academic institutions worldwide.
Application Procedure: Application forms are available from the Research Council of the Swiss National Science Foundation at the end of each calendar year.
Closing Date: February 1st.

Fellowships for Prospective Researchers

Subjects: All subjects.
Eligibility: Promising young scholars under the age of 33 who are Swiss nationals or permanent residents of Switzerland, hold an MA or PhD and can demonstrate at least one years experience in active research. An exception to the age

restriction (to a maximum of two years) can be made for candidates from clinical disciplines, or candidates who have interrupted their scientific careers due to family obligations. The main condition for such an exception is that the candidate has reached a high scientific level and will in the future pursue an active career in science and research. A high priority will be given to candidates who plan to return to Switzerland.
Level of Study: Postdoctorate, Predoctorate.
Purpose: To promote holders of MA or PhD degrees, who have had at least one year's experience in active research after the completion of their degree.
Type: A variable number of Fellowships.
No. of awards offered: Varies.
Frequency: Annual.
Value: Varies.
Length of Study: Varies.
Study Establishment: Universities worldwide.
Country of Study: Any country.
Application Procedure: Application forms are available from the Local Research Commission. Candidates with a degree from a Swiss university should contact the Research Commission of their institution. Candidates with Italian as their native language, who have completed their studies in a foreign country should contact the Research Commission for the Italian speaking part of Switzerland. Swiss candidates who are residents of foreign countries, hold a degree from a foreign university, but who have concrete of returning to Switzerland should contact the Swiss scientific academy responsible for their area of research.
Closing Date: Please write for details.
Additional Information: For further information please contact Benno Frey or Laurence Bohren at the Office for Fellowship and Exchange Programs, or refer to the website: http://www.snf.ch.

Marie Heim-Vögtlin Programme

Subjects: Engineering, mathematics and computer science, medical sciences, natural sciences.
Eligibility: Promising female researchers up to the age of 45, who are Swiss nationals or permanent residents of Switzerland.
Level of Study: Doctorate, Postdoctorate, Postgraduate.
Purpose: To aid women wishing to return to their scientific activities after having interrupted their career for family reasons.
Type: A variable number of Fellowships.
No. of awards offered: Varies.
Frequency: Annual.
Value: Dependent on the local salary scale.
Length of Study: 1-3 years.
Study Establishment: Universities or research institutions in Switzerland.
Country of Study: Switzerland.
Application Procedure: Submission of an application which includes a 3-5 page research proposal, a detailed curriculum vitae, a copy of degree certificate, a letter of acceptance from the university or research institution of the candidate's choice and a letter stating the candidate's reason for interrupting their academic career. Application forms are available from

the Department of Biology and Medicine (Dr E Steiner) or the Department of Mathematics, Natural Sciences and Engineering (Dr M Kullin) at the SNSF.
Closing Date: May 1st.

PROSPER Fellowship Programme

Subjects: Social and preventive medicine.
Eligibility: Open to promising young researchers at postdoctoral level, up to the age of 40. Applicants must have outstanding qualifications in social and preventive medicine and be Swiss nationals or permanent residents of Switzerland.
Level of Study: Postdoctorate.
Purpose: To promote and encourage young researchers at postdoctoral level.
Type: A variable number of Fellowships.
No. of awards offered: Varies.
Frequency: Annual.
Value: Varies.
Length of Study: 3-6 years.
Study Establishment: Swiss universities or academic institutions.
Country of Study: Switzerland.
Application Procedure: Please contact Dr Benno Frey or Laurence Bohren at the Office for Fellowship and Exchange Programmes of the SNSF.
Closing Date: July 1st.

SCORE Fellowship Programme

Subjects: Clinical medicine.
Eligibility: Promising young researchers at postdoctoral level who are Swiss nationals or permanent residents of Switzerland. The age limit for the beginners level is 35, the age limit for the advanced level is 40.
Level of Study: Postdoctorate.
Purpose: To promote and encourage promising young researchers at postdoctoral level. The SCORE programme operates on both a beginners and an advanced level.
Type: A variable number of Fellowships.
No. of awards offered: Varies.
Frequency: Annual.
Value: Varies.
Length of Study: 3 years for beginner level; up to 5 years for advanced level.
Study Establishment: Swiss universities or academic institutions.
Country of Study: Switzerland.
Application Procedure: For details please contact Dr Benno Frey or Laurence Bohren at the Office for Fellowship and Exchange Programmes, or refer to the website: http://www.snf.ch.
Closing Date: July 1st.

SYRACUSE UNIVERSITY

SU Graduate School
303 Bowne Hall, Syracuse, NY, 13244-1200, United States of America
Tel: (1) 315 443 4492
Fax: (1) 315 443 3423
Email: kmsciort@syr.edu
www: http://cwis.syr.edu
Contact: Ms Kristin Sciortino, Graduate Awards Co-ordinator

Syracuse University is a non-profit, private student research university.

Syracuse University Fellowship

Subjects: All subjects.
Eligibility: Open to nationals of any country.
Level of Study: Unrestricted.
Purpose: To provide a full support package during a student's term of study.
Type: Fellowship.
No. of awards offered: 101.
Frequency: Annual.
Value: US$27,597.
Length of Study: 1-6 years.
Study Establishment: Syracuse University.
Country of Study: USA.
Application Procedure: Application for fellowship is done through admission application.
Closing Date: July 2nd.

THOURON-UNIVERSITY OF PENNSYLVANIA FUND FOR BRITISH-AMERICAN STUDENT EXCHANGE

Thouron Awards
University of Glasgow, Glasgow, G12 8QQ, Scotland
Tel: (44) 141 330 3628
Fax: (44) 141 307 4920
Email: jmblack@mis.gla.ac.uk
www: http://www.upenn.edu
Contact: Mr J M Black, Secretary

The University of Glasgow is host to the UK operation of the Thouron Awards and organises the annual competition for the selection of UK graduates applying for awards tenable at the University of Pennsylvania, Philadelphia, USA.

Thouron Awards

Subjects: All subjects.
Eligibility: Open to British citizens who are graduates and unmarried. Postdoctoral candidates are ineligible unless their proposed study is in a field different from that in which they

undertook their previous postgraduate study. No application will be considered from a student already in the USA.

Level of Study: Postgraduate.

Purpose: To promote better understanding between the people of the UK and the USA.

Type: Award.

No. of awards offered: Approx. 10.

Frequency: Annual.

Value: US$1,247 per month, plus tuition and fees.

Length of Study: 1 or 2 years.

Study Establishment: The University of Pennsylvania, Philadelphia.

Country of Study: USA.

Application Procedure: Two application forms with two passport size photographs and three referee forms must be submitted.

Closing Date: October 20th.

Additional Information: American citizens interested in studying in the UK should write to the University of Pennsylvania for further details.

THRASHER RESEARCH FUND

50 East North Temple, Salt Lake City, UT, 84150-6840, United States of America
Tel: (1) 801 240 4753
Fax: (1) 801 240 1625
Email: bussej@ldschurch.org
Contact: Ms Melissa Davies, Project Co-ordinator

Thrasher Research and Field Demonstration Project Grants

Subjects: Child health.

Eligibility: Open to research scientists and private voluntary organisations. Pre and postdoctoral students may be employed on Thrasher-funded projects, but the principal investigator is expected to take an active role in the project and assume full responsibility for it. The principal investigator must have a connection with a university, research institution, or appropriate private voluntary organisation.

Level of Study: Postdoctorate.

Purpose: To promote international and national child health research and child health-related projects. Emphasis is on practical and applied interventions with the potential to improve the health of children worldwide.

Type: Grant.

No. of awards offered: Varies.

Frequency: Twice a year.

Value: Up to US$50,000 per year.

Length of Study: Up to 3 years.

Country of Study: Any country.

Application Procedure: Instructions for sending initial prospectus available upon request. Applicants are encouraged to consult with Fund staff prior to submitting a prospectus.

Closing Date: Proposals for which review is complete at the time of the semi-annual meetings are considered at those meetings.

Additional Information: The Thrasher Research Fund supports two programmes. The Scientific Programme supports research primarily in the areas of maternal and child health, infectious and parasitic diarrheal diseases, acute respiratory disease, and major nutritional deficiency. The Innovative Programme supports projects that bridge the gap between formal research in the areas of children's health and field application of research findings. Research in the areas of abortion, reproductive physiology, contraceptive technology, and sexually transmitted disease is not supported. Grants are not given for conferences, workshops, or symposia; general operations; or construction or renovation of buildings. Material detailing the policy guidelines, application procedures, and the review process are available on request. Investigators are encouraged to call or write to consult with Fund staff before submitting a prospectus.

TIERÄRZTLICHE HOCHSCHULE HANNOVER

Postfach 71 11 80, Hannover, D-30545, Germany
Tel: (49) 511 9536
Fax: (49) 511 953 8050
Email: bhuesch@vw.tiho-hannover.de
www: http://www.tiho-hannover.de
Contact: Mr Hans Linneman

Karl-Enigk-Stipendium

Subjects: Parasitology, mainly veterinary parasitology.

Eligibility: Applicants must not be aged more than 32 and must be from European countries where German is spoken.

Level of Study: Postdoctorate.

Purpose: To support research in experimental parasitology, mainly veterinary parasitology.

Type: Scholarship.

No. of awards offered: 2.

Frequency: Annual.

Value: DM2,490/DM2,590 per month according to the age of the applicant.

Length of Study: 1-2 years.

Country of Study: Any country.

Application Procedure: Please submit CV, publication list, short research proposal and references from the head of the research institute.

Closing Date: Applicantions are welcome at any time.

TOURETTE SYNDROME ASSOCIATION, INC.

42-40 Bell Boulevard, Bayside, NY, 11361-2874, United States of America
Tel: (1) 718 224 2999
Fax: (1) 718 279 9596
Email: tourette@ix.netcom.com
www: http://tsa.mgh.harvard.edu
Contact: Ms Sue Levi-Pearl, Liaison for Medical and Scientific Programs

Tourette Syndrome Association (TSA), founded in 1972, is the only national voluntary non-profit membership organisation dedicated to identifying the cause; finding the cure; and controlling the effects of Tourette syndrome. Members include individuals with the disorder, their relatives and other interested, concerned people. The Association develops and disseminates educational material to individuals, professionals and to agencies in the fields of health care, education and government; co-ordinates support services to help people and their families cope with the problems that occur with Tourettes; funds research that will ultimately find the cause of and cure for it and, at the same time, lead to improved medications and treatments.

Tourette Syndrome Association Research Grants

Subjects: Grants are awarded in three categories - basic neuroscience specifically relevant to Tourette Syndrome, clinical studies, training of postdoctoral Fellows.
Eligibility: Open to candidates who have an MD, PhD or equivalent qualifications. Previous experience in the field of movement disorders is desirable, but not essential. Fellowships are intended for young postdoctoral investigators in the early stages of their careers.
Level of Study: Doctorate.
Purpose: To foster basic and clinical research related to the causes or treatment of Tourette Syndrome.
Type: Research Grant.
No. of awards offered: Varies.
Frequency: Annual.
Value: Varies depending upon category, and experience within that category: US$5,000-US$40,000.
Length of Study: 1-2 years.
Study Establishment: Any institution with adequate facilities.
Country of Study: Any country.
Application Procedure: Please submit a letter of intent briefly describing the scientific basis of the proposed project.
Closing Date: October.
Additional Information: The association provides up to 10% of overhead or indirect costs within the total amount budgeted.

UNION OF JEWISH WOMEN OF SOUTH AFRICA

PO Box 87556
Houghton, Johannesburg, 2041, South Africa
Tel: (27) 11 646 3402
Fax: (27) 11 646 3424
Email: ujwexec@netactive.co.za
Contact: The Bursary Officer

The Union of Jewish Women of South Africa is committed to: the needs and ideals of the Jewish community; the enrichment of the peoples of South Africa; the promotion of the rights and status of women; the strengthening of links with Israel; and the maintenance of an affiliation to the International Council of Jewish Women.

The Toni Saphra Bursary and the Fanny and Shlomo Backon Bursary

Subjects: Those subject areas in which the graduate can make a positive contribution to the community and South African society.
Eligibility: Open to any female student who already holds an undergraduate degree and whose proposed postgraduate course of study will qualify her to render some form of social service in the South African community. Applicants who have not completed a first degree but are in the final year of study may also apply. These applicants will only be considered for the bursary once they have provided their final year marks. Applicants must be South African citizens.
Level of Study: Postgraduate.
Purpose: To enable women graduates to upgrade their qualifications in order to continue rendering service to their communities.
Type: Bursary.
No. of awards offered: 2.
Frequency: Annual.
Value: The Toni Saphra Bursary amount fluctuates according to the prevailing interest rates and the amount is divided between 2-3 applicants. The Backon Bursary remains static and is awarded to two students.
Length of Study: 1 year; renewable.
Study Establishment: A university.
Country of Study: South Africa.
Application Procedure: Applicants must apply in writing for the bursary in the year preceding their proposed year of study. An application form with an allocated reference number will be sent to the student for completion. Any photocopied application forms will be disqualified. Proof of acceptance by the university for the proposed course must be submitted.
Closing Date: Closing date for written applications: July 31st. All other relevant documentation: August 31st.

UNIVERSITY OF ALBERTA

Faculty of Graduate Studies & Research
105 Administration Building, Edmonton, AB, T6G2M7,
Canada
Tel: (1) 403 492 3499
Fax: (1) 403 492 0692
Email: grad.mail@ualberta.ca
www: http://www.ualberta.ca/~graduate/graduate.html
Contact: Ms T J Retson-Spalding, Graduate Awards
Assistant

Opened in 1908, the University of Alberta has a long tradition of scholarly achievements and commitment to excellence in teaching, research and service to the community. It is one of Canada's five largest research-intensive universities, with an annual research income from external sources of more than C$112 million. It participates in all fourteen of the Federal Networks of Centres of Excellence which link industry, universities and government in applied research and development.

Izaak Walton Killam Memorial Postdoctoral Fellowships

Subjects: All subjects.
Eligibility: Open to candidates of any nationality who have recently completed a PhD programme or will do so in the immediate future. Applicants who have received their PhD degree from the University of Alberta, or who will be on sabbatical leave, or who have held (or will have held) postdoctoral fellowships at other institutions for two years are not eligible. Tenable at the University of Alberta.
Level of Study: Postdoctorate.
Purpose: To attract scholars of superior research ability who have graduated within the last three years.
Type: Fellowship.
No. of awards offered: 5.
Frequency: Annual.
Value: C$35,000 per year. A non-renewable, one-time research grant of C$3,000 accompanies the award, plus incoming and return airfare.
Length of Study: 2 years.
Study Establishment: University of Alberta.
Country of Study: Canada.
Application Procedure: Application information is available from university departments.
Closing Date: January 2nd.

Izaak Walton Killam Memorial Scholarships

Subjects: All subjects.
Eligibility: Open to candidates of any nationality who are registered in, or are admissible to, a doctoral programme at the University. Scholars must have completed at least one year of graduate work prior to beginning the Scholarship. Applicants must be nominated by the department in which they plan to pursue their doctoral studies.
Level of Study: Doctorate, Postgraduate.
Type: Scholarship.
No. of awards offered: Approx. 13.

Frequency: Annual.
Value: C$16,200 per year, a non-renewable, one-time C$1,500 research grant, plus tuition and fees.
Length of Study: 2 years (from May 1st or September 1st); subject to review after the first year.
Study Establishment: University of Alberta.
Country of Study: Canada.
Application Procedure: Application information is available from university departments.
Closing Date: February 1st for submission of nominations from departments. Check with the department for internal deadline.

Province of Alberta Graduate Fellowships

Subjects: All subjects.
Eligibility: Open to Canadian citizens or permanent residents at the date of application who have completed at least one year of graduate study and are registered in a full time doctoral programme at the University of Alberta.
Level of Study: Doctorate, Postgraduate.
Type: Fellowship.
No. of awards offered: Approx. 35.
Frequency: Annual.
Value: C$10,500 (May commencement); C$7,000 (September commencement).
Length of Study: 1 year (from May 1st or September 1st).
Study Establishment: University of Alberta.
Country of Study: Canada.
Application Procedure: Applicants must be nominated by the department in which they plan to pursue their doctoral studies.
Closing Date: February 1st for submission of nominations from departments. Check with the department for internal deadline.
Additional Information: Recipients must carry out a full-time research programme during the summer months.

Province of Alberta Graduate Scholarships

Subjects: All subjects.
Eligibility: Open to Canadian citizens or permanent residents at the date of application who are entering or continuing in a full-time Master's programme at the University of Alberta. Applicants must be nominated by the department in which they plan to pursue their studies. Students registered as qualifying graduate students are not eligible.
Level of Study: Postgraduate.
Type: Scholarship.
No. of awards offered: Approx. 38.
Frequency: Annual.
Value: C$9,300 (May commencement); C$6,200 (September commencement).
Length of Study: 12 months (from 1 May) or for 8 months (from September 1st); partial awards may be recommended at a reduced value and the award may be terminated earlier by either the student or the university and the amount reduced proportionately.
Study Establishment: University of Alberta.
Country of Study: Canada.

Application Procedure: Application forms are available from university departments.

Closing Date: February 1st for submission of nominations from departments. Check with the department for internal deadline.

UNIVERSITY OF AUCKLAND

Private Bag 92019, Auckland, 1000, New Zealand
Tel: (64) 9 373 7999
Fax: (64) 9 373 7400
Email: appointments@auckland.ac.nz
www: http://www.auckland.ac.nz
Contact: Mr M V Lellman, Assistant Registrar

The University of Auckland has a commitment to conserving, advancing and disseminating knowledge through teaching of the highest standard provided by scholars who are among the foremost researchers in New Zealand. The University aims to be a university of high international standing and a leader in the Asia-Pacific region.

UARC Postdoctoral Fellowships

Subjects: Any academic discipline represented at this University.
Eligibility: Applicants must have completed a PhD not more than four years previously. Open to any suitably qualified applicant who has been the holder of a doctorate from an institution other than the University of Auckland for not more than four years.
Level of Study: Postdoctorate.
Purpose: To foster research.
Type: Fellowship.
No. of awards offered: 4 or 5.
Frequency: Annual.
Value: NZ$46,250 per year, plus allowance for air fare of up to NZ$4,000.
Length of Study: 2 years; not renewable.
Study Establishment: Auckland University.
Country of Study: New Zealand.
Application Procedure: All vacancies are advertised and application details are given in the advertisement.
Closing Date: Around June.
Additional Information: Fellowships are assigned to university staff members on a competitive basis. Graduates of the University of Auckland are not eligible for the Fellowships.

University of Auckland Foundation Visiting Fellowships

Subjects: Any subject offered by the University.
Eligibility: Open to suitably qualified scholars of high academic standing.
Level of Study: Postdoctorate, Professional development.
Purpose: To bring visiting scholars of high standing in their academic field, to the University of Auckland.

Type: Fellowship.
No. of awards offered: Up to 15.
Frequency: Annual.
Value: Varies, up to NZ$5,000.
Length of Study: Variable periods of up to 1 year.
Study Establishment: University of Auckland.
Country of Study: New Zealand.
Application Procedure: Recipients must be nominated by a staff member at the University of Auckland.
Closing Date: June 30th.

UNIVERSITY OF BATH

Graduate Office
Claverton Down, Bath, BA2 7AY, England
Tel: (44) 1225 826826
Fax: (44) 1225 826366
Email: grad-office@bath.ac.uk
www: http://www.bath.ac.uk/
Contact: Dr Lisa Isted, Graduate Office Administrator

The University, which occupies a beautiful greenfield site just outside the world hertitage city of Bath, specialises in engineering and design, science, humanities and social sciences, and management. The University of Bath came sixth in the 1996 research assessment exercise, with 12 out of 21 units achieving grade 5.

University Research Studentships

Subjects: All subjects offered by the University.
Eligibility: Open to candidates of any nationality with a first or good second class honours degree or equivalent. Candidates must have applied, or been accepted, for study for a research degree.
Level of Study: Doctorate, Postdoctorate.
Purpose: To provide funds for well-qualified candidates to pursue full-time research leading to a research degree.
Type: 1 Scholarship.
No. of awards offered: Approx. 20.
Frequency: Annual, if funds are available.
Value: Home fees plus maintenance at level equivalent to research councils.
Length of Study: Up to 3 years.
Study Establishment: University of Bath.
Country of Study: United Kingdom.
Application Procedure: Those wishing to be considered should state this when applying for a higher degree and should contact the appropriate academic department or the graduate office.
Closing Date: August 1st.
Additional Information: Other studentships are available at the University of Bath. Please contact the graduate office for further details.

UNIVERSITY OF BRISTOL

Student Finance Office
Students Union
Queen's Road, Bristol, BS8 1LN, England
Tel: (44) 117 954 5886
Fax: (44) 117 923 9085
Email: judith.tyler@bristol.ac.uk
www: http://www.bristol.ac.uk
Contact: Ms J Tyler, Overseas Recruitment & Liaison Director

University Postgraduate Scholarships

Subjects: Any research topic which is covered in the work of the Department within the University.
Eligibility: New research students with normally at least an upper second class honours degree or equivalent. Full-time students or part-time students who are not in full-time employment. All University scholars must be registered and in attendance for a research degree at the University.
Level of Study: Postgraduate.
Purpose: To help the University to recruit high quality research students.
Type: Scholarship.
No. of awards offered: 90.
Frequency: Annual.
Value: £5,455-£7,910 plus home tuition fees of £2,610.
Length of Study: 3 years.
Study Establishment: University of Bristol.
Country of Study: United Kingdom.
Application Procedure: Students must apply on the appropriate form to the Department of their field of interest.
Closing Date: Normally May 1st.
Additional Information: Overseas students need to find the difference between home and overseas fees. To do this they can apply for an overseas research scholarship.

For further information contact:

Postgraduate Admissions
University of Bristol
Senate House
Tyndall Avenue
Clifton, Bristol, BS8 1TH, England

UNIVERSITY OF BRITISH COLUMBIA

Faculty of Graduate Studies
180-6371 Crescent Road, Vancouver, BC, V6T 1Z2, Canada
Tel: (1) 604 822 4556
Fax: (1) 604 822 5802
Email: gradawards@mercury.ubc.ca
www: http://www.grad.ubc.ca/awards/top.htm
Contact: Graduate Awards Officer

The University of British Columbia is one of North America's major research universities. The faculty of Graduate Studies has 6,500 students and is a national leader in interdisciplinary study and research, with 88 departments, 17 research centres, 6 graduate programmes, 2 residential colleges and a school.

Izaak Walton Killam Postdoctoral Fellowships

Subjects: All subjects.
Eligibility: Open to candidates who show superior ability in research and have obtained, within two academic years of the anticipated commencement date of the Fellowship, a doctorate at a university other than the University of British Columbia. Graduates of the University of British Columbia are not normally eligible.
Level of Study: Postdoctorate.
Purpose: To support all areas of academic research.
Type: Fellowship.
No. of awards offered: 8.
Frequency: Annual.
Value: C$32,000.
Length of Study: 2 years, subject to satisfactory progress at the end of the first year.
Study Establishment: UBC.
Country of Study: Canada.
Application Procedure: Application form, academic transcripts and three reference letters must be submitted to the appropriate department.
Closing Date: November 15th.
Additional Information: Candidates are responsible for contacting the appropriate department at the University to ensure their proposed research project is acceptable and may be undertaken under the supervision of a member of the department. Travel/research grant of C$3,000 is available during the tenure of the fellowship. (Email: killam@mercury.ubc.ca).

Killam Predoctoral Fellowship

Subjects: Full-time study and/or research leading to a doctoral degree in any subject.
Eligibility: Open to students of any nationality, discipline, age or sex. This award is given at PhD level only and is strictly based on academic merit. Students must have a first class standing in their last two years of study.
Level of Study: Doctorate.
Purpose: To assist doctoral students to devote full time to their studies and research.
Type: Fellowship.
No. of awards offered: Approx. 20.
Frequency: Annual.
Value: C$22,000 per year.
Study Establishment: UBC.
Country of Study: Canada.
Application Procedure: Top-ranked students are selected from the University Graduate Fellowship competition. Application forms can be obtained from departments or the Faculty of Graduate Studies.
Closing Date: January 26th.
Additional Information: Students must submit their applications to the departments, not to Graduates Studies; please check for internal departmental deadlines.

University of British Columbia Graduate Fellowship

Subjects: Full-time study and/or research leading to a masters or doctoral degree in any discipline.
Eligibility: Open to students of any nationality, discipline, age or sex. This award is strictly based on academic merit. Students must have a first class standing in their last two years of study.
Level of Study: Postgraduate.
Purpose: To assist graduate students to devote full time to their studies and research.
Type: Fellowship.
No. of awards offered: Approx. 400.
Frequency: Annual.
Value: C$16,000 per year for full renewable UGFs; or C$8,000 for one-year UGF's.
Study Establishment: UBC.
Country of Study: Canada.
Application Procedure: Applicants are nominated by their departments based on academic merit. Students must submit their applications to the UBC Department, not to The Faculty of Graduate Studies.
Closing Date: End of January or mid-March.
Additional Information: Please check for internal departmental deadlines.

THE UNIVERSITY OF CALGARY

Earth Sciences Building
Room 720
2500 University Drive NW, Calgary, AB, T2N 1N4, Canada
Tel: (1) 403 220 5690
Fax: (1) 403 289 7635
Email: cbusch@acs.ucalgary.ca
www: http://www.ucalgary.ca
Contact: Ms Connie Busch, Graduate Scholarship Assistant

Davies (William H) Medical Research Scholarship

Subjects: Medicine.
Eligibility: Open to qualified graduates of any recognised university who will be registered in the Faculty of Graduate Studies at the University of Calgary.
Level of Study: Postgraduate.
Type: Scholarship.
No. of awards offered: 1+.
Value: C$3,000 to C$11,000 depending on qualifications, experience and graduate program.
Length of Study: 4-12 months.
Study Establishment: University of Calgary.
Country of Study: Canada.
Application Procedure: Applicants should apply to the Assistant Dean (Medical Science) in the first instance. The Graduate Scholarship Committee will make the final decison based on departmental recommendations.

Closing Date: April 1st.
Additional Information: Successful candidates must conduct their research programme within the Faculty of Medicine; others cannot be considered. Awards are made solely on the basis of academic excellence. Renewable in open competition.

Izaak Walton Killam Memorial Scholarships

Subjects: All subjects.
Eligibility: Open to qualified graduates of any university who are admissible to a doctoral programme at the University of Calgary. Applicants must have completed at least one year of graduate study prior to taking up the award.
Level of Study: Doctorate, Postgraduate.
Type: Scholarship.
No. of awards offered: 4-5.
Frequency: Annual.
Value: C$19,500. If approved, award holders may also receive up to C$2,100 over the full term of appointment for special equipment and/or travel in direct connection with the PhD research.
Length of Study: 1 year.
Study Establishment: University of Calgary.
Country of Study: Canada.
Application Procedure: Apply for application from The Graduate Scholarship Secretary at the university.
Closing Date: February 1st annually.
Additional Information: One year duration renewable once upon presentation of evidence of satisfactory progress. Further renewal in open competition.

Province of Alberta Graduate Scholarships and Fellowships

Subjects: All subjects.
Eligibility: Candidates for the scholarships or fellowships must be registered in or admissible to a programme leading to a Master's or Doctoral degree respectively. Eligible to Canadian citizens and landed immigrants.
Level of Study: Doctorate, Postgraduate.
Type: Fellowship, Scholarship.
No. of awards offered: 60-70.
Frequency: Annual.
Value: Scholarship: C$9,300 per year. Fellowship: C$10,500 per year.
Length of Study: 1 year.
Study Establishment: University of Calgary.
Country of Study: Canada.
Application Procedure: Application forms are available from the Directors of Graduate Studies of the regarded departments.
Closing Date: February 1st.
Additional Information: One year, renewable in open competition. Students whose awards begin in May are expected to carry out a full-time research programme during the summer months.

University of Calgary Dean's Special Entrance Scholarship

Subjects: All subjects.
Eligibility: Open to women admissible to the Faculty of Graduate Studies in a programme of study leading to either the Master's or Doctoral degree.
Level of Study: Doctorate, Postgraduate.
Type: Scholarship.
No. of awards offered: 4.
Frequency: Annual.
Value: C$8,000.
Length of Study: 1 year; not renewable.
Study Establishment: University of Calgary.
Country of Study: Canada.
Application Procedure: Candidates should apply to the chairperson of the Graduate Scholarship Committee, Room 720 Earth Sciences Building, The University of Calgary, using the Graduate Scholarship Application Form. In addition, the description of the family responsibilities, no longer than one page, must be appended to the application.
Closing Date: February 1st.
Additional Information: Applicants must be entering a first year of graduate work after an absence from full-time study at a university for a minimum of three years for the purposes of raising children, caring for elderly parents or other demanding family responsibilities. Applicants must include a description of those responsibilities.

University of Calgary Dean's Special Master's Scholarship

Subjects: Disciplines where the Master's degree is the terminal degree at the University of Calgary.
Eligibility: Open to candidates who are or will be registered in a full-time thesis-based MA programme in a discipline where the MA-degree is the terminal degree at the University of Calgary.
Level of Study: Postgraduate.
Type: Scholarship.
No. of awards offered: Up to 15.
Frequency: Annual.
Value: C$5,000.
Length of Study: 1 year.
Study Establishment: University of Calgary.
Country of Study: Canada.
Application Procedure: Candidates must apply to the regarded departments at the University of Calgary.
Closing Date: February 1st.
Additional Information: One-year duration, renewable in open competition.

University of Calgary Silver Anniversary Graduate Fellowships

Subjects: All subjects.
Eligibility: Open to qualified graduates of any recognised university who are registered in or admissible to a doctoral programme at the University of Calgary. Canadian residents only.
Level of Study: Doctorate.

Type: Fellowship.
No. of awards offered: Minimum of 2.
Frequency: Annual.
Value: Up to C$20,000 but in no case less than C$16,000.
Length of Study: 1 year.
Study Establishment: University of Calgary.
Country of Study: Canada.
Application Procedure: Candidates should apply to their department.
Closing Date: February 1st.
Additional Information: One year duration, renewable once upon presentation of evidence of satisfactory progress. Awards are granted on the basis of academic standing and demonstrated potential for advanced study and research.

UNIVERSITY OF CAMBRIDGE

University Registry
The Old Schools, Cambridge, CB2 1TN, England
Tel: (44) 1223 332 317
Fax: (44) 1223 332 332
Email: mrf25@admin.cam.ac.uk
Contact: Ms Melanie Foster, Scholarships Clerk

The University of Cambridge is a loose confederation of faculties, colleges and other bodies. The Colleges are mainly concerned with the teaching of their undergraduate students (through tutorials and supervisions) and the academic support of both graduate and undergraduate students, while the University employs Professors, Readers, Lecturers and other teaching and administrative staff who provide the formal teaching (in lectures seminars and practical classes). The University also administers the University Library.

Churchill College Research Studentships

Subjects: Any subject for which research supervision can be provided at the university.
Eligibility: Open to any person who has graduated from a university or, if not a graduate, can show evidence of exceptional qualifications for research.
Level of Study: Doctorate.
Purpose: To assist research for candidates who intend to register for the degree of PhD at the University of Cambridge.
Type: Studentship.
No. of awards offered: Varies, depending on funds available.
Frequency: Annual.
Value: University and college fees, plus maintenance (based on recommended rates).
Length of Study: 3 years.
Study Establishment: Churchill College.
Country of Study: United Kingdom.
Application Procedure: Application forms are available from the given address.
Closing Date: February 15th.

For further information contact:

Churchill College, Cambridge, CB3 0DS, England
Tel: (44) 1223 336157
Fax: (44) 1223 336177
Contact: Mr Henry Hurst, Tutor for Advanced Students

Clare Hall Foundation Fellowship

Subjects: All subjects.
Eligibility: Open to persons who already hold academic posts in their own country, have not previously studied in the UK or North America, and are able to demonstrate that a period of study in Cambridge would be of special benefit. There is no restriction as to sex or age, although preference may be given to applicants under the age of 40.
Level of Study: Postdoctorate.
Purpose: To help a rising scholar from either a developing country, a centrally planned economy, or a country in transition to a market economy.
Type: Fellowship.
No. of awards offered: 1.
Frequency: Annual.
Value: Normally sufficient for three months residence in Cambridge.
Length of Study: 3 months; although by supplementing other funds the Fellowship would possibly permit a longer stay of up to 6 months.
Study Establishment: Normally Clare Hall, but probably attached to one of the university departments.
Country of Study: United Kingdom.
Application Procedure: Applications, accompanied by a curriculum vitae, should be addressed to the Chairman of the Fellowship Committee at the College, to whom three referees should write direct. One reference should be from a referee whose work is recognized in the UK.
Closing Date: Application are accepted at any time.
Additional Information: The Fellowship is awarded on the grounds of academic suitability.

For further information contact:

Clare Hall
Herschel Road, Cambridge, CB3 9AL, England
Tel: (44) 1223 332360
Fax: (44) 1223 332333
Contact: Ms Elizabeth Ramsden, College Secretary

Corpus Christi College Research Scholarships

Subjects: All subjects.
Eligibility: Open to holders of a first class honours degree or equivalent. Candidates eligible for UK state awards are not eligible.
Level of Study: Doctorate.
Purpose: To enable the successful candidate to pursue, as a member of the College, a course of study in any subject leading to a research-based higher degree, normally the PhD, at the University of Cambridge.
Type: Scholarship.
No. of awards offered: 1+.
Frequency: Annual.

Value: Awards are made usually in collaboration with the Cambridge Commonwealth and Overseas Trusts. The amount of the awards varies but substantial contributions (£6,000) towards fees or maintenance costs are made.
Length of Study: Usually 3 years.
Study Establishment: Corpus Christi College.
Country of Study: United Kingdom.
Application Procedure: All applications to the Board of Graduate Studies which name Corpus Christi College as their first preference on CIGAS Form A will be considered for these scholarships, provided they reach the College by the closing date. Separate application to the College is not required.
Closing Date: End of March.

For further information contact:

Corpus Christi College, Cambridge, CB2 1RH, England
Tel: (44) 1223 338038
Fax: (44) 1223 338057
Contact: Dr C J B Brookes, The Tutor for Advanced Students

E D Davies Scholarship

Subjects: All subjects.
Eligibility: Open to graduates of any university who have been admitted to a course of research.
Level of Study: Doctorate.
Purpose: To enable graduates to undertake a course of research in any subject area.
Type: Scholarship.
No. of awards offered: 1.
Frequency: Annual.
Value: £1,250 per year. The award is designed to supplement funding from other sources.
Length of Study: 3 years.
Study Establishment: Fitzwilliam College.
Country of Study: England.
Application Procedure: Application forms are available on request.
Closing Date: June 13th.

For further information contact:

Fitzwilliam College, Cambridge, CB3 ODG, England
Tel: (44) 1223 332 035
Fax: (44) 1223 332 082
Contact: Dr W Alison, Tutor for Graduate Students

Fitzwilliam College Research Fellowship

Subjects: To be advised in further particulars.
Eligibility: Open to candidates who are carrying out research for a PhD at any British or Irish university, or who have recently completed their course of study for this degree. Candidates should not have completed four years of full-time research by the April preceding the commencement of the fellowship.
Level of Study: Doctorate.
Purpose: To enable scholars to carry out a programme of new research.
Type: Fellowship.
No. of awards offered: Varies.

Frequency: Annual.
Value: Varies. Non-stipendiary also offered.
Study Establishment: Fitzwilliam College.
Country of Study: United Kingdom.
Application Procedure: Please write for details.
Closing Date: Early September.
Additional Information: Fellowships are awarded for new research only, not to enable candidates to complete their PhD dissertation.

For further information contact:

Fitzwilliam College, Cambridge, CB3 0DG, England
Tel: (44) 1223 332 035
Fax: (44) 1223 332 082
Contact: Dr W Alison, Tutor for Graduate Students

Gonville and Caius College Gonville Bursary

Subjects: Any offered by the University.
Eligibility: Open to candidates who have been accepted by the College through its normal admissions procedures, and who are classified as overseas students for fees purposes. A statement of financial circumstances is required.
Level of Study: Doctorate, Postgraduate, Undergraduate.
Purpose: To help outstanding students from outside the EC to meet the costs of degree courses at the University of Cambridge.
Type: Bursary.
No. of awards offered: Up to 6.
Frequency: Annual.
Value: Reimbursement of College fees.
Length of Study: Up to 3 years, (renewable dependent on satisfactory progress).
Study Establishment: Gonville and Caius College.
Country of Study: United Kingdom.
Application Procedure: There are no application forms. For further information please contact the admissions tutor.
Closing Date: The same as for the University's courses.

For further information contact:

Gonville and Caius College, Cambridge, CB2 1TA, England
Tel: (44) 1223 332447
Fax: (44) 1223 332456
Contact: The Admissions Tutor

Magdalene College Leslie Wilson Research Scholarships

Subjects: Any subject offered by the University.
Eligibility: Open to graduates from the UK and overseas who will be studying at Cambridge for a PhD degree. Consideration is normally restricted to those who have obtained, or who have a strong prospect of obtaining, a first class honours (Bachelor's) degree. Preference is given to those nominating Magdalene as their first choice college.
Level of Study: Doctorate.

Purpose: To assist study leading to the degree of Doctor of Philosophy.
Type: Scholarship.
No. of awards offered: 1.
Frequency: Annual.
Value: A maximum of £10,787 (1998-99 values) for a scholar who has no other sources of finance (maintenance grant £6,455, university fees £2,610, and college fees £1,772). Rented accommodation in or near Magdalene College will be made available during the first year of residence for unmarried scholars. Married scholars will be offered rented accommodation near to the college.
Length of Study: Up to 3 years.
Study Establishment: Magdalene College and the University of Cambridge.
Country of Study: United Kingdom.
Application Procedure: Leslie Wilson Scholarship applicants should obtain a CIGAS form from the Board of Graduate Studies, 4 Mill Lane, Cambridge. UK candidates are expected to apply, if eligible, for State or Research Council Studentships. Overseas candidates are expected to apply for UK government support as well as Overseas Student Bursaries awarded by the University of Cambridge and administered by the Board of Graduate Studies. In addition, all candidates should obtain a Leslie Wilson Research Scholarship form from the address below.
Closing Date: May 1st.

For further information contact:

Magdalene College
University of Cambridge, Cambridge, CB3 0AG, England
Tel: (44) 1223 332135
Fax: (44) 1223 462589
Contact: Admissions Tutor for Graduates

Pembroke College Graduate Awards

Subjects: Any subject offered by the University.
Eligibility: Open to candidates of any nationality who are accepted by Pembroke College, and who intend to register for a PhD degree at the University of Cambridge. Candidates must make Pembroke their first choice college.
Level of Study: Doctorate, Postgraduate.
Type: Studentship.
No. of awards offered: 1.
Frequency: Annual.
Value: Full support.
Length of Study: 3 years.
Study Establishment: Pembroke College.
Country of Study: United Kingdom.
Closing Date: April 1st.
Additional Information: There are also a number of scholarships (fees only) and bursaries available.

For further information contact:

Pembroke College, Cambridge, CB2 1RZ, England
Tel: (44) 1223 338115
Fax: (44) 1223 338163
Contact: Ms Jenny Davis, Graduate Admissions Tutor

Queen's College Research Fellowships

Subjects: Subjects announced each year.
Eligibility: Open to graduates of any university who should normally be under 30 years of age and who are well advanced in their doctoral research or who have recently begun postdoctoral research.
Level of Study: Postdoctorate.
Purpose: To provide the opportunity for postdoctoral research in various fields of study.
Type: Fellowship.
No. of awards offered: 2.
Frequency: Annual.
Value: Approximately £10,000.
Length of Study: 3 years.
Study Establishment: Queen's College.
Country of Study: United Kingdom.
Application Procedure: Application form must be completed and research proposal submitted. Written work will be requested from short-listed candidates.
Closing Date: Usually October 8th.

For further information contact:

Queens' College, Cambridge, CB3 9ET, England
Tel: (44) 1223 335601
Fax: (44) 1223 335522
Contact: Dr K J I Thorne, Senior Tutor

St John's College Benefactors' Scholarships for Research

Subjects: Any subject offered by the University.
Eligibility: Open to candidates of any nationality with a first class honours or equivalent degree.
Level of Study: Postgraduate.
Purpose: To fund candidates for the PhD and MPhil degrees.
Type: Scholarship.
No. of awards offered: 6.
Frequency: Annual.
Value: £5,295; plus approved college & university fees, book allowance of £310 and other expenses.
Length of Study: Up to 3 years.
Study Establishment: St John's College.
Country of Study: United Kingdom.
Application Procedure: For further particulars see the Cambridge University Graduate Studies Prospectus.
Closing Date: May 1st.

For further information contact:

St John's College, Cambridge, CB2 1TP, England
Tel: (44) 1223 338612
Fax: (44) 1223 766419
Contact: Tutor for Graduate Affairs

UNIVERSITY OF DUNDEE

Dundee, DD1 4HN, Scotland
Tel: (44) 1382 23 181
Fax: (44) 1382 345 515
Email: j.e.nicholson@dundee.ac.uk
www: http://www.dundee.ac.uk
Contact: Postgraduate Office

The mission of the University is to provide education of the highest quality coupled with a leading contribution to the advancement of knowledge, thereby developing in its students the imagination, talents, creativity and skills necessary for the varied and rapidly changing requirements of modern life.

University of Dundee Research Awards

Subjects: Medicine, dentistry, science, engineering, law, arts, social sciences, environmental studies, town planning, architecture, management and consumer studies, nursing, fine art, television & imaging.
Eligibility: Open to holders of a first class or upper second class honours degree or equivalent.
Level of Study: Postgraduate.
Purpose: To assist full-time research leading to a PhD.
Type: Studentship.
No. of awards offered: Approx. 4-6 depending on funds available.
Frequency: Annual.
Value: £5,400 plus tuition fees at the home rate.
Length of Study: 1 year; renewable annually for up to a maximum of 2 additional years.
Study Establishment: University of Dundee, Tayside.
Country of Study: United Kingdom.
Application Procedure: Write for information.
Closing Date: February 26th.

UNIVERSITY OF EXETER

Northcote House
The Queen's Drive, Exeter, Devon, EX4 4QJ, England
Tel: (44) 1392 263 263
Fax: (44) 1392 263 108
Email: pgao@exeter.ac.uk
www: http://www.ex.ac.uk/
Contact: Postgraduate Admissions Office

The University of Exeter is representative of the best of British University education. It combines research of international standing across all departments with excellence in education, and is one of the most popular in the country among applicants.

University of Exeter Postgraduate Scholarships

Subjects: Any subject offered by the university if the School has scholarship funding available. Graduate Teaching Assistantships and Graduate Research Assistantships may also be available in certain schools.
Eligibility: Open to candidates for research degrees who have obtained at least an upper second class honours degree or its equivalent.
Level of Study: Doctorate, Postgraduate.
Purpose: To study for a higher degree, ie. MPhil or PhD.
Type: Scholarship.
No. of awards offered: 5-20.
Frequency: Annual, if funds are available.
Value: Home fees plus maintenance at similar level to research council level awards.
Length of Study: Up to 3 years.
Study Establishment: University of Exeter.
Country of Study: United Kingdom.
Application Procedure: Those wishing to be considered should state this when applying for a higher degree and should contact the appropriate academic department direct.
Additional Information: The following named Scholarships are included in this scheme: Sir Arthur Reed Graduate Scholarship; Fuller Scholarship; Anning Morgan Bursary; Sir Henry Lopes Scholarship; Eden Phillpotts Scholarship; Exeter Research Scholarship; Devon Graduate Scholarship; St Cyres Scholarship; G T J James Postgraduate Scholarship; Wreford Clark Scholarship; Frank Southerden Scholarship; Andrew Simons Graduate Scholarship. Scholarships may not be held in conjunction with other major awards or sources of income. Not every scholarship is available every year.

UNIVERSITY OF GLASGOW

Glasgow, G12 8QQ, Scotland
Tel: (44) 141 330 4515
Fax: (44) 141 330 4413
Email: pgadmissions@mis.gla.ac.uk
Contact: Ms Hazel Sydeserff, Graduate Admissions Officer

The University of Glasgow is a major research-led university operating in an international context which aims to: provide education through the development of learning in a research environment; undertake fundamental, strategic and applied research; and to sustain and add value to Scottish culture, to the natural environment and to the national economy.

University of Glasgow Postgraduate Scholarships

Subjects: All subjects.
Eligibility: Open to candidates of any nationality who are proficient in English and who have obtained a first or an upper second class honours or equivalent degree.
Level of Study: Postgraduate.
Purpose: To assist with research toward a PhD degree.
Type: Scholarship.
No. of awards offered: 26.
Frequency: Annual.
Value: £6,456 maintenance allowance, plus home fees of £2,610.
Length of Study: 3 years; subject to satisfactory progress.
Study Establishment: University of Glasgow.
Country of Study: Scotland.
Application Procedure: Applicants should use the University's form, Application for Graduate Studies, which covers application for admission and for the scholarship. For the address to send the application form to please refer to Notes for Applicants booklet issued with the application form.
Closing Date: Faculties of Medicine and Science, January 31st; Arts, Divinity, and Veterinary Medicine, February 28th; Engineering, Law and Financial Studies, and Social Sciences, March 31st.
Additional Information: Scholars from outside the European Union will be expected to make up the difference between the home fee and the overseas fee.

UNIVERSITY OF KENT

Canterbury, Kent, C2T 7NZ, England
Tel: (44) 1227 827 656
Fax: (44) 1227 762 811
www: http://www.ukc.ac.uk
Contact: Postgraduate Office

Tizard Centre Departmental Scholarships

Subjects: Mental health.
Eligibility: Candidate for scholarships should hold or expect to obtain a first or second class honours degree. They must also be a citizen of one of the European Union countries.
Level of Study: Postgraduate.
Purpose: To support research studies in mental health or learning disabilities; one award in each.
Type: Studentship.
No. of awards offered: 2.
Frequency: Dependent on funds available.
Value: Home tuition fees plus a maintenance bursary at the same rate as the EPSRC.
Length of Study: 3 years.
Study Establishment: University of Kent.
Country of Study: United Kingdom.
Application Procedure: An application form must be completed.

UNIVERSITY OF LEEDS

Research Degrees & Scholarships Office, Leeds, West Yorkshire, LS2 9JT, England
Tel: (44) 113 233 4007
Fax: (44) 113 233 3941
Email: rsdnh@central.admin.leeds.ac.uk
www: http://www.leeds.ac.uk
Contact: Mrs J Y Findlay

Iceland - Leeds University - FCO Chevening Scholarships

Subjects: All subjects.
Eligibility: Open to candidates who have obtained a first degree of similar standard to at least a UK second class honours degree. Candidates must be nationals of Iceland.
Level of Study: Postgraduate.
Type: Scholarship.
No. of awards offered: 1.
Frequency: Annual.
Value: To cover academic fees and living expenses, books, equipment, arrival and departure allowance, economy return airfares and production of dissertation.
Length of Study: 1 year taught mastership course.
Study Establishment: University of Leeds.
Country of Study: United Kingdom.
Application Procedure: By application form and acceptance on to a taught course. Application forms are available from the British Embassy in Ireland.
Closing Date: January 10th.

For further information contact:

British Embassy, Reykjavik, Iceland
Contact: HM Ambassador

Kulika-Leeds University FCO Chevening Scholarships

Subjects: All subjects.
Eligibility: Open to candidates who have obtained a first degree of similar standard to at least a second UK second class honours degree. Candidates must be a national of Uganda.
Level of Study: Postgraduate.
Purpose: To provide postgraduate scholarships to students of a high academic calibre.
Type: Scholarship.
No. of awards offered: 3.
Frequency: Annual.
Value: To cover academic fees and living expenses, books equipment, arrival and departure allowance, economy return airfares and production of dissertation.
Length of Study: 1 year taught mastership course.
Study Establishment: University of Leeds.
Country of Study: United Kingdom.
Application Procedure: By application form and acceptance on to a taught course. Application forms are available from the university.
Closing Date: To be announced.

For further information contact:

British Council in Uganda
IPS Building
Parliament Avenue
PO Box 7070, Kampala, Uganda

Tetley and Lupton Scholarships for Overseas Students

Subjects: All subjects.
Eligibility: Open to candidates liable to pay tuition fees for Master's degrees and research degrees at the full-cost rate for overseas students. Applicants must be of a high academic standard.
Level of Study: Doctorate, Postgraduate.
Purpose: To provide awards to overseas students of high academic calibre.
Type: Scholarship.
No. of awards offered: 70.
Frequency: Annual.
Value: £3,000 per year to be credited towards academic fees.
Length of Study: 1 year; may be renewed for second or third year according to duration of course. May be held concurrently with other awards except those providing full payment of fees.
Study Establishment: University of Leeds.
Country of Study: United Kingdom.
Application Procedure: Apply for a course and then apply for scholarship. Research candidates need to apply with national ORS competition.

UNIVERSITY OF LONDON

Senate House
Malet Street, London, WC1E 7HU, England
Tel: (44) 171 636 8000
Fax: (44) 171 636 0373
www: http://www.qmw.ac.uk
Contact: Grants Management Officer

Queen Mary and Westfield College Research Studentships

Subjects: Arts (except French), sciences, engineering, social sciences, law, medicine and denstistry.
Eligibility: Open to suitably qualified candidates who hold at least an upper second class honours at first degree level.
Level of Study: Research.
Purpose: To provide the opportunity for full-time research leading towards an MPhil or PhD.
Type: Studentship.
No. of awards offered: Approx. 50.
Frequency: Annual.
Value: Maintenance at the current research council rate, plus tuition fees at the home level (successful overseas apllicants must provide the difference).
Length of Study: 3 years full-time, subject to satisfactory academic report.
Study Establishment: Queen Mary and Westfield College.

Country of Study: United Kingdom.
Application Procedure: Please write to the Admission and Research Student Office for details.
Closing Date: June 25th.
Additional Information: These studentships are open only to research students commencing their studies in the 1999/200 session. They are not available to existing research students.

For further information contact:

Queen Mary and Westfield College
University of London
Mile End Road, London, E1 4NS, England
Tel: (44) 171 975 3657
Fax: (44) 171 975 5588
Contact: Mr Peter Smith, Admissions Assistant

UNIVERSITY OF MANCHESTER

Oxford Road, Manchester, M13 9PL, England
Tel: (44) 161 275 2736
Fax: (44) 161 275 2445
www: http://www.man.ac.uk
Contact: Office of the Academic Registrar

The University of Manchester is an international provider of quality research and graduate education across a wide variety of disciplines.

Frederick Craven Moore Awards

Subjects: Clinical medicine.
Eligibility: Open to graduates of any approved university, or other suitably qualified persons, who can furnish satisfactory evidence of their qualifications to pursue research in clinical medicine.
Level of Study: Postgraduate.
Purpose: Principally to support postgraduate research.
Type: Scholarships, Fellowships.
No. of awards offered: Varies.
Frequency: As funds permit; scholarships are awarded annually.
Value: The value of the scholarship varies, but is normally not less than the annual value of a State or Research Council Postgraduate Award in Medicine. The value of the fellowship is determined on an individual basis in accordance with the qualifications and experience of the Fellow.
Length of Study: 1 year; the scholarships only are renewable for up to a maximum of 2 additional years.
Study Establishment: Manchester University.
Country of Study: United Kingdom.
Application Procedure: Please contact Graduate School of Science, Engineering and Medicine.
Closing Date: May 1st.

University of Manchester Research Studentships or Scholarships

Subjects: Any area of study within the purview of the Graduate Schools of Arts, Social Sciences, Education, Science, Engineering and Medicine.

Eligibility: Open to graduates of any approved university, or other suitably qualified persons, who can furnish satisfactory evidence of their qualifications to pursue research. Applicants must hold at least an upper second class degree to be eligible.
Level of Study: Postgraduate.
Purpose: To support postgraduate research, and provide funding for high quality UK, European and overseas graduates wishing to study for PhD.
Type: Studentship/Scholarship.
No. of awards offered: Up to 50.
Frequency: Annual.
Value: Varies. Some full studentships (maintenance and UK fees), also part scholarships.
Length of Study: Normally 3 years.
Study Establishment: Manchester University.
Country of Study: United Kingdom.
Application Procedure: Application forms available on request from Research and Graduate Support Unit.
Closing Date: May 1st.

UNIVERSITY OF MANITOBA

Faculty of Graduate Studies
500 University Centre, Winnipeg, MB, R3T 2N2, Canada
Tel: (1) 204 474 9836
Fax: (1) 204 474 7553
Email: ilse_krentz@umanitoba.ca
www:
http://www.umanitoba.ca/faculties/graduate_studies/awards
Contact: Ms Ilse Krentz, Awards Officer

University of Manitoba Graduate Fellowships

Subjects: Any discipline taught at the graduate level at the University.
Eligibility: At the time of application, students do not need to have been accepted by the Department/Faculty, but at the time of taking up the award must be regular full-time graduate students who have been admitted to and registered in advanced degree programmes (Master's or PhD, but not pre-Master's) in any field of study or Faculty of the University of Manitoba. Students beyond the second year in the Master's programme or beyond the fourth year in the PhD programme are not eligible to apply for or hold a University of Manitoba Graduate Fellowship. Students whose previous study at the Master's level has been part-time will be eligible for a University of Manitoba Graduate Fellowship for a period of one year from the date of registration as full-time students.
Level of Study: Doctorate, Postgraduate.
Purpose: To award academic excellence for graduate study.
Type: Fellowship.
No. of awards offered: 100-110.
Frequency: Annual.
Value: C$16,000 for PhD; C$10,000 for Master's.
Study Establishment: The University of Manitoba in either a Master's (not pre-Master's) or a PhD program.
Country of Study: Canada.

Application Procedure: Application forms may be requested from the department to which applicants are applying at the University of Manitoba and must be returned to that department. Forms are available from the beginning of December and can be requested either by phoning or writing or from the website at: http://www.umanitoba.ca/faculties/graduate_studies/forms.
Closing Date: February 15th, with earlier departmental deadline.

UNIVERSITY OF MELBOURNE

Parkville, VIC, 3052, Australia
Tel: (61) 3 344 8747
Fax: (61) 3 349 1760
Email: postgrad@scholarships.unimelb.edu.au
www: http://www.unimelb.edu.au
Contact: Ms Janet White, Melbourne Scholarships Office

The University of Melbourne has a long and distinguished tradition of excellence in teaching and research. It is the leading research institution in Australia and enjoys a reputation for the high quality of its research programs, consistently winning the largest share of national competitive research funding.

University of Melbourne Research Scholarships

Subjects: Any subject offered by the University.
Eligibility: Open to candidates from Australia and foreign countries.
Level of Study: Doctorate, Postgraduate.
Purpose: To enable graduates to undertake research.
Type: Scholarship.
No. of awards offered: 232 (of which up to 50 may be awarded to international students).
Frequency: Annual.
Value: A$15,600 per year, payable fortnightly.
Length of Study: Up to 2 years at the Master's level; up to 3 years at the PhD level, with the possibility of extension for an additional 6 months.
Study Establishment: The University of Melbourne.
Country of Study: Australia.
Application Procedure: Application form must be completed. Please contact the Melbourne Scholarships Office.
Closing Date: October 31st for Australian citizens and residents (main selection round); September 15th for international students (a small number of scholarships may be available throughout the year subject to availabilty).
Additional Information: Further information can be accessed through the internet site.

UNIVERSITY OF NEW ENGLAND

Research Services, Armidale, NSW, 2351, Australia
Tel: (61) 2 6773 3571
Fax: (61) 2 6773 3543
Email: aharris@metz.une.edu.au
www: http://research.une.edu.au/home/
Contact: Postgraduate Scholarships Officer

The University of New England is Australia's oldest regional university. UNE has a reputation for quality research with students undertaking research in the arts, education, environmental engineering, health studies, rural science, and science. The UNE PhD is over 40 years old and has 550 PhD students currently enrolled.

University of New England Research Scholarships

Subjects: Arts, education, economics, sciences, social science, resource sciences, archaeology, and environmental engineering.
Eligibility: Open to candidates of any nationality having at least a Bachelor's degree with first class honours or equivalent, and English test for candidates from non-English speaking countries.
Level of Study: Postgraduate.
Purpose: To provide assistance toward the completion of a research Master's degree, PhD, or EdD.
Type: Scholarship.
No. of awards offered: 20.
Frequency: Annual.
Value: Approximately A$16,000.
Length of Study: 2 years (Master's degree) or for an initial period of 3 years which may be renewed for 6 months (PhD).
Study Establishment: University of New England.
Country of Study: Australia.
Application Procedure: Application form with certified copies of academic transcripts and academic referees.
Closing Date: October 31st.
Additional Information: Candidates who are not permanent residents or citizens of Australia must provide evidence of additional financial support of at least A$10,000. The research proposal must be approved by the head of the relevant department. Initial enquiries from overseas students should be directed to the International Students Officer at the university.

UNIVERSITY OF NOTTINGHAM

Graduate School
University Park, Nottingham, NG7 2RD, England
Tel: (44) 115 951 4664
Fax: (44) 115 951 4668
Email: graduateschool@nottingham.ac.uk
www: http://www.nottingham.ac.uk
Contact: Dr Richard Masterman, Director of Research Policy
Administration

University of Nottingham Graduate Studentships

Subjects: Any subject from a prescribed list.
Level of Study: Postgraduate.
Purpose: To provide promising students with home and EU fees only studentships for one year full-time (or equivalent) taught Master's courses.
Type: Studentship.
No. of awards offered: Approx. 20.
Frequency: Annual.
Value: Home/EU fees only.
Length of Study: Usually 1 year full-time (or part-time equivalent).
Study Establishment: University of Nottingham.
Country of Study: United Kingdom.
Application Procedure: Applications must be submitted to the individual schools. Please contact schools offering studentships for details.
Closing Date: Applications are accepted at anytime.

University of Nottingham Postgraduate Scholarships

Subjects: Any subject offered by the University.
Eligibility: Open to graduates of all nationalities. The scholarships are allocated to schools/institutes, to whom students should apply for further information.
Level of Study: Postgraduate, Predoctorate.
Purpose: To promote research.
Type: Scholarship.
No. of awards offered: 75.
Frequency: Annual.
Value: £6,455 per year maintenance and payment of fees at home/EU rate.
Length of Study: 3 years leading to PhD submission given adequate academic progress.
Study Establishment: University of Nottingham.
Country of Study: United Kingdom.
Application Procedure: Please contact the individual schools for information.
Closing Date: Please contact the individual schools for information.
Additional Information: The scholarships are awarded internally to the schools and/or institutes that bid for them. It is then up to those schools receiving awards to advertise the scholarship and set an application deadline.

UNIVERSITY OF OXFORD

University Offices
Wellington Square, Oxford, OX1 2JD, England
Tel: (44) 1865 270 000
Fax: (44) 1865 270 708
www: http://www.oxford.ac.uk
Contact: Information Officer

Brasenose Hector Pilling Scholarship

Subjects: All subjects.
Eligibility: Open to graduates of any Commonwealth university; preference will be given to applicants who are serving or who have served in the Royal Air Force or the Air Force of a Commonwealth country or to the children or dependents of such persons, but this qualification is not essential.
Level of Study: Postgraduate.
Type: Scholarship.
No. of awards offered: 1.
Frequency: Varies.
Value: Fees plus maintenance equal to a state maintenance grant, plus college room for the first year.
Length of Study: 1 year plus 2 further years.
Study Establishment: Brasenose College.
Country of Study: United Kingdom.
Closing Date: Please write for details.
Additional Information: Not available very year, the next time it will be available will be October 2000.

For further information contact:

Brasenose College, Oxford, OX1 4AJ, England
Contact: Tutor for Graduates

Brasenose Senior Germaine Scholarship

Subjects: All subjects.
Eligibility: Candidates must have graduated from a university or institution of similar standing in the UK, or be expected to graduate by October 1st in the year in which they make their application; candidates should normally be below the age of 27 on October 1st of the year in which they apply.
Level of Study: Postgraduate.
Type: Scholarship.
No. of awards offered: 1.
Frequency: Annual.
Value: Fees plus maintenance equal to the state maintenance grant, plus college room for the first year of the course.
Length of Study: 1 year; being annually renewable for a maximum of 2 further years.
Study Establishment: Brasenose College.
Country of Study: United Kingdom.
Application Procedure: Please write for details.
Additional Information: Not available every year, the next year it is available is 2000; check availability with the Tutor for Graduates.

For further information contact:

Brasenose College, Oxford, OX1 4AJ, England
Contact: The Tutor for Graduates

Canon Collins Educational Trust/Chevening Scholarships

Subjects: Social anthropology, economics for development, educational research methodology, educational studies, comparitive and social research, sociology, environmental change and management, forestry and its relation to land use, applied statistics, computation, human biology, neurosciences.
Eligibility: Students from South Africa, Zimbabwe, Namibia, Lesotho and Botswana.
Level of Study: Postgraduate.
Purpose: To assist candidates studying for Masters degrees in certain subjects.
No. of awards offered: 5.
Value: University and College fees and maintenance costs.
Length of Study: 1 year.
Study Establishment: University of Oxford.
Country of Study: United Kingdom.
Application Procedure: Candidates must apply separately for admission to Oxford through the Graduate Admissions Office.
Closing Date: April 1st.

For further information contact:

International Office
University Offices
Wellington Square, Oxford, OX1 2JD, England

Chevening Oxford-Australia Scholarships

Subjects: All subjects.
Eligibility: Open to Australians.
Level of Study: Postgraduate.
Purpose: To assist Australians with overseas study.
Type: Travel Grant.
No. of awards offered: 2.
Value: £11,000.
Length of Study: 1 year.
Study Establishment: University of Oxford.
Country of Study: United Kingdom.
Application Procedure: Please write for details.
Additional Information: The alternative address can be contacted for details as can Oxford University International Office.

For further information contact:

Research school for Chemistry
Australian National University
GPO Box 414, Canberra, ACT, 2601, Australia
Tel: (61) 6 249 3637
Fax: (61) 6 249 4903

Christ Church Hugh Pilkinton Scholarship

Subjects: All subjects.
Eligibility: Open to graduate students from the European Union.
Level of Study: Postgraduate.
Type: Scholarship.
Value: £3,000 per annum.
Length of Study: 1 year.
Study Establishment: Christ Church.
Country of Study: United Kingdom.
Application Procedure: Please write to the Dean's secretary at Christ Church College for further information. Applications should be made when applying for admission.

For further information contact:

Christ Chutch College, Oxford, OX1 1DP, England
Contact: Dean's Secretary

Christ Church ODA Shared Scholarship

Subjects: All subjects.
Eligibility: Citizens of developing Commonwealth countries only.
Level of Study: Postgraduate.
Type: Scholarship.
No. of awards offered: 1.
Frequency: Annual.
Value: £7,000 per annum.
Length of Study: Up to 3 years.
Study Establishment: Christ Church.
Country of Study: England.
Application Procedure: Please write for details.

For further information contact:

University Offices
Wellington Square, Oxford, OX1 2JD, England
Contact: International Office

Christ Church Senior Scholarships

Subjects: All subjects.
Eligibility: Open to candidates who will have been reading for a higher degree in the University of Oxford for at least one year, but not more than two years, by October 1st of the year in which the award is sought.
Level of Study: Postgraduate.
Purpose: To enable graduate scholars to undertake some definite course of literary, educational, scientific or professional study or training.
Type: Scholarship.
No. of awards offered: 2.
Frequency: Annual.
Value: Rooms and maintenance at Research Council level.
Length of Study: 2 years; renewable for a further year.
Study Establishment: Christ Church, University of Oxford.
Country of Study: United Kingdom.
Application Procedure: Please write for details, Applications should be made in February.
Closing Date: The date is fixed each year, but usually during April.

Additional Information: Normally, the Scholarship is held in conjunction with an award from a government agency which pays the university fees.

For further information contact:

The Deanery
Christ Church, Oxford, OX1 1DP, England
Contact: The Dean's Secretary

Christ Church The American Friends Scholarship

Subjects: All subjects.
Eligibility: Open to graduate students from the USA only.
Level of Study: Postgraduate.
Type: Scholarship.
No. of awards offered: Varies.
Frequency: Annual.
Value: $7,000 per annum.
Length of Study: 1 year.
Study Establishment: Christ Church.
Country of Study: United Kingdom.
Closing Date: Please write for details.
Additional Information: Subject to deduction of grants from other sources.

For further information contact:

Christ Church, Oxford, OX1 1DP, England
Contact: The Senior Censor

Exeter College Usher-Cunningham Senior Studentship

Subjects: Alternately awarded for a graduate degree in medical science, or for any graduate from an Irish University studying for a graduate degree in medieval or modern history. Next available for modern history in 2000.
Eligibility: The Modern History Studentship is only open to graduates of Irish Universities. Enquiries should be addressed to the College Secretary.
Level of Study: Postgraduate.
Purpose: To support graduate study.
Type: Studentship.
No. of awards offered: 1.
Frequency: Every three years.
Value: Full fees plus maintenance up to the equivalent of a Research Council Studentship.
Length of Study: 1 year, renewable for up to 2 additional years.
Study Establishment: Exeter College.
Country of Study: United Kingdom.
Closing Date: Please write for details.

For further information contact:

Exeter College, Oxford, OX1 3DP, England
Tel: (44) 1865 279660
Fax: (44) 1865 279630
Contact: Tutor for Graduates

Felix Scholarships

Subjects: All subjects.
Eligibility: Indian nationals under 30 years of age and must have at least a first class Bachelor's degree from an Indian university or comparable institution. Those who already hold degrees from universities outside India are not eligible to apply.
Level of Study: Postgraduate.
Purpose: To enable Indian graduates accepted for entry to Oxford to read for taught graduate courses or for a Master's or DPhil degree by research, who would be unable, without financial assistance, to take up their place.
No. of awards offered: Up to 6.
Value: University and college fees and maintenance costs.
Length of Study: For 2 years in the first instance, with a possible extension for 3 years for those initially registered for a DPhil degree.
Study Establishment: University of Oxford.
Country of Study: United Kingdom.
Application Procedure: Candidates must apply separately for admission to Oxford through the Graduate Admissions Office. Please write for further details. Applicants for Felix Scholarships are expected to apply for an Overseas Research Students (ORS) award if the course they intend to take makes them eligible.
Closing Date: March 1st.

For further information contact:

International Office
University Offices
Wellington square, Oxford, OX1 2JD, England

Fulbright Oxford University Scholarships

Subjects: All subjects.
Level of Study: Postgraduate.
Value: Full funding (round trip travel, maintenance allowance and approved tuition fees). The value of bursaries will be determined according to individual need with a maximum of £3,245 (at 1999-2000 rates). A candidate gaining 3 awards (Fulbright, ORS and Oxford bursary) will have adequate funding for 2 years..
Length of Study: 2-3 years.
Study Establishment: University of Oxford.
Country of Study: United Kingdom.
Application Procedure: An application form must be completed.
Closing Date: October 23rd; those enrolled in US institutions must file applications with their Fulbright Programme Advisor by the deadline set by the campus advisor.
Additional Information: The course must lead to a higher degree and qualify for funding under the Overseas Research Students (ORS) award scheme. Candidates must apply for the ORS award.

For further information contact:

US Student Programs
Institute of International Education (IIE)
809 United Nations Plaza, New York, NY, 10017-3580, United States of America

Hertford College Senior Scholarships

Subjects: All subjects.
Eligibility: Restricted to students about to commence a new research degree course or those about to upgrade their current course.
Level of Study: Postgraduate.
Type: Scholarship.
Value: £500 per annum, plus priority for housing.
Length of Study: 2 years in the first instance renewable for a further year.
Study Establishment: Hertford College.
Country of Study: United Kingdom.
Application Procedure: Please write to the college for further details.

For further information contact:

Hertford College, Oxford, OX1 3BW, England
Contact: College Secretary

Hong Kong Oxford Scholarship Fund Bursaries

Subjects: All subjects.
Eligibility: National's of the People's Republic of China. It is a condition of the award that students should be planning to return to and to benefit their home country on completion of their studies.
Level of Study: Postgraduate.
Value: Up to £4,000.
Study Establishment: University of Oxford.
Country of Study: United Kingdom.
Application Procedure: Candidates must apply for admission to Oxford through the Graduate Admissions Office. Please write for further details.
Closing Date: July.

For further information contact:

International Office
University Offices
WellingtonSquare, Oxford, OX1 2JD, England

James Fairfax and Oxford-Australia Fund

Subjects: Oxford-Australia Fund scholarships are open to any discipline, James Fairfax Scholarships are intended for those wishing to study for a second undergraduate or a graduate degree in the arts or social sciences.
Level of Study: Postgraduate.
No. of awards offered: 2.
Value: University and college fees and living allowance of the order of A$11,000 per annum.
Length of Study: Oxford-Australia Fund scholarships- 2 years or in the case of MPhil, for 3 years; James Fairfax Scholarships will generally be 2 years duration.

Study Establishment: University of Oxford.
Country of Study: United Kingdom.
Application Procedure: Please write for details.
Closing Date: March 20th.
Additional Information: Candidates are also expected to apply for an Overseas Research Students (ORS) award if the course they intend to follow makes them eligible.

For further information contact:

International Office
University Offices
Wellington Square, Oxford, OX1 2JD, England

K C Wong Scholarships

Subjects: All subjects.
Eligibility: Residents of the People's Republic of China. (It should be noted that it is a requirement for the award of K C Wong Scholarships that candidates should currently be resident in the People's Republic of China).
Level of Study: Doctorate.
Purpose: To assist students studying at doctorate level.
No. of awards offered: 3.
Value: University and college fees and maintenance for a maximum of 3 years.
Study Establishment: University of Oxford.
Country of Study: United Kingdom.
Application Procedure: Please write for further details and an application form.
Closing Date: April 1st.
Additional Information: Applicants for the K C Wong scholarships are also expected to apply for an Overseas Research Students (ORS) award.

For further information contact:

International Office
University Offices
Wellington Square, Oxford, OX1 2JD, England

Karim Rida Said Foundation Scholarships

Subjects: All subjects.
Eligibility: Students from countries in the Arab League.
Level of Study: Postgraduate.
Purpose: To assist students from the Arab League with either a taught Master's degree, a Master's degree by research or for the DPhil degree.
No. of awards offered: Varies.
Value: University and college fees plus maintenance grant for the duration of the student's course.
Study Establishment: University of Oxford.
Country of Study: United Kingdom.
Application Procedure: Candidates must apply separately for admission to Oxford through the Graduate Admissions Office. Please write for further details.
Closing Date: July.

For further information contact:

International Office
University Offices
Wellington square, Oxford, OX1 2JD, England

Keble College Gwynne-Jones Scholarship

Subjects: All subjects.
Eligibility: Eligible to nationals of Sierra Leone, or among the Yoruba-speaking people of Nigeria.
Level of Study: Postgraduate.
Type: Scholarship.
No. of awards offered: Varies.
Frequency: Annual.
Value: Up to £4,000 per annum.
Length of Study: 2 years.
Study Establishment: Keble College.
Country of Study: United Kingdom.
Closing Date: Late May.

For further information contact:

Keble College, Oxford, OX1 3PG, England
Contact: Tutor for Graduates

Keble College Keble Association Graduate Scholarship

Subjects: All subjects.
Level of Study: Postgraduate.
Type: Scholarship.
No. of awards offered: At least 1.
Frequency: Annual.
Value: To the value of College fees.
Length of Study: Up to 2 years.
Study Establishment: Keble College.
Country of Study: United Kingdom.
Closing Date: Late February.

For further information contact:

Keble College, Oxford, OX1 3PG, England
Contact: Tutor for Graduates

Keble College Water Newton and Gosden Graduate Scholaraship

Subjects: All subjects.
Eligibility: Restricted to students admitted to study for a research degree in the University of Oxford and intending to seek ordination in a church or communion with the Church of England.
Level of Study: Postgraduate.
Type: Scholarship.
Value: Up to £5,000 per annum.
Length of Study: 2 years.
Study Establishment: Keble College.
Country of Study: United Kingdom.
Application Procedure: Contact the Tutor for Graduate, in the first instance at Keble College.
Closing Date: Late February.

For further information contact:

Keble College, Oxford, OX1 3PG, England
Contact: Tutor for Graduates

Kellogg College Kellogg Scholarships

Subjects: All subjects.
Eligibility: Restricted to those offered a place at Kellogg College, Oxford.
Level of Study: Postgraduate.
Type: Scholarship.
Value: Approximately £300 per annum.
Length of Study: 2 years or more.
Study Establishment: Keble College.
Country of Study: United Kingdom.
Application Procedure: Contact the Tutor for Admissions in the first instance at Kellog College.

For further information contact:

Kellogg College, Oxford, OX1 2JA, England
Contact: Tutor for Admissions

Lady Noon/Oxford University Press Scholarship

Subjects: All subjects.
Eligibility: Nationals of Pakistan.
Level of Study: Postgraduate.
No. of awards offered: 1 partial award.
Value: Approx £10,500.
Study Establishment: University of Oxford.
Country of Study: United Kingdom.
Application Procedure: Candidates must apply separately for admission to Oxford through the Graduate Admissions Office. Please write for further details.
Closing Date: April 1st.

For further information contact:

International Office
University Offices
Wellington Square, Oxford, OX1 2JD, England

Linacer College Lloyd African Scholarship DFID Scholarships

Subjects: A subject which will be beneficial in aiding the economic and/or social development of the student's country.
Eligibility: Open to qualified graduate students from African universities.
Level of Study: Postgraduate.
Purpose: To enable a qualified graduate student from an African university to pursue a one or two year taught Master's course.
Type: Scholarship.
No. of awards offered: 2.
Frequency: Annually or bi-annual.
Value: University and college fees; stipend; return air travel.
Length of Study: 1 or 2 years.
Study Establishment: Linacre College.

Country of Study: England.
Application Procedure: Please write for details.

For further information contact:

Linacre College, Oxford, OX1 3JA, England
Contact: The Tutor of Admissions

Linacre College Domus Studentships

Subjects: All subjects.
Eligibility: Open to students with a good first degree, who intend to begin reading for a higher degree, or to current members of Linacre College.
Level of Study: Postgraduate.
Purpose: To assist postgraduate study.
Type: Studentship.
No. of awards offered: Varies.
Frequency: Annual.
Value: £250 per year.
Length of Study: Up to 3 years.
Study Establishment: Linacre College.
Country of Study: United Kingdom.
Closing Date: Please write for details.

For further information contact:

Linacre College
St Cross Road, Oxford, OX1 3JA, England
Tel: (44) 1865 271657
Fax: (44) 1865 271668
Contact: The Tutor for Admissions

Linacre College European Blaschko Visiting Research Scholarship

Subjects: Pharmacology, neuropharmacology.
Eligibility: Open to students with a doctorate or equivalent degree.
Level of Study: Postgraduate.
Purpose: To enable European students to carry out research for one year in the department of Pharmacology or the MRC Anatomical Neuropharmacology Unit.
Type: Scholarship.
Frequency: Annual.
Value: College and university fees for visiting student status, stipend and the cost of return travel from the scholars home country.
Length of Study: 1 year.
Study Establishment: Linacre College.
Country of Study: United Kingdom.
Closing Date: Please write for details.

For further information contact:

Department of Pharmacology
Mansfield Road, Oxford, OX1 3QT, England
Contact: Professor A D Smith

Lincoln College Berrow Scholarship

Subjects: All subjects.
Eligibility: Open to graduates of the following Swiss universities: Berne, Geneva, Lausanne, Fribourg, Neuchâtel, or the Ecole Polytechnique Fédérale de Lausanne.
Level of Study: Doctorate, Postgraduate.
Purpose: To permit graduates of Swiss universities to undertake postgraduate study at Oxford.
Type: Scholarship.
No. of awards offered: 3.
Frequency: Annual.
Value: All university and college fees are covered, plus a generous maintenance allowance.
Length of Study: 2 years, with possible renewal for 1 year.
Study Establishment: Lincoln College, Oxford.
Country of Study: United Kingdom.
Application Procedure: Please write for details.
Closing Date: Please write for details.

For further information contact:

Lincoln College, Oxford, OX1 3DR, England
Tel: (44) 1865 279836
Fax: (44) 1865 279802
Contact: Tutor for Graduates

Lincoln College Dresdner Kleinwort Benson Senior Scholarships

Subjects: Any area of study.
Eligibility: Restricted to students from Studienstiftung des deutschen Volkes wishing to study at Lincoln. Such students come to Oxford as Visiting Graduate Students.
Level of Study: Postgraduate.
Type: Scholarship.
No. of awards offered: 2.
Frequency: Annual.
Value: Sufficient to cover College fees and proven academic supervision at a high level.
Length of Study: 1 year only.
Study Establishment: Lincoln College.
Country of Study: United Kingdom.
Application Procedure: Students form the Studienstiftong who place Lincoln College as first choice are eligible; no separate application is necessary.
Closing Date: Please write for details.

For further information contact:

Lincoln College, Oxford, OX1 3DR, England
Contact: Tutor for Graduates

Lincoln College Keith Murray Senior Scholarship

Subjects: Varies from year to year.
Eligibility: Open to holders of a very good first degree, who are citizens of any country outside the EC.
Level of Study: Doctorate, Postgraduate.
Purpose: To permit students from outside the EU to undertake postgraduate study at Oxford University.
Type: Scholarship.

No. of awards offered: 1+, depending on funds available.
Frequency: Dependent on funds available.
Value: All university and college fees are covered, plus a generous maintenance allowance.
Length of Study: 2 years with the possibility of a 3rd year.
Study Establishment: Lincoln College, Oxford.
Country of Study: United Kingdom.
Application Procedure: Please write for details.
Closing Date: December of the year preceding commencement of study.

For further information contact:

Lincoln College, Oxford, OX1 3DR, England
Tel: (44) 1865 279836
Fax: (44) 1865 279802
Contact: Tutor for Graduates

Lincoln College Overseas Graduate Entrance Scholarships

Subjects: Crewe Scholarship may be held in any area of study, Paul Shuffrey Scholarship in history of art and related subjects, two EPA fund-supported scholarships are for medicine and the medical sciences.
Eligibility: Restricted to those offered a place at Lincoln College.
Level of Study: Postgraduate.
Type: Scholarship.
No. of awards offered: 4.
Value: £1,500.
Length of Study: 1 year.
Study Establishment: Lincoln College.
Country of Study: United Kingdom.
Application Procedure: For further information contact the Tutor for Graduates, Lincoln College.

For further information contact:

Lincoln College, Oxford, OX1 3DR, England
Contact: Tutor for Graduates

Magdalen College Hichens Scholarship

Subjects: All subjects.
Level of Study: Postgraduate.
Value: Cost of college accomodation.
Length of Study: 1 year.
Study Establishment: Mansfield college.
Country of Study: United Kingdom.
Application Procedure: For further information contact the Tutor for Graduates in the first instance at Magdalen College.

For further information contact:

Magdalen College, Oxford, OX1 4UA, England
Contact: Tutor for Graduates

Merton College Graduate Entrance Scholarships

Subjects: Any subject accepted by the college.
Eligibility: Open to non-UK citizens.
Level of Study: Postgraduate.

Type: Scholarship.
No. of awards offered: 2.
Frequency: Annual.
Value: Fees; housing and maintenance.
Length of Study: 3.
Study Establishment: Merton College.
Country of Study: United Kingdom.
Closing Date: Late January.

For further information contact:

Merton College, Oxford, OX1 4JD, England
Contact: Assistant Tutorial Secretary

Merton College Greendale Senior Scholarships

Subjects: All subjects.
Eligibility: Open to nationals and permanent residents of Switzerland who have a degree from a Swiss university.
Level of Study: Postgraduate.
Type: Scholarship.
No. of awards offered: 1.
Frequency: Annual.
Value: Fees, housing and maintenance.
Length of Study: For length of course up to 3 years.
Study Establishment: Merton College.
Country of Study: United Kingdom.
Closing Date: Early December- please check with the college.

For further information contact:

Merton College, Oxford, OX1 4JD, England
Contact: Assistant Tutorial Secretary

Merton College Senior Scholarships

Subjects: All subjects.
Eligibility: Candidates from any country may apply.
Level of Study: Postgraduate.
Type: Scholarship.
Frequency: Annual.
Value: Fees, housing and maintenance.
Length of Study: 2 years.
Study Establishment: Merton College.
Country of Study: United Kingdom.
Application Procedure: For further datils contact the Assistant Tutorial Secretary in the first instance at Merton College.
Closing Date: Beginning of April.

For further information contact:

Merton College, Oxford, OX1 4JD, England
Contact: Assistant Tutorial Secretary

New Century Scholarships

Subjects: All subects.
Eligibility: Nationals of Japan. Candidates should be completing or have completed a first degree course and should be between the ages of 21 and 30.
Level of Study: Postgraduate.

Purpose: To assist postgraduate study leading to a degree or for a one year period of study as a visiting student.
No. of awards offered: Varies.
Study Establishment: University of Oxford.
Country of Study: United Kingdom.
Application Procedure: Please write for further details.

For further information contact:

International Office
University Offices
Wellington Square, Oxford, OX1 2JD, England

Oriel College Graduate Scholarships

Subjects: Arts or sciences.
Eligibility: Open to all graduates in residence in the College reading for a higher degree.
Level of Study: Postgraduate.
Type: Scholarship.
Value: £1,250.
Length of Study: 2 years.
Study Establishment: Oriel College.
Country of Study: United Kingdom.
Application Procedure: For further information contact the Tutor for Graduates in the first instance at Oriel College.

For further information contact:

Oriel College, Oxford, OX1 4EW, England
Contact: Tutor for Graduates

Overseas Research Student (ORS) Awards Scheme

Subjects: All subjects.
Level of Study: Postgraduate.
No. of awards offered: Varies.
Value: Equivalent to the difference between home and overseas fees.
Length of Study: Renewable for as long as a student is liable for University fees.
Study Establishment: University of Oxford.
Country of Study: United Kingdom.
Application Procedure: Please write for further details.
Additional Information: ORS awards can be held in conjunction with many other scholarships, and can be seen as an element of a package of financial support assembled by a prospective student. The degrees at Oxford which qualify as research courses for ORS support are: DPhil, MLitt, MSc by research, BPhil, MPhil (where an applicant intends to submit a dissertation), and those MSt's in Research or Research Methods which are an integral part of a research programme in a particular subject. Therefore, students who are applying for admission as a Probationer Research Student (leading to a degree of DPhil, MLitt or MSc by research) or as a BPhil or MPhil are eligible to apply. Students applying for an MSt (other than the research MSt's defined above), MBA, MSc by coursework, MJur, BCL, Diploma or Certificate, or who will not submit a dissertation as part of an MPhil, are not eligible for an ORS award. Competition for ORS awards is severe, and candidates should be aware that

acceptance for study at Oxford does not necessarily mean the University will nominate them for an ORS award, and that nomination by the University does not guarantee success in the national ORS competition. Candidates who gain an ORS award may take it up at any time in the academic year for which it is initially awarded, but cannot defer the award for a full academic year.

For further information contact:

International Office
University Offices
Wellington Square, Oxford, OX1 2JD, England

Pembroke College Australian Graduate Scholarship

Subjects: Classics, law, medicine, philosophy, theology.
Eligibility: Open to male graduates of Melbourne University.
Level of Study: Postgraduate.
Type: Scholarship.
No. of awards offered: Varies.
Frequency: Annual.
Value: £4,000 per annum.
Length of Study: 2 years.
Study Establishment: Pembroke College.
Country of Study: United Kingdom.
Application Procedure: Please write for details.

For further information contact:

Pembroke College, Oxford, OX1 1DW, England
Contact: Dean of Graduate Students

Pembroke College Jose Gregorio Hernandez Award of the Venezuelan National Academy of Medicine

Subjects: Medicine or the biological sciences.
Eligibility: Open to nationals of Venezuela.
Level of Study: Postgraduate.
Type: Scholarship.
No. of awards offered: Varies.
Frequency: Annual.
Value: Full fees and maintenance.
Length of Study: 1 year; renewable.
Study Establishment: Pembroke College.
Country of Study: United Kingdom.
Application Procedure: Please write for details.

For further information contact:

Pembroke College, Oxford, OX1 1DW, England
Contact: The Dean of Graduate Students

Peter Jenks Vietnam Scholarship

Subjects: All subjects.
Eligibility: Nationals of Vietnam.
Level of Study: Postgraduate.
Purpose: To assist students studying for a taught Master's degree, a Master's degree by research, or the DPhil degree.
No. of awards offered: 1.

Value: University and college fees and maintenance costs for the duration of the student's course.
Study Establishment: University of Oxford.
Country of Study: United Kingdom.
Application Procedure: Candidates must apply separately for admission to Oxford through the Graduate Admissions Office. Please write for further particulars and an application form.
Closing Date: April 1st.
Additional Information: For further details please contact the International Office.

Pirie-Reid Scholarships

Subjects: All subjects.
Level of Study: Postgraduate, Undergraduate.
Purpose: To enable persons, who would otherwise be prevented by lack of funds, to begin a course of study at Oxford.
Type: Scholarship.
No. of awards offered: Up to 2.
Frequency: Annual.
Value: University and College fees plus maintenance grant; subject to assessment of income from other sources.
Length of Study: Renewable from year to year, subject to satisfactory progress and continuance of approved full-time study.
Study Establishment: University of Oxford.
Country of Study: United Kingdom.
Application Procedure: Please write for application forms.
Closing Date: May 1st.
Additional Information: Preference will be given to candidates applying from other universities i.e. not matriculated at Oxford, and to those domiciled or educated in Scotland. Candidates not fulfilling these criteria are unlikely to be successful. For further information please contact Mrs J M Brown, at the University Offices.

Prendergast Bequest

Subjects: All subjects.
Eligibility: Candidates must be men or women born in the Republic of Ireland whose parents are citizens of the Republic of Ireland.
Level of Study: Postgraduate, Undergraduate.
No. of awards offered: 1.
Frequency: Annual.
Value: Varies; in the region of £500 - £2,000 (means tested).
Length of Study: 1 year.
Study Establishment: University of Oxford.
Country of Study: United Kingdom.
Application Procedure: Applicants who intend to follow a postgraduate course must have been accepted by both a college and the faculty board concerned before a grant can be awarded. Please write for further information and application forms.
Closing Date: July.

For further information contact:

Prendegast Bequest
University Offices
Wellington Square, Oxford, OX1 2JD, England
Contact: The Secretary to the Board of Management

Queen's College Florey EPA Scholarship

Subjects: Medical, biological or chemical sciences.
Eligibility: EU countries (excluding UK and Ireland); Finland, Norway, or Sweden.
Level of Study: Postgraduate.
Type: Scholarship.
No. of awards offered: Varies.
Frequency: Annual.
Value: £1,436 per annum (under review); assistance may also be given with fees (maximum of half cost).
Length of Study: 1 year; renewable for second and third years.
Study Establishment: The Queen's College.
Country of Study: United Kingdom.
Closing Date: Please write for details.

For further information contact:

The Queen's College, Oxford, OX1 4AW, England
Contact: The Tutor for Admissions

The Queen's College Hastings Senior Studentship

Subjects: All subjects.
Eligibility: For graduates (with first class Honours) of the Universities of Bradford, Hull, Leeds, Sheffield and York.
Level of Study: Postgraduate.
Type: Scholarship.
Value: £1,436 per annum (under review); assistance may be given with fees if holder not eligible for Research Council or British Academy Studentships.
Length of Study: 1 year, renewable for 2nd and 3rd years.
Study Establishment: The Queen's College.
Country of Study: United Kingdom.
Application Procedure: For further details contact the Tutor for Admissions, in the first instance, at Queen's College.

For further information contact:

Queen's College, Oxford, OX1 4AW, England
Contact: Tutor for Admissions

Queen's College Wendell Herbruck Studentship

Subjects: All subjects.
Eligibility: Preference given to residents of Ohio, although open to other US residents; no older than 26 when appointed.
Level of Study: Postgraduate.
Type: Studentship.
No. of awards offered: Varies.
Frequency: Annual.
Value: £1,425 per annum (under review).

Length of Study: 1 year; renewable for 2nd or 3rd year.
Study Establishment: The Queen's College.
Country of Study: United Kingdom.
Application Procedure: Please write for details.

For further information contact:

The Queen's College, Oxford, OX1 4AW, England
Contact: The Tutor for Admissions

Radhakrishnan/British Chevening Scholarships

Subjects: All subjects.
Eligibility: Nationals of India.
Level of Study: Postgraduate.
No. of awards offered: Varies.
Value: University and colleges fees and maintenance for the duration of the student's course.
Study Establishment: University of Oxford.
Country of Study: United Kingdom.
Application Procedure: Please write for further information and an application form.
Closing Date: April 1st.
Additional Information: For further details please contact the International Office.

Regent's Park College (Permanent Private Hall) J W Lord Scholarship

Subjects: Medicine or theology.
Eligibility: Open to men and women preparing to serve Christian churches in India, Hong Kong and China, or otherwise in Asia, Africa, Central and South America and the Carribean; also available for in-service training or sabbatical study for similar candidates.
Level of Study: Postgraduate.
Type: Scholarship.
No. of awards offered: Varies.
Frequency: Annual.
Value: Up to £1,500 per annum.
Length of Study: Up to 3 years.
Study Establishment: Regent's Park College (Permanent Private Hall).
Country of Study: United Kingdom.
Application Procedure: Please contact the college for further information.

Regent's Park College (Permanent Private Hall) Organ Scholarship

Subjects: All subjects.
Eligibility: Open to suitably qualified candidates in any subject, but with preference to a graduate student in music.
Level of Study: Postgraduate.
Type: Scholarship.
No. of awards offered: Varies.
Frequency: Annual.
Value: £2,000 per annum.
Length of Study: Up to 3 years; renewable annually.
Study Establishment: Regent's Park College (Permanent Private Hall).

Country of Study: United Kingdom.
Application Procedure: Please contact the college for further information.
Additional Information: Includes duties as musical director at New Road Baptist Church.

Rhodes Scholarships

Subjects: All subjects.
Eligibility: Candidates must be between the ages of 19 and 25 (in Kenya the upper age limit is 27). Rhodes scholars must have graduated from a university and have resided for a number of years in their country of origin. Annual distribution of awards - Australia 9, Bermuda 1, Commonwealth Caribbean 2, Canada 11, Germany 4, Hong Kong 1, India 6, Jamaica 1, Kenya 2, Malaysia 1, New Zealand 3, Pakistan 2, Singapore 1, South Africa 9, USA 32, Zambia 1, Zimbabwe 2.
Level of Study: Postgraduate.
No. of awards offered: 88.
Value: University and college fees and maintenance stipend.
Length of Study: 2-3 years.
Study Establishment: University of Oxford.
Country of Study: United Kingdom.
Application Procedure: Rhodes scholars are chosen by local Selection Committees in each constituency. There is no formal written examination; scholars are chosen for their academic all-round qualities on the evidence of testimonials from responsible persons, and after personal interview (which is dispensible) by the Selection Committee concerned. Elections usually take place in November and December, and the Scholars come into residence the following October. After election, application is made on behalf of Scholars for admission to individual colleges and faculties in Oxford, and the election is not confirmed by the Rhodes Trustees until the Scholar-elect has been accepted for admission by the college.
Additional Information: All applications should be made to the Secretary of the local Selection Committee. A separate memorandum explaining the regulations in detail is published for each country and may be obtained from the local secretaries whose names and addresses are below: Australia: Professor G L Hutchinson, Civil and Environmental Engineering Department, University of Melbourne, Parkville, Victoria 3052. Bermuda: J C Collins Esq, c/o Conyers, Dill & Pearmen, Clarendon House, Church Street, Hamilton HM 11. Canada: A R A Scace Esq, QC, General Secretary Rhodes Scholarship Trust, PO Box 48, Toronto, Ontario, M5K 1E6. Commonwelath Caribbean & Jamaica: Mr Peter S Goldson, Secretary, Rhodes Scholarship Selection Committee, PO Box 417, Kingston 6. Germany: Herr T F M Böcking, Scherneck, Alteschlossstrasse 9, 8621 Untersiemau. Hong Kong: Mrs C Lee, Rhodes Scholarship Selection Committee, Office of Student Affairs, The Chinese University of Hong Kong, Shatin, NT, Hong Kong. India: Professor V S Chauhan, International Centre for Genetice Engineering and Biotechnology, Aruna Asaf Ali Marg, New Delhi 110067 Kenya: J D M Silvester Esq, PO Box 30333, Nairobi. Malaysia: Mr P Slinn, Scholarships and Training Officer, The British Council, Jalan Bukit Aman, PO Box 10539, 50916 Kuala Lumpur. New Zealand: The Scholarships Officer, The New Zealand Vice Chancellors' Committee, PO Box 11-915, Manners Street, Wellington.

Pakistan: Rhodes Scholarship Selection Committee, PO Box 2939, Islamabad. Singapore: Dr Ong Teck Chin, c/o Department of Physiology, National University of Singapore, Lower Kent Ridge Road, Singapore 0511. South Africa: The General Secretary, Rhodes Scholarships in South Africa, PO Box 41468, Craighall, Tranvaal 2024. USA: Mr E F Gerson, The Rhodes Scholarship Trust, 700 14th St NW, Suite 500, Washington DC 20005-2010. Zambia: Professor A S Saasa, Director, Institute for African Studies, University of Zambia, PO Box 30900, Lusaka. Zimbabwe: Mr D L L Morgan, The Secretary of the Selection Committee, Rhodes Scholarships, PO Box 53, Harare.

Somerville College Graduate Scholarships

Subjects: Any subject offered at the College.
Eligibility: Open to students of any nationality who are reading for a higher degree.
Level of Study: Postgraduate.
Type: Scholarship.
No. of awards offered: 2.
Value: £1,500 per annum.
Length of Study: 2 years; with the possibility of renewal for a third year.
Study Establishment: Somerville College.
Country of Study: United Kingdom.
Application Procedure: Please contact the college Secretary in the first instance.

For further information contact:

Somerville College, Oxford, OX2 6HD, England
Contact: The College Secretary

Somerville College Oxford Bursary for American Graduates (Janet Watson Bursary)

Subjects: All subjects.
Eligibility: For those reading for a higher degree or diploma.
Level of Study: Postgraduate.
Type: Bursary.
Value: Approximately one quarter of total fees to a maximum of £3,500 per annum.
Length of Study: 2 years.
Study Establishment: Somerville College.
Country of Study: United Kingdom.
Application Procedure: Please contact the college Secretary.

For further information contact:

Somerville College, Oxford, OX2 6HD, England
Contact: College Secretary

St Anne's College Overseas Scholarship

Subjects: Any subject offered by the University.
Eligibility: Open to graduates of any university who are not UK or EC citizens. All candidates must be accepted by the University of Oxford to read for a higher degree of at least two years' duration, and by the college, by June 1st.
Level of Study: Postgraduate.

Purpose: To fund graduate research.
Type: Scholarship.
No. of awards offered: 3.
Frequency: Annual.
Value: Equal to the College fee.
Length of Study: 1 year; renewable for a further year.
Study Establishment: St Anne's College.
Country of Study: United Kingdom.
Closing Date: June 20th.

For further information contact:

St Anne's College, Oxford, OX2 6HS, England
Tel: (44) 1865 274825
Fax: (44) 1865 274899
Contact: Registrar

St Catherine's College Overseas Graduate Scholarship

Subjects: All subjects (see the University Graduate Studies Prospectus).
Eligibility: Open to qualified individuals who are citizens of non EC countries.
Level of Study: Postgraduate.
Purpose: To assist graduates studying for a research degree, usually in their first year at the University of Oxford.
Type: Scholarship.
No. of awards offered: 1.
Frequency: Annual.
Value: £1,500.
Length of Study: 2 years in the first instance; current holders may reapply for a 3rd year.
Study Establishment: St Catherine's College, University of Oxford.
Country of Study: United Kingdom.
Application Procedure: Please write for details.
Closing Date: July 1st.

For further information contact:

St Catherine's College, Oxford, OX1 3UJ, England
Tel: (44) 1865 271732
Fax: (44) 1865 271768
Contact: Tutor for Graduates

St Cross College Major College Scholarships

Subjects: All subjects.
Eligibility: Open to students from Oxford or from other institutions of higher education who intend to study or are studying for a postgraduate degree.
Level of Study: Postgraduate.
Purpose: To support postgraduate study.
Type: Scholarship.
No. of awards offered: Up to 2.
Frequency: Annual.
Value: £1,675 per annum.
Length of Study: 1 to 3 year.
Study Establishment: St Cross College.
Country of Study: United Kingdom.
Closing Date: March.

For further information contact:

St Cross College, Oxford, OX1 3LZ, England
Tel: (44) 1865 278490
Contact: Tutor for Admissions

St Cross College Paula Soans O'Brian Scholarships

Subjects: All subjects.
Eligibility: Open to students from Oxford or from other institutions of higher education who intend to study or are studying for a postgraduate degree.
Level of Study: Postgraduate.
Purpose: To support postgraduate study.
Type: Scholarship.
Frequency: Varies.
Value: £1,675 per year.
Length of Study: 1-3 years.
Study Establishment: St Cross College.
Country of Study: United Kingdom.
Application Procedure: Forms are available from the Tutor for Admissions in January and February.
Closing Date: Please write for details.

For further information contact:

St Cross College, Oxford, OX1 3LZ, England
Tel: (44) 1865 278490
Contact: Tutor for Admissions

St Edmund Hall William R Miller Graduate Awards

Subjects: All subjects.
Level of Study: Postgraduate.
No. of awards offered: 3.
Frequency: Annual.
Value: Free accomodation.
Length of Study: 2 years.
Study Establishment: St Edmund Hall.
Country of Study: United Kingdom.
Application Procedure: Please contact the Tutor for Graduates, St Edmund Hall for further information.
Closing Date: May 1st.

For further information contact:

St Edmund Hall, Oxford, OX1 4AR, England
Contact: Tutor for Graduates

St Hilda's College Graduate Scholarships

Subjects: Any subject offered by the University.
Eligibility: Open to women graduates from any country working for a higher research degree.
Level of Study: Postgraduate.
Type: Scholarship.
No. of awards offered: Normally 4.
Frequency: Annual.
Value: Up to £1,000 per year.
Length of Study: 1 year; renewable.

Study Establishment: St Hilda's College.
Country of Study: United Kingdom.
Application Procedure: Applicants must have been accepted by the relevant university faculty before applying for a scholarship.
Closing Date: August 1st.
Additional Information: The award amalgamates the previous Graduate Studentships and Overseas Bursaries.

For further information contact:

St Hilda's College, Oxford, OX4 1DY, England
Tel: (44) 1865 276815
Fax: (44) 1865 276816
Contact: Academic Office

St Hilda's College New Zealand Bursaries

Subjects: Any subject offered by the University.
Eligibility: Open to women students who are New Zealand citizens, who have been accepted for a graduate research degree.
Level of Study: Postgraduate.
Purpose: To enable women educated and resident in New Zealand to study at Oxford.
Type: Bursary.
No. of awards offered: Varies.
Frequency: Annual.
Value: Up to £1,700 per annum.
Length of Study: 1-3 years.
Study Establishment: St Hilda's College.
Country of Study: United Kingdom.
Application Procedure: Application forms will be sent after the candidates have been accepted by Oxford University.
Closing Date: August 1st.
Additional Information: Available for undergraduate or postgraduate degrees. The main criteria for the award is academic merit; financial circumstances are also considered. Applicants must show evidence of sufficient funding to complete their course.

For further information contact:

St Hilda's College, Oxford, OX4 1DY, England
Tel: (44) 1865 276815
Fax: (44) 1865 276816
Contact: Academic Office

St Hugh's College Bursaries for Students from PRC

Subjects: Any subject offered at the College.
Eligibility: Open to nationals of the People's Republic of China.
Level of Study: Postgraduate.
Type: Scholarship.
Value: £2,000 per annum.
Length of Study: 2 years, with the possibility of renewal for the fee-paying duration of the course.
Study Establishment: St Hugh's College.
Country of Study: United Kingdom.

Application Procedure: Please contact the College Secretary in the first instance.

For further information contact:

St Hugh's College, Oxford, OX2 6LE, England
Contact: The College Secretary

St Hugh's College Graduate Scholarships

Subjects: All subjects.
Eligibility: Open to British nationals and candidates from overseas.
Level of Study: Postgraduate.
Purpose: To provide financial support to graduates reading for a degree by research.
Type: Scholarship.
No. of awards offered: Up to 12.
Frequency: Annual.
Value: £2,000 per annum, plus accommodation and some dining rights.
Length of Study: For the fee-paying duration of the course.
Study Establishment: St Hugh's College.
Country of Study: United Kingdom.
Application Procedure: Please contact the College Secretary in the first instance.
Closing Date: March 1st.

For further information contact:

St Hugh's College, Oxford, OX2 6LE, England
Tel: (44) 1865 274918
Fax: (44) 1865 274912
Contact: The College Secretary

St John's College I Beeston Scholarships

Subjects: All subjects, but particularly Middle Eastern Studies.
Eligibility: Normally restricted to graduates with UK degrees, who have already begun research; advertised in November/December and tenable from following October; no deferment of commencement of scholarships is permitted.
Level of Study: Postgraduate.
Type: Scholarship.
Value: Fees and accomodation and equivalent of a Research Council grant when the candidate's grant expires.
Length of Study: Normally 2 years.
Study Establishment: St John's College.
Country of Study: United Kingdom.
Application Procedure: Please contact the Senior Tutor, St John's College in the first instance.

For further information contact:

St John's College, Oxford, OX1 3JP, England
Contact: Senior Tutor

St Peter's College Leonard J Theberge Memorial Scholarship

Subjects: Any subject offered at the College.
Eligibility: Open to US citizens; preference is to mature students over 30, or those who have been employed for five years.
Level of Study: Postgraduate.
Type: Scholarship.
Value: A substantial contribution to maintenance and personal expenses.
Length of Study: 1-2 years.
Study Establishment: St Peter's College.
Country of Study: United Kingdom.
Application Procedure: Please contact the Tutor for Graduates in the first instance.

For further information contact:

St Peter's College, Oxford, OX1 2DL, England
Contact: Tutor for Graduates

Wadham College Norwegian Scholarship

Subjects: All subjects.
Eligibility: Open to registered students or graduates of Oslo University who are Norwegian citizens.
Level of Study: Postgraduate, Undergraduate.
Type: Scholarship.
Frequency: Annual.
Value: Fees and maintenance.
Length of Study: 1 year.
Study Establishment: Wadham College, Oxford.
Country of Study: United Kingdom.
Application Procedure: Applications in August of each year to the committee for the Norsk Oxford-Stipendium ved Wadham College at the University of Oslo.
Closing Date: August.

Wolfson College Department for International Development Shared Scholarship Scheme (formerly ODASSS)

Subjects: All subjects.
Eligibility: Developing Commonwealth countries only.
Type: Scholarship.
Value: Full fees and maintenance.
Length of Study: Normally 1 year.
Study Establishment: Wolfson College.
Country of Study: United Kingdom.
Application Procedure: Please write for details.

For further information contact:

International Office
University Offices
Wellington Square, Oxford, OX1 2JD, England

THE UNIVERSITY OF QUEENSLAND

Office of Research and Postgraduate Studies, QLD, 4072, Australia
Tel: (61) 7 3365 2033
Fax: (61) 7 3365 4455
www: http://www.uq.edu.au
Contact: Ms Jan Massey, The Scholarships Officer

University of Queensland Postdoctoral Research Fellowship

Subjects: Any subject offered by the University.
Eligibility: Open to candidates of any nationality. An applicant must not have had more than five years' full-time professional experience since the award of a Doctoral degree as at June 30th of the year before the fellowship commences. Fellowships may be offered to applicants who do not hold a doctoral degree provided that evidence is given that a doctoral thesis has been submitted by June 30th (for candidates from Australia, New Zealand or Papua New Guinea) or September 1st (for all other candidates), and that the selection committee is satisfied that the degree will be awarded by June 30th of the fellowship year.
Level of Study: Postdoctorate, Professional development.
Type: Fellowship.
No. of awards offered: Approx. 9.
Frequency: Annual.
Value: A$41,199-A$45,910 per year, plus excursion return air fare for the recipient only.
Length of Study: 2 years; sometimes extendable by 1 year.
Study Establishment: The University.
Country of Study: Australia.
Application Procedure: Application forms are available from the heads of the relevant departments or from the Director, Research Services. They can also be downloaded from the university website.
Closing Date: May 17th of the year preceding the award.

University of Queensland Postgraduate Research Scholarships

Subjects: All subjects.
Eligibility: Open to candidates of any nationality who are acceptable as full-time internal students for a postgraduate research degree at the University. Applicants should hold an Australian first class honours or Master's degree, or the equivalent. Candidates must have a sound knowledge of both written and spoken English.
Level of Study: Doctorate, Postgraduate.
Type: Scholarship.
No. of awards offered: Approx. 75.
Frequency: Annual.
Value: A$15,000.
Length of Study: 2 years for the Master's degree, and for up to 3 years for the PhD degree.
Study Establishment: The University.
Country of Study: Australia.

Application Procedure: International students must apply through the university's International Education Office, email ieoenquiries@mailbox.uq.edu.au; Australian students must apply through The Scholarships Officer, email m.schmidt@research.uq.edu.au.
Closing Date: September 30th.
Additional Information: To assist with tuition fee expenses international students may apply for the Overseas Postgraduate Research Scholarships (OPRS) which are administered through the International Education Office.

University of Queensland Travel Scheme for International Collaborative Research

Subjects: Any subject offered by the University.
Eligibility: Open to any suitably qualified scholar actively engaged in academic work at a university or internationally recognised research institution, who will be able to contribute substantially to research activity in the department to which he or she is attached at the University of Queensland.
Level of Study: Postdoctorate.
Purpose: To facilitate visits by scholars from institutions in other countries.
Type: Grant.
No. of awards offered: Approx. 15.
Frequency: Annual.
Value: Return economy air fare.
Length of Study: 8 weeks or longer during semester periods in the year of the award.
Study Establishment: The University.
Country of Study: Australia.
Application Procedure: Application forms are available from the head of the relevant department or from the Director, Research Services, at the University of Queensland. Details and application forms may also be downloaded from the university website.
Closing Date: August 1st of the year preceding the award year.

THE UNIVERSITY OF READING

Whiteknights
PO Box 217, Reading, Berkshire, RG6 6AU, England
Tel: (44) 118 931 8373
Fax: (44) 118 935 2063
Email: d.a.stannard@reading.ac.uk
www: http://www.rdg.ac.uk/
Contact: Mr D A Stannard, Senior Administrative Assistant

The University of Reading is one of the UK's foremost institutions of higher education. It offers undergraduate and postgraduate taught and research degree courses in all the traditional subject areas, except medical sciences. Many other, more vocational courses are also offered. Research work in many areas is of international renown.

The University of Reading Postgraduate Studentship

Subjects: There are no restrictions on subject area, subject to availability of appropriate supervision at the University.
Eligibility: Candidates must hold a first degree qualification.
Level of Study: Doctorate, Postgraduate.
Purpose: To enable students to obtain a doctoral degree.
Type: Studentship.
No. of awards offered: 4.
Frequency: Annual.
Value: Composition fee (at home standard rate), plus maintenance award as for Research Council Postgraduate Studentships, plus £1,000.
Length of Study: Up to 3 years.
Study Establishment: University of Reading.
Country of Study: United Kingdom.
Application Procedure: An application form (available from Mr D A Stannard) should be completed, and a confidential academic reference should also be submitted.
Closing Date: A date to be arranged in March of the year of entry.
Additional Information: At present the Studentships are awarded on the nomination of the Head of Department.

UNIVERSITY OF REGINA

Faculty of Graduate Studies & Research, Regina, SK, S4S OA2, Canada
Tel: (1) 306 585 4161
Fax: (1) 306 585 4893
Email: grad.studies@leroy.cc.uregina.ca
www: http://www.uregina.ca/gradstudies/
Contact: Ms Chris Blair

Founded as Regina College and granted a provincial charter in 1911, the University of Regina became an affiliated junior college of the University of Saskatchewan in 1925, and acquired degree-granting status in 1959. The University achieved academic autonomy in 1974.

Regina Graduate Scholarships

Subjects: Any graduate programme offered at the University of Regina.
Eligibility: Applicants must be accepted by the Graduate Faculty as fully-qualified for admission to Master's or PhD degree programme at the University of Regina. Must be registered as full-time student and must not receive any other scholarship(s).
Level of Study: Doctorate, Postgraduate.
Purpose: These scholarships are awarded to students of high academic standing who wish to work full-time on programme requirements.
Type: Scholarship.
No. of awards offered: Approx. 120.
Frequency: Three times each year.
Value: Master's level: C$3,800 per semester; Doctoral level: C$4,000 per semester.

Length of Study: Varies.
Study Establishment: University of Regina.
Country of Study: Canada.
Application Procedure: Application forms are available from the Faculty of Graduate Studies and Research.
Closing Date: February 28th, June 15th, October 15th.

Regina Teaching Assistantships

Subjects: Any graduate programme offered at the University of Regina.
Eligibility: Candidates must meet appropriate qualifications to participate in the instructional programme in the assigned academic unit. Must be accepted by the Graduate Faculty at the University of Regina as fully qualified for admission to Master's or PhD degree.
Level of Study: Doctorate, Postgraduate.
Purpose: Teaching assistants to assist with the instructional programme of undergraduate courses or laboratories.
Type: Assistantship.
No. of awards offered: Approx. 88.
Frequency: Twice a year.
Value: Master's level: C$3,660 per semester; Doctoral level C$4,182 per semester.
Length of Study: Varies.
Study Establishment: University of Regina.
Country of Study: Canada.
Application Procedure: Application forms are available from the Faculty of Graduate Studies and Research.
Closing Date: June 15th, October 15th.

UNIVERSITY OF SOUTHAMPTON

Highfield, Southampton, Hampshire, SO17 1BJ, England
Tel: (44) 1703 594741
Fax: (44) 1703 593037
Contact: Academic Registrar

The University of Southampton was founded as the Hartley Institute in the mid 19th Century, and was granted its royal charter in 1952. Today, the university offers a range of postgraduate courses in 8 faculties: arts, engineering and applied science, law mathematics, medicine, health and biological science, science, social sciences and education.

University of Southampton Studentships

Subjects: All subjects offered by the University.
Eligibility: Open to candidates who hold a good honours first degree and are eligible for admission to the department in which they intend to study.
Level of Study: Postgraduate.
Purpose: To support postgraduate research study.
Type: Studentship.
No. of awards offered: Varies.
Frequency: Annual.
Value: Based on Research Council Studentship rates.
Length of Study: The duration of the course of study and research.

Study Establishment: University of Southampton.
Country of Study: United Kingdom.
Application Procedure: Initial enquiries should be directed to the head of the academic department in which research is to be undertaken.
Closing Date: Varies; enquiries should be made by January for the following October.

UNIVERSITY OF SOUTHERN CALIFORNIA (USC)

University Park
Mail Code 4012, Los Angeles, CA, 90089, United States of America
Tel: (1) 213 740 5294
Fax: (1) 213 740 8607
www: http://www.usc.edu/dept/las/faculty/mellon.htm
Contact: Mr Joseph Aonn, Dean of Faculty

Located near the heart of Los Angeles, the University of Southern California is a private research university. It maintains a tradition of academic strength at all levels - from the earliest explorations of the undergraduate to the advanced scholarly research of the postdoctoral Fellow.

USC All-University Predoctoral Diversity Fellowships

Subjects: All subjects.
Eligibility: Consideration for a fellowship through the graduate school is contingent upon a completed application for admission to a PhD programme, and completion of a fellowship application. Open to incoming PhD applicants who are US citizens and members of the following under-represented minority groups: American Indians and Alaskan Natives (Eskimo or Aleut), Black/African Americans, US Hispanic/Latinos, and Native Pacific Islanders (Micronesians and Polynesians).
Level of Study: Postgraduate.
Purpose: The graduate school announces a programme of diversity fellowships for students aiming toward the PhD at USC and planning a career in university teaching and research.
Type: Fellowship.
No. of awards offered: Varies.
Frequency: Annual.
Value: US$14,000 per year, plus full tuition and mandatory fees.
Length of Study: 3 years eligibility, awarded annually with automatic renewal for a second and third year with continued superior performance.

Study Establishment: University of Southern California.
Country of Study: USA.
Application Procedure: A completed application must include: fellowship application form including statement of purpose; one transcript from each college or university; photocopy of scores from the Graduate Record Examination, and three academic letters of recommendation. Photocopies for all of the above are acceptable.
Closing Date: February 1st.

For further information contact:

University of Southern California
3601 Watt Way
GFS 315, Los Angeles, CA, 90089-1695, United States of America
Contact: The Graduate School

UNIVERSITY OF STIRLING

Research Office, Stirling, FK9 4LA, Scotland
Tel: (44) 1786 407041
Fax: (44) 1786 466688
Email: research@stir.ac.uk
www: http://www.stir.ac.uk/
Contact: Administrative Assistant

The University of Stirling offers postgraduate awards for research degrees on a full-time or part-time basis.

University of Stirling Research Studentships

Subjects: Awards are available in the arts and humanities, human sciences (applied, psychology and education) management studies including marketing, and natural sciences including aquaculture.
Eligibility: No restrictions.
Level of Study: Doctorate, Postgraduate.
Purpose: To support postgraduate study.
Type: Studentship.
No. of awards offered: 40.
Frequency: Annual.
Value: £6,500 per annum.
Length of Study: Up to 3 years.
Study Establishment: University of Stirling.
Country of Study: Scotland.
Application Procedure: Application forms for the individual faculties must be completed. The address to write to is the same as the main address including the name of the faculty being applied to.
Closing Date: Ongoing.

THE UNIVERSITY OF SYDNEY

The Research and Scholarships Office
Main Quadrangle A14, Sydney, NSW, 2006, Australia
Tel: (61) 2 9351 3250
Fax: (61) 2 9351 3256
Email: scholars@reschols.usyd.edu.au
www: http://www.usyd.edu.au/rescols/welcome.html
Contact: Grants Management Officer

Australian Postgraduate Award (APA)

Subjects: All subjects.
Eligibility: Open to Australian citizens & permanent residents (resident in Australia continuously for 12 months prior to the closing date of each year).
Level of Study: Doctorate, Postgraduate.
Purpose: To enable candidates with exceptional research potential to undertake a higher degree.
Type: Scholarship.
No. of awards offered: Varies from year to year (147 in 1999).
Frequency: Annual.
Value: Stipend is A$16,135 (in 1999).
Length of Study: 2 year for Masters by research candidate; 3 years with possible 6 month extension for PhD candidate.
Study Establishment: University of Sydney.
Country of Study: Australia.
Application Procedure: Forms are available from the Scholarships Office between August and October. Can be downloaded from website or emailed on request.
Closing Date: October 31st.

University of Sydney International Postgraduate Research Scholarships (IPRS) and International Graduate Awards (IPA)

Subjects: All subjects.
Eligibility: Open to suitably qualified graduates from any country eligible to commence a higher degree by research. Australia and New Zealand citizens and Australian permanent residents are not eligible to apply.
Level of Study: Doctorate, Postgraduate.
Purpose: To fund study.
Type: Scholarship.
No. of awards offered: Varies from year to year.
Frequency: Annual.
Value: IPRS - tuition fees; IPA A$16,135 in 1999.
Study Establishment: University of Sydney.
Country of Study: Australia.
Application Procedure: Application forms are available between May and August from the International Office.
Closing Date: August 31st.

For further information contact:

International Office
Margaret Telfer Building K07, Sydney, NSW, 2006, Australia
Tel: (61) 2 9351 4161
Fax: (61) 2 9351 4013
Contact: Grants Management Officer

University of Sydney Postgraduate Award (UPA)

Subjects: All subjects.
Eligibility: Open to Australian citizens and permanent residents, and New Zealand citizens.
Level of Study: Doctorate, Postgraduate.
Purpose: To enable candidates with exceptional research potential to undertake a higher degree.
Type: Scholarship.
No. of awards offered: Varies from year to year (40 in 1999).
Frequency: Annual.
Value: A$16,135 per year (in 1999).
Length of Study: 2 years for Masters by research candidate; 3 years with possible 6 month extension for PhD candidate.
Study Establishment: University of Sydney.
Country of Study: Australia.
Application Procedure: Forms are available from the Scholarships Office between August and October. Can be downloaded from website or emailed on request.
Closing Date: October 31st.

UNIVERSITY OF TASMANIA

GPO Box 252-45, Hobart, TAS, 7001, Australia
Tel: (61) 2 6226 2766
Fax: (61) 2 6226 7497
www: http://www.research.utas.edu.au
Contact: Office for Research

Merle Weaver Postgraduate Scholarship

Subjects: All subjects.
Eligibility: Open to women graduates from South East Asia and the Pacific region.
Level of Study: Postgraduate.
Purpose: To fund research leading to a higher degree.
Type: Scholarship.
No. of awards offered: 1.
Frequency: Dependent on funds available.
Value: A$16,135 per year.
Length of Study: Up to 3 years.
Study Establishment: University of Tasmania.
Country of Study: Australia.
Application Procedure: Please write for details.
Closing Date: October 31st.

UNIVERSITY OF THE WITWATERSRAND

Private Bag 3, Wits, 2050, South Africa
Tel: (27) 11 716 1111
Fax: (27) 11 339 4387
www: http://www.wits.ac.za
Contact: Mr Haydn Johnson

E P Bradlow/John Lemmer Scholarship

Subjects: All subjects.
Eligibility: Open to candidates showing appropriate academic merit. A student who accepts a scholarship shall be required to remain in South Africa for a period of time equal to that for which the scholarship was held after completing all the requirements for the postgraduate degree.
Level of Study: Doctorate, Postgraduate.
Purpose: To assist with full-time Master's or PhD degree study.
Type: Scholarship.
Frequency: Annual.
Value: At the discretion of the Committee.
Study Establishment: University of the Witwatersrand.
Country of Study: South Africa.
Application Procedure: Please write for details.
Closing Date: January 10th.

Freda Lawenski Scholarship Fund Grants

Subjects: All fields of study offered at the University.
Eligibility: Open to distinguished graduates of approved universities in South Africa.
Level of Study: Postgraduate.
Purpose: To assist with full-time postgraduate studies.
Type: Scholarship.
Frequency: Annual.
Value: At the discretion of the Committee.
Length of Study: 1 year of full-time study.
Study Establishment: University of the Witwatersrand.
Country of Study: South Africa.
Application Procedure: Please write for details.
Closing Date: January 10th.

Henry Bradlow Scholarship

Subjects: Not restricted.
Eligibility: Open to distinguished graduates of approved universities in South Africa.
Level of Study: Postgraduate.
Purpose: To assist in postgraduate study towards a full-time Master's or PhD degree.
Type: Scholarship.
Frequency: Annual.
Value: At the discretion of the Committee.
Length of Study: 1 year of full-time study.
Study Establishment: University of the Witwatersrand.
Country of Study: South Africa.
Application Procedure: Please write for details.
Closing Date: January 10th.

UNIVERSITY OF WALES, ABERYSTWYTH

Old College
King Street, Aberystwyth, Ceredigion, SY23 2AX, Wales
Tel: (44) 1970 622 270
Fax: (44) 1970 622 921
Email: postgraduate-admissions@aber.ac.uk
www: http://www.aber.ac.uk
Contact: Dr Russell Davies, Marketing Manager

The University of Wales, Aberystwyth was established in 1872 and is situated in an area of outstanding natural beauty on the west coast of Wales, providing a rich academic and cultural environment. The postgraduate student population is about 800 and approximately thirty per cent of these are international students.

University of Wales (Aberystwyth) Postgraduate Research Studentships

Subjects: Any full-time research course (MPhil/PhD/LLM by research).
Eligibility: Open to UK/EU candidates who have obtained at least upper second class honours or equivalent in their degree examination and who wish to study full-time.
Level of Study: Doctorate, Postgraduate.
Purpose: To enable UK/EU students to undertake full-time postgraduate research at University of Wales, Aberystwyth.
Type: Studentship.
No. of awards offered: Usually 12.
Frequency: Annual.
Value: UK fees plus a subsistence allowance based on research council rates.
Length of Study: 1 year; usually renewable for up to 2 additional years, subject to satisfactory academic progress.
Study Establishment: The College.
Country of Study: United Kingdom.
Application Procedure: Completion of application form is required. Application forms are available from the Postgraduate Admissions Office.
Closing Date: March 1st.
Additional Information: For all enquiries, please contact the Postgraduate Admissions Office.

UNIVERSITY OF WALES, BANGOR

Academic Registry
College Road, Bangor, Gwynedd, LL57 2DG, Wales
Tel: (44) 1248 382025
Fax: (44) 1248 370451
Email: aos057@bangor.ac.uk
Contact: Dr John C T Perkins, Assistant Registrar

The University of Wales, Bangor is the principal seat of learning, scholarship and research in North Wales. It was established in 1884 and is a constituent institution of the

Federal University of Wales. The University attaches considerable importance to research training in all disciplines and offers research studentships of a value similar to those of the research councils.

Mr and Mrs David Edward Roberts Memorial Award

Subjects: Any subject offered at University of Wales, Bangor.
Eligibility: Open to holders of relevant first or, exceptionally, upper second class honours degree, who are of any nationality classified as a home/EC student for fees purposes.
Level of Study: Doctorate, Postgraduate.
Purpose: To support doctoral studies in any subject area.
Type: Research Studentship.
No. of awards offered: 1.
Frequency: Dependent on funds available.
Value: No less than that of a Research Council or British Academy Research Studentship, including fees.
Length of Study: 1 year; renewable for a further 2 years if satisfactory progress is maintained.
Study Establishment: University of Wales, Bangor.
Country of Study: Wales.
Application Procedure: Application forms may be obtained from the Postgraduate Admissions Office at UWB.
Closing Date: June 1st.

University of Wales (Bangor) Postgraduate Studentships

Subjects: Any subject offered by the University.
Eligibility: Open to candidates classified as home/EC for fees payment purposes who have attained a first or exceptional upper second class honours degree (or equivalent).
Level of Study: Doctorate, Postgraduate.
Purpose: To fund research training to PhD level.
Type: Research Studentship.
No. of awards offered: 12-15.
Frequency: Annual.
Value: Equal to that of a British public-funded Research Studentship.
Length of Study: 1 year; renewable for up to 2 additional years.
Study Establishment: University of Wales, Bangor.
Country of Study: Wales.
Application Procedure: Expressions of interest should be made to the relevant department of proposed study. The department will nominate the most worthy eligible students.
Closing Date: June 1st.

University of Wales Bangor (UWB) Research Studentships

Subjects: All subjects covered within UWB.
Eligibility: Recent graduates classified at the lower (EU) rate, or for payment purposes hold a first or upper second class honours degree (or equivalent) in a relevant subject.
Level of Study: Postgraduate.
Purpose: To support students for the duration of a PhD programme.

Type: Studentship.
No. of awards offered: 10-14.
Frequency: Annual, if funds are available.
Value: Same basic value as a research council studentship.
Length of Study: 3 years.
Study Establishment: University of Wales, Bangor.
Country of Study: United Kingdom.
Application Procedure: An initial approach should be made to the Senior Postgraduate Tutor in the department of the proposed research programme. (See Postgraduate Prospectus).
Closing Date: 30th June. Those interested should make enquiries well before this date.
Additional Information: In exceptional circumstances and award may be made to an international student classified for the full cost fee. In such a case, the student would be required to pay the difference between the full cost fee and the home/EU fee.

UNIVERSITY OF WALES, CARDIFF

Postgraduate Registry
University of Wales College of Cardiff
PO Box 495, Cardiff, CF1 3XD, Wales
Tel: (44) 1222 874413
Fax: (44) 1222 874130
Contact: Senior Assistant Registrar

Cardiff University is one of Britain's major centres of higher education; its origins date back to 1883. The University currently has some 14,500 students of whom more than 3,000 are postgraduates. Cardiff is a research-led university, ranked 15th out of 102 UK universities for research activity, with 23 subject areas recognised as undertaking research of national and international excellence.

Cardiff University Postgraduate Research Studentships

Subjects: All subjects offered by the University.
Eligibility: Candidates must possess at least an upper second class honours degree from an approved university. For purposes of fee payment, applicants must be a home student ordinarily resident in the UK (or the European Community provided he or she is an EC national) throughout the period of three years immediately preceding the date on which the course of study is due to begin. Heads of department at the University select recipients from among the applicants for admission.
Level of Study: Postgraduate.
Purpose: To enable nominated students to pursue doctoral research to PhD level.
Type: Studentship.
No. of awards offered: 10.
Frequency: Annual.
Value: £2,610 (fees), plus up to £6,455 maintenance allowance.

Length of Study: 1 year; renewable annually to a maximum of 3 years.
Study Establishment: The University.
Country of Study: United Kingdom.
Application Procedure: Please write for details.
Closing Date: June 30th.

UNIVERSITY OF WESTERN AUSTRALIA

Nedlands, Perth, WA, 6009, Australia
Tel: (61) 9 380 2490
Fax: (61) 9 380 1919
www: http://www.uwa.edu.au
Contact: Ms Margaret Edwards, Senior Administrative Officer

Richard Walter Gibbon Medical Research Fellowship

Subjects: Research into the causes and treatment of cancer and Parkinson's disease.
Eligibility: Open to Australian residents who are medical graduates of a recognised tertiary institution.
Level of Study: Postgraduate.
Purpose: To promote research by facilitating and encouraging students to pursue postgraduate research in the Faculty of Medicine at the University.
Type: Fellowship.
No. of awards offered: Varies.
Frequency: Varies, depending on funds available and standard of the applications.
Value: $15,100 per annum.
Length of Study: Up to 3 years.
Study Establishment: UWA.
Country of Study: Australia.
Closing Date: June 30th.
Additional Information: Except by permission a Fellow may not engage in any work during tenure of the fellowship other than that for which it was awarded. A full report is required at the end of tenure. Resulting publications must acknowledge that the work was done under a Gibbon Fellowship.

Saw Medical Research Fellowship

Subjects: The causation, prevention and cure of disease, primarily diabetes mellitus.
Eligibility: Candidates need not have medical qualifications.
Level of Study: Doctorate, Postgraduate.
Purpose: To promote personal research.
Type: Fellowship.
No. of awards offered: 1.
Frequency: Annually, or as vacancies occur.
Value: Up to A$37,345 per year depending on qualifications. May not be held concurrently with other awards.
Length of Study: 1 year; renewable for 1 further year.
Study Establishment: UWA.
Country of Study: Australia.

Closing Date: June 30th of the year preceding tenure.
Additional Information: During the tenure of the fellowship a Fellow may not engage in any work other than that for which the fellowship has been awarded except by permission of the Vice-Chancellor.

University of Western Australia Postdoctoral Research Fellowship

Subjects: All areas covered by UWA departments. Please see UWA WWW home page for details.
Eligibility: Open to all nationalities. Applicants should hold a PhD for all appointments. The appointment of an overseas Fellow is subject to Australian Department of Immigration and Ethnic Affairs' approval of UWA's sponsorship for residence, and the Fellow's successful application for appropriate visa.
Level of Study: Postdoctorate.
Purpose: To provide a two-year appointment to a postdoctoral Research Fellow bringing special new expertise and a high level of relevant experience which is not otherwise available at the UWA department, to carry out a research project in a UWA department.
Type: Fellowship.
No. of awards offered: 3.
Frequency: Annual.
Value: A$37,345-A$40,087 per year salary plus A$3,500-A$5,000 per year fellowship support grant. A relocation allowance is also included.
Length of Study: 2 years.
Study Establishment: UWA.
Country of Study: Australia.
Application Procedure: Applications are accepted from UWA departments only.
Closing Date: Usually March 1st.

University of Western Australia Postgraduate Awards

Subjects: Any subject offered by the University.
Eligibility: Open to Australian citizens who are graduates with at least an upper second class honours degree, or a small number of overseas graduates who possess a first class honours or equivalent.
Level of Study: Postgraduate.
Purpose: To enable students to conduct research leading to a Master's or doctoral degree.
Type: Studentship.
No. of awards offered: Varies.
Frequency: Annual.
Value: A$15,100 per year (tax free); plus travel costs; relocation allowance within Australia of up to A$1,270; thesis allowance of A$400 (Master's) or A$800 (doctoral).
Length of Study: 1 year; renewable for 1 year (Master's) or for 2 years (doctoral).
Study Establishment: The University.
Country of Study: Australia.
Application Procedure: Please write for details.
Closing Date: August 31st for overseas applicants, October 31st for Australian applicants.

Additional Information: Scholarships may not be held concurrently with other awards of a similar nature. Employment is permitted to a maximum of 240 hours in a calendar year and no more than 8 hours in any one week.

UNIVERSITY OF WESTERN SYDNEY

Nepean Research Office
PO Box 10, Kingswood, NSW, 2747, Australia
Tel: (61) 2 4736 0052
Fax: (61) 2 4736 0013
Email: h.holmes@nepean.uws.edu.au
www: http://www.uws.edu.au
Contact: Ms Helen Holmes, Research Scholarships Officer

Nepean Postgraduate Research Award

Subjects: All subjects offered at the university.
Eligibility: Applicants must hold or be eligible for the award of B(Hons) Degree Class 1, from an Australian university, or an equivalent award.
Level of Study: Doctorate.
Purpose: To support students of high academic merit in undertaking postgraduate research degrees at UWS Nepean.
Type: Scholarship.
No. of awards offered: 10.
Frequency: Annual.
Value: A$16,135 stipend plus allowances.
Length of Study: 2 years for the Master's and 3 years for the doctorate.
Study Establishment: University of Western Sydney, Nepean.
Country of Study: Australia.
Application Procedure: Please submit application form, certified copies of all academic records and two academic referee reports (submitted by referees).
Closing Date: October 31st.

UNIVERSITY OF WOLLONGONG

Northfields Avenue, Wollongong, NSW, 2522, Australia
Tel: (61) 2 4221 3555
Contact: Ms Sharon Hughes

Wollongong sits between the dramatic Illawarra escarpment and the Pacific Ocean just one hour away from Sydney, Australia's largest city. The University of Wollongong enjoys a significant international research profile attracting more Australian Research Council funding per student in 1999 than any other Australian university. Over 3,000 postgraduate students are enrolled (30% overseas).

University of Wollongong Postgraduate Awards

Subjects: Any postgraduate research subject offered by the University.
Eligibility: Open to graduates with at least a second class honours degree.
Level of Study: Postgraduate.
Purpose: To provide financial support for full-time study leading to a Master's or PhD degree.
No. of awards offered: Varies.
Frequency: Annual.
Value: A$16,135.
Length of Study: 2 years for the Master's or 3 years for the PhD; renewable subject to satisfactory progress.
Study Establishment: University of Wollongong.
Country of Study: Australia.
Application Procedure: Application forms are available from the Office of Research in July/August each year.
Closing Date: October 31st.
Additional Information: Holders of the Award must pursue studies on a full-time basis and submit an annual report.

UNIVERSITY OF YORK

Graduate Schools Office
Heslington, York, YO1 5DD, England
Tel: (44) 1904 432 143
Fax: (44) 1904 432 092
Email: graduate@york.ac.uk
www: http://www.york.ac.uk/admin/gso/gsp/
Contact: Mr Philip Simison

The University of York offers postgraduate degree courses in archaeology, architectural and conservation studies, art history, biology, biochemistry, chemistry, computer science, economics, educational studies, electronics, english, environment, health sciences, health studies, history, language and linguistics, mathematics, medieval studies, music, philosophy, physics, politics, psychology, social policy, social work, sociology, and women's studies.

University of York Master's Scholarships

Subjects: All subjects.
Eligibility: Open to full-time candidates for Master's degrees (MA/MSc/MRes).
Level of Study: Postgraduate.
Purpose: To assist candidates of high academic standards to complete Master's degrees.
Type: Scholarship.
No. of awards offered: Approx. 10.
Frequency: Annual.
Value: Fee-waiver of up to £2,000.
Length of Study: 1 year.
Study Establishment: University of York.
Country of Study: England.
Application Procedure: Application forms are available from the Graduate Schools Office.
Closing Date: May 29th.

University of York Research Studentships/Scholarships

Subjects: All subjects.
Eligibility: Open to full-time candidates for research degrees (MPhil/DPhil).
Level of Study: Doctorate, Postgraduate.
Purpose: To assist candidates of a high academic standard to complete research degrees.
Type: Scholarship.
No. of awards offered: Approx. 24.
Frequency: Annual.
Value: Fees (at home/EU rate) plus up to £6,200.
Length of Study: Up to 3 years.
Study Establishment: University of York.
Country of Study: England.
Application Procedure: Application forms are available from Graduate Schools Office.
Closing Date: May 29th.

University of York Scholarships for Overseas Students

Subjects: Any full-time degree (graduate or undergraduate), diploma or certificate of the University.
Eligibility: Open to students who have been accepted for registration as a full-time student for a degree, diploma or certificate course of the University of York and are liable to pay tuition fees at the full-cost rate for overseas (non-EC) students.
Level of Study: Postgraduate, Undergraduate.
Purpose: To assist overseas candidates of high academic standard.
Type: Scholarship.
No. of awards offered: Approx. 30.
Frequency: Annual.
Value: One-third or one-sixth of the value of tuition fees.
Length of Study: Up to 3 years.
Study Establishment: University of York.
Country of Study: United Kingdom.
Application Procedure: Application form available for completion, contact the International office.
Closing Date: May 1st.

US-ISRAEL BINATIONAL SCIENCE FOUNDATION

PO Box 7677, Jerusalem, 91076, Israel
Tel: (972) 2 561 7314
Fax: (972) 2 563 3287
Email: bsf@vms.huji.ac.il
www: http://www.bsf.org.il
Contact: Grants Management Officer

US-Israel BSF Research Grants

Subjects: Health sciences, life sciences, physics, chemistry, mathematical sciences, atmospheric and earth sciences, oceanography and limnology, materials research, environmental research, energy research, biomedical engineering, economics, sociology, anthropology, social and developmental psychology.
Eligibility: Applicants must hold tenured positions in the US or in Israel. Scientists who wish to apply for grants must submit their applications through an institution or agency with legal status. The BSF accepts research proposals from institutions of higher learning, government research institutions, hospitals and other non-profit research organisations. Proposals originating in industry are not considered. Although proposals cannot be submitted by for-profit or industrial organisations, the US principal investigator may be affiliated with such an organisation. In such cases the investigators must be familiar with BSF patent policy before completing the collaborative arrangements. Israeli and American principal investigators must hold a doctoral degree or its equivalent. Graduate students are not eligible to submit applications.
Level of Study: Postdoctorate.
Purpose: To encourage co-operation between US and Israeli scientists.
Type: Research Grant.
No. of awards offered: Approx. 100-1140.
Frequency: Annual.
Value: Approx. US$50,000.
Length of Study: up to 3 years.
Study Establishment: Appropriate Research Institutions in the US or Israel.
Country of Study: USA or Israel.
Application Procedure: Prior to formal submission, the proposal may be discussed with the BSF staff either by letter, telephone or in person. Application forms are available on the website.
Closing Date: November 15th.
Additional Information: Investigators may submit only one proposal to each annual competition. Further, since an investigator may hold only one BSF award at a time, a grantee may submit a new proposal only during the last year of the award.

THE US-UK FULBRIGHT COMMISSION

Fulbright House
62 Doughty Street, London, WC1N 2LS, England
Tel: (44) 171 404 6880
Fax: (44) 171 404 6834
Email: education@fulbright.co.uk
www: http://www.fulbright.co.uk
Contact: Ms E Davey, Programme Director

The US-UK Fulbright Commission has a programme of awards offered annually to citizens of the UK and USA. The Commission's Educational Advisory Service deals with enquiries from the public on all aspects of US education.

Fulbright Fellowship in Cancer Research

Subjects: Oncology.
Eligibility: Open to British scientists or clinicians.
Level of Study: Postdoctorate.
Purpose: To enable a scientist or clinician to carry out research into cancer.
Type: Fellowship.
No. of awards offered: 1.
Frequency: Annual.
Value: £15,000.
Length of Study: A minimum of 6 months.
Study Establishment: An approved US institution.
Country of Study: USA.
Application Procedure: Formal application is required.
Closing Date: March/April.
Additional Information: Short listed candidates will be interviewed (usually in June).

Fulbright Graduate Student Awards

Subjects: All subjects. Some special funding exists for MBA or related studies. Other special funding available for software or electronic engineering, bioscience, teaching of English as a second language.
Eligibility: Open to US citizens, normally resident in the USA. Minimum GPA: 3.5; must demonstrate evidence of leadership qualities.
Level of Study: Postgraduate.
Purpose: To enable US students to follow postgraduate study or research in the UK.
No. of awards offered: Approx. 20.
Frequency: Annual.
Value: Maintenance allowance, approved tuition fees and round-trip travel are covered.
Length of Study: A minimum of 9 months.
Study Establishment: Any approved UK institution of higher education.
Country of Study: United Kingdom.
Application Procedure: Formal application is required, with four references and a telephone interview for shortlisted candidates.
Closing Date: October - to be confirmed.

For further information contact:

Institute of International Education
809 United Nations Plaza, New York, NY, 10017, United States of America
Tel: (1) 212 984 5466
Fax: (1) 212 984 5465
Contact: Student Program Division

Fulbright Louise Buchanan Fellowship in Cancer Research

Subjects: Oncology.
Eligibility: Open to British scientists or clinicians.
Level of Study: Postdoctorate.
Purpose: To enable a scientist or clinician to carry out research into cancers of the lymph glands.
Type: Fellowship.

No. of awards offered: 1 depending on funds available.
Frequency: Annual.
Value: £4,000 plus round-trip travel.
Length of Study: A minimum of 3 months.
Study Establishment: An approved US institution of higher education.
Country of Study: USA.
Application Procedure: Formal application is required.
Closing Date: March/April - to be confirmed.
Additional Information: Shortlisted candidates will be interviewed (usually in June).

Fulbright Scholar Grants

Subjects: Any subject, with particular interest in topics which address problems shared by the USA and UK.
Eligibility: Open to US scholars who took their first degree more than five years ago.
Level of Study: Postdoctorate.
Purpose: To enable US scholars to carry out lecturing and research in the UK.
No. of awards offered: 4 Distinguished Scholars.
Frequency: Annual.
Value: Distinguished Scholar: £15,000 (round trip travel inclusive).
Length of Study: 1 full academic year.
Study Establishment: Any approved UK institution of higher education.
Country of Study: United Kingdom.
Application Procedure: Application and four references should be submitted to the CIES.
Closing Date: August 1st.

For further information contact:

Council for International Exchange of Scholars
3007 Tilden Street NW
Suite 5M, Washington, DC, 20008-3009, United States of America
Tel: (1) 202 686 6245
Contact: Grants Management Officer

US-UK Fulbright Commission Postdoctoral Research Scholarship at De Montfort University

Subjects: All subjects offered by the University.
Eligibility: Open to US nationals only.
Level of Study: Postdoctorate.
Purpose: To enable a scholar to undertake postdoctoral research at De Montfort University, Leicester.
Type: Scholarship.
No. of awards offered: 1.
Frequency: Annual.
Value: £5,000 plus round-trip travel.
Length of Study: 12 months.
Study Establishment: De Montfort University.
Country of Study: United Kingdom.
Application Procedure: Application forms are available from: CIES, 3007 Tilden Street NW, Suite 5M, Washington, DC 2008-3009.
Closing Date: August 1st.

US-UK Fulbright Commission Postgraduate Student Awards

Subjects: All subjects.
Eligibility: Applicants must: be UK citizens normally resident in the UK; hold, prior to departure, a minimum of an upper second class honours degree; and demonstrate outstanding leadership qualities.
Level of Study: Postgraduate.
Purpose: To enable students to carry out postgraduate study or research in the USA.
No. of awards offered: 10-12.
Frequency: Annual.
Value: Tuition and maintenance for nine months and round-trip travel.
Length of Study: A minimum of 9 months.
Study Establishment: An approved US institution of higher education.
Country of Study: USA.
Application Procedure: Please submit a formal application with two references.
Closing Date: Usually early November - to be confirmed.
Additional Information: Shortlisted candidates will be interviewed.

US-UK Fulbright Commission Scholarship Grants

Subjects: All subjects - although subjects where there is an opportunity for collaborative innovation of international significance or a focus on Anglo-American relations are preferred.
Eligibility: Candidates must demonstrate academic or artistic excellence.
Level of Study: Postdoctorate, Professional development.
Purpose: To enable lecturers, junior and senior postdoctoral research scholars, to lecture or carry out research in the USA for a minimum of three months.
Type: Scholarship.
No. of awards offered: 3.
Frequency: Annual.
Value: £15,000; proof of additional dollar support is required.
Length of Study: 10 moths minimum.
Study Establishment: An approved US institution of higher education or similar.
Country of Study: USA.
Application Procedure: Please submit a formal application and two references.
Closing Date: March/April - exact date to be confirmed.
Additional Information: Shortlisted candidates will be interviewed (usually in April/May).

USIA FULBRIGHT PROGRAMMES

Institute of International Education
809 United Nations Plaza, New York, NY, 10017-3580, United States of America
Tel: (1) 212 984 5330
www: http://www.usia.gov
Contact: US Student Programs

USIA Fulbright Study and Research Grants for US Citizens

Subjects: Study and research in all fields, as well as professional training in the creative and performing arts.
Eligibility: Open to US citizens who have a Bachelor's degree or equivalent qualification. Candidates must have a high scholastic record, have an acceptable plan of study, demonstrate proficiency in the language of the host country, and be in good health. In some cases special language training is provided as part of a grant. Preference is given to persons who have not had prior experience of, or opportunity for, extended foreign study, residence or travel.
Level of Study: Postgraduate.
Purpose: To increase mutual understanding between the people of the USA and the people of other countries by means of educational and cultural exchange.
No. of awards offered: Varies.
Frequency: Annual.
Value: Full grants cover international transportation, language or orientation course (where appropriate), tuition, book, and maintenance allowances, and health and accident insurance. Travel grants will consist of travel expenses supplementing students personal funds or maintenance allowances and tuition scholarships which are granted to students by universities and other organisations.
Length of Study: 1 academic year.
Study Establishment: Institutions of higher learning.
Country of Study: Outside USA. A list of participating countries in a given year may be obtained from the Institute of International Education.
Application Procedure: Applicants enrolled in a college or university should apply to the Fulbright Programme Adviser on their campus. Applicants not enrolled in a college or university should apply to the Institute of International Education. Applications should be requested at least 15 days prior to the closing date.
Closing Date: October 23rd.

VAN SLYKE SOCIETY

2101 L Street NW
Ste 202, Washington, DC, 20037-1526, United States of
America
Tel: (1) 202 857 0717
Fax: (1) 202 887 5093
Email: jgrimes@aacc.org
www: http://www.aacc.org
Contact: Research Grant Program

The Van Slyke Society is part of a Washington DC-based,
non-profit, professional association with a membership of
10,500 clinical chemists, pathologists, medical technologists
and others in related fields. Through educational services and
publications, the society works to improve and advance
laboratory services to enhance public health and patient care.

Van Slyke Society Research Grant in Clinical Chemistry

Subjects: Clinical laboratory science.
Eligibility: Applicant should be no more than five years past
his or her most recently earned degree, or no more than five
years past postdoctoral training.
Level of Study: Unrestricted.
Purpose: To provide support to those clinical laboratory
scientists who need limited research funds to explore new
ideas in areas where funds are not normally available.
Type: Research Grant.
No. of awards offered: Dependent on funds received.
Frequency: Annual.
Value: US$10,000.
Country of Study: Any country.
Application Procedure: Application form must be
completed.
Closing Date: March 15th.

VISITING NURSE ASSOCIATION OF CENTRAL JERSEY

141 Bodman Place, Red Bank, NJ, 07701, United States of
America
Tel: (1) 732 224 6756
Fax: (1) 732 747 2822
www: http://www.vnacj.org
Contact: Ms Cherie M Lamont, Annual Fund and Campaign
Manager

Marcia Granucci Memorial Scholarship

Subjects: Psychiatric/mental health or community health
nursing.
Eligibility: Open to New Jersey state residents only. There is
a part-time and full-time student consideration. Current
licensure. Demonstrate acceptance to a graduate program.
Must have a 3.0 GPA. Must attend a National League of
Nursing (NLN) accredited educational institution.

Level of Study: Postgraduate.
Purpose: To provide scholarships for nursing students
interested in pursuing an educational concentration in
psychiatric and mental health or community health nursing.
Type: Scholarship.
No. of awards offered: 1.
Frequency: Annual.
Value: Up to US$2,000.
Length of Study: 1 academic year.
Country of Study: Any country.
Application Procedure: Applicants must complete an
application form, and submit with recommendation forms,
transcripts, GRE scores and a personal statement. Final
applicant may be required to appear for a personal interview.
Closing Date: May 15th.

For further information contact:

VNA of Central Jersey
141 Bodman Place, Red Bank, NJ, 07701, United States of
America
Contact: Director of Development

WACKER FOUNDATION

10848 Strait Lane, Dallas, TX, 75229, United States of
America
Tel: (1) 214 368 0150
Fax: (1) 214 373 3308
Email: wackerjohn@aol.com
www: http://www.crime-times.org
Contact: Mr John Wacker, President

The Wacker Foundation funds research and dissemination of
research information which targets the proving, diagnosing or
treating of biologically-based disordered behaviour. Areas of
special interest include nutrition, food and chemical
intolerance, neurochemistry, and genetics.

Research Grant

Subjects: Neurology, paediatrics, psychiatry and mental
health, biomedicine, biophysics and molecular biology,
genetics, neurosciences, toxicology, cognitive sciences.
Purpose: To provide funds for research and dissemination of
research information which targets the proving, diagnosing or
treating of biologically-based disordered behaviour.
Value: Varies.
Application Procedure: Submit a brief letter giving a
description of the proposed project and stating appropriate
cost.
Closing Date: None.

WASHINGTON UNIVERSITY

Graduate School of Arts & Sciences
Campus Box 1187
1 Brookings Drive, St Louis, MO, 63130, United States of
America
Tel: (1) 314 935 6821
Fax: (1) 314 935 4887
Email: c43000je@wuvmd.wustl.edu
www: http://www.artsci.wustl.edu/gsas
Contact: Ms Joyce Edwards, Graduate Student Affairs and
Services Co-ordinator

Mr and Mrs Spencer T Olin Fellowships for Women

Subjects: Any graduate discipline or professional school in
the University.
Eligibility: Open to female graduates of a baccalaureate
institution in the USA who plan to prepare for a career in
higher education or the professions. Applicants must meet
the admission requirements of the graduate or professional
school of Washington University. Preference will be given to
those who wish to study for the highest earned degree in their
chosen field, do not already hold an advanced degree, and
who are not currently enrolled in a graduate or professional
degree programme.
Level of Study: Doctorate, Postgraduate.
Purpose: To encourage women of exceptional promise to
prepare for professional careers.
Type: Fellowship.
No. of awards offered: Approx. 6.
Frequency: Annual.
Value: Full tuition and, in some cases, a living expense
stipend.
Length of Study: 1 year; renewable up to 4 years, or until
completion of degree program, whichever comes first.
Study Establishment: Washington University in St Louis.
Country of Study: USA.
Application Procedure: Application form must be
completed. Candidates must be interviewed on campus at
the expense of the University. Applications should be
addressed to Dr Nancy P Pope.
Closing Date: February 1st.
Additional Information: Candidates must also make
concurrent application to the department or school of
Washington University in which they plan to study.

Washington University Chancellor's Graduate Fellowship Programme for African Americans

Subjects: Any of Washington University's PhD or DSc
programs in arts and sciences, business, engineering, or
social work. The fellowship includes other Washington
University programs providing final disciplinary training for
prospective college professors.
Eligibility: Open to African-American doctoral candidates.
Level of Study: Doctorate.

Purpose: To encourage African Americans who are interested
in becoming college or university professors.
Type: Fellowship.
No. of awards offered: 5-6.
Frequency: Annual.
Value: Doctoral candidates will receive full tuition plus
US$16,000 stipend and allowances.
Length of Study: 5 years, subject to satisfactory academic
progress.
Study Establishment: Washington University.
Country of Study: USA.
Application Procedure: Application form must be
completed.
Closing Date: January 25th.

WELLBEING

27 Sussex Place, London, NW1 4SP, England
Tel: (44) 171 262 5337
Fax: (44) 171 724 7725
Email: mary.stanton@wellbeing.org.uk
www: http://www.wellbeing.demon.co.uk
Contact: Research Administrator

WellBeing is the research arm of the Royal College of
Obstetricians and Gynaecologists, funding medical and
scientific research in hospitals and universities around the UK.
Wellbeing is involved in research into all aspects of women's
health, as well as the health of new babies.

WellBeing Project Grants

Subjects: Obstetrics, gynaecology, and related disciplines.
Eligibility: There are no eligibility restrictions. Open to all
qualified candidates, with the emphasis on clinicians.
Level of Study: Unrestricted.
Purpose: For research into all matters of women's obstetric
and gynaecological health and the health of their babies;
particularly all aspects of pregnancy, birth and care of
newborns; gynaecological cancers including ovarian, cervical
and endometrial cancer; and quality of life issues such as
menstrual problems, the menopause, infertility and
incontinence.
Type: Grant.
No. of awards offered: 15-20.
Frequency: Annual, if funds are available.
Value: Varies; up to £80,000.
Length of Study: 1-3 years.
Study Establishment: Approved institutions.
Country of Study: No restrictions but usually United
Kingdom.
Application Procedure: Application form and full instructions
are available from the Research Administrator.
Closing Date: First Monday of December.

THE WELLCOME TRUST

183 Euston Road, London, NW1 2BE, England
Tel: (44) 171 611 8888
Fax: (44) 171 611 8545
www: http://www.wellcome.ac.uk
Contact: Ms Rebecca Christon, Grants Information Officer

The Trust aims to support research in the biomedical sciences, the history of medicine and the implications of medicine in society. It supports the work of academic staff in universities, medical and veterinary schools and other institutions of higher education from the basic sciences related to medicine to the clinical aspects of medicine and veterinary medicine.

Wellcome Trust Awards, Fellowships and Studentships

Subjects: Biomedical sciences, from the basic sciences related to medicine to the clinical aspects of medicine and veterinary medicine. The Trust also operates a portfolio of schemes to support research in the history of medicine, the public appreciation of sciences and bioethics.
Eligibility: Open to academic staff in universities, medical and veterinary schools and other institutions of higher education, who are engaged in all types of research.
Level of Study: Postdoctorate, Professional development, Research.
Purpose: The Trusts aims to support and maintain the strength of biomedical research by providing individual researchers of the highest quality with the resources they need to pursue their subject.
Type: Project and programme grants, fellowships and travel grants.
No. of awards offered: Varies.
Frequency: Annual.
Value: Varies.
Length of Study: Varies.
Country of Study: Mostly United Kingdom and Republic of Ireland, but also schemes available for overseas, particularly in the developing or restructuring countries.
Application Procedure: Submit a written preliminary outline consisting of: brief CV's of applicant(s) including their source of salary, outline of proposed research project and approx cost of project. Outline preliminary application forms are available for some schemes. Information can be obtained from the Trust's website.
Closing Date: Preliminary applications are accepted at any time.
Additional Information: The Wellcome Trust is the most richly endowed of all charitable institutions that fund general medical research in the UK. The Governors review their policy annually in response to proposals from their advisory panels and professional staff.

THE WINGATE SCHOLARSHIPS

38 Curzon Street, London, W1Y 8EY, England
Tel: (44) 171 465 1521
Fax: (44) 171 499 2018
Email: reid@win-sch.demon.co.uk
www: http://www.win-sch.demon.co.uk
Contact: Ms Jane Reid, Administrator

Wingate Scholarships are awarded to individuals (over 24) of great potential or proven excellence who need financial support to undertake creative or original work of intellectual, scientific, artistic, social or environmental value, and to outstanding musicians for advanced training.

Wingate Scholarships

Subjects: Almost any subject, except fine arts and taught courses of any kind, including courses of drama, art or business, or courses leading to professional qualifications and electives.
Eligibility: Open to British, Commonwealth, Irish or Israeli and European Union country citizens provided that they are, and have been for at least five years, resident in the United Kingdom. Applicants must be over 24 years of age and resident in British Isles when applying. No qualifications are necessary.
Level of Study: Doctorate, Postdoctorate, Postgraduate.
Purpose: To fund creative or original work of intellectual, scientific, artistic, social or environmental value and advanced music study. Need is also taken into account.
Type: Scholarship.
No. of awards offered: Approx. 40.
Frequency: Annual.
Value: Costs of a project which may last for up to 3 years. Average of £6,500 total and the maximum in any one year is £10,000.
Length of Study: 1-3 years.
Study Establishment: Any or none.
Country of Study: Any country.
Application Procedure: Application forms available from the Administrator. Applicants must be: able to satisfy the Scholarship Committee that they need financial support to undertake the work projected; able to show why the propsed work (if it takes the form of academic research) is unlikely to attract Research Council, British Academy or major agency funding; citizens of the United Kingdom.
Closing Date: February 1st.
Additional Information: The scholarships are not intended for professional qualifications, taught courses or electives. Musicians are eligible for advanced training, but apart from that all applicants must have projects which are personal to them and involve either creative or orginal work.

WINSTON CHURCHILL MEMORIAL TRUST (AUS)

218 Northbourne Avenue, Braddon, ACT, 2612, Australia
Tel: (61) 6 2478333
www: http://sunsite.anu.edu.au/churchill_fellowships
Contact: Ms Margaret Bell, Finance Officer

The principal object of the Trust is to perpetuate and honour the memory of Sir Winston Churchill by the awarding of Memorial Fellowships known as Churchill Fellowships.

Churchill Fellowships

Subjects: All subjects.
Eligibility: Open to all Australian residents over the age of 18 years. There are no prescribed qualifications academic or otherwise for the award of most Churchill Fellowships. Merit is the primary test, whether based on past achievement or demonstrated ability for future achievements in any walk of life. Fellowships will not be awarded to enable the applicant to obtain higher academic or formal qualifications. The only criteria for the awarding of a Fellowship is that the applicant has gone as far as they can go in Australia and now needs to go overseas to obtain information not available in Australia.
Level of Study: Unrestricted.
Purpose: To enable Australians from all walks of life to undertake overseas study or an investigative project of a kind that is not fully available in Australia.
Type: Fellowship.
No. of awards offered: Approx. 100.
Frequency: Annual.
Value: Approximately A$15,000. Return economy air fare to country/countries to be visited. Living allowance plus fees if necessary.
Length of Study: 4-10 weeks (but this may be longer or shorter depending upon the project).
Country of Study: Any country.
Application Procedure: Application form must be completed. Please send a self address envelope to 'Application Forms' at the main address. Applications open on November 1st.
Closing Date: Last day of February.

THE WOLFSON FOUNDATION

8 Queen Anne Street, London, W1M 9LD, England
Tel: (44) 171 323 5730
Fax: (44) 171 323 3241
Contact: Executive Secretary

The aims of the Wolfson Foundation are the advancement of health, education, arts and humanities. Grants are given to act as a catalyst, to back excellence and talent and provide support for promising projects which may be underfunded, particularly for renovation and equipment. The emphasis is on science and technology, research, education, health and the arts.

Wolfson Foundation Grants

Subjects: Areas supported by the Trustees are - medicine and health care, including the prevention of disease and the care and treatment of the sick, disadvantaged and disabled; research, science, technology and education, particularly where benefits may accrue to the development of industry or commerce in the UK; arts and the humanities, including libraries, museums, galleries, theatres, academies and historic buildings.
Eligibility: Open to registered charities and to exempt charities such as universities. Eligible applications from registered charities for contributions to appeals will normally be considered only when at least 50% of that appeal has already been raised. Grants to universities for research and scholarship are normally made under the umbrella of designated competitive programmes in which vice-chancellors and principals are invited to participate from time to time. Applications from university researchers are not considered outside these programmes. Grants are not made to private individuals.
Level of Study: Postgraduate.
Type: Grant.
No. of awards offered: Varies.
Frequency: The trustees meet twice a year.
Value: The Trustees make several types of grant which are not necessarily independent of each other. Capital Projects: grants may contribute towards the cost of erecting a new building or extension, or of renovating and refurbishing existing buildings; Equipment Grants: the supply of equipment for specific purposes, and/or furnishing and fittings; Recurrent Costs: grants in this category are not normally provided unless they form part of a designated programme.
Country of Study: Any country.
Application Procedure: Before embarking on a detailed proposal, prospective applicants are encouraged to explore its eligibility by submitting in writing a brief outline of the project with one copy of the organisation's most recent audited accounts.
Closing Date: March 15th and September 15th.

WORLD CANCER RESEARCH FUND (WCRF)

105 Park Street, London, W1Y 3FB, England
Tel: (44) 171 343 4200
Fax: (44) 171 343 4201
Email: science@wcrf.org.uk
Contact: Grant Administrator

WCRF is the only major UK registered charity dedicated solely to the prevention of cancer by means of healthy diets and associated lifestyles. WCRF's education and science programmes are now based on the recommendations of the report: 'Food, Nutrition and the Prevention of Cancer: a global perspective', published in 1997.

WCRF Research Grant

Subjects: Social and preventive medicine, public health, epidemiology, diet and cancer prevention.
Eligibility: Open to qualified researchers of any nationality.
Level of Study: Unrestricted.
Purpose: To fund innovative research science designed to increase knowledge of the effects of diet and nutrition on the origins, causes, prevention and treatment of cancer.
Type: Research Grant.
No. of awards offered: Varies.
Frequency: Annual.
Value: Up to a maximum of £100,000 over three years.
Length of Study: 1-3 years.
Country of Study: Any country, although priority is currently given to UK research.
Application Procedure: The programme is advertised in 'Nature' and 'Lancet' in August/September each year. Application pack is available from WCRF.
Closing Date: Mid-December, as specified in journal advertisements/application pack.

WORLD HEALTH ORGANIZATION (WHO)

Regional Office for the Americas/Pan-American Sanitary Bureau
525 23rd Street NW, Washington, DC, 20037, United States of America
Tel: (1) 202 974 3000
Fax: (1) 202 974 3680
Email: rgp@paho.org
www: http://www.paho.org
Contact: Grants Management Officer

WHO Fellowships, Research Training Grants and Visiting Scientist Grants

Subjects: Medical and health studies. The most common subjects of study are in the various areas of public health, teacher training in health sciences, postgraduate studies in medicine and surgery. Fellowships are awarded to attend formal courses or to study the services and practice in other countries. As a general rule, WHO does not organize regular courses.
Eligibility: Open to nationals of Member States and Associate Members of WHO and to nationals of trust and other territories for whose international relations WHO Member States are responsible, or which are administered by international authorities established by the United Nations.
Level of Study: Postgraduate.
Purpose: To promote the international exchange of scientific knowledge and techniques relating to health, for the purpose of improving standards of teaching and training in the health, medical and related fields; and to strengthen national health services.
Type: Grant, Fellowship.
No. of awards offered: Varies.

Frequency: As required.
Value: To cover the cost of travel, maintenance, tuition fees and other expenses in special cases.
Study Establishment: For attendance of formal courses or to study the services and practices of the countries concerned.
Country of Study: As appropriate, according to the subject of study and the origin of the candidate.
Application Procedure: The World Health Organization only awards Fellowships through the governments of its Member States, and candidates should contact the Ministry of Health, or the corresponding national health administration, of their country of origin, which will advise them on the procedure for application. Applicants are discouraged from applying to the Geneva address. At the Headquarters level, the World Health Organization only awards Research Training Grants and Visiting Scientist Grants to candidates from institutions working in collaboration with the Special Programme of Research, Development and Research Training in Human Reproduction, and the Special Programme for Research and Training in Tropical Diseases. However, the WHO regional offices award grants in other fields and further information can be requested from the WHO regional office of the region of origin of the candidate.
Closing Date: At least six months prior to study.

For further information contact:

Regional Office for Africa
PO Box No 6, Brazzaville, Congo
Tel: (242) 83 38 60 64
Fax: (242) 83 18 79
Contact: Research Training Grants
or
Regional Office for Europe
8 Scherfigsvej, Copenhagen, DK-2100, Denmark
Tel: (45) 39 17 17 17
Fax: (45) 39 17 18 18
Contact: Grants Management Officer
or
Regional Office for the Eastern Mediterranean
PO Box No 1517, Alexandria, 21511, Egypt
Tel: (20) 3 48 202 23
Fax: (20) 3 48 38 916
Contact: Grants Management Officer
or
Regional Office for South-East Asia
Indraprastha Estate, Mahatma Gandhi Road, New Delhi, 110002, India
Tel: (91) 11 331 7804
Fax: (91) 11 331 8607
Contact: Grants Management Officer
or
Regional Office for the Western Pacific
PO Box 2932, Manila, Laguna, 1099, Philippines
Tel: (63) 2 521 8421
Fax: (63) 2 591 1036
Contact: Grants Management Officer
or
Regional Office for the Americas/Pan-American Sanitary Bureau
525 23rd Street NW, Washington, DC, 20037, United States of America

Tel: (1) 202 861 3200
Fax: (1) 202 223 5971
Contact: Grants Management Officer

WORLD UNIVERSITY SERVICE (WUS)

14 Dufferin Street, London, EC1Y 8PD, England
Tel: (44) 171 426 5800
Fax: (44) 171 251 1314
Contact: The Small Grants Programme

WUS Adaption Grants

Subjects: Subjects leading to professional requalification.
Eligibility: Open to refugees, including asylum seekers who wish to requalify in the UK.
Level of Study: Unrestricted.
Purpose: To assist refugees, including people with exceptional leave to remain and asylum seekers. WUS also offers an educational advisory service.
No. of awards offered: Varies.
Frequency: Dependent on funds available.
Value: A one-off payment not normally exceeding £500. Cheques will normally be made out in the name of the educational institution.
Country of Study: United Kingdom.
Application Procedure: Prospective applicants should visit WUS offices on Tuesdays and Thursdays between 10.00am-12.30pm.

SUBJECT AND ELIGIBILITY
GUIDE TO AWARDS

SUBJECT CATEGORIES

MEDICAL SCIENCES

General
Public health and hygiene
  Social/preventive medicine
  Dietetics
  Sports medicine
Health administration
Medicine and surgery
  Anaesthesiology
  Cardiology
  Dermatology
  Endocrinology
  Epidemiology
  Gastroenterology
  Geriatrics
  Gynaecology and obstetrics
  Haematology
  Hepatology
  Nephrology
  Neurology

Oncology
Ophthalmology
Otorhinolaryngology
Parasitology
Pathology
Paediatrics
Plastic surgery
Pneumology
Psychiatry and mental health
Rheumatology
Urology
Virology
Tropical medicine
Venereology
Rehabilitation medicine and therapy
Nursing
Medical auxiliaries
Midwifery
Radiology
Treatment techniques

Medical technology
Dentistry and stomatology
  Oral pathology
  Orthodontics
  Periodontics
  Community dentistry
Dental technology
  Prosthetic dentistry
Pharmacy
Biomedicine
Optometry
Podiatry
Forensic medicine and dentistry
Acupuncture
Homeopathy
Chiropractic
Osteopathy
Traditional eastern medicine

ANY SUBJECT

Any Country

AACR Career Development Awards in Cancer Research, 19

AAUW/IFUW International Fellowships, 70

AFUW Victoria Endowment Scholarship, Lady Leitch Scholarship, 58

The AFUW-SA Inc Trust Fund Bursary, 59

AIEJ Honors Scholarships, 55

Alexander Graham Bell Scholarship Awards, 12

Alexander von Humboldt Research Fellowships, 156

Anglo-Jewish Association Bursary, 45

ANU Masters Degree Scholarships (The Faculties), 62

ANU PhD Scholarships, 62

Barbara Crase Bursary, 59

Bernhard Baron Travelling Scholarships, 256

BFWG Charitable Foundation and Emergency Grants, 66

BFWG Scholarships, 71

Brasenose Senior Germaine Scholarship, 300

The British Federation Crosby Hall Fellowship, 175

Bunting Fellowship, 82

Bunting Institute Affiliation, 83

Caledonian Scholarship, 84

Carnegie Grants, 121

Carnegie Scholarships, 121

Cartmel College Scholarship Fund, 191

Cathy Candler Bursary, 59

Christ Church Senior Scholarships, 301

Churchill College Research Studentships, 292

CIMO Scholarships for Young Researchers and University Teaching Staff, 124

Colombo Plan Scholarships, Fellowships and Training Awards, 127

Corpus Christi College Research Scholarships, 293

DAAD Information Visits, 157

DAAD Research Grants for Recent PhDs and PhD Candidates, 157

DAAD Study Visit Research Grants for Faculty, 157

DAAD/AICGS Grant, 157

Datatel Scholars Foundation Scholarship, 133

Diamond Jubilee Bursary, 59

Doreen McCarthy Bursary, 59

E D Davies Scholarship, 293

Eden Travelling Fellowship, 256

Fitzwilliam College Research Fellowship, 293

GET Grants, 158

Gilchrist Expedition Award, 158

Gonville and Caius College Gonville Bursary, 294

Graduate Colleges, 139

Graduate School Scholarships, 62

Green-Armytage and Spackman Travelling Scholarship, 257

Griffith University Postgraduate Research Scholarships, 160

Henry Bradlow Scholarship, 317

Hermon Dunlap Smith Center for the History of Cartography Fellowships, 239

Hertford College Senior Scholarships, 303

HIAS Scholarship Awards, 166

Humboldt Research Award for Foreign Scholars, 13

Ian Karten Scholarship, 169

Ida Smedley Maclean, CFUW/A Vibert Douglas, IFUW and Action Fellowship, 175

IFUW International Fellowships, 71

Institute of Irish Studies Research Fellowships, 171

Institute of Irish Studies Senior Visiting Research Fellowship, 171

Izaak Walton Killam Memorial Postdoctoral Fellowships, 288

Izaak Walton Killam Memorial Scholarships, 288, 291

Izaak Walton Killam Memorial Scholarships, 288, 291

Izaak Walton Killam Postdoctoral Fellowships, 290

James Cook University Postgraduate Research Scholarship, 181

JAUW International Fellowships, 72

Keble College Keble Association Graduate Scholarship, 304

Killam Predoctoral Fellowship, 290

L B Wood Travelling Scholarship, 238

La Trobe University Postdoctoral Research Fellowship, 190

Lancaster University County College Awards, 192

Learn 'German in Germany' for Faculty, 158

Linacre College Domus Studentships, 305

Magdalene College Leslie Wilson Research Scholarships, 294

Margaret K B Day Memorial Scholarships, 72

Max-Planck Award for International Co-operation, 13

Menopause Travel Award, 258

Mental Health Foundation Grants in Aid of Travel During Medical Students Elective Periods, 203

Merton College Senior Scholarships, 306

Michigan Society of Fellows Postdoctoral Fellowships, 203

Mr and Mrs Spencer T Olin Fellowships for Women, 325

National Black MBA Association Scholarships, 212

NCAA Postgraduate Scholarship, 216

Newby Trust Awards, 239

NSERC New Faculty Support Grants, 234

Ontario Graduate Scholarship Programme, 242

Overseas Postgraduate Research Scholarships (OPRS), 137

Peel Awards, 192

Pembroke College Graduate Awards, 294

Peterhouse Research Fellowship, 247

Peterhouse Research Studentship, 247

Pirie-Reid Scholarships, 308

Postdoctoral Humboldt Research Fellowships, 14

Queen's College Research Fellowships, 295

Queen's University of Belfast Visiting Fellowships, 250

Queen's University of Belfast Visiting Studentships, 250

Queensland University of Technology Postdoctoral Research Fellowship, 250

Regent's Park College (Permanent Private Hall) Organ Scholarship, 309

Regina Graduate Scholarships, 314

Regina Teaching Assistantships, 314

Rotary Foundation Academic Year Ambassadorial Scholarships, 254

Rotary Foundation Multi-Year Ambassadorial Scholarships, 255

Rotary Grants for University Teachers to Serve in Developing Countries, 255

SAAUW International Fellowship, 277

Scholarships for International Students Only, 63

Sidney Sussex College Research Studentship, 267

SOEID Personal Research Fellowships, 262

SOEID/RSE Support Research Fellowships, 263

African Nations

Australia

Fellowships and Grants for Study and Research in Scandinavia, 44
Fulbright Graduate Student Awards, 322
Fulbright Scholar Grants, 322
John Dana Archbold Fellowship, 210, 240
John Dana Archbold Fellowship Program, 240
Kosciuszko Foundation Graduate and Postgraduate Studies and Research in Poland Program, 189
Lincoln College Keith Murray Senior Scholarship, 305
Merton College Graduate Entrance Scholarships, 306
North Dakota Indian Scholarship, 239
Queen's College Wendell Herbruck Studentship, 308
Rhodes Scholarships, 309
Somerville College Oxford Bursary for American Graduates (Janet Watson Bursary), 310
The SSRC Soviet Union and Successor States Graduate Training Fellowships, 274
St Andrew's Society of the State of New York Scholarship, 281
St Anne's College Overseas Scholarship, 310
St Catherine's College Overseas Graduate Scholarship, 310
St Peter's College Leonard J Theberge Memorial Scholarship, 312

US-UK Fulbright Commission Postdoctoral Research Scholarship at De Montfort University, 322
USC All-University Predoctoral Diversity Fellowships, 315
USIA Fulbright Study and Research Grants for US Citizens, 323

West European Countries

AAUW International Fellowships Program, 3
British-German Academic Research Collaboration (ARC) Programme, 68
Canon Foundation Visiting Research Fellowships/Professorships, 120
Christ Church Hugh Pilkinton Scholarship, 301
CIMO Bilateral Scholarships, 124
CIMO Nordic Scholarship Scheme for the Baltic Countries and Northwest Russia, 124
Clare Hall Foundation Fellowship, 293
Denmark-America Foundation Grants, 135
Department of Education and Science (Ireland) Exchange Scholarships and Postgraduate Scholarships Exchange Scheme, 136
DoE (Ireland) Summer School Exchange Scholarships, 136
ERASMUS Grants, 128
Feodor Lynen Research Fellowships for German Scholars, 13

Japan Society for the Promotion of Science (JSPS) Research Fellowships, 13
John Dana Archbold Fellowship Program, 240
Lincoln College Berrow Scholarship, 305
Lincoln College Dresdner Kleinwort Benson Senior Scholarships, 305
Merton College Graduate Entrance Scholarships, 306
Merton College Greendale Senior Scholarships, 306
Mr and Mrs David Edward Roberts Memorial Award, 318
Norwegian Government Scholarship for Foreign Students, 252
PEO International Peace Scholarship, 178
Prendergast Bequest, 308
Scholarships for Postgraduate Studies in Greece, 282
Science and Technology Agency (STA) Research Fellowships, 14
St Anne's College Overseas Scholarship, 310
St Catherine's College Overseas Graduate Scholarship, 310
University of Wales (Bangor) Postgraduate Studentships, 318
Wadham College Norwegian Scholarship, 312

MEDICAL SCIENCES

GENERAL

Any Country

AACR Gerald B Grindley Memorial Young Investigator Award, 20
AACR Peczoller International Award for Cancer Research, 20
AACR Susan G Komen Breast Cancer Foundation Career Development Award, 21
Action Research Programme Grants, 4
Action Research Project Grants, 4
Action Research Training Fellowship, 4
AHA Grant-in-Aid, 34
AIATSIS Research Grants, 61
Airey Neave Trust Award, 9
Alberta Heritage Clinical Fellowships, 9
Alberta Heritage Clinical Investigatorships, 10

Alberta Heritage Full-Time Fellowships, 10
Alberta Heritage Full-Time Studentships, 10
Alberta Heritage Medical Scholarships, 10
Alberta Heritage Medical Scientist Awards, 10
Alberta Heritage Part-Time Fellowships, 11
Alberta Heritage Part-Time Studentship, 11
Alzheimer's Association Investigator-Initiated Research Grants, 14
Alzheimer's Association Pilot Research Grants, 14
American Cancer Society Award for Research Excellence in Cancer Epidemiology and Prevention, 21
American Lung Association Career Investigator Awards, 36

American Lung Association Clinical Research Grants, 37
American Lung Association Research Grants, 37
American Lung Association Research Training Fellowships, 37
Apex Foundation Annual Research Grants, 45
APMA Research Grant Program, 41
ASHA Research Fellowship Fund, 42
Asthma Society of Canada Research Grants, 57
Basic Clinical and Translational Breast Cancer Research, 282
Basil O'Connor Starter Scholar Research Award Program, 196
British Diabetic Association Equipment Grant, 69
British Diabetic Association Project Grants, 69

South African MRC Travel Grants to International Scientific Meetings, 281
South African MRC Travel Grants to Local Scientific Meetings, 281

South America

AACR Research Fellowships, 21
Fulbright Postdoctoral Research and Lecturing Awards for Non-US Citizens, 155
International Fellowships in Medical Education, 143
Pembroke College Jose Gregorio Hernandez Award of the Venezuelan National Academy of Medicine, 307
Pew Latin American Fellows Program, 247
Richard and Hinda Rosenthal Foundation Award, 22

United Kingdom

BHF Research Awards, 75
CFRT Research Grants, 133
Frank Knox Fellowships at Harvard University, 154
Fulbright Postdoctoral Research and Lecturing Awards for Non-US Citizens, 155
Green-Armytage Anglo American Lectureship, 257
The Grundy Educational Trust, 160
Harkness Fellowships in Health Care Policy, 128
Huntingtons Disease Association Research Grant, 168
Insole Research Award, 79
International Fellowships in Medical Education, 143
Joan Dawkins Fellowship, 79
John Fyffe Memorial Fellowship, 76
Kennedy Scholarships, 187
Medical Missionary Association Grants, 197
Moynihan Travelling Fellowship, 56
Nathaniel Bishop Harman Research Award, 79
Polish Embassy Short-Term Bursaries, 248
Regent's Park College (Permanent Private Hall) J W Lord Scholarship, 309
Royal Society Research Grants, 261
Sir Charles Hastings and Charles Oliver Hawthorne Research Awards, 80
Smith and Nephew Foundation Medical Research Fellowships, 273
Wingate Scholarships, 326

USA

AACR EN Young Investigator Awards for Asian Scientists, 20

AACR HBCU Faculty Award in Cancer Research, 20
AACR Research Fellowships, 21
AHA Established Investigator Grant, 34
AHA Scientist Development Grant, 35
Alcohol Beverage Medical Research Foundation Research Project Grant, 12
ASLHF Graduate Student Scholarship, 42
ASLHF New Investigator Research Grant, 42
ASLHF Student Research in Clinical Rehabilitative Audiology, 43
ASLHF Student Research in Early Childhood Language Development, 43
ASLHF Young Scholars Award for Minority Students, 43
Belgian-American Educational Foundation Graduate Fellowships for Study in Belgium, 65
British Schools and Universities Foundation, Inc. Scholarships, 82
CFF Research Programmes in Cystic Fibrosis, 132
CFF Training Programmes in Cystic Fibrosis, 133
Duke University Center Postdoctoral Training in Ageing Research, 142
Federal Chancellor Scholarship, 13
Fellowship of the Flemish Community, 149
Fulbright Scholar Awards for Research and Lecturing Abroad, 131
Gertrude B Elion Cancer Research Award, 22
Green-Armytage Anglo American Lectureship, 257
IFEBP Grants for Research, 177
John P Utz Postdoctoral Fellowship in Medical Mycology, 217
Joseph Collins Foundation Grants, 186
Kala Singh Graduate Scholarship, 43
Leslie Isenberg Award, 43
Mount Desert Island New Investigator Award, 206
Native American Scholarship Program, 234
New Investigator Matching Grants, 217
NFID Fellowship in Infectious Diseases, 217
NFID New Investigator Matching Grants, 218
NFID Postdoctoral Fellowship in Nosocomial Infection Research and Training, 218
NLM Fellowship in Applied Informatics, 228
NLM Investigator Initiated Project Grant, 229
NLM Publication Grant Programme, 229
NORD Clinical Research Grants, 231

Parker B Francis Fellowship Program, 246
Postdoctoral Training Programme in Addiction and Mental Health, 124
Richard and Hinda Rosenthal Foundation Award, 22

West European Countries

Belgian-American Educational Foundation Graduate Fellowships for Study in the USA, 65
Fulbright Postdoctoral Research and Lecturing Awards for Non-US Citizens, 155
Henry Dryerre Scholarship, 262
International Fellowships in Medical Education, 143
Postgraduate Fellowships for Study in the USA, 66
Queen's College Florey EPA Scholarship, 308
Scholarship Foundation of the League for Finnish-American Societies, 266
Wingate Scholarships, 326

PUBLIC HEALTH AND HYGIENE

Any Country

The BNF/Nestlé Bursary Scheme, 80
CIAR Postdoctoral Fellowships, 122
CIAR Research Contract, 122
Dissertation Research Award, 283
Dr Sydney Segal Research Grants, 115
Grants-in-Aid, 274
IARC Fellowships for Research Training in Cancer, 172
Mobil-NUS Postgraduate Medical Research Scholarship, 233
Population Council Fellowships in Population and Social Sciences, 249
Postdoctoral Fellowship in Breast Cancer Research, Public Health or Epidemiology, 283
Roche Research Foundation, 254
The Sir Allan Sewell Visiting Fellowship, 160
Thrasher Research and Field Demonstration Project Grants, 286
University of Glasgow Postgraduate Scholarships, 296
University Postgraduate Scholarships, 290
WCRF Research Grant, 328

Australia

Biomedical and Medical Postgraduate
Research Scholarships, 57
Dora Lush (Biomedical) and Public
Health Postgraduate Scholarships, 220
Medical Research Project Grant, 57
New South Wales Cancer Council
Research Programme Grant, 237
New South Wales Cancer Council
Research Project Grants, 237
NHMRC Medical and Dental and Public
Health Postgraduate Research
Scholarships, 221
Wingate Scholarships, 326

British Commonwealth

Wingate Scholarships, 326

Canada

Alcohol Beverage Medical Research
Foundation Research Project Grant, 12
Canadian Window on Instrumental
Development, 174
Frank Knox Memorial Fellowships at
Harvard University, 56
Personnel Awards, 137
Wingate Scholarships, 326

East European Countries

AAAS Travel Fellowships for Young
Scientists on Problems of Environment
and Health, 40

Indian Sub-Continent

Wingate Scholarships, 326

Middle East

Wingate Scholarships, 326

South Africa

South African MRC Staff Development
and Credentialling Grants, 280

United Kingdom

Brackenbury Research Award, 78
Wingate Scholarships, 326

USA

Alcohol Beverage Medical Research
Foundation Research Project Grant, 12
Atlantic Fellowships in Public Policy,
128
Grants for Innovative Methods for
Control of Tick-Borne Diseases, 37
NIH Research Grants, 227
NLM Fellowship in Applied Informatics,
228

Wyeth Ayerst Scholarship for Women in
Graduate Medical and Health Business
Programs, 83

West European Countries

Scholarship Foundation of the League
for Finnish-American Societies, 266
Wingate Scholarships, 326

SOCIAL/PREVENTIVE MEDICINE

Any Country

American Cancer Society International
Fellowships for Beginning
Investigators, 25, 212
ASBAH Research Grant, 54
The BNF/Nestlé Bursary Scheme, 80
Collaborative Research Projects, 274
Dr Sydney Segal Research Grants, 115
IARC Fellowships for Research Training
in Cancer, 172
International Cancer Research
Technology Transfer Project (ICRETT),
179
National Back Pain Association
Research Grants, 212
Queen Elizabeth the Queen Mother
Fellowship Award, 252
Research Grant, 39, 324
Research into Ageing Prize
Studentships, 253
Research into Ageing Research Grants,
253
Services to Academia, 274
Translational Cancer Research
Fellowships (TRCF), 180
University Postgraduate Scholarships,
290
WCRF Research Grant, 328

Australia

Biomedical and Medical Postgraduate
Research Scholarships, 57
Medical Research Project Grant, 57
Nepean Postgraduate Research Award,
320
Wingate Scholarships, 326

British Commonwealth

Wingate Scholarships, 326

Canada

Canadian Window on Instrumental
Development, 174
IFEBP Grants for Research, 177

The Kidney Foundation of Canada Allied
Health Doctoral Fellowship, 187
The Kidney Foundation of Canada Allied
Health Research Grant, 187
The Kidney Foundation of Canada Allied
Health Scholarship, 187
KidsAction Research Fellowships and
Grants, 188
Wingate Scholarships, 326

East European Countries

AAAS Travel Fellowships for Young
Scientists on Problems of Environment
and Health, 40

Indian Sub-Continent

Wingate Scholarships, 326

Middle East

Wingate Scholarships, 326

New Zealand

National Heart Foundation of New
Zealand Fellowships, 224
National Heart Foundation of New
Zealand Grants-in-Aid, 224
National Heart Foundation of New
Zealand Project Grants, 224
National Heart Foundation of New
Zealand Travel Grants, 224
Nepean Postgraduate Research Award,
320

United Kingdom

Brackenbury Research Award, 78
Katherine Bishop Harman Research
Award, 79
T P Gunton Research Award, 80
Wingate Scholarships, 326

USA

The Arc of the United States Research
Grant, 46
Arthritis Investigator Award, 48
Grants for Innovative Methods for
Control of Tick-Borne Diseases, 37
IFEBP Grants for Research, 177

West European Countries

Wingate Scholarships, 326

DIETETICS

Any Country

The Bio-Serv Award in Experimental
Animal Nutrition, 35
The BNF/Nestlé Bursary Scheme, 80
The Cenrium Center for Nutritional
Science Award, 35
The Conrad A Elvehjem Award for
Public Service in Nutrition, 36
The E L R Stokstad Award, 36
The Mead Johnson Award, 36
The Osborne and Mendel Award, 36
Queen Elizabeth the Queen Mother
Fellowship Award, 252
Research into Ageing Prize
Studentships, 253
Research into Ageing Research Grants,
253
Royal Irish Academy National
Committee for Nutritional Sciences
Award, 261

Australia

Wingate Scholarships, 326

British Commonwealth

Wingate Scholarships, 326

Canada

The Kidney Foundation of Canada Allied
Health Doctoral Fellowship, 187
The Kidney Foundation of Canada Allied
Health Research Grant, 187
The Kidney Foundation of Canada Allied
Health Scholarship, 187
Wingate Scholarships, 326

Indian Sub-Continent

Wingate Scholarships, 326

Middle East

Wingate Scholarships, 326

New Zealand

National Heart Foundation of New
Zealand Fellowships, 224
National Heart Foundation of New
Zealand Grants-in-Aid, 224
National Heart Foundation of New
Zealand Project Grants, 224
National Heart Foundation of New
Zealand Travel Grants, 224

United Kingdom

Wingate Scholarships, 326

West European Countries

Wingate Scholarships, 326

SPORTS MEDICINE

Any Country

APMA Research Grant Program, 41
Bristol-Myers Squibb/Zimmer Research
Grant for Excellence in Orthapedaedic
Treatment, 244
NSCA Challenge Scholarship, 232
NSCA Student Grant Research Grant,
232
OREF Career Development Award, 244
OREF Prospective Clinical Research,
244
OREF Research Grants, 244
OREF Resident Research Award, 244
Queen Elizabeth the Queen Mother
Fellowship Award, 252
Research into Ageing Prize
Studentships, 253
Research into Ageing Research Grants,
253
University of Glasgow Postgraduate
Scholarships, 296
University Postgraduate Scholarships,
290

Australia

Wingate Scholarships, 326

British Commonwealth

Wingate Scholarships, 326

Canada

AAOS/OREF Fellowship in Health
Services Research, 243
OREF Clinical Research Award, 244
Wingate Scholarships, 326

Indian Sub-Continent

Wingate Scholarships, 326

Middle East

Wingate Scholarships, 326

United Kingdom

Duke of Edinburgh Prize for Sports
Medicine, 171
The Robert Atkins Award, 171
Wingate Scholarships, 326

USA

AAOS/OREF Fellowship in Health
Services Research, 243
Arthritis Foundation Biomedical Science
Grant, 46
Arthritis Foundation Clinical Science
Grant, 47
Arthritis Foundation New Investigator
Grant, 47
Arthritis Investigator Award, 48
OREF Clinical Research Award, 244

West European Countries

Wingate Scholarships, 326

HEALTH
ADMINISTRATION

Any Country

Roche Research Foundation, 254
Savoy Foundation Post Doctoral and
Clinical Research Fellowships, 266
Savoy Foundation Research Grants,
266
Savoy Foundation Studentships, 266
The Sir Allan Sewell Visiting Fellowship,
160
University of Glasgow Postgraduate
Scholarships, 296
University of New England Research
Scholarships, 299
University Postgraduate Scholarships,
290

Australia

New South Wales Cancer Council
Research Project Grants, 237
Wingate Scholarships, 326

British Commonwealth

Wingate Scholarships, 326

Canada

Albert W Dent Student Scholarships,
153
Foster G McGaw Student Scholarships,
154
Wingate Scholarships, 326

Indian Sub-Continent

Wingate Scholarships, 326

Middle East

Wingate Scholarships, 326

South Africa

South African MRC Staff Development and Credentialling Grants, 280

United Kingdom

Wingate Scholarships, 326

USA

Albert W Dent Student Scholarships, 153

Arthritis Foundation Clinical Science Grant, 47

Arthritis Foundation New Investigator Grant, 47

Arthritis Investigator Award, 48

Foster G McGaw Student Scholarships, 154

New York Life Foundation Scholarship for Women in the Health Professions Program, 83

NLM Fellowship in Applied Informatics, 228

Wyeth Ayerst Scholarship for Women in Graduate Medical and Health Business Programs, 83

West European Countries

Scholarship Foundation of the League for Finnish-American Societies, 266

Wingate Scholarships, 326

MEDICINE AND SURGERY

Any Country

AAFPRS Investigator Development Grant, 17

APMA Research Grant Program, 41

Bristol-Myers Squibb/Zimmer Research Grant for Excellence in Orthapedaedic Treatment, 244

British Lung Foundation Project Grants, 77

British Medical and Dental Students' Trust Scholarships and Travel Grants, 77

CAMS Scholarship, 126

Canadian Cystic Fibrosis Foundation Research Grants Scholarships for Research in Cystic Fibrosis, 112

Canadian Cystic Fibrosis Foundation Studentships, 113

Ethicon Foundation Fund, 257, 260

FRAXA Postdoctoral Fellowship, 155

Grants-in-Aid, 274

Humanitarian Trust Awards, 168

ISH Postdoctoral Fellowship, 152

John of Arderne Medal, 263

Lee Foundation and Tan Sri Dr Runme Shaw Foundation Fellowships in Orthopaedic Surgery, 233

Lionel Colledge Memorial Fellowship in Otolaryngology, 260

Lister Institute Senior Research Fellowships, 195

Medical Insurance Agency Prize, 264

Michael Geisman Memorial Fellowship Fund, 245

Mobil-NUS Postgraduate Medical Research Scholarship, 233

National Back Pain Association Research Grants, 212

Norman Capener Travelling Fellowships, 260

Norman Tanner Medal and Prize, 264

Novartis Foundation Symposium Bursaries, 241

OREF Career Development Award, 244

OREF Prospective Clinical Research, 244

OREF Research Grants, 244

OREF Resident Research Award, 244

Osteogenesis Imperfecta Foundation Seed Research Grant, 245

Roche Research Foundation, 254

Savoy Foundation Post Doctoral and Clinical Research Fellowships, 266

Savoy Foundation Research Grants, 266

Savoy Foundation Studentships, 266

Sir Richard Stapley Educational Trust Grants, 272

University of Glasgow Postgraduate Scholarships, 296

University Postgraduate Scholarships, 290

Visiting Scientist Awards, 113

WellBeing Project Grants, 325

Zeneca Pharmaceuticals Underserved Healthcare Grant, 39

Australia

Biomedical and Medical Postgraduate Research Scholarships, 57

Foundation for High Blood Pressure Research Postdoctoral Fellowship, 151

Medical Research Project Grant, 57

NHMRC Medical and Dental and Public Health Postgraduate Research Scholarships, 221

Postgraduate Scholarship (sponsored by BioMérieux-Vitek Australia and AIMS), 61

Wingate Scholarships, 326

British Commonwealth

Wingate Scholarships, 326

Canada

AAFPRS Resident Research Grants, 17

AAOS/OREF Fellowship in Health Services Research, 243

Bernstein Grant, 17

Canadian Cystic Fibrosis Foundation Fellowships, 112

Canadian Cystic Fibrosis Foundation Research Grants, 112

KidsAction Research Fellowships and Grants, 188

OREF Clinical Research Award, 244

Postdoctoral Training Programme in Addiction and Mental Health, 124

Wingate Scholarships, 326

East European Countries

Salzburg Seminars for Physicians, 242

Indian Sub-Continent

Wingate Scholarships, 326

Middle East

Wingate Scholarships, 326

New Zealand

Foundation for High Blood Pressure Research Postdoctoral Fellowship, 151

United Kingdom

Moynihan Travelling Fellowship, 56

Polish Embassy Short-Term Bursaries, 248

Wingate Scholarships, 326

USA

AAFPRS Resident Research Grants, 17

AAOS/OREF Fellowship in Health Services Research, 243

Bernstein Grant, 17

NLM Fellowship in Applied Informatics, 228

OREF Clinical Research Award, 244

Postdoctoral Training Programme in Addiction and Mental Health, 124

Wyeth Ayerst Scholarship for Women in Graduate Medical and Health Business Programs, 83

West European Countries

Wingate Scholarships, 326

ANAESTHESIOLOGY

Any Country

Mobil-NUS Postgraduate Medical
Research Scholarship, 233
National Back Pain Association
Research Grants, 212
Queen Elizabeth the Queen Mother
Fellowship Award, 252
Research into Ageing Prize
Studentships, 253
Research into Ageing Research Grants,
253
University Postgraduate Scholarships,
290

Australia

Wingate Scholarships, 326

British Commonwealth

Wingate Scholarships, 326

Canada

Wingate Scholarships, 326

Indian Sub-Continent

Wingate Scholarships, 326

Middle East

Wingate Scholarships, 326

United Kingdom

Wingate Scholarships, 326

USA

NORD Clinical Research Grants, 231

West European Countries

Wingate Scholarships, 326

CARDIOLOGY

Any Country

AHA Grant-in-Aid, 34
AHAF National Heart Foundation, 33
BHF PhD Studentships, 75
Collaborative Research Projects, 274
Lister Institute Senior Research
Fellowships, 195
Services to Academia, 274
University Postgraduate Scholarships,
290

African Nations

BHF Overseas Visiting Fellowships, 74
Warren McDonald International
Fellowship, 223

Australia

BHF Overseas Visiting Fellowships, 74
National Heart Foundation of Australia
Overseas Research Fellowships, 223
National Heart Foundation of Australia
Postgraduate (Non-Medical) Research
Scholarship, 223
National Heart Foundation of Australia
Postgraduate Medical Research
Scholarship, 223
National Heart Foundation of Australia
Research Grants-in-Aid, 223
Wingate Scholarships, 326

British Commonwealth

Wingate Scholarships, 326

Canada

Alcohol Beverage Medical Research
Foundation Research Project Grant, 12
BHF Overseas Visiting Fellowships, 74
Warren McDonald International
Fellowship, 223
Wingate Scholarships, 326

Caribbean Countries

Warren McDonald International
Fellowship, 223

East European Countries

BHF Overseas Visiting Fellowships, 74
Warren McDonald International
Fellowship, 223

Far East

BHF Overseas Visiting Fellowships, 74
Warren McDonald International
Fellowship, 223

Indian Sub-Continent

BHF Overseas Visiting Fellowships, 74
Warren McDonald International
Fellowship, 223
Wingate Scholarships, 326

Middle East

BHF Overseas Visiting Fellowships, 74
Warren McDonald International
Fellowship, 223
Wingate Scholarships, 326

New Zealand

BHF Overseas Visiting Fellowships, 74
National Heart Foundation of New
Zealand Fellowships, 224
National Heart Foundation of New
Zealand Grants-in-Aid, 224
National Heart Foundation of New
Zealand Project Grants, 224
National Heart Foundation of New
Zealand Travel Grants, 224
Warren McDonald International
Fellowship, 223

South Africa

BHF Overseas Visiting Fellowships, 74
Warren McDonald International
Fellowship, 223

South America

BHF Overseas Visiting Fellowships, 74
Warren McDonald International
Fellowship, 223

United Kingdom

BHF Clinical Science Fellowships, 73
BHF Intermediate Research
Fellowships, 74
BHF Junior Research Fellowships, 74
BHF Senior Research Fellowships, 75
BHF Travelling Fellowships, 75
Geoffrey Holt, Ivy Powell and Edith
Walsh Research Awards, 78
Warren McDonald International
Fellowship, 223
Wingate Scholarships, 326

USA

AHA Established Investigator Grant, 34
AHA Scientist Development Grant, 35
Alcohol Beverage Medical Research
Foundation Research Project Grant, 12
American Society of
Hypertension/Hoechst Marion Roussel
Clinical Fellowship in Hypertension, 42
BHF Overseas Visiting Fellowships, 74
NORD Clinical Research Grants, 231
Warren McDonald International
Fellowship, 223

West European Countries

BHF Overseas Visiting Fellowships, 74
Warren McDonald International
Fellowship, 223
Wingate Scholarships, 326

DERMATOLOGY

Any Country

DEBRA Medical Research Grant
Scheme, 134
LEPRA Grants, 193
Lister Institute Senior Research
Fellowships, 195
University Postgraduate Scholarships,
290

Australia

New South Wales Cancer Council
Research Programme Grant, 237
New South Wales Cancer Council
Research Project Grants, 237
Wingate Scholarships, 326

British Commonwealth

Wingate Scholarships, 326

Canada

Wingate Scholarships, 326

Indian Sub-Continent

Wingate Scholarships, 326

Middle East

Wingate Scholarships, 326

United Kingdom

Wingate Scholarships, 326

USA

NORD Clinical Research Grants, 231

West European Countries

Wingate Scholarships, 326

ENDOCRINOLOGY

Any Country

British Diabetic Association Equipment
Grant, 69
British Diabetic Association Project
Grants, 69
British Diabetic Association Research
Fellowships, 70
British Diabetic Association Research
Studentships, 70
British Diabetic Association Small Grant
Scheme, 70
Collaborative Research Projects, 274

Diabetes Development Project, 70
Grants-in-Aid, 274
Lister Institute Senior Research
Fellowships, 195
OFAS Grants, 243
Services to Academia, 274
University Postgraduate Scholarships,
290
WellBeing Project Grants, 325

Australia

Wingate Scholarships, 326

British Commonwealth

Wingate Scholarships, 326

Canada

Alcohol Beverage Medical Research
Foundation Research Project Grant, 12
KidsAction Research Fellowships and
Grants, 188
Wingate Scholarships, 326

Indian Sub-Continent

Wingate Scholarships, 326

Middle East

Wingate Scholarships, 326

United Kingdom

Wingate Scholarships, 326

USA

Alcohol Beverage Medical Research
Foundation Research Project Grant, 12
NIH Research Grants, 227
NORD Clinical Research Grants, 231

West European Countries

Wingate Scholarships, 326

EPIDEMIOLOGY

Any Country

AHAF National Heart Foundation, 33
Alzheimer's Disease Research Grant, 34
American Cancer Society International
Fellowships for Beginning
Investigators, 25, 212
ASHA Research Fellowship Fund, 42
Basic Clinical and Translational Breast
Cancer Research, 282
CIAR Postdoctoral Fellowships, 122
CIAR Research Contract, 122
Collaborative Research Projects, 274

Dissertation Research Award, 283
Dr Sydney Segal Research Grants, 115
Grants-in-Aid, 274
Health Research Board Grants,
Fellowships and Projects, 163
IARC Fellowships for Research Training
in Cancer, 172
ICR Research Studentships, 170
Imaging Technology, 283
International Cancer Research
Technology Transfer Project (ICRETT),
179
Lister Institute Senior Research
Fellowships, 195
National Back Pain Association
Research Grants, 212
OFAS Grants, 243
Population Council Fellowships in
Population and Social Sciences, 249
Population Specfic Research Project,
283
Postdoctoral Fellowship in Breast
Cancer Research, Public Health or
Epidemiology, 283
Queen Elizabeth the Queen Mother
Fellowship Award, 252
Research into Ageing Prize
Studentships, 253
Research into Ageing Research Grants,
253
Services to Academia, 274
University of Dundee Research Awards,
295
University Postgraduate Scholarships,
290
WCRF Research Grant, 328

Australia

Asthma Victoria Research Grants, 57
Lilian Roxon Memorial Research Trust
Travel Grant, 58
New South Wales Cancer Council
Research Programme Grant, 237
New South Wales Cancer Council
Research Project Grants, 237
Wingate Scholarships, 326

British Commonwealth

Wingate Scholarships, 326

Canada

Alcohol Beverage Medical Research
Foundation Research Project Grant, 12
CNF Scholarships and Fellowships, 116
Heritage Health Research Career
Renewal Awards, 11
KidsAction Research Fellowships and
Grants, 188
Wingate Scholarships, 326

East European Countries

AAAS Travel Fellowships for Young
Scientists on Problems of Environment
and Health, 40

Indian Sub-Continent

Wingate Scholarships, 326

Middle East

Wingate Scholarships, 326

New Zealand

National Heart Foundation of New
Zealand Fellowships, 224
National Heart Foundation of New
Zealand Grants-in-Aid, 224
National Heart Foundation of New
Zealand Project Grants, 224
National Heart Foundation of New
Zealand Travel Grants, 224

United Kingdom

Parkinson's Disease Society Medical
Research Project Grant, 246
Wingate Scholarships, 326

USA

Alcohol Beverage Medical Research
Foundation Research Project Grant, 12
American Society of
Hypertension/Hoechst Marion Roussel
Clinical Fellowship in Hypertension, 42
NFID Postdoctoral Fellowship in
Emerging Infectious Diseases, 218
NORD Clinical Research Grants, 231

West European Countries

Wingate Scholarships, 326

GASTROENTEROLOGY

Any Country

Collaborative Research Projects, 274
Elsevier Research Initiative Award, 29
Endoscopic Multicenter/Comparative
Trials Award, 29
Grants-in-Aid, 274
Industry Research Scholar Awards, 30
Innovative Seed Grants in Basic
Research in Liver Diseases, 30
Lister Institute Senior Research
Fellowships, 195
Miles and Shirley Fiterman Foundation
Basic Research Awards, 30

Miles and Shirley Fiterman Foundation
Clinical Research in Gastroenterology
or Hepatology/Nutrition Awards, 31
Olympus Endoscopic Career
Enhancement Awards, 31
Outcomes Research Training Awards,
31
Queen Elizabeth the Queen Mother
Fellowship Award, 252
R Robert and Sally D Funderburg
Research Scholar Award in Gastric
Biology Related to Cancer, 31
Research into Ageing Prize
Studentships, 253
Research into Ageing Research Grants,
253
Services to Academia, 274
Student Research Fellowship Awards,
32
TAP Pharmaceuticals, Inc. Outcomes
Research Awards, 32
Thrasher Research and Field
Demonstration Project Grants, 286
University Postgraduate Scholarships,
290
Wilson-Cook Endoscopic Research
Career Development Awards, 32

Australia

Wingate Scholarships, 326

British Commonwealth

Wingate Scholarships, 326

Canada

Alcohol Beverage Medical Research
Foundation Research Project Grant, 12
Wingate Scholarships, 326

Indian Sub-Continent

Wingate Scholarships, 326

Middle East

Wingate Scholarships, 326

United Kingdom

Digestive Disorders Foundation
Fellowships and Grants, 141
Wingate Scholarships, 326

USA

Alcohol Beverage Medical Research
Foundation Research Project Grant, 12
NORD Clinical Research Grants, 231

West European Countries

Wingate Scholarships, 326

GERIATRICS

Any Country

Grants-in-Aid, 274
Lister Institute Senior Research
Fellowships, 195
Queen Elizabeth the Queen Mother
Fellowship Award, 252
Research into Ageing Prize
Studentships, 253
Research into Ageing Research Grants,
253
University Postgraduate Scholarships,
290
Wilson-Fulton and Robertson Awards in
Ageing Research, Cecille Gould
Memorial Fund Award in Cancer
Research, Richard Shepherd
Fellowship, 33

Australia

Wingate Scholarships, 326

British Commonwealth

Wingate Scholarships, 326

Canada

Alcohol Beverage Medical Research
Foundation Research Project Grant, 12
Wingate Scholarships, 326

Indian Sub-Continent

Wingate Scholarships, 326

Middle East

Wingate Scholarships, 326

South Africa

Zerilda Steyn Memorial Trust, 277

United Kingdom

Parkinson's Disease Society Medical
Research Project Grant, 246
Wingate Scholarships, 326

USA

Alcohol Beverage Medical Research
Foundation Research Project Grant, 12
NIH Research Grants, 227
NORD Clinical Research Grants, 231

West European Countries

Wingate Scholarships, 326

GYNAECOLOGY AND OBSTETRICS

Any Country

Edgar Research Fellowship, 257
Grants-in-Aid, 274
Lister Institute Senior Research
  Fellowships, 195
Mobil-NUS Postgraduate Medical
  Research Scholarship, 233
National Back Pain Association
  Research Grants, 212
University of Dundee Research Awards,
  295
University Postgraduate Scholarships,
  290
WellBeing Project Grants, 325

African Nations

Young Obstetrician/Gynaecologist
  Fellowship, 259

Australia

New South Wales Cancer Council
  Research Programme Grant, 237
New South Wales Cancer Council
  Research Project Grants, 237
Wingate Scholarships, 326

British Commonwealth

Wingate Scholarships, 326

Canada

ACOG/3M Pharmaceuticals Research
  Award in Lower Genital Infections, 25
ACOG/Cytyc Corporation Research
  Award for the Prevention of Cervical
  Cancer, 26
ACOG/Ethicon Research Award for
  Innovations in Gynecological Surgery,
  26
ACOG/Merck Award for Research in
  Migraine Management in Women's
  Healthcare, 26
ACOG/Organon, Inc. Research Award in
  Contraception, 27
ACOG/Ortho-McNeil Academic Training
  Fellowships in Obstetrics and
  Gynecology, 27
ACOG/Parke-Davis Research Award to
  Advance the Management of Women's
  Healthcare, 27
ACOG/Pharmacia and Upjohn Research
  Award in Urogynecology of the
  Postreproductive Woman, 27

ACOG/Searle Research Award in
  Gynecologic Infections and Their
  Complications, 28
ACOG/Solvay Pharmaceuticals
  Research Award in Menopause, 28
KidsAction Research Fellowships and
  Grants, 188
Warren H Pearse/Wyeth-Ayerst
  Women's Health Policy Research
  Award, 28
Wingate Scholarships, 326

East European Countries

Young Obstetrician/Gynaecologist
  Fellowship, 259

Indian Sub-Continent

Wingate Scholarships, 326
Young Obstetrician/Gynaecologist
  Fellowship, 259

Middle East

Wingate Scholarships, 326

United Kingdom

Green-Armytage Anglo American
  Lectureship, 257
Katherine Bishop Harman Research
  Award, 79
Nichols Fellowship, 264
Wingate Scholarships, 326

USA

ACOG/3M Pharmaceuticals Research
  Award in Lower Genital Infections, 25
ACOG/Cytyc Corporation Research
  Award for the Prevention of Cervical
  Cancer, 26
ACOG/Ethicon Research Award for
  Innovations in Gynecological Surgery,
  26
ACOG/Merck Award for Research in
  Migraine Management in Women's
  Healthcare, 26
ACOG/Novartis Pharmaceuticals
  Fellowship for Research in
  Endocrinology of the Postreproductive
  Woman, 26
ACOG/Organon, Inc. Research Award in
  Contraception, 27
ACOG/Ortho-McNeil Academic Training
  Fellowships in Obstetrics and
  Gynecology, 27
ACOG/Parke-Davis Research Award to
  Advance the Management of Women's
  Healthcare, 27
ACOG/Pharmacia and Upjohn Research
  Award in Urogynecology of the
  Postreproductive Woman, 27

ACOG/Searle Research Award in
  Gynecologic Infections and Their
  Complications, 28
ACOG/Solvay Pharmaceuticals
  Research Award in Menopause, 28
Green-Armytage Anglo American
  Lectureship, 257
NORD Clinical Research Grants, 231
Warren H Pearse/Wyeth-Ayerst
  Women's Health Policy Research
  Award, 28

West European Countries

Wingate Scholarships, 326

HAEMATOLOGY

Any Country

Cooley's Anemia Foundation Research
  Fellowship Grant, 131
Gordon Piller Studentships, 193
ICR Research Studentships, 170
Lady Tata Memorial Trust Scholarships,
  191
Leukaemia Research Fund Clinical
  Research Fellowship, 193
Leukaemia Research Fund Clinical
  Training Fellowship, 193
Leukaemia Research Fund Grant
  Programme, 194
Leukaemia Research Fund Grant
  Project, 194
Leukemia Research Fund Awards, 194
Lister Institute Senior Research
  Fellowships, 195
Queen Elizabeth the Queen Mother
  Fellowship Award, 252
Research into Ageing Prize
  Studentships, 253
Research into Ageing Research Grants,
  253
University of Dundee Research Awards,
  295
University Postgraduate Scholarships,
  290

Australia

New South Wales Cancer Council
  Research Programme Grant, 237
New South Wales Cancer Council
  Research Project Grants, 237
Postgraduate Scholarship (sponsored
  by BioMérieux-Vitek Australia and
  AIMS), 61
Wingate Scholarships, 326

British Commonwealth

Wingate Scholarships, 326

Canada

Alcohol Beverage Medical Research Foundation Research Project Grant, 12
Wingate Scholarships, 326

Indian Sub-Continent

Wingate Scholarships, 326

Middle East

Wingate Scholarships, 326

United Kingdom

Wingate Scholarships, 326

USA

Alcohol Beverage Medical Research Foundation Research Project Grant, 12
NORD Clinical Research Grants, 231

West European Countries

Wingate Scholarships, 326

HEPATHOLOGY

Any Country

Elsevier Research Initiative Award, 29
Endoscopic Multicenter/Comparative Trials Award, 29
Industry Research Scholar Awards, 30
Innovative Seed Grants in Basic Research in Liver Diseases, 30
Lister Institute Senior Research Fellowships, 195
Miles and Shirley Fiterman Foundation Basic Research Awards, 30
Miles and Shirley Fiterman Foundation Clinical Research in Gastroenterology or Hepatology/Nutrition Awards, 31
Olympus Endoscopic Career Enhancement Awards, 31
Outcomes Research Training Awards, 31
R Robert and Sally D Funderburg Research Scholar Award in Gastric Biology Related to Cancer, 31
Student Research Fellowship Awards, 32
TAP Pharmaceuticals, Inc. Outcomes Research Awards, 32
Wilson-Cook Endoscopic Research Career Development Awards, 32

Australia

Wingate Scholarships, 326

British Commonwealth

Wingate Scholarships, 326

Canada

Alcohol Beverage Medical Research Foundation Research Project Grant, 12
Canadian Liver Foundation Establishment Grants, 115
Canadian Liver Foundation Fellowships, 115
Canadian Liver Foundation Graduate Studentships, 116
Canadian Liver Foundation Operating Grant, 116
Wingate Scholarships, 326

Indian Sub-Continent

Wingate Scholarships, 326

Middle East

Wingate Scholarships, 326

United Kingdom

Wingate Scholarships, 326

USA

Alcohol Beverage Medical Research Foundation Research Project Grant, 12
NORD Clinical Research Grants, 231

West European Countries

Wingate Scholarships, 326

NEPHROLOGY

Any Country

Charlotte Roberts Trust Kidney Research Award, 227
Lister Institute Senior Research Fellowships, 195
NKRF Research Project Grants, 227
NKRF Senior Fellowships, 227
NKRF Special Project Grants, 228
NKRF Studentships, 228
NKRF Training Fellowships, 228

Australia

Wingate Scholarships, 326

British Commonwealth

Wingate Scholarships, 326

Canada

The Kidney Foundation of Canada Allied Health Doctoral Fellowship, 187
The Kidney Foundation of Canada Allied Health Research Grant, 187
The Kidney Foundation of Canada Allied Health Scholarship, 187
The Kidney Foundation of Canada Biomedical Fellowship, 188
The Kidney Foundation of Canada Biomedical Research (Operating) Grant, 188
The Kidney Foundation of Canada Biomedical Scholarship, 188
Wingate Scholarships, 326

Indian Sub-Continent

Wingate Scholarships, 326

Middle East

Wingate Scholarships, 326

United Kingdom

Elizabeth Wherry Research Award, 78
Wingate Scholarships, 326

USA

American Society of Hypertension/Hoechst Marion Roussel Clinical Fellowship in Hypertension, 42
NORD Clinical Research Grants, 231

West European Countries

Wingate Scholarships, 326

NEUROLOGY

Any Country

AHAF National Heart Foundation, 33
Alzheimer's Disease Research Grant, 34
ASBAH Research Grant, 54
Ataxia Research Grant, 211
Collaborative Research Projects, 274
Grants-in-Aid, 274
HDSA Fellowships, 169
HDSA Research Grants, 169
HDSA Research Initiative Grants, 169
Henry R Viets Medical/Graduate Student Research Fellowship, 209
Jeanne Timmins Costello Fellowships, 206
JP Cordeau Fellowship, 123
Lister Institute Senior Research Fellowships, 195
Migraine Trust Grants, 204

Multiple Sclerosis Society Research Grants, 207

Muscular Dystrophy Association Grant Programs, 208

National Back Pain Association Research Grants, 212

National Multiple Sclerosis Society Pilot Research Grants, 230

National Multiple Sclerosis Society Postdoctoral Fellowships, 230

National Multiple Sclerosis Society Research Grants, 231

Osserman Research Fellowship, 209

Preston Robb Fellowship, 206

Queen Elizabeth the Queen Mother Fellowship Award, 252

Research Grant, 39, 324

Research Grant, 39, 324

Research into Ageing Prize Studentships, 253

Research into Ageing Research Grants, 253

Royal Society of Medicine President's Prize, 265

Savoy Foundation Post Doctoral and Clinical Research Fellowships, 266

Savoy Foundation Research Grants, 266

Savoy Foundation Studentships, 266

Services to Academia, 274

Tourette Syndrome Association Research Grants, 287

University Postgraduate Scholarships, 290

African Nations

Canon Collins Educational Trust/Chevening Scholarships, 301

Australia

Wingate Scholarships, 326

British Commonwealth

Wingate Scholarships, 326

Canada

Alcohol Beverage Medical Research Foundation Research Project Grant, 12

Herbert H Jasper Fellowship, 123

KidsAction Research Fellowships and Grants, 188

Paralyzed Veterans of America Research Grants, 245

Wingate Scholarships, 326

East European Countries

Linacre College European Blaschko Visiting Research Scholarship, 305

Indian Sub-Continent

Wingate Scholarships, 326

Middle East

Wingate Scholarships, 326

South Africa

Canon Collins Educational Trust/Chevening Scholarships, 301

United Kingdom

Doris Hillier Research Award, 78

Linacre College European Blaschko Visiting Research Scholarship, 305

Parkinson's Disease Society Medical Research Project Grant, 246

REMEDI Research Grants, 251

Vera Down Research Award, 80

Wingate Scholarships, 326

USA

Alcohol Beverage Medical Research Foundation Research Project Grant, 12

National Multiple Sclerosis Society Junior Faculty Awards, 230

NIH Research Grants, 227

NORD Clinical Research Grants, 231

Paralyzed Veterans of America Research Grants, 245

West European Countries

Linacre College European Blaschko Visiting Research Scholarship, 305

Wingate Scholarships, 326

ONCOLOGY

Any Country

American Cancer Society International Fellowships for Beginning Investigators, 25, 212

American Cancer Society International Fellowships for Beginning Investigators (ACBSI), 212

American Institute for Cancer Research Investigator Initiator Grants, 35

Anti-Cancer Foundation Research Grants, 45

Cancer Association of South Africa Research Grants, 118

Cancer Research Campaign Research Grant, 119

Cancer Research Society, Inc. (Can) Research Grants, 120

Collaborative Research Projects, 274

CRC Studentship, 247

Gordon Piller Studentships, 193

Grants-in-Aid, 274

IARC Fellowships for Research Training in Cancer, 172

ICR Research Studentships, 170

Imperial Cancer Research Fund Clinical Research Fellowships, 170

Imperial Cancer Research Fund Graduate Studentships, 170

Imperial Cancer Research Fund Research Fellowships, 170

Instituto Nacional de Cancerologia Postgraduate Training in Oncologic Topics, 172

International Cancer Research Technology Transfer Project (ICRETT), 179

International Cancer Technology Transfer (ICRETT) Fellowships, 213

Jane Coffin Childs Memorial Fund for Medical Research Fellowships, 182

Latin America COPES Training and Education Fellowships (LACTEF), 180

Leukaemia Research Fund Clinical Research Fellowship, 193

Leukaemia Research Fund Clinical Training Fellowship, 193

Leukaemia Research Fund Grant Programme, 194

Leukaemia Research Fund Grant Project, 194

Leukemia Research Fund Awards, 194

Leukemia Society of America Scholarships, Special Fellowships and Fellowships, 194

Leukemia Society of America Translational Research Award, 195

Lister Institute Senior Research Fellowships, 195

NCIC Research Fellowships, 214

NCIC Research Grants to Individuals, 214

NCIC Research Scientist Awards, 214

OFAS Grants, 243

Services to Academia, 274

Sylvia Lawler Prize, 265

Translational Cancer Research Fellowships (TRCF), 180

University of Dundee Research Awards, 295

University Postgraduate Scholarships, 290

WCRF Research Grant, 328

WellBeing Project Grants, 325

Wilson-Fulton and Robertson Awards in Ageing Research, Cecille Gould Memorial Fund Award in Cancer Research, Richard Shepherd Fellowship, 33

Yamagiwa-Yoshida Memorial
International Cancer Study Grants,
181, 216
Yamagiwa-Yoshida Memorial
International Cancer Study Grants,
181, 216

Australia

New South Wales Cancer Council
Research Programme Grant, 237
New South Wales Cancer Council
Research Project Grants, 237
Postgraduate Scholarship (sponsored
by BioMérieux-Vitek Australia and
AIMS), 61
Richard Walter Gibbon Medical
Research Fellowship, 319
Wingate Scholarships, 326

British Commonwealth

Wingate Scholarships, 326

Canada

Alcohol Beverage Medical Research
Foundation Research Project Grant, 12
CCS Feasibility Grants, 213
CCS Grants for Molecular
Epidemiologic/Clinical Correlative
Studies, 213
CCS Student Travel Award, 213
CCS Travel Award for Senior Level PhD
Students, 213
CNF Scholarships and Fellowships, 116
NCIC Clinical Research Fellowships,
213
Terry Fox Equipment Grants for New
Investigators, 215
Terry Fox Post-PhD and Post-MD
Research Fellowships, 215
Terry Fox Research Grants for New
Investigators, 215
Terry Fox Research Studentships, 215
Wingate Scholarships, 326

East European Countries

International Oncology Nursing
Fellowships, 180

Far East

Asia-Pacific Cancer Society Training
Grants (APCASOT), 179

Indian Sub-Continent

Wingate Scholarships, 326

Middle East

Wingate Scholarships, 326

South Africa

Cancer Association of South Africa
Travel and Subsistence (Study) Grants,
119
Lady Cade Memorial Fellowship, 119

United Kingdom

Albert McMaster and Helen Tomkinson
Research Awards, 77
Fulbright Fellowship in Cancer
Research, 322
Fulbright Louise Buchanan Fellowship in
Cancer Research, 322
T P Gunton Research Award, 80
Wingate Scholarships, 326

USA

Alcohol Beverage Medical Research
Foundation Research Project Grant, 12
NORD Clinical Research Grants, 231
Ruth Estrin Goldberg Memorial for
Cancer Research, 265

West European Countries

Wingate Scholarships, 326

OPHTHALMOLOGY

Any Country

AHAF Macular Degeneration Research,
33
Fight for Sight Grants-in-Aid, 149
Fight for Sight Postdoctoral Research
Fellowships, 149
Fight for Sight Student Research
Fellowships, 149
International Eye Foundation (Colombia)
Fellowship, 174
Lister Institute Senior Research
Fellowships, 195
Mobil-NUS Postgraduate Medical
Research Scholarship, 233
National Glaucoma Research, 34
Ophthalmology Travelling Fellowship,
265
Queen Elizabeth the Queen Mother
Fellowship Award, 252
Research into Ageing Prize
Studentships, 253
Research into Ageing Research Grants,
253
University Postgraduate Scholarships,
290

African Nations

Shaffer International Fellowship
Program, 159

Australia

Wingate Scholarships, 326

British Commonwealth

Wingate Scholarships, 326

Canada

Alcohol Beverage Medical Research
Foundation Research Project Grant, 12
E A Baker Fellowship/Grant, 116
KidsAction Research Fellowships and
Grants, 188
Wingate Scholarships, 326

Caribbean Countries

Shaffer International Fellowship
Program, 159

East European Countries

Shaffer International Fellowship
Program, 159

Far East

Shaffer International Fellowship
Program, 159

Indian Sub-Continent

Shaffer International Fellowship
Program, 159
Wingate Scholarships, 326

Middle East

Shaffer International Fellowship
Program, 159
Wingate Scholarships, 326

South America

Shaffer International Fellowship
Program, 159

United Kingdom

Iris Fund Award, 181
Iris Fund Grants for Research and
Equipment (Ophthalmology), 181
John William Clark Research Award, 79
Middlemore Research Award, 79
Wingate Scholarships, 326

USA

Alcohol Beverage Medical Research
Foundation Research Project Grant, 12

Clinician-Scientist Fellowship, 159
Heed Award, 166
NORD Clinical Research Grants, 231

West European Countries

Wingate Scholarships, 326

OTORHINOLARYNGOLOGY

Any Country

Karl Storz Travelling Scholarship, 264
Lister Institute Senior Research
  Fellowships, 195

Canada

DRF Otological Research Fellowship,
  134
DRF Research Grants, 134

United Kingdom

Norman Gamble Fund and Research
  Prize, 264

USA

ATA Scientific and Medical Research
  Grants, 44
DRF Otological Research Fellowship,
  134
DRF Research Grants, 134
NORD Clinical Research Grants, 231

PARASITOLOGY

Any Country

Lister Institute Senior Research
  Fellowships, 195
Thrasher Research and Field
  Demonstration Project Grants, 286

African Nations

AHRI African Fellowship, 46

Australia

Postgraduate Scholarship (sponsored
  by BioMérieux-Vitek Australia and
  AIMS), 61

USA

Grants for Innovative Methods for
  Control of Tick-Borne Diseases, 37
NORD Clinical Research Grants, 231

West European Countries

Karl-Enigk-Stipendium, 286

PATHOLOGY

Any Country

AHAF National Heart Foundation, 33
Gillson Scholarship in Pathology, 275
Linnean Macleay Fellowship, 195
Lister Institute Senior Research
  Fellowships, 195
Mobil-NUS Postgraduate Medical
  Research Scholarship, 233
Queen Elizabeth the Queen Mother
  Fellowship Award, 252
Research into Ageing Research Grants,
  253
University Postgraduate Scholarships,
  290

Australia

New South Wales Cancer Council
  Research Programme Grant, 237
New South Wales Cancer Council
  Research Project Grants, 237
Postgraduate Scholarship (sponsored
  by BioMérieux-Vitek Australia and
  AIMS), 61

Canada

Alcohol Beverage Medical Research
  Foundation Research Project Grant, 12

United Kingdom

Musgrave Research Studentships, 250
Parkinson's Disease Society Medical
  Research Project Grant, 246

USA

Alcohol Beverage Medical Research
  Foundation Research Project Grant, 12
American Society of
  Hypertension/Hoechst Marion Roussel
  Clinical Fellowship in Hypertension, 42
Hilgenfeld Foundation Grant, 167
NORD Clinical Research Grants, 231

PAEDIATRICS

Any Country

AAP Resident Research Grants, 19
Arthritis Foundation Postdoctoral
  Fellowship, 48

ASBAH Research Grant, 54
Charles H Hood Foundation Child
  Health Research Grant, 125
Dr Sydney Segal Research Grants, 115
FRAXA Postdoctoral Fellowship, 155
FSID Research Grant Award, 153
FSID Short Term Training Fellowship,
  153
ICR Research Studentships, 170
Michael Geisman Memorial Fellowship
  Fund, 245
Mobil-NUS Postgraduate Medical
  Research Scholarship, 233
National Back Pain Association
  Research Grants, 212
Osteogenesis Imperfecta Foundation
  Seed Research Grant, 245
Paediatric AIDS Foundation Student
  Intern Awards, 144
Research Grant, 39, 324
Research Grants One-Year and Two-
  Year, 144
Savoy Foundation Post Doctoral and
  Clinical Research Fellowships, 266
Savoy Foundation Research Grants,
  266
Savoy Foundation Studentships, 266
Scholar Awards, 144
Thrasher Research and Field
  Demonstration Project Grants, 286
University of Dundee Research Awards,
  295
University Postgraduate Scholarships,
  290

African Nations

Heinz Fellowships (Types A and C), 259

Australia

Heinz Fellowships (Types A and C), 259

Canada

AAP Residency Scholarships, 19
Duncan L Gordon Fellowships, 167
Heinz Fellowships (Types A and C), 259
Hospital for Sick Children Foundation
  External Grants, 167
KidsAction Research Fellowships and
  Grants, 188
Physician Scientist Development Award,
  49

Indian Sub-Continent

Heinz Fellowships (Types A and C), 259

New Zealand

Heinz Fellowships (Types A and C), 259

South Africa

Heinz Fellowships (Types A and C), 259

United Kingdom

Heinz Fellowships (Types A and C), 259

USA

AAP Residency Scholarships, 19
American Society of
  Hypertension/Hoechst Marion Roussel
  Clinical Fellowship in Hypertension, 42
Arthritis Investigator Award, 48
NORD Clinical Research Grants, 231
Physician Scientist Development Award,
  49

PLASTIC SURGERY

Any Country

AAFPRS Investigator Development
  Grant, 17
BAPS European Travelling Scholarship,
  67
BAPS Travelling Bursary, 67
Paton/Maser Memorial Fund, 67
Student Bursaries, 67

African Nations

BAPS Fellowship, 67

Canada

AAFPRS Resident Research Grants, 17
Bernstein Grant, 17
KidsAction Research Fellowships and
  Grants, 188

Far East

BAPS Fellowship, 67

Indian Sub-Continent

BAPS Fellowship, 67

Middle East

BAPS Fellowship, 67

USA

AAFPRS Resident Research Grants, 17
Bernstein Grant, 17
NORD Clinical Research Grants, 231

PNEUMOLOGY

Australia

Asthma Victoria Research Grants, 57
Lilian Roxon Memorial Research Trust
  Travel Grant, 58

Canada

Alcohol Beverage Medical Research
  Foundation Research Project Grant, 12
Parker B Francis Fellowship Program,
  246

United Kingdom

H C Roscoe Fellowship, 78
T V James Research Fellowship, 80

USA

Alcohol Beverage Medical Research
  Foundation Research Project Grant, 12
NORD Clinical Research Grants, 231
Parker B Francis Fellowship Program,
  246

PSYCHIATRY AND MENTAL HEALTH

Any Country

Collaborative Research Projects, 274
Diabetes Development Project, 70
FRAXA Postdoctoral Fellowship, 155
HDSA Fellowships, 169
HDSA Research Grants, 169
HDSA Research Initiative Grants, 169
Mental Health Foundation Essay Prize,
  264
NARSAD Distinguished Investigator
  Awards, 210
NARSAD Independent Investigator
  Award, 210
NARSAD Young Investigator Awards,
  210
National Back Pain Association
  Research Grants, 212
Queen Elizabeth the Queen Mother
  Fellowship Award, 252
Research Grant, 39, 324
Research into Ageing Prize
  Studentships, 253
Research into Ageing Research Grants,
  253
Savoy Foundation Post Doctoral and
  Clinical Research Fellowships, 266
Savoy Foundation Research Grants,
  266

Savoy Foundation Studentships, 266
Services to Academia, 274
Tourette Syndrome Association
  Research Grants, 287
University Postgraduate Scholarships,
  290

British Commonwealth

Doris Odlum Research Award, 78

Canada

Alcohol Beverage Medical Research
  Foundation Research Project Grant, 12
APA/Glaxo Wellcome Fellowship, 41
Postdoctoral Training Programme in
  Addiction and Mental Health, 124

United Kingdom

Doris Odlum Research Award, 78
Margaret Temple Fellowship, 79
Mental Health Foundation Research
  Grant, 203
Mental Health Foundation Studentship,
  203
Parkinson's Disease Society Medical
  Research Project Grant, 246
Tizard Centre Departmental
  Scholarships, 296

USA

Alcohol Beverage Medical Research
  Foundation Research Project Grant, 12
APA/CMHS and Zeneca Minority
  Fellowship Programme in Psychiatry,
  122
APA/Glaxo Wellcome Fellowship, 41
APA/Zeneca Fellowship, 122
Arthritis Foundation Biomedical Science
  Grant, 46
Arthritis Foundation Clinical Science
  Grant, 47
Arthritis Investigator Award, 48
James Comer Minority Research
  Fellowship for Medical Students, 16
Jeanne Spurlock Minority Medical
  Student Clinical Fellowship in Child
  and Adolescent Psychiatry, 16
Jeanne Spurlock Research Fellowship
  in Drug Abuse and Addiction for
  Minority Medical Students, 17
Marcia Granucci Memorial Scholarship,
  324
NORD Clinical Research Grants, 231
Postdoctoral Training Programme in
  Addiction and Mental Health, 124

West European Countries

Tizard Centre Departmental
  Scholarships, 296

RHEUMATOLOGY

Any Country

AFA Grants-in-Aid, 49
Arthritis Foundation Postdoctoral
Fellowship, 48
Arthritis Society Industry Program, 52
Arthritis Society Research Fellowships,
52
Bristol-Myers Squibb/Zimmer Research
Grant for Excellence in Orthapedaedic
Treatment, 244
Geoff Carr Lupus Fellowship, 53
Lister Institute Senior Research
Fellowships, 195
National Back Pain Association
Research Grants, 212
OREF Career Development Award, 244
OREF Prospective Clinical Research,
244
OREF Research Grants, 244
OREF Resident Research Award, 244
Philip Benjamin Memorial Grant, 51
University Postgraduate Scholarships,
290
Wilson-Fulton and Robertson Awards in
Ageing Research, Cecille Gould
Memorial Fund Award in Cancer
Research, Richard Shepherd
Fellowship, 33

African Nations

Metro A Ogryzlo International
Fellowship, 53

Australia

AFA Special Project Grants, 50
AFA/ARA Heald Fellowship, 50
Frank G Spurway Scholarship and
Arthritis Foundation of NSW Branches,
50
Mary Paxton Gibson Scholarships, 50
McGill Domestic Fellowship, 50
Metro A Ogryzlo International
Fellowship, 53
Michael Mason Fellowship, 50

British Commonwealth

ARC Postdoctoral Research
Fellowships, 51

Canada

AAOS/OREF Fellowship in Health
Services Research, 243
Alcohol Beverage Medical Research
Foundation Research Project Grant, 12
Arthritis Society Clinical Fellowships, 52
Arthritis Society Research Grants, 53

Arthritis Society Research Scholarships,
53
Arthritis Society Research Scientist
Awards, 53
KidsAction Research Fellowships and
Grants, 188
OREF Clinical Research Award, 244
Physician Scientist Development Award,
49

East European Countries

Metro A Ogryzlo International
Fellowship, 53

Far East

Metro A Ogryzlo International
Fellowship, 53

Indian Sub-Continent

Metro A Ogryzlo International
Fellowship, 53

Middle East

Metro A Ogryzlo International
Fellowship, 53

New Zealand

Metro A Ogryzlo International
Fellowship, 53

South Africa

Metro A Ogryzlo International
Fellowship, 53

South America

Metro A Ogryzlo International
Fellowship, 53

United Kingdom

ARC Clinical Research Fellowships, 51
ARC Project Grants, 51
ARC Travelling Fellowships, 51
Doris Hillier Research Award, 78
REMEDI Research Grants, 251
Senior ARC Fellowships, 52

USA

AAOS/OREF Fellowship in Health
Services Research, 243
Alcohol Beverage Medical Research
Foundation Research Project Grant, 12
Arthritis Foundation Biomedical Science
Grant, 46
Arthritis Foundation Clinical Science
Grant, 47
Arthritis Foundation New Investigator
Grant, 47

Arthritis Investigator Award, 48
NORD Clinical Research Grants, 231
OREF Clinical Research Award, 244
Physician Scientist Development Award,
49

West European Countries

Metro A Ogryzlo International
Fellowship, 53

UROLOGY

Any Country

ASBAH Research Grant, 54
ICR Research Studentships, 170
Lister Institute Senior Research
Fellowships, 195
Queen Elizabeth the Queen Mother
Fellowship Award, 252
Research Grant, 39, 324
Research into Ageing Prize
Studentships, 253
Research into Ageing Research Grants,
253
Royal Society of Medicine Travelling
Fellowship, 265
WellBeing Project Grants, 325

Canada

The Kidney Foundation of Canada Allied
Health Doctoral Fellowship, 187
The Kidney Foundation of Canada Allied
Health Research Grant, 187
The Kidney Foundation of Canada Allied
Health Scholarship, 187
The Kidney Foundation of Canada
Biomedical Fellowship, 188
The Kidney Foundation of Canada
Biomedical Research (Operating)
Grant, 188
The Kidney Foundation of Canada
Biomedical Scholarship, 188
Paralyzed Veterans of America
Research Grants, 245

USA

NORD Clinical Research Grants, 231
Paralyzed Veterans of America
Research Grants, 245

VIROLOGY

Any Country

Collaborative Research Projects, 274

Grants-in-Aid, 274

Lister Institute Senior Research Fellowships, 195

Queen Elizabeth the Queen Mother Fellowship Award, 252

Research into Ageing Research Grants, 253

Services to Academia, 274

University of Dundee Research Awards, 295

Wilson-Fulton and Robertson Awards in Ageing Research, Cecille Gould Memorial Fund Award in Cancer Research, Richard Shepherd Fellowship, 33

Australia

Postgraduate Scholarship (sponsored by BioMérieux-Vitek Australia and AIMS), 61

Wingate Scholarships, 326

British Commonwealth

Wingate Scholarships, 326

Canada

Wingate Scholarships, 326

Indian Sub-Continent

Wingate Scholarships, 326

Middle East

Wingate Scholarships, 326

United Kingdom

H C Roscoe Fellowship, 78
Wingate Scholarships, 326

USA

NORD Clinical Research Grants, 231

West European Countries

Wingate Scholarships, 326

TROPICAL MEDICINE

Any Country

Lister Institute Senior Research Fellowships, 195

African Nations

AHRI African Fellowship, 46

Australia

Postgraduate Scholarship (sponsored by BioMérieux-Vitek Australia and AIMS), 61

Wingate Scholarships, 326

British Commonwealth

Wingate Scholarships, 326

Canada

Wingate Scholarships, 326

Indian Sub-Continent

Wingate Scholarships, 326

Middle East

Wingate Scholarships, 326

United Kingdom

Wingate Scholarships, 326

USA

NORD Clinical Research Grants, 231

West European Countries

Wingate Scholarships, 326

VENEREOLOGY

Any Country

Lister Institute Senior Research Fellowships, 195

Australia

Postgraduate Scholarship (sponsored by BioMérieux-Vitek Australia and AIMS), 61

Wingate Scholarships, 326

British Commonwealth

Wingate Scholarships, 326

Canada

Wingate Scholarships, 326

Indian Sub-Continent

Wingate Scholarships, 326

Middle East

Wingate Scholarships, 326

United Kingdom

Wingate Scholarships, 326

USA

NORD Clinical Research Grants, 231

West European Countries

Wingate Scholarships, 326

REHABILITATION MEDICINE AND THERAPY

Any Country

Agnes Storar/Constance Owens Fund, 127

Arthritis Foundation Postdoctoral Fellowship, 48

British Lung Foundation Project Grants, 77

Farrer-Brown Professional Development Fund, 127

Margaret Dawson Fund, 127

Michael Geisman Memorial Fellowship Fund, 245

Osteogenesis Imperfecta Foundation Seed Research Grant, 245

Queen Elizabeth the Queen Mother Fellowship Award, 252

Research Grant, 39, 324

Research into Ageing Research Grants, 253

Roche Research Foundation, 254

Savoy Foundation Post Doctoral and Clinical Research Fellowships, 266

Savoy Foundation Research Grants, 266

Savoy Foundation Studentships, 266

Sigma Theta Tau International Rehabilitation Nursing Foundation Grant, 270

Australia

Nepean Postgraduate Research Award, 320

The Sir Robert Menzies Memorial Research Scholarships in the Allied Health Sciences, 273

Wingate Scholarships, 326

British Commonwealth

Wingate Scholarships, 326

Canada

CNF Scholarships and Fellowships, 116
KidsAction Research Fellowships and
   Grants, 188
Paralyzed Veterans of America
   Research Grants, 245
Wingate Scholarships, 326

Indian Sub-Continent

Wingate Scholarships, 326

Middle East

Wingate Scholarships, 326

New Zealand

National Heart Foundation of New
   Zealand Fellowships, 224
National Heart Foundation of New
   Zealand Grants-in-Aid, 224
National Heart Foundation of New
   Zealand Project Grants, 224
National Heart Foundation of New
   Zealand Travel Grants, 224
Nepean Postgraduate Research Award,
   320

United Kingdom

Doris Hillier Research Award, 78
Parkinson's Disease Society Welfare
   Research Project Grant, 246
REMEDI Research Grants, 251
Wingate Scholarships, 326

USA

Arthritis Foundation Clinical Science
   Grant, 47
Arthritis Foundation Doctoral
   Dissertation Award, 47
Arthritis Foundation New Investigator
   Grant, 47
Arthritis Investigator Award, 48
New Investigator Fellowships Training
   Initiative (NIFTI), 152
New York Life Foundation Scholarship
   for Women in the Health Professions
   Program, 83
NIH Research Grants, 227
NLM Fellowship in Applied Informatics,
   228
Paralyzed Veterans of America
   Research Grants, 245
Promotion of Doctoral Studies (PODS),
   152

West European Countries

Wingate Scholarships, 326

NURSING

Any Country

ANF Nursing Research Grants, 38
Dr Sydney Segal Research Grants, 115
HP/AACN Critical Care Nursing
   Research Grant, 166
ICR Research Studentships, 170
Massey Doctoral Scholarship, 196
Myasthenia Gravis Nursing Fellowship,
   209
Queen Elizabeth the Queen Mother
   Fellowship Award, 252
Research into Ageing Research Grants,
   253
Roche Research Foundation, 254
Sigma Theta Tau International American
   Association of Critical Care Nurses,
   267
Sigma Theta Tau International American
   Association of Diabetes Educators
   Grant, 267
Sigma Theta Tau International American
   Nephrology Nurses Association Grant,
   268
Sigma Theta Tau International American
   Nurses Foundation Grant, 268
Sigma Theta Tau International
   Emergency Nursing Foundation Grant,
   269
Sigma Theta Tau International Glaxo
   Wellcome New Investigator Mentor
   Grant, 269
Sigma Theta Tau International Glaxo
   Wellcome Prescriptive Practice Grant,
   269
Sigma Theta Tau International Mead
   Johnson Nutritionals Perinatal Grant,
   270
Sigma Theta Tau International Oncology
   Nursing Society Grant, 270
Sigma Theta Tau International Research
   Grant Opportunities, 271
The Sir Allan Sewell Visiting Fellowship,
   160
University of Dundee Research Awards,
   295
University of Glasgow Postgraduate
   Scholarships, 296
University of Stirling Research
   Studentships, 315

Australia

Nepean Postgraduate Research Award,
   320
The Sir Robert Menzies Memorial
   Research Scholarships in the Allied
   Health Sciences, 273
Wingate Scholarships, 326

British Commonwealth

Wingate Scholarships, 326

Canada

CNF Scholarships and Fellowships, 116
The Kidney Foundation of Canada Allied
   Health Doctoral Fellowship, 187
The Kidney Foundation of Canada Allied
   Health Research Grant, 187
The Kidney Foundation of Canada Allied
   Health Scholarship, 187
Wingate Scholarships, 326

East European Countries

Scholarships for Émigrés in the Health
   Professions, 183

Indian Sub-Continent

Wingate Scholarships, 326

Middle East

Wingate Scholarships, 326

New Zealand

Nepean Postgraduate Research Award,
   320

South Africa

DENOSA Bursaries, Scholarships and
   Grants, 134

United Kingdom

Mental Health Foundation Research
   Grant, 203
Mental Health Foundation Studentship,
   203
Parkinson's Disease Society Welfare
   Research Project Grant, 246
Smith and Nephew Nursing Research
   Fellowships and Scholarships, 273
University of Wales Bangor (UWB)
   Research Studentships, 318
Wingate Scholarships, 326

USA

Arthritis Foundation Clinical Science
   Grant, 47
Arthritis Foundation Doctoral
   Dissertation Award, 47
Arthritis Foundation New Investigator
   Grant, 47
Arthritis Investigator Award, 48
Marcia Granucci Memorial Scholarship,
   324
New York Life Foundation Scholarship
   for Women in the Health Professions
   Program, 83

NLM Fellowship in Applied Informatics, 228
Nurses' Educational Funds Fellowships and Scholarships, 241

West European Countries

University of Wales Bangor (UWB) Research Studentships, 318
Wingate Scholarships, 326

MEDICAL AUXILIARIES

Any Country

Roche Research Foundation, 254

Australia

Wingate Scholarships, 326

British Commonwealth

Wingate Scholarships, 326

Canada

Wingate Scholarships, 326

Indian Sub-Continent

Wingate Scholarships, 326

Middle East

Wingate Scholarships, 326

United Kingdom

Wingate Scholarships, 326

West European Countries

Wingate Scholarships, 326

MIDWIFERY

Any Country

Dr Sydney Segal Research Grants, 115
Massey Doctoral Scholarship, 196
Roche Research Foundation, 254
University of Dundee Research Awards, 295
University of Glasgow Postgraduate Scholarships, 296
University of Stirling Research Studentships, 315

Australia

Nepean Postgraduate Research Award, 320

Wingate Scholarships, 326

British Commonwealth

Wingate Scholarships, 326

Canada

Wingate Scholarships, 326

Indian Sub-Continent

Wingate Scholarships, 326

Middle East

Wingate Scholarships, 326

New Zealand

Nepean Postgraduate Research Award, 320

United Kingdom

University of Wales Bangor (UWB) Research Studentships, 318
Wingate Scholarships, 326

West European Countries

University of Wales Bangor (UWB) Research Studentships, 318
Wingate Scholarships, 326

RADIOLOGY

Any Country

British Institute of Radiology Travel Bursary, 76
Flude Memorial Prize, 76
Grants-in-Aid, 274
Mobil-NUS Postgraduate Medical Research Scholarship, 233
National Back Pain Association Research Grants, 212
Nic McNally Memorial Prize, 76
Nycomed Amersham Fellowship, 76
Roche Research Foundation, 254
Stanley Melville Memorial Award, 76

Australia

New South Wales Cancer Council Research Programme Grant, 237
New South Wales Cancer Council Research Project Grants, 237
Wingate Scholarships, 326

British Commonwealth

Wingate Scholarships, 326

Canada

Wingate Scholarships, 326

Indian Sub-Continent

Wingate Scholarships, 326

Middle East

Wingate Scholarships, 326

United Kingdom

University of Wales Bangor (UWB) Research Studentships, 318
Wingate Scholarships, 326

USA

New York Life Foundation Scholarship for Women in the Health Professions Program, 83

West European Countries

University of Wales Bangor (UWB) Research Studentships, 318
Wingate Scholarships, 326

TREATMENT TECHNIQUES

Any Country

American Cancer Society International Fellowships for Beginning Investigators, 25, 212
APMA Research Grant Program, 41
Arthritis Foundation Postdoctoral Fellowship, 48
Bristol-Myers Squibb/Zimmer Research Grant for Excellence in Orthapedaedic Treatment, 244
Collaborative Research Projects, 274
Cooley's Anemia Foundation Research Fellowship Grant, 131
CSMLS Founders' Fund Award, 117
DEBRA Medical Research Grant Scheme, 134
Diabetes Development Project, 70
HDSA Fellowships, 169
HDSA Research Grants, 169
HDSA Research Initiative Grants, 169
National Headache Foundation Research Grant, 219
OREF Career Development Award, 244
OREF Prospective Clinical Research, 244
OREF Research Grants, 244
OREF Resident Research Award, 244
Research Grant, 39, 324

Roche Research Foundation, 254
Services to Academia, 274
Translational Cancer Research
Fellowships (TRCF), 180

Australia

Asthma Victoria Research Grants, 57
Lilian Roxon Memorial Research Trust
Travel Grant, 58
Nepean Postgraduate Research Award,
320
New South Wales Cancer Council
Research Programme Grant, 237
New South Wales Cancer Council
Research Project Grants, 237
The Sir Robert Menzies Memorial
Research Scholarships in the Allied
Health Sciences, 273
Wingate Scholarships, 326

British Commonwealth

Wingate Scholarships, 326

Canada

AAOS/OREF Fellowship in Health
Services Research, 243
KidsAction Research Fellowships and
Grants, 188
OREF Clinical Research Award, 244
Paralyzed Veterans of America
Research Grants, 245
Wingate Scholarships, 326

Indian Sub-Continent

Wingate Scholarships, 326

Middle East

Wingate Scholarships, 326

New Zealand

Nepean Postgraduate Research Award,
320

United Kingdom

Nathaniel Bishop Harman Research
Award, 79
Parkinson's Disease Society Welfare
Research Project Grant, 246
Wingate Scholarships, 326

USA

AAOS/OREF Fellowship in Health
Services Research, 243
American Society of
Hypertension/Hoechst Marion Roussel
Clinical Fellowship in Hypertension, 42
Arthritis Foundation Clinical Science
Grant, 47

Arthritis Foundation Doctoral
Dissertation Award, 47
Arthritis Foundation New Investigator
Grant, 47
ATA Scientific and Medical Research
Grants, 44
OREF Clinical Research Award, 244
Paralyzed Veterans of America
Research Grants, 245

West European Countries

Wingate Scholarships, 326

MEDICAL TECHNOLOGY

Any Country

British Lung Foundation Project Grants,
77
Collaborative Research Projects, 274
Diabetes Development Project, 70
Hastings Center International Scholars
Program, 161
Roche Research Foundation, 254
Services to Academia, 274

Australia

Postgraduate Scholarship (sponsored
by BioMérieux-Vitek Australia and
AIMS), 61
Wingate Scholarships, 326

British Commonwealth

Wingate Scholarships, 326

Canada

Quebec CE Fund Grants, 117
Wingate Scholarships, 326

East European Countries

Hastings Center Eastern European
Program, 160

Indian Sub-Continent

Wingate Scholarships, 326

Middle East

Wingate Scholarships, 326

United Kingdom

Wingate Scholarships, 326

West European Countries

Wingate Scholarships, 326

DENTISTRY AND STOMATOLOGY

Any Country

AADR Student Research Fellowships,
23
ADHA Institute Scholarship Program, 6
British Medical and Dental Students'
Trust Scholarships and Travel Grants,
77
CAMS Scholarship, 126
Colyer Prize, 263
DCF Biennial Research Award, 135
DCF/Wrigley Dental Student Research
Awards, 136
Dentsply Scholarship Fund, 69
Dr Alfred C Fones Scholarship, 6
Dr Harold Hillenbrand Scholarship, 7
Eastman Dental Center Clinical
Fellowships, 143
Irene E Newman Scholarship, 7
John O Butler Graduate Scholarships, 7
Lever Pond's Postgraduate Fellowship,
277
Margaret E Swanson Scholarship, 7
National Association of Dental
Assistants Annual Scholarship Award,
211
Queen Mary and Westfield College
Research Studentships, 297
Roche Research Foundation, 254
Sigma Phi Alpha Graduate Scholarship,
7
Sir Richard Stapley Educational Trust
Grants, 272
Tylman Research Program, 18
University of Dundee Research Awards,
295
University of Glasgow Postgraduate
Scholarships, 296
University Postgraduate Scholarships,
290
The Winifred E Preedy Postgraduate
Bursary, 60

Australia

NHMRC Medical and Dental and Public
Health Postgraduate Research
Scholarships, 221
Wingate Scholarships, 326

British Commonwealth

Wingate Scholarships, 326

Canada

DCF Fellowships for
Teacher/Researcher Training, 135

Frank Knox Memorial Fellowships at
  Harvard University, 56
Heritage Dental Fellowships, 11
Wingate Scholarships, 326

East European Countries

Scholarships for Émigrés in the Health
  Professions, 183

Indian Sub-Continent

Wingate Scholarships, 326

Middle East

Wingate Scholarships, 326

South Africa

South African MRC Dentistry
  Scholarships, 278

United Kingdom

Wingate Scholarships, 326

USA

Dental Student Scholarship, 5
Minority Dental Student Scholarship, 5

West European Countries

Scholarship Foundation of the League
  for Finnish-American Societies, 266
Wingate Scholarships, 326

ORAL PATHOLOGY

Any Country

Colyer Prize, 263
Grants-in-Aid, 274

Australia

Wingate Scholarships, 326

British Commonwealth

Wingate Scholarships, 326

Canada

Wingate Scholarships, 326

Indian Sub-Continent

Wingate Scholarships, 326

Middle East

Wingate Scholarships, 326

United Kingdom

Wingate Scholarships, 326

West European Countries

Wingate Scholarships, 326

ORTHODONTICS

Any Country

BOS Research and Audit Fund, 81
Chapman Prize, 81
Eastman Dental Center Clinical
  Fellowships, 143
Houston Research Scholarship, 81
University of Dundee Research Awards,
  295
University Postgraduate Scholarships,
  290

Australia

Wingate Scholarships, 326

British Commonwealth

Wingate Scholarships, 326

Canada

Wingate Scholarships, 326

Indian Sub-Continent

Wingate Scholarships, 326

Middle East

Wingate Scholarships, 326

United Kingdom

Wingate Scholarships, 326

USA

NLM Fellowship in Applied Informatics,
  228

West European Countries

Wingate Scholarships, 326

PERIODONTICS

Any Country

Eastman Dental Center Clinical
  Fellowships, 143
University of Dundee Research Awards,
  295

University Postgraduate Scholarships,
  290

Australia

Wingate Scholarships, 326

British Commonwealth

Wingate Scholarships, 326

Canada

Wingate Scholarships, 326

Indian Sub-Continent

Wingate Scholarships, 326

Middle East

Wingate Scholarships, 326

United Kingdom

Wingate Scholarships, 326

West European Countries

Wingate Scholarships, 326

COMMUNITY DENTISTRY

Any Country

University of Dundee Research Awards,
  295

Australia

Wingate Scholarships, 326

British Commonwealth

Wingate Scholarships, 326

Canada

Wingate Scholarships, 326

Indian Sub-Continent

Wingate Scholarships, 326

Middle East

Wingate Scholarships, 326

United Kingdom

Wingate Scholarships, 326

West European Countries

Wingate Scholarships, 326

DENTAL TECHNOLOGY

Any Country

Colyer Prize, 263
Roche Research Foundation, 254
University of Dundee Research Awards, 295
University of Glasgow Postgraduate Scholarships, 296

USA

Allied Dental Health Scholarship (Dental Hygiene, Dental Assisting, Dental Laboratory Technology), 5

PROSTHETIC DENTISTRY

Any Country

Eastman Dental Center Clinical Fellowships, 143
University of Dundee Research Awards, 295
University Postgraduate Scholarships, 290

Australia

Wingate Scholarships, 326

British Commonwealth

Wingate Scholarships, 326

Canada

Wingate Scholarships, 326

Indian Sub-Continent

Wingate Scholarships, 326

Middle East

Wingate Scholarships, 326

United Kingdom

Wingate Scholarships, 326

West European Countries

Wingate Scholarships, 326

PHARMACY

Any Country

Collaborative Research Projects, 274
Grants-in-Aid, 274
HDSA Fellowships, 169
HDSA Research Grants, 169
HDSA Research Initiative Grants, 169
Roche Research Foundation, 254
Services to Academia, 274

Australia

Biomedical and Medical Postgraduate Research Scholarships, 57
Medical Research Project Grant, 57
Wingate Scholarships, 326

British Commonwealth

Wingate Scholarships, 326

Canada

CPhA Canada Centennial Scholars Award, 117
Wingate Scholarships, 326

East European Countries

Scholarships for Émigrés in the Health Professions, 183

Indian Sub-Continent

Wingate Scholarships, 326

Middle East

Wingate Scholarships, 326

United Kingdom

Parkinson's Disease Society Medical Research Project Grant, 246
Wingate Scholarships, 326

West European Countries

Wingate Scholarships, 326

BIOMEDICINE

Any Country

AHAF Macular Degeneration Research, 33
AHAF National Heart Foundation, 33
Alzheimer's Disease Research Grant, 34
Arthritis Foundation Postdoctoral Fellowship, 48

British Diabetic Association Project Grants, 69
British Diabetic Association Research Fellowships, 70
British Diabetic Association Research Studentships, 70
British Diabetic Association Small Grant Scheme, 70
Collaborative Research Projects, 274
Diabetes Development Project, 70
FRAXA Postdoctoral Fellowship, 155
Grants-in-Aid, 274
Hastings Center International Scholars Program, 161
HDSA Fellowships, 169
HDSA Research Grants, 169
HDSA Research Initiative Grants, 169
ICR Research Studentships, 170
John E Fogarty International Research Fellowship Program, 184
MRC Career Development Award, 198
MRC Clinical Scientist Fellowship, 198
MRC Clinical Training Fellowships, 198
MRC Research Fellowship, 199
MRC Senior Clinical Fellowship, 199
MRC Senior Non-Clinical Fellowship, 200
MRC Special Training Fellowship in Bioinformatics, 200
MRC/Joint MRC Health Regions Special Training Fellowship in Health Services Research, 200
National Glaucoma Research, 34
NIH Visiting Program, 185
OFAS Grants, 243
Paediatric AIDS Foundation Student Intern Awards, 144
Queen Elizabeth the Queen Mother Fellowship Award, 252
Research Assistant or Technician, 141
Research Fellowship, 141
Research Grant, 39, 324
Research into Ageing Research Grants, 253
Roche Research Foundation, 254
Services to Academia, 274
University of Glasgow Postgraduate Scholarships, 296
Wellcome Trust Awards, Fellowships and Studentships, 326
Wilson-Fulton and Robertson Awards in Ageing Research, Cecille Gould Memorial Fund Award in Cancer Research, Richard Shepherd Fellowship, 33

African Nations

AHRI African Fellowship, 46

Australia

Burnet Fellowships, 219
C J Martin Fellowships, 219
Dora Lush (Biomedical) and Public
  Health Postgraduate Scholarships, 220
Eccles Awards, 220
NHMRC/INSERM Exchange
  Fellowships, 222
Peter Doherty Fellowships, 222
R Douglas Wright Awards, 222
Wingate Scholarships, 326

British Commonwealth

Wingate Scholarships, 326

Canada

Alcohol Beverage Medical Research
  Foundation Research Project Grant, 12
MRS Wellcome Trust Agreement, 202
Wingate Scholarships, 326

East European Countries

Hastings Center Eastern European
  Program, 160

Indian Sub-Continent

Wingate Scholarships, 326

Middle East

Wingate Scholarships, 326

South Africa

South African MRC Research
  Supplements for Disadvantaged
  Students, 279

South America

Pew Latin American Fellows Program,
  247

United Kingdom

MRC Research Studentships, 199
MRS Wellcome Trust Agreement, 202
Muscular Dystrophy Programme Grant,
  208
Muscular Dystrophy Project Grant, 208
Muscular Dystrophy Research Grants,
  209
Wingate Scholarships, 326

USA

Alcohol Beverage Medical Research
  Foundation Research Project Grant, 12
Arthritis Foundation Biomedical Science
  Grant, 46
Arthritis Investigator Award, 48

John E Fogarty Senior International
  Fellowship Program, 185
MARC Faculty Predoctoral Fellowships,
  225
NIGMS Fellowship Awards for Minority
  Students, 225
NIGMS Fellowship Awards for Students
  With Disabilities, 226
NIGMS Postdoctoral Awards, 226
NIGMS Research Project Grants, 226
NIGMS Research Supplements for
  Underrepresented Minorities, 226
Pew Scholars Programme in the
  Biomedical Sciences, 248

West European Countries

MRC Research Studentships, 199
Wingate Scholarships, 326

OPTOMETRY

Any Country

Roche Research Foundation, 254
University Postgraduate Scholarships,
  290

Australia

The Sir Robert Menzies Memorial
  Research Scholarships in the Allied
  Health Sciences, 273
Wingate Scholarships, 326

British Commonwealth

Wingate Scholarships, 326

Canada

Wingate Scholarships, 326

Indian Sub-Continent

Wingate Scholarships, 326

Middle East

Wingate Scholarships, 326

United Kingdom

Wingate Scholarships, 326

USA

AFVA Research Grant, 33

West European Countries

Wingate Scholarships, 326.

PODIATRY

Any Country

APMA Research Grant Program, 41
National Back Pain Association
  Research Grants, 212
Roche Research Foundation, 254

Australia

Wingate Scholarships, 326

British Commonwealth

Wingate Scholarships, 326

Canada

KidsAction Research Fellowships and
  Grants, 188
Wingate Scholarships, 326

Indian Sub-Continent

Wingate Scholarships, 326

Middle East

Wingate Scholarships, 326

United Kingdom

Wingate Scholarships, 326

West European Countries

Wingate Scholarships, 326

FORENSIC MEDICINE AND DENTISTRY

Any Country

Roche Research Foundation, 254
University of Dundee Research Awards,
  295
University of Glasgow Postgraduate
  Scholarships, 296

Australia

Wingate Scholarships, 326

British Commonwealth

Wingate Scholarships, 326

Canada

Wingate Scholarships, 326

Indian Sub-Continent

Wingate Scholarships, 326

Middle East

Wingate Scholarships, 326

United Kingdom

C H Milburn Research Award, 78
Wingate Scholarships, 326

West European Countries

Wingate Scholarships, 326

ACUPUNCTURE

Any Country

HDSA Fellowships, 169
HDSA Research Grants, 169
HDSA Research Initiative Grants, 169
National Back Pain Association
  Research Grants, 212
Roche Research Foundation, 254

HOMEOPATHY

Any Country

Roche Research Foundation, 254

CHIROPRACTIC

Any Country

FCER Fellowships, 151

FCER Research Grants, 151
FCER Residencies, 151
National Back Pain Association
  Research Grants, 212
Research Grant, 39, 324
Roche Research Foundation, 254

OSTEOPATHY

Any Country

National Back Pain Association
  Research Grants, 212
Roche Research Foundation, 254

Canada

Alcohol Beverage Medical Research
  Foundation Research Project Grant, 12

USA

Alcohol Beverage Medical Research
  Foundation Research Project Grant, 12
AOA Research Grants, 38

TRADITIONAL EASTERN MEDICINE

Any Country

Roche Research Foundation, 254

INDEX OF AWARDS

A

AAAS Travel Fellowships for Young Scientists on Problems of Environment and Health, 40
AACN Clinical Practice Grant, 23
AACN Critical Care Research Grant, 23
AACN Sigma Theta Tau Critical Care Grant, 23
AACR Career Development Awards in Cancer Research, 19
AACR EN Young Investigator Awards for Asian Scientists, 20
AACR Gerald B Grindley Memorial Young Investigator Award, 20
AACR HBCU Faculty Award in Cancer Research, 20
AACR Peczoller International Award for Cancer Research, 20
AACR Research Fellowships, 21
AACR Susan G Komen Breast Cancer Foundation Career Development Award, 21
AADR Student Research Fellowships, 23
AAFPRS Investigator Development Grant, 17
AAFPRS Resident Research Grants, 17
AAOS/OREF Fellowship in Health Services Research, 243
AAP Residency Scholarships, 19
AAP Resident Research Grants, 19
AAUW Educational Foundation American Fellowships, 3
AAUW International Fellowships Program, 3
AAUW/IFUW International Fellowships, 70
Aboriginal and Torred Strait Islander Scholarship, 61
ACOG/3M Pharmaceuticals Research Award in Lower Genital Infections, 25
ACOG/Cytyc Corporation Research Award for the Prevention of Cervical Cancer, 26
ACOG/Ethicon Research Award for Innovations in Gynecological Surgery, 26
ACOG/Merck Award for Research in Migraine Management in Women's Healthcare, 26
ACOG/Novartis Pharmaceuticals Fellowship for Research in Endocrinology of the Postreproductive Woman, 26
ACOG/Organon, Inc. Research Award in Contraception, 27
ACOG/Ortho-McNeil Academic Training Fellowships in Obstetrics and Gynecology, 27

ACOG/Parke-Davis Research Award to Advance the Management of Women's Healthcare, 27
ACOG/Pharmacia and Upjohn Research Award in Urogynecology of the Postreproductive Woman, 27
ACOG/Searle Research Award in Gynecologic Infections and Their Complications, 28
ACOG/Solvay Pharmaceuticals Research Award in Menopause, 28
Action Research Programme Grants, 4
Action Research Project Grants, 4
Action Research Training Fellowship, 4
ADHA Institute Minority Scholarship, 6
ADHA Institute Scholarship Program, 6
AFA Grants-in-Aid, 49
AFA Special Project Grants, 50
AFA/ARA Heald Fellowship, 50
Africa Educational Trust Emergency Grants, 8
Africa Educational Trust Scholarships, 8
AFUW Georgina Sweet Fellowship, 71
AFUW Victoria Endowment Scholarship, Lady Leitch Scholarship, 58
The AFUW-SA Inc Trust Fund Bursary, 59
AFVA Research Grant, 33
Agnes Storar/Constance Owens Fund, 127
AHA Established Investigator Grant, 34
AHA Grant-in-Aid, 34
AHA Scientist Development Grant, 35
AHAF Macular Degeneration Research, 33
AHAF National Heart Foundation, 33
AHRI African Fellowship, 46
AIATSIS Research Grants, 61
AIDS International Training and Research Programme (AITRP), 183
AIEJ Honors Scholarships, 55
Airey Neave Trust Award, 9
Albert McMaster and Helen Tomkinson Research Awards, 77
Albert W Dent Student Scholarships, 153
Alberta Heritage Clinical Fellowships, 9
Alberta Heritage Clinical Investigatorships, 10
Alberta Heritage Full-Time Fellowships, 10
Alberta Heritage Full-Time Studentships, 10
Alberta Heritage Medical Scholarships, 10
Alberta Heritage Medical Scientist Awards, 10
Alberta Heritage Part-Time Fellowships, 11
Alberta Heritage Part-Time Studentship, 11

Alcohol Beverage Medical Research Foundation Research Project Grant, 12
Alexander Graham Bell Scholarship Awards, 12
Alexander von Humboldt 'Bundeskanzler' Scholarships, 156
Alexander von Humboldt Research Fellowships, 156
Alice Creswick and Sheila Kimpton Foundation Scholarship, 58
Alice E Wilson Awards, 113
Allied Dental Health Scholarship (Dental Hygiene, Dental Assisting, Dental Laboratory Technology), 5
Alzheimer's Association Investigator-Initiated Research Grants, 14
Alzheimer's Association Pilot Research Grants, 14
Alzheimer's Disease Research Grant, 34
America-Norway Heritage Fund, 240
American Cancer Society Award for Research Excellence in Cancer Epidemiology and Prevention, 21
American Cancer Society International Fellowships for Beginning Investigators, 25, 212
American Cancer Society International Fellowships for Beginning Investigators (ACBSI), 212
American Institute for Cancer Research Investigator Initiator Grants, 35
American Lung Association Career Investigator Awards, 36
American Lung Association Clinical Research Grants, 37
American Lung Association Research Grants, 37
American Lung Association Research Training Fellowships, 37
American Nurses Foundation Research Grant, 24
American Society of Hypertension/Hoechst Marion Roussel Clinical Fellowship in Hypertension, 42
American-Scandinavian Foundation, 44, 240
ANF Nursing Research Grants, 38
The Anglo-Danish (London) Scholarships, 44
Anglo-Jewish Association Bursary, 45
Anti-Cancer Foundation Research Grants, 45
ANU Alumni Association Country Specific PhD Scholarships, 62
ANU Masters Degree Scholarships (The Faculties), 62
ANU PhD Scholarships, 62
AOA Research Grants, 38
APA/CMHS and Zeneca Minority Fellowship Programme in Psychiatry, 122

GrantFinder - Medicine

GrantFinder - Medicine

V

W

Y

Z

INDEX OF AWARDING
ORGANISATIONS

A

AAUW Educational Foundation, *USA*, 3

Action Research, *England*, 4

The ADA Endowment and Assistance Fund, Inc., *USA*, 5

ADHA Institute for Oral Health, *USA*, 6

Africa Educational Trust, *England*, 8

Afro-Asian Institute in Vienna and Catholic Women's League of Austria, *Austria*, 8

Airey Neave Trust, *England*, 9

Alberta Heritage Foundation for Medical Research (AHFMR), *Canada*, 9

Alcohol Beverage Medical Research Foundation, *USA*, 12

Alexander Graham Bell Association for the Deaf, *USA*, 12

Alexander von Humboldt Foundation, *Germany*, 12

Alzheimer's Association, *USA*, 14

Alzheimer's Disease Society, *England*, 16

American Academy of Child and Adolescent Psychiatry, *USA*, 16

The American Academy of Facial Plastic and Reconstructive Surgery (AAFPRS Foundation), *USA*, 17

American Academy of Family Physicians (AAFP), *USA*, 18

The American Academy of Fixed Prosthodontics, *USA*, 18

American Academy of Pediatrics (AAP), *USA*, 19

American Association for Cancer Research, *USA*, 19

American Association for Dental Research (AADR), *USA*, 23

American Association of Critical-Care Nurses (AACN), *USA*, 23

American Cancer Society, *USA*, 25

American College of Obstetricians and Gynecologists (ACOG), *USA*, 25

American Digestive Health Foundation, *USA*, 29

American Foundation for Ageing Research, *USA*, 32

American Foundation for Vision Awareness (AFVA), *USA*, 33

American Health Assistance Foundation (AHAF), *USA*, 33

American Heart Association, Inc (AHA), *USA*, 34

American Institute for Cancer Research, *USA*, 35

American Institute of Nutrition, *USA*, 35

American Lung Association, *USA*, 36

The American Lyme Disease Foundation, Inc., *USA*, 37

American Nurses Foundation (ANF), *USA*, 38

American Osteopathic Association (AOA), *USA*, 38

American Osteopathic Foundation (AOF), *USA*, 38

American Paralysis Association, *USA*, 39

American Philosophical Society, *USA*, 39

American Physiological Society, *USA*, 40

American Podiatric Medical Association (APMA), *USA*, 41

American Psychiatric Association, *USA*, 41

American Social Health Association, *USA*, 41

American Society of Hypertension, *USA*, 42

American Speech-Language-Hearing Foundation (ASLHF), *USA*, 42

American Tinnitus Association (ATA), *USA*, 44

The American-Scandinavian Foundation (ASF), *USA*, 44

The Anglo-Danish Society, *England*, 44

Anglo-Jewish Association, *England*, 45

The Anti-Cancer Foundation of South Australia, *Australia*, 45

The Apex Foundation for Research into Intellectual Disability Ltd, *Australia*, 45

The Arc of the United States, *USA*, 46

Armauer Hansen Research Institute (AHRI), *Ethiopia*, 46

Arthritis Foundation, *USA*, 46

Arthritis Foundation of Australia (AFA), *Australia*, 49

Arthritis Research Campaign (ARC), *England*, 51

The Arthritis Society, *Canada*, 52

Association for Spina Bifida and Hydrocephalus (ASBAH), *England*, 54

Association of African Universities, *Ghana*, 54

Association of Commonwealth Universities, *England*, 55

Association of International Education, Japan (AIEJ), *Japan*, 55

Association of Rhodes Scholars in Australia, *Australia*, 55

Association of Surgeons of Great Britain and Ireland, *England*, 56

Association of Universities and Colleges of Canada, *Canada*, 56

The Asthma Foundation of New South Wales, *Australia*, 57

Asthma Society of Canada, *Canada*, 57

Asthma Victoria, *Australia*, 57

Australian Early Childhood Association, Inc., *Australia*, 58

Australian Federation of University Women - Victoria, *Australia*, 58

The Australian Federation of University Women, South Australia, Inc Trust Fund (AFUW), *Australia*, 59

The Australian Government, *Australia*, 60

Australian Institute of Aboriginal and Torres Strait Islander Studies, *Australia*, 61

Australian Institute of Medical Scientists, *Australia*, 61

Australian National University, *Australia*, 61

Australian-American Educational Foundation, *Australia*, 63

B

Beit Memorial Fellowships, *England*, 65

Beit Trust (Zimbabwe, Zambia & Malawi), *Zimbabwe*, 65

Belgian-American Educational Foundation, Inc., *USA*, 65

BFWG Charitable Foundation (formerly Crosby Hall), *England*, 66

Board of Trustees for the Award of the Heinrich Wieland Prize, *Germany*, 66

British Association of Plastic Surgeons (BAPS), *England*, 67

The British Council, *Germany*, 68

The British Council, *USA*, 68

British Dental Association, *England*, 69

British Diabetic Association, *England*, 69

British Federation of Women Graduates (BFWG), *England*, 70

British Heart Foundation (BHF), *England*, 73

British Institute of Radiology, *England*, 76

British Lung Foundation, *England*, 77

British Medical and Dental Students' Trust, *Scotland*, 77

British Medical Association (BMA), *England*, 77

The British Nutrition Foundation (BNF), *England*, 80

British Orthodontic Society, *England*, 81

The British Schools and Universities Foundation, Inc. (BSUF), *England*, 81

BUNAC, *England*, 82

The Bunting Institute of Radcliffe College, *USA*, 82

Business and Professional Women's Foundation, *USA*, 83

GrantFinder - Medicine

GrantFinder - Medicine